OXFORD MEDICAL PUBLICATIONS

Infection in Surgical Practice

Infection in Surgical Practice

Edited by

Eric W. Taylor

Consultant Surgeon
Vale of Leven Hospital
Alexandria
Dunbartonshire
Scotland

OXFORD NEW YORK TOKYO
OXFORD UNIVERSITY PRESS
1992

Oxford University Press, Walton Street, Oxford 0X2 26DP
Oxford New York Toronto
Delhi Bombay Calcutta Madras Karachi
Petaling Jaya Singapore Hong Kong Tokyo
Nairobi Dar es Salaam Cape Town
Melbourne Auckland
and associated companies in
Berlin Ibadan

Oxford is a trade mark of Oxford University Press

Published in the United States
by Oxford University Press, New York

A catalogue record for this book is available from the British Library

Library of Congress Cataloging in Publication Data
Infection in surgical practice / edited by Eric W. Taylor
(Oxford medical publications)
Includes bibliographical references and index.
1. Surgical wound infections. I. Taylor, Eric W. II. Series.
[DNLM: 1. Surgical Wound Infection—prevention & control. WO 185 I425]
RD98.3.I54 1992 617'.01—dc20 91-27040
ISBN 0-19-262023-1

Set by Colset Pte Ltd, Singapore
Printed and bound in Hong Kong

Foreword

by M.R.B. KEIGHLEY, MS, FRCS

Infection remains an important cause of morbidity in surgical practice. The subject is of particular importance with worldwide budgeting constraints in the provision of medical care. Thus, the prevention of infection is not only a subject of importance to doctors but to medical economists as well.

Mr Eric Taylor must be congratulated on the wide spectrum of clinical practice covered in his book. He has successfully combined a thorough review of the biology and immunology of infection with the principles of infection control. The text covers audit, definition, quality assurance, and surgical principles, as well as antimicrobial agents. The spectrum of surgical activity is wide, including trauma, general surgery, vascular surgery, urology, neurosurgery, ENT, cardiothoracic surgery, obstetrics and gynaecology, orthopaedics, and surgery in the immuno-compromised host.

Although there have been many textbooks on surgical infection, this surely is the most comprehensive account so far produced. It is thoroughly up-to-date and beautifully referenced. The contributors are all internationally respected in their own fields. Mr Taylor's book provides a fresh approach to surgical infection and I am sure it will have a wide appeal.

We are left in the hands of generations (of doctors) which, having heard of microbes, . . . suddenly concluded that the whole art of healing could be summed up in the formula: Find the microbe and kill it.

George Bernard Shaw.
The Devil's Disciple (1906)

Preface

Infection is the cause of much surgical pathology and remains a common complication after most operative procedures. Postoperative nosocomial infection is frequently implicated in the death of patients. We live in a symbiotic relationship with bacteria, and it has been estimated that each of us plays host to some 10^{14} bacteria of over 500 different species (1,2); indeed there may be more bacteria in and on our bodies than cells forming our body. The symbiotic balance which exists can be disturbed by modern antibiotic therapy, which allows colonization by new or more pathogenic species, or it may be disturbed by an operation when the barriers between the body and the bacteria are broken allowing the bacteria access to areas where they can behave in a different, pathogenic role. The world of surgery is changing rapidly and, in particular, an increasing number of implant procedures are performed which has given new opportunities of pathogenesis to bacteria previously considered harmless.

Whilst many technical barriers have been broken down to allow surgeons to perform dramatic new operations, immunological frontiers have also been pushed back. Our understanding of host resistance and the role of the body's defence mechanisms in response to transplanted tissue, foreign bodies, and bacteria continues to develop. At the same time political changes are demanding that surgeons be more responsible with the resources that they utilize. Audit has become the key word. Surgeons must audit their work by cataloguing the short and long term complications, thus ensuring that the operations they perform are properly done, with the minimal use of resource, and are of the greatest benefit to the patient.

Audit is a complicated and multifaceted exercise which can embrace analysis of activity, methods, resources, and outcome. As audit systems have developed there has been an increasing awareness that, if clinical results are to be compared between surgeons, hospitals, or countries it is essential for preoperative risk criteria and outcome definitions to be standardized, agreed, and utilized.

The definition of infection and its diagnosis can be difficult. Whilst the infective pathology may not have changed a great deal, new investigative techniques are now available and, in addition, there have been many developments in the pharmaceutical world leading to the marketing of new antibiotics. Surgeons are traditionally conservative and it is sometimes difficult to make sense of these developments. It is particularly difficult to keep up to date with the literature relating to the plethora of new antimicrobial drugs as many papers are published in journals beyond the reading scope of most surgeons.

I trust readers will find this book a useful review of the microbiology and clinical management of the infective pathology that presents in surgical practice, as well as an update in the basic science of the body's response to infection. New concepts of pathology such as abacterial sepsis and of prophylaxis and therapy such as selective decontamination of the digestive tract have been reviewed, as have the problems posed to both surgeon and patient by HIV infection.

It has been a privilege to edit this book and I have learnt a great deal in doing so. Although my name appears on the spine of the book as the editor, this is very much a joint effort and I can only express my profound gratitude to all the contributors who have given of their time and experience to make this book possible.

References

1. Williams R. E. O. (1973). Benefit and mischief from commensal bacteria. *J. Clin. Path.*, **26**, 811–18.
2. Moore, W. E. C. and Holdeman, L. V. (1974). Human fecal flora: the normal flora of 20 Japanese-Hawaiians. *Applied Microbiology*, **27**, 961–79.

E. W. T.

1991

Acknowledgements

There are many people involved in the production of a multi-author book such as this. I am most grateful to all the authors who have contributed to the book. I am grateful to them all and particularly to their secretaries who have not only coped with my frequent telephone calls, but have had to suffer my requests for correction or retyping of their manuscript. It is impossible to acknowledge each by name, but I trust all will know that I am most grateful for their efforts and wish to express my sincere thanks.

The staff at Oxford University Press have been a source of great help and encouragement from the initial commissioning of this book through to publication and to sales, and I would wish to thank them all.

This book would not have come about had it not been for my experience with *Surgical Infection*, the six-monthly abstracting journal produced by the Surgical Infection Study Group, many of whom are contributors to this book. I would like to thank them for the opportunity they gave me and for their constant help and support. Similarly my thanks are due to the many surgeons and microbiologists working in the West of Scotland who have contributed to the clinical trials and subsequent publications achieved by the West of Scotland Surgical Infection Study Group Trust. In particular I wish to thank Dr Gavin Lindsay, Consultant Microbiologist at the Southern General Hospital, Glasgow who has taught me a great deal of microbiology, and has been a constant source of advice on the microbiology in this book.

I wish to thank my colleagues at the Vale of Leven Hospital, in particular Mr John Ross Maccallum and Mr Philip Shouler MBE, for their help and support, for their tolerance of my apparent distraction and not infrequent absence from the hospital. The help of Mrs Elizabeth Aitchison, Librarian, has been invaluable in chasing up the details of many of the references, and my special gratitude goes to my secretary, Miss Rita Major, who has coped magnificently with the inordinate workload of typing, retyping, and redrafting that I have placed upon her, and most of all for the tolerance and understanding she has shown to my impatient wish to have everything done yesterday.

Lastly I must thank my wife Judy and my children Sarah, William, Katie, and Peter who have often wondered why I spent so much time closeted in my office, and have been available so infrequently to join family activities. Without their love, understanding, and support this book would not have come into being.

I ask all who have made this book possible to accept my thanks.

Contents

List of contributors

John R. Babb, FIMLS, Laboratory Manager, Hospital Infection Research Laboratory, Dudley Road Hospital, Birmingham

Thomas Beattie, BA, DCH, FRCS (A/E), Consultant Accident & Emergency Surgeon, Royal Infirmary, Aberdeen

Paul H.B. Blair, FRCS (Eng), Surgical Research Fellow and Senior Surgical Registrar, Queen's University of Belfast, Northern Ireland

C. Joseph Cahill, MChir, FRCS (Eng), Lecturer in Surgery, Westminster Hospital, London

Peter J.E. Cruse, MB, ChB, FRCS (Ed), FRCSC, FACS, Professor of Surgery, Foothills Hospital, Calgary, Alberta, Canada

E. Paxton Dewar, OBE, FRCS (Eng) Surgeon Captain RN, Consultant Surgeon, Royal Naval Hospital, Plymouth, Devon

J. Michael Dixon, BSc, MD, FRCS (Eng), FRCS (Ed), Senior Lecturer in Surgery, University Department of Surgery, Edinburgh

David L. Easty, MD, FRCS (Eng), Professor of Ophthalmology, University of Bristol

Michael Emmerson, BSc, FRCPath, FRCP (G), Professor of Microbiology, University of Nottingham

Simon Harrison, MA, MChir, FRCS (Eng), Senior Urological Registrar, Taunton and Somerset Hospital, Taunton

Denis F. Hawkins, PhD, DSc, FRCOG, Professor of Obstetrics & Gynaecology, Royal Postgraduate Medical School, Hammersmith Hospital, London

Sean P.F. Hughes, MS, FRCS (Ed), FRCS (Eng), FRCS (I), Professor of Orthopaedic Surgery, Royal Postgraduate Medical School, Hammersmith Hospital, London

Harry R. Ingham, FRCPath, Consultant Microbiologist, Newcastle General Hospital

Stephen J. Karran, MA, MChir, FRCS (Eng), FRCS (Ed) Reader in Surgery and Consultant Surgeon, University Surgical Unit, Southampton

D. Frank P. Larkin, MRCPI, FCOphth, Lecturer in Ophthalmology, University of Bristol

David J. Leaper, MD, ChM, FRCS (Eng), Consultant & Senior Lecturer in Surgery, University of Bristol, Southmead Hospital, Bristol

Valerie J, Lewington, BM, MSc, MRCP, Senior Registrar in Nuclear Medicine, The General Hospital, Southampton

A. Christine McCartney, BSc, PhD, MRCPath, Top Grade Microbiologist, Royal Infirmary, Glasgow

Allan B. Maclean, BMedSc, MD, FRCOG, Senior Lecturer, Department of Midwifery, Queen Mother's Hospital, Glasgow

Michael J. McMahon, ChM, PhD, FRCS (Eng), Reader in Surgery and Consultant Surgeon, University of Leeds

Alan Maynard, BA, BPhil, Professor of Economics and Director of the Centre for Health Economics, University of York

Jonathan L Meakins, MD, DSc, FRCSC, FACS, Professor, Department of Surgery and Microbiology, Royal Victoria Hospital, McGill University, Montreal, Canada

Shaheen Mehtar, FRCPath, Consultant Microbiologist, North Middlesex Hospital, London

Arthur McG Morris, MA, FRCS (Ed), FRCS (Eng), Consultant Plastic Surgeon, Royal Infirmary, Dundee

Per Olof Nyström, MD, PhD, Consultant Surgeon, Department of Surgery, Linköping University, Sweden

Patrick J. O'Boyle, ChM, FRCS (Eng), Consultant Urologist, Taunton & Somerset Hospital, Musgrove Park, Taunton

Michael S. Owen-Smith, MS, FRCS (Ed), FRCS (Eng), Consultant Surgeon, Hinchingbrooke Hospital, Huntingdon, Cambridgeshire

Graham Page, ChM, FRCS (Ed), Consultant Accident & Emergency Surgeon, Royal Infirmary, Aberdeen

Anthony L.G. Peel, MA, MChir, FRCS (Eng), Consultant Surgeon, North Tees General Hospital, Stockton-on-Tees, U.K.

Dennis Raahave, MD, DSc, Associate Professor of Surgery, University of Copenhagen, Horsholm, Denmark

Graham Ramsay, MD, FRCS (Glasg), Senior Lecturer in Surgery, University Department of Surgery, Western Infirmary, Glasgow

Geoffrey L. Ridgway, MD, BSc, FRCPath, Consultant Microbiologist, Department of Clinical Microbiology, University College Hospital, London

Brian J. Rowlands, MD, FRCS (Eng), FACS, Professor of Surgery, Queen's University of Belfast, Northern Ireland

Stuart D. Scott, MS, FRCS (Eng), Senior Surgical Registrar, The General Hospital, Southampton

Penelope R. Sisson, BSc, Principal Microbiologist, Department of Microbiology, Newcastle General Hospital

John A.R. Smith, PhD, FRCS (Ed), FRCS (Eng), Consultant Surgeon, Northern General Hospital, Sheffield

Colin J.L. Strachan, MD, FRCS (Ed), FRCS (Glas), Consultant Vascular Surgeon, Royal Sussex County Hospital, Brighton

Andrew C. Swift, ChM, FRCS (Eng), FRCS (Ed) Consultant ENT Surgeon, Walton Hospital, Liverpool

David P. Taggart, MD, FRCS (Glas), Senior Registrar in Cardiothoracic Surgery. Brompton Hospital, and National Heart Hospital, London

Eric W. Taylor, FRCS (Eng), FRCS (Glas), Consultant Surgeon, Vale of Leven Hospital, Alexandria, Dunbartonshire, Scotland

T. Vincent Taylor, MD, ChM, FRCS (Eng) Consultant Surgeon, Department of Surgical Gastroenterology, Royal Infirmary, Manchester

Jean I. Tchervenkov, MD, FRCSC, Department of Surgery, Royal Victoria Hospital, McGill University, Montreal, Canada

Michael J. Turner, MAO, MRCPI, MRCOG, Consultant Obstetrician and Gynaecologist, Coombe, Meath and Adelaide Hospitals, Dublin, Ireland

David J. Wheatley, MD, ChM, FRCS (Ed), FRCS (Glas), British Heart Foundation Professor of Cardiac Surgery, Royal Infirmary, Glasgow

A. Peter R. Wilson, MA, MD, MRCPath, Consultant Microbiologist, Department of Clinical Microbiology, University College Hospital, London

Margaret A. Worsley, BSc, RGN, DN, FETC, Senior Nurse Infection Control, North Manchester General Hospital, Manchester

1

Classification of operations and audit of infection

PETER J.E. CRUSE

Introduction

The ideal operation results in primary healing, an uneventful recovery, and the cure of the disease. When an operation fails to achieve these objectives because of complications it becomes expensive: the price tag includes human suffering, hospital utilization, as well as the patient's loss of income and productivity.

In spite of the advances of the twentieth century, surgical infection remains the principal cause of the prolonged and debilitating complications of surgery.

This chapter will emphasize four points: *First*, that a wound classification allows for the isolation of a 'clean wound' category. *Second*, the clean wound infection rate is a simple measure of the worth of procedures and drugs used in the daily practice of surgery. *Third*, surveillance of the wound infection rate remains the best form of quality control or audit in a department of surgery because the clean wound infection rate is a direct reflection of the surgeon's operating technique. *Fourth*, when motivated surgeons are regularly informed of their infection rates, these rates are markedly reduced. Put another way, personal statistics will modify the behaviour of the motivated surgeon.

The development of the concepts which led to wound classification

In 1861, Louis Pasteur showed bacteria to be responsible for the putrefaction of meat. Four years later, Joseph Lister applied this concept to 'wound putrefaction', and used carbolic acid to prevent exogenous contamination and infection in a compound fracture of the tibia. This discovery, far more than the discovery of anaesthesia (1846), was the turning point for the rapid advance of surgery. The Listerian concept of antisepsis was not instantly accepted; in the Franco-Prussian War of 1870, for example, von Nussbaum reported a 100 per cent mortality in the performance of 34 through the knee amputations.

Furthermore, Lawson Tait and others argued that they obtained as good results as Lister with scrupulous cleanliness. This controversy was finally resolved with the introduction of autoclaves and *aseptic* surgery in the 1880s by Von Bergmann.

Theodore Kocher of Berne, Switzerland in the 1890s perfected the meticulous, bloodless, and unhurried surgical technique. His safeguarding of the body tissues was a remarkable advance and by 1899 he was able to report a 2.3 per cent infection rate in his thyroid surgery. Halsted championed Kocher's operating technique in North America.

In spite of these advances it became obvious that certain operations, notably those involving the colon, were associated with a prohibitive morbidity and mortality because of sepsis. The danger of contamination by the patient's own bacteria—endogenous contamination—came to be recognized as the most serious risk in the causation of surgical infection. This concept led to the National Research Council Classification of wounds based on the extent of endogenous and exogenous contamination at operation (1).

The Foothills Hospital wound study

In 1965 we decided to use *wound infection* as the yardstick by which to measure all infections on the surgical services. The reason for this decision is that the wound remains the common denominator of all surgeons. Two years later, we began the prospective audit of all surgical wounds at Foothills Hospital with four aims in mind:

1. To obtain an accurate monthly infection rate to be used as a continuing audit of the efficiency of the operating theatres, the surgical wards and the surgeons.
2. To obtain a bank of statistics with which future variables could be compared.
3. To determine and audit the factors which influence our infection rate.
4. To reduce the surgical wound infection rate at our hospital.

Method

A full-time surgical surveillance nurse personally observed all wounds throughout each patient's hospital stay and telephoned the surgeons' offices 28 days after the operation for a final report on the wound. A protocol was used to collect 80 items of information on each patient. This information was then coded and stored in a computer. The computer provides monthly and yearly infection reports, as well as an annual report to each surgeon showing the rate of infection of his or her clean wounds compared with the average clean wound infection rate of the peer surgical division. Rectal and vaginal operations, burns, and circumcision are excluded from the study because of the difficulties involved in inspecting the wounds.

Definitions

We used the definitions of the 1964 National Research Council Study on wound infection and the influence of ultraviolet light (1) so that our results could be compared (2).

Wound infections are difficult to define (3) (see Chapter 9). Discharges may be sterile on culture—even from infected wounds—and conversely pathogens may be recovered from wounds that are healing without infection. For the purposes of the study a wound is defined as *infected* if it discharges pus; *uninfected* if it heals *per primum* without discharge; and *possibly infected* if it develops the Celsian signs of inflammation or a serous discharge. The possibly infected wound is followed daily until it resolves (uninfected) or discharges pus (infected).

Wound classification

The circulating nurse in the theatre assigns every wound to one of four categories of contamination.

Clean

Clean wounds are those from operations in which the gastrointestinal, genitourinary, or respiratory tract is not entered, no apparent inflammation is encountered, and no break in aseptic technique occurs; however, three operations—cholecystectomy, appendicectomy in passing, and hysterectomy—are usually included in this category if no acute inflammation is present.

Clean contaminated

Clean contaminated wounds are from clean operations in which the gastrointestinal or respiratory tract was entered but no significant spillage occurred.

Contaminated

Contaminated wounds are from operations in which acute inflammation without pus formation is encountered or in which gross spillage from a hollow viscus occurs; fresh traumatic wounds and operation wounds in which a major break in aseptic technique occurs are included in this category.

Dirty

Dirty wounds are created by operations in which pus is encountered or a perforated viscus is found; traumatic wounds more than four hours old are included in this group.

The results of the Foothills Hospital wound audit

In this chapter the first 100 000 wounds studied will be analysed. Of these 4412 became infected for an infection rate of 4.4 per cent. We have not found the overall infection rate to be of epidemiologic value. If mostly clean operations are performed in an institution (e.g. hernia repairs) then the overall infection rate will be much lower than in the hospital where much bowel surgery is done.

Table 1.1 shows the influence of contamination on the infection rates for various types of wounds. The rate of infection of clean wounds was 1.4 per cent; for dirty wounds, where pus was found at operation, the infection rate was 39.9 per cent. This difference in the rates is a reminder that endogenous contamination at operation is the single most important factor in the production of subsequent wound infection.

The clean wound infection rate

The clean infection rate has proved to be our most useful figure. We use the clean wound infection rate for surveillance research and quality assurance. *The clean wound infection rate is the most valuable reflection of surgical care in any hospital.* Endogenous bacterial contamination is at a minimum in these wounds and the influence of the other factors such as hand scrubs, skin preparation and patient resistance—such as age and obesity—can be accurately assessed. The clean wound infection rate allows for a comparison among hospitals, among the various surgical divisions in each hospital, and among individual surgeons.

A number of Foothills surgeons have, over a 10-year period, achieved a clean wound infection rate of less than one per cent. Since surgeons in each discipline perform the same operations on similar patients, and use the same operating rooms and wards, the variation in the clean wound infection rate must be attributed to differences in operating technique.

The Foothills Hospital audit standard

This experience with the clean wound infection rate established a practice standard at Foothills Hospital: a clean wound infection rate of less than 1 per cent is considered exemplary; 1 to 2 per cent acceptable; and more than 2 per cent unacceptable and requires an investigation. The monthly report of the clean wound infection rate is measured against this standard.

Factors which influence the infection rate

Two factors determine whether a wound becomes infected: the dose of bacterial contamination introduced at operation and the patient's ability to resist that contamination.

Contamination

Bacterial contamination can originate from extraneous sources (exogenous contamination) or from the patient's own bacteria (endogenous contamination). Table 1.1 shows the overriding importance of endogenous contamination which proves to be more important than all the exogenous factors combined. In the operating room ritual, ironically, most time and money are devoted to reducing exogenous contamination and little attention is paid to the endogenous risk.

Table 1.1. Incidence of infection, Foothills Hospital

Category	No. of patients	No. infected	Percentage
Clean	73 589	1002	1.4
Clean contaminated	14 018	879	6.3
Contaminated	9 085	1211	13.3
Dirty	3 308	1310	39.9
Total	100 000	4412	4.4

Exogenous contamination

The surgeons' hands

In the Foothills Hospital, the clean wound infection rate was not affected by the type of scrub antiseptic used. Most surgeons at our institution now use chlorhexidine as it is effective against Gram-negative and Gram-positive organisms and a residue of the antiseptic remaining on the hand provides a prolonged antiseptic action.

Duration of the hand scrub

To reduce the ritual ten minutes scrub to our present two to three minute scrub proved to be remarkably difficult as it went against the grain of generations of nurses' training. The unchanged figures of the monthly clean wound infection audit eventually carried the day—with a great saving of time, water, and hand epithelium.

Gloves

In 1958 Penikett and Gorrill (4) described a simple device to detect glove punctures. One pole of a battery is connected to a metal scrub basin and the other to a terminal that the surgeon can touch with his or her forehead. A glove puncture completes the circuit and fired the alarm. The Electronics Department at Foothills Hospital constructed a glove tester based on this principle. We tested 1209 pairs of gloves and found 141 gloves to be punctured (11.6 per cent) at the end of the operation (5). Somewhat to our surprise not a single wound infection developed. It would seem that with the use of an antiseptic hand scrub insufficient viable bacteria escape through a puncture to produce an infection.

The patient's skin

Pre-operative shower

In the early part of the Foothills Study, it appeared that a shower using hexachlorophene soap was of value in reducing infection (6). The infection rate was 2.3 per cent if the patient did not shower, 2.1 per cent if the patient showered using bath soap before operation. When hexachlorophene was used the infection rate fell to 1.3 per cent. At present all patients booked for operation at our hospital are given two chlorhexidine impregnated scrub sponges to use in the shower the night before and the morning of operation. Ayliffe and co-workers (7) found that pre-operative washing with an antiseptic did not reduce the infection rate in Birmingham.

Shaving the site of operation

In patients who were shaved more than 2 hours before operation, the clean wound infection rate was 2.3 per cent; in patients who had no shave but only had their body hair clipped, the infection rate fell to 1.7 per cent; and in patients who had neither shave nor clipping, the infection rate was 0.9 per cent (8). Seropian and Reynolds (9) also reported on the deleterious effects of body shaving on the wards. Altemeier *et al.* (10) showed the importance of shaving immediately before an operation to prevent bacterial multiplication in the serum oozing from the razor nicks. At Foothills Hospital we recommend that the surgeon or the registrar shave the operation site—if shaving is considered essential—and that this shaving be done once the patient is anaesthetized.

Preparation of the patient's skin

Based on the work of Lowbury *et al.* (11) who showed that 1 per cent iodine in 70 per cent alcohol and 0.5 per cent chlorhexidine in 70 per cent alcohol were the two most effective skin antiseptics we have used the chlorhexidine in alcohol solution for the last 15 years. This would be an ideal skin antiseptic were it not for the single defect of *inflammability*. During this year (1990) three fires have occurred in operating rooms in Calgary. These accidents happened when the operation site had to be enlarged during the course of the operation and the alcohol skin preparation had soaked into the drapes and ignited with a spark from the electrocautery. As a consequence of these events we have now *removed all inflammable antiseptics from the theatre* and prepare the patients skin at present with povidone iodine (Betadine). To date there has been no increase in the clean wound infection rate.

Draping

Drapes demarcate and isolate the area of the operation and each hospital should develop a standard technique. The type of drapes in use are (1) the conventional double thickness cotton sheets, (2) disposable prefabricated drapes, and (3) plastic adhesive skin drapes.

1. *Cotton drapes* At Foothills Hospital we use square draping with cotton drapes. To prevent a 'bacterial strike through' when the drapes become soaked from wet instruments, we cover the patient's thighs with a layer of sterile plastic before we spread the drapes. This inexpensive method to prevent strike through is just as effective as using expensive waterproof disposable drapes.

2. *Disposable prefabricated drapes* have been intensively promoted and claims made that the clean wound infection rate falls with their use. In a year's study at Foothills Hospital alternating between cotton drapes and gowns during one week and disposable drapes and gowns during the other weeks, the clean wound infection rate was not altered by one decimal point. A hospital decision to use cotton or disposable drapes should be based exclusively on cost, convenience, and the environment. Considerations are the laundry and sterilization procedures associated with cotton drapes versus the expense of prepackaged disposable drapes including the environmental penalties of deforestation to produce the cellulose and the incineration problems and air pollution.

3. *Plastic adhesive drapes* when introduced appeared to be the ideal method of covering the exposed skin at operation. It was a disappointment to see the reports of increasing wound infection when these drapes are used (12) because of sweating and bacterial proliferation beneath the plastic. Further, Raahave in Copenhagen (13) compared quantitative cultures from herniorrhaphy wounds draped alternately with plastic adhesive drapes and cloth. The colony counts proved to be the same. (see Chapter 5).

At Foothills Hospital, the use of cotton drapes was associated with a 1.5 per cent clean wound infection rate (405 of 26 303) while the addition of plastic adhesive drapes increased the rate to 2.3 per cent (214 of 9252) (5). A recent outbreak of clean wound infection which occurred in cardiac surgery at Foothills Hospital confirmed the hazard of plastic adhesive drapes. The problem was traced to the plastic adhesive windows built into the whole-body disposable drapes used by the cardiac surgeons. Plastic adhesive drapes are as a consequence, not used at Foothills Hospital—a considerable economy.

Pre-operative hospitalization

The longer the patient stays in hospital before an operation, the greater becomes the likelihood of succeeding wound infection. With a one day pre-operative stay the infection rate is 1.1 per cent; with a one-week pre-operative stay 2.1 per cent; and if the patient stays in the hospital for more than two weeks before operation, 3.4 per cent.

This finding becomes an additional incentive for every hospital to establish a pre-operative assessment clinic (POAC). In this clinic, staffed by anaesthetists and internists, sick and elderly patients are thoroughly investigated, prepared and educated, and are then admitted on the night before operation or even on the morning of operation. The POAC at Foothills Hospital has been successful in providing the imperative of 'better care at reduced cost' in these straitened economic times. The patients particularly appreciate the additional care and attention they received in the POAC whereas the cost of hospitalization and the wound infection rate is reduced (14).

Theatres and anaesthetists

There is no difference in the clean wound infection rate in the various operating theatres; further, there is no difference in the clean wound infection rate involving individual anaesthetists. Although bacterial carriers are uncommon, they are quickly detected with a wound surveillance programme. At Foothills Hospital we do not exclude personnel with upper respiratory infections but do not permit those with a staphylococcal infection into the operating rooms. In general, the less the people, the talk, the movement and the shorter the hair in the operating room the greater the margin of safety.

Duration of operation

There is a direct relation between the length of the operation and the infection rate. The clean wound infection rate roughly doubles with every hour. Other studies have also shown a rise in the infection rate associated with prolongation of the operating time (1, 15) There are four explanations:

1. Bacterial contamination increases with time.
2. The tissues in the operative area are damaged by drying and retractors.
3. A longer operation is usually associated with increased use of sutures and electrocoagulation which reduce the local resistance of the wound.
4. Longer procedures are more likely to be associated with blood loss and shock, thereby reducing the general resistance of the patient.

Surgical wards

The clean wound infection rate did not differ among the four wards to which ten general surgeons admitted patients. The same dressing and isolation techniques were used. However, the clean wound infection rate of the individual surgeons differed a great deal We concluded that the surgeon was responsible for his or her infection rate and that post-operative ward care played an insignificant part in the development of wound infections.

This finding led to a relaxation of ward regulations: nurses do not wear gloves or masks during the performance of wound dressings, clean wounds are left exposed after 48 h and the infected wound isolation technique has been simplified. Patients whose wound discharge can be contained in dressings are allowed to walk in the wards and in the hospital. These modifications, carried out under the umbrella of a surveillance system, have saved much needless effort and expense.

Endogenous contamination

The overriding importance of endogenous contamination is clear from the analysis of the wound categories (Table 1.1). Endogenous contamination is the main risk because of the large dose of organisms available from the bowel and other hollow muscular organs. Krizek and Robson (16) found that traumatic wounds were likely to become infected if they contained more than 500 000 organisms per gram of tissue; no wound became infected if the bacterial count was less than 10. Methods to reduce the dose of endogenous contamination in large bowel surgery are mechanical bowel preparation and the use of oral antibiotics. These methods and the use of prophylactic systemic antibiotics will be described in other chapters of this book.

The resistance of the patient

Culbertson *et al.* (17) stated that the risk of wound infection varies according to the equation:

$$\frac{\textit{Dose of bacterial contamination} \times \text{Virulence}}{\text{Host resistance}}$$

This concept explains why the heavily contaminated wound will often heal without infection in a patient with normal host defence mechanisms. Because all wounds are contaminated to some extent, it also explains the high infection rate among the immunocompromised patients. The concept of assisting the resistance of the patient is as old as Hippocrates, whose essential tenet in patient management was to assist the *vis medicatrix naturae* (the healing power of nature). Host resistance can be classified into general and local factors.

General factors

Age

All studies have shown an increase in the wound infection rate with advancing age (5). The same trend is seen in the Foothills statistics.

Sex

The clean wound infection rate is the same in male and female patients.

Diabetes, obesity, and malnutrition

These are also associated with an increase in the clean wound infection rate. Among malnourished patients undergoing clean operations at Foothills, 16 per cent developed post-operative wound infection (6). Nineteenth-century statistics from the Glasgow Royal Infirmary showed that in the 1860s the average family income improved and that with better nutrition there was an associated fall in the number of patients with typhus and patients with scurvy ulcers (18). Hamilton's hypothesis is that the reduction in the surgical wound infection rate at the

Royal Infirmary was as much due to better nourishment as to the application of carbolic acid to the wounds after 1865! This theory reinforces the well known concept of stabilizing diabetics before operation, weight reduction in the obese, and correction of malnutrition before operation.

The local resistance of the wound

Operative technique

The local resistance of the wound far exceeds in importance the general resistance of the patient. In 1537, Ambroise Paré rediscovered the gentle management of wounds when he found that gunshot wounds healed better when treated with bland irrigations rather than with boiling oil. In the 1890s Kocher demonstrated the low wound infection rate attainable by gentle technique and meticulous haemostasis. Halsted extolled Kocher's technique and proclaimed the principles of wound care: complete haemostasis, adequate blood supply, removal of all devitalized tissue, obliteration of dead space, use of fine non-absorbable sutures, and wound closure without tension.

Foreign bodies in wounds

In 1957, Elek and Conen (19) measured the deleterious effect of foreign bodies on local resistance by injecting the forearms of British medical students at St. George's Hospital with measured numbers of staphylococci. The investigators found that a dose of 6.5 million staphylococci was required to produce a subcuticular abscess, whereas only 100 organisms were necessary if they were injected into the area of a previously placed subcutaneous silk suture. The silk foreign body reduced the local resistance by a factor of 10 000!

The authors concluded that the bacteria could multiply in the interstices of the suture while being protected from the tissue defences in the wound, but Edlich and his colleagues have demonstrated similar pernicious effects with monofilament sutures (20). Howe and Marston (21) showed that the infective dose of bacteria could be further reduced if tissue were included with the ligated blood vessel—necrosis and foreign body joining forces.

Haematoma

Haematoma in the surgical wound is, however, the single most important factor in reducing local resistance at operation. Hemostasis can be achieved by electrocoagulation. Provided only the bleeding vessel is coagulated, leaving a minimal amount of necrotic tissue, no difference is seen in the clean wound infection rate with or without the use of the electrocoagulation unit.

Closed wound suction drains

The development of suction drains has been a great advance in reducing the occurrence of wound haematomata. Stagnant wound fluid, deficient in opsonin, is evacuated allowing fresh wound fluid complete with opsonin to enter the wound (22). At Foothills we have found closed wound suction drains to be of value in wounds in which hematoma formation is likely (e.g. in spinal fusion operations) (5). McIlrath and colleagues (23) demonstrated the benefit of placing closed wound suction drains subcutaneously in abdominal operations. The use of Penrose drains in the wound on the other hand is harmful. Nora (24) has shown that these drains afford ingress for bacteria down to the tip of the drain. Penrose drains provide the double jeopardy of a direct route of contamination combined with a foreign body in the wound. It is not surprising that the wound infection rate in cholecystectomies managed with Penrose drains through the wounds, increased to 6.6 per cent.

Wound closure

Sutures, staples, clips, and tapes

Any foreign material in the wound reduces local host defences. In this regard, clips and adhesive tapes have an obvious advantage. Edlich and associates (20) have shown that wounds closed with tape are more resistant to infection, followed by stapled wounds and least, wounds closed by sutures. Fine skin clips (autoclips) provide the most perfect skin edge approximation, allowing rapid epithelial closure to close the narrow gap. The clips are removed after 48 h and wound tapes are applied for 7 to 10 days to relieve the strain from the wound edges. These wounds are left exposed once the tapes are applied.

Delayed primary closure

John Hunter first fostered open wound management in the Belle Isle campaign of 1761. His method has had to be rediscovered with every war since that time, including the recent Falklands War. All wounds made by missiles or contaminated by saliva, faeces, pus, or soil should be considered for delayed primary closure. The wound edges can usually be approximated with tape after 4 days when there is no evidence of infection and healthy granulations are present.

Conclusion

The findings in this study have led to the following conclusions:

1. By categorizing operations on the basis of endogenous contamination, clean operations can be isolated and studied.
2. Clean wounds constitute about 75 per cent of a general hospital's workload. The main factor determining the development of infection in a clean wound is the local resistance of the wound. Poor operative technique reduces the local resistance by drying of the wound surface, implantation of excessive sutures, leaving dead tissue from electrocoagulation and ligatures, and haematoma formation. As a consequence, the clean wound infection rate is a direct reflection of operative technique and thus remains the best measure of the quality of surgery in an institution, in a department and of the individual surgeon.
3. Once a department accepts this concept of accountability

then regular information to all the surgeons of their own infection rates compared with the average of their peers provides strong motivation and results in a 50 per cent reduction in the clean wound infection rate.

References

1. National Research Council Division of Medical Sciences, Ad Hoc Committee of the Committee of Trauma (1964) Post-operative wound infections: The influence of ultraviolet irradiation of the operating room and various other factors. *Ann. Surg.* **160** (suppl 2), 1.
2. Cruse, P.J.E. (1975). Incidence of wound infection on the surgical services. *Surg. Clin. North Am.*, **55**, 1269.
3. Altemeier, W.A., Burke, J.F., Pruitt, B.A., Jr., and Sandusky, W.R. (eds) (1976). Definitions and classifications of surgical infections. In *Manual on control of infection in surgical patients*, p. 20. Lippincott, Philadelphia, Penn.
4. Penikett, E.J.K. and Gorill, R.H. (1958). The integrity of surgical gloves tested during use. *Lancet*, **2**, 1042.
5. Cruse, P.J.E. and Foord, R. (1980). The epidemiology of wound infection: A 10-year prospective study of 62 939 wounds. *Surg. Clin. North Am.*, **60**, 1.
6. Cruse, P.J.E. (1970). Surgical wound sepsis. *Can. Med. Assoc. J.*, **102**, 251.
7. Ayliffe, G.A.J. Noy, M.F., Babb, J.R. *et al.* (1983). A comparison of pre-operative bathing with chlorohexidine—detergent and nonmedicated soap in the prevention of wound infection. *J. Hosp. Infect.*, **4**, 237.
8. Cruse, P.J.E. and Foord, R. (1983). A five year prospective study of 23 649 surgical wounds. *Arch. Surg.*, **107**, 206.
9. Seropian, R. and Reynolds, B.M. (1971). Wound infections after pre-operative depilatory versus razor preparation. *Am. J. Surg.*, **121**, 251.
10. Incidence and cost of infection. In *Manual on control of infection in surgical patients* (ed. W.A. Altemeier, J.F. Bushe, B.A. Pruitt, Jr., and W.R. Sandusky) Lippincott, Philadelphia, Penn.
11. Lowbury, E.J.L., and Lilly, H.A. (1960). Disinfection of the hands of surgeons and nurses. *Br. Med. J.*, **1**, 1445.
12. Paskin, D.L. and Lerner, H.J. (1969). A prospective study of wound infections. *Am. Surg.*, **35**, 627.
13. Raahave, D. (1976). Effect of plastic skin and wound drapes on the density of bacteria in operation wounds. *Br. J. Surg.*, **64**, 421.
14. Cruse, P.J.E. (1988). Pre-operative Patient Assessment and Education. *Proceedings of International Conference on Hospital Infection*, Harrogate.
15. Public Health Laboratory Service (1960). Incidence of surgical wound infection in England and Wales: A report of the Public Health Laboratory Service, Great Britain. *Lancet*, **2**, 658.
16 Krizek, T.J. and Robson, M.C. (1975). Biology of surgical infection. *Surg. Clin. North Am.*, **55**, 1261.
17. Culbertson, W.R. *et al.* (1961). Studies on the epidemiology of post-operative infection of clean operative wounds. *Ann. Surg.*, **154**, 599.
18. Hamilton, D. (1982). The nineteenth century surgical revolution —Antisepsis or better nutrition. *Bull. Hist. Med.*, **56**, 30.
19. Elek, S.D., and Conen, P.E. (1957). The virulence of Staphylococcus pyogenes for man: A study of the problems of wound infection. *Br. J. Exp. Pathol.*, **38**, 573.
20. Edlich, R.F., Panek, P.H., Rodeheaver, G.T., *et al.* (1973). Physical and chemical configuration of sutures in the development of surgical infection. *Ann. Surg.*, **117**, 679.
21. Howe, C.W. and Marston, A.T. (1962). A study on sources of post-operative staphylococcal infection. *Surg. Gynecol. Obstet.*, **115**, 266.
22. Alexander, J.W., Korelitz, J., and Alexander, N.S. (1976). Prevention of wound infections: A case for closed suction drainage to remove wound fluids deficient in opsonic proteins. *Am. J. Surg.*, **132**, 59.
23. McIlrath, D.C., van Heerden, J., and Edis, A.J. (1976). Closure of abdominal incisions with subcutaneous catheters. *Surgery*, **4**, 4112.
24. Nora P.F. (1973). In discussion of paper by Cruse, P.J.E. and Foord, R. A five year prospective study of 23 649 surgical wounds. *Arch. Surg.*, **107**, 206.

2

Environmental factors influencing infection

MICHAEL EMMERSON

Introduction

Patients who are admitted to hospital and undergo surgical operations risk acquiring one or more nosocomial infections. In order to prevent surgical wound infections all necessary precautions must be taken; the most important of which is good surgical technique.

Pathogens that infect surgical wounds can be part of the patient's normal flora (endogenous source) or acquired from the hospital environment, other infected patients or the patient's attendees (exogenous source). Endogenous sources appear to be responsible for most post-operative infections especially if clean operations are excluded. However, the operating environment has to be controlled and this chapter deals with the environmental factors which in one way or another influence surgical wound infection. At the extremes of clean surgery, e.g. total hip replacement, environmental control becomes paramount and surgical staff must learn to respect these constraints.

Ventilation in operation suites

In 1972, a joint working party consisting of members from the Department of Health and Social Security (DHSS), the Medical Research Council (MRC) and Regional Engineers reported on the requirements for air ventilation in Operation Suites (1). The purpose of ventilation in the operation suite is to provide an environment that is safe for the patient and comfortable for the surgical team. This report also considered the ways in which anaesthetic gases were removed.

The purpose of ventilation is primarily to prevent infection of the patient's wound – and possibly the respiratory tract – by micro-organisms that are transported about the operation room on airborne particles. There is ample evidence that contamination, in the form of skin scales with attendant bacteria, is generated through the physical activity of humans.

Most healthy people disperse bacteria with low pathogenicity such as *Staphylococcus epidermidis*, diphtheroids, and propionibacteria spp. but about 10 per cent of males and 1 per cent of women also disperse *Staphylococcus aureus*. In total, some 10^7 skin scales are disseminated per day, of which it is estimated that 10 per cent of the skin squames (mean diameter 20 microns) carry viable micro-organisms. Carriage rates and dispersal problems will be discussed in a later section.

Information on the relative contributions of the airborne route as a cause of wound infection is limited, although recent work by Lidwell *et al.* in 1983 demonstrated a good correlation between air contamination and joint infection rate (2). In this respect the message seems quite clear; the presence of micro-organisms in the air of operating rooms is relevant to the production of deep post-operative infection in the special circumstances of prosthetic orthopaedic surgery. It may also seem relevant to extend this concept to other implant surgery involving prosthetic material, e.g. heart valves, central nervous system shunts. However, it may *not* be appropriate to impune the airborne route as a cause of wound infection following contaminated surgery such as colo-rectal or genito-urinary surgery. Other factors, such as bowel preparation and appropriate chemo-prophylaxis may be more relevant.

Microbiological requirements. These may be broadly stated as the prevention of airborne infection from sources outside the hospital, from hospital sources outside the operation room, and from sources in the operation room.

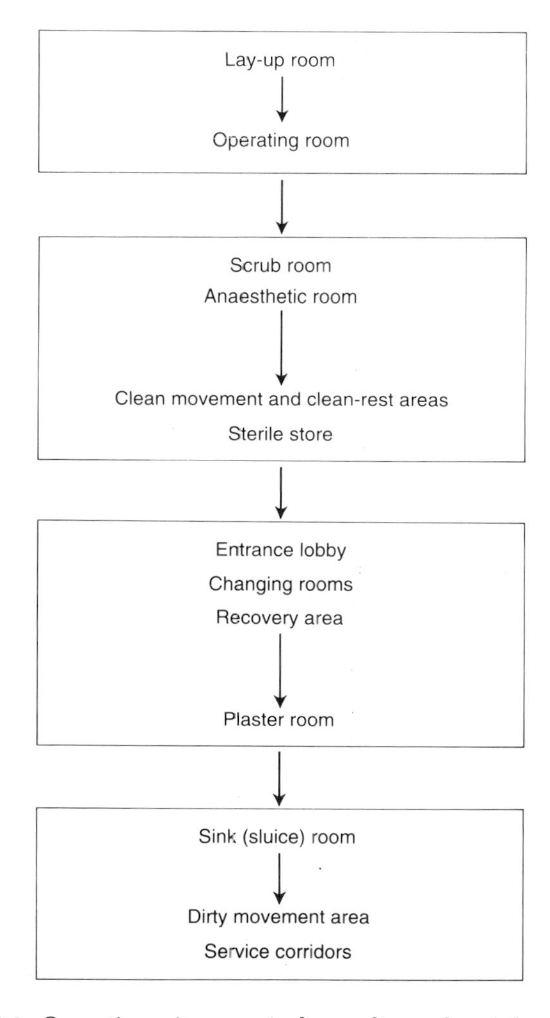

Fig. 2.1. Operation suite areas in descending order of cleanliness. (Adapted from ref. 1.)

Air movement control

The supply of air to an operating room has three main functions:

(a) To control the air movement within the suite such that transfer of airborne bacteria from less clean to cleaner areas is minimized.

(b) To reduce airborne bacterial contamination.

(c) To control the temperature and humidity of the space.

In a conventional operating theatre air is maintained under positive pressure (plenum) by an inflow of air filtered to remove particles above 5 microns. This air is introduced at high level through diffusers that give a general mixing to the total air volume. The air flow is turbulent and is lost by low-level extraction. Air flow is maintained from clean to less clean areas even when a door is opened (Fig. 2.1). Baffles may have to be fitted to doors to prevent back flow of air should other doors, e.g. corridor doors, be opened. It may be necessary to balance the ventilation system or fit air locks to prevent back-flow of air from 'dirtier' areas. Plenum ventilation works most efficiently when all doors are closed and opened infrequently. Whilst all windows should be sealed and portable fans prohibited, it is important that windows allowing in natural light be present. 'Stimulus deprivation' in windowless operating rooms is a well known phenomenon in hard working surgeons!

Bacterial content of air. Air delivered to the suite by the ventilation equipment should not contain more than 1 colony of *Clostridium perfringens* or *Staph. aureus* in a sample of 30 m^3 (1060 ft^3) of air. Aerobic cultures on non-selective medium should indicate not more than 35 bacteria carrying particles in 1 m^3 (1 per ft^3) of circulating air. In the past, agar plates (settle plates) were placed on the floor of quiet (unused) theatres and bacterial counts made after 24 hours. This rather haphazard method has now been replaced with set air volume sampling using the Casella slit sampler. Portable systems (Biotest RCS Centrifugal air sampler) are now available which are quieter and can be used during surgical operations to detect *Staph. aureus* skin dispersers. Air sampling is a complex procedure and needs to be performed by trained operators. It is done as part of the theatre commissioning programme and after any major overhaul of the ventilation system. The coarse pre-filters and the final filters are changed routinely by service engineers according to pre-determined resistance patterns and not as a result of air sampling. Air sampling may be needed if the clean wound infection rate increases and a disperser of *Staph. aureus* is suspected after case controlled studies.

Air temperature and humidity control

There is a wide variation in individual temperature preferences and there is also a substantial difference between temperatures preferred by surgeons and other members of the operation team, e.g. the 'sedentary' anaesthetist. The conflict of preference can be resolved only by those who feel cold at the temperatures most acceptable to the surgeon, wearing warmer clothing. The temperature controls should allow settings in the range 15–25 °C and should be accessible to the operation-room staff. A temperature of 21 °C (70 °F) will be warm enough for all but about 2 per cent of surgeons and 24 °C (75 °F) is warm enough for more than 98 per cent of anaesthetists.

Relative humidity should be held within the range 40 to 60 per cent. Since filtered and pre-warmed air needs to be humidified, the water source, often steam, must be free of water borne pathogens such as *Pseudomonas* spp. and *Legionella* spp. There must be easy access for routine cleaning and maintenance of all mechanical components.

Ultra clean air (UCA)

In a conventional operating theatre air is brought in from outside at a steady flow, changing not less than 20 times per hour. This gives a volume change in the range of 30 to 60 m^3 per minute. A further reduction of airborne contaminants can be achieved by improving the air filtration by high efficiency particulate air (HEPA) filters, and by increasing the air turnover rates around the operating site to achieve maximum positive pressure flushing effects. By altering the pattern of air movements so that the air passes in a non-turbulent fashion over the operating site an additional flushing mechanism comes into play. Such unidirectional flow can be either downwards, as in the vertical laminar flow, or from a side wall as in horizontal laminar flow. The rate of air change is 40 times per hour with a specified air flow of 50 to 100 ft/min. The first clean-air operating enclosure was introduced into service in 1964 by Charnley (3). A further reduction of airborne contaminants was achieved by the operational staff wearing special protective clothing consisting of overalls, full head coverings, and helmets with visors and body exhaust systems. This system will be discussed later.

Air is sucked from the operating room and enclosure which serves as a lock and is mixed with absolute filtered and conditioned fresh air. It is subsequently pushed by fans built into the ceiling of the adjacent room, via sound attenuators, into the ultrafilter ceiling system and is thus recirculated. There are advantages of vertical laminar flow compared with horizontal laminar systems. The Charnley–Howarth ventilated enclosure used in association with special exhaust ventilated clothing or the Trexler isolator (large plastic bubble) for the patient enables the contaminated-particle count to be reduced to 1/10–1/100 of that in a conventionally ventilated room. There are reports of substantial falls in the incidence of infection after the adoption of systems such as these. However, other surgeons have reported equally low infection rates after operations performed in rooms with good conventional ventilation and without special clothes.

In an attempt to resolve this difference of opinion the MRC, on behalf of the DHSS have conducted a multicentre controlled study in which some 8000 hip and knee replacement operations have been performed in rooms with conventional or UCA ventilation (4). When the operations were performed in an UCA environment the incidence of deep periarticular infection was reduced from 3.4 per cent to 1.6 per cent. When the team wore coverall exhaust ventilated, suits in addition, the rate of deep infection fell to 0.9 per cent. However, the available data suggest that prophylactic antibiotics are at least as effective as UCA and exhaust-ventilated suits in reducing deep infection. A rational appraisal suggests that the benefit to be derived from this very much cheaper alternative should be exhausted before any of the substantially more expensive provisions are considered (5).

Economies of use can be achieved without jeopardizing safety by simply switching off the main theatre ventilation during quiet periods. This was the conclusion from a recent detailed air study on plenum systems (6). Ventilation can be reduced or turned off at night and during weekends and cleaning can also be carried out without increased risk of infection if full flow is restored at least one hour prior to surgery. If these findings can be shown to apply under the very rigorous conditions of laminar downflow systems the cost savings should encourage the installation of many more for the increasingly demanding procedures of modern surgery.

Theatre wear

Theatre gowns

'A surgeon who is comfortably dressed in light cool theatre clothing is less likely to make an error of judgment than one who is perspiring in a heavy, airless gown'. Mitchell *et al.* in 1978 (7) compared conventional loose-weave cotton operating garments with clothing made of non-woven fabric to test their efficacy in reducing the dispersal of skin bacteria into theatre air. A substantial reduction (72 per cent) in the dispersal of skin bacteria was achieved when the men wore operating suits made of the non-woven material. Hill *et al.* in 1974 (8) had shown that dispersal of *Staph. aureus* into the air was fairly common during physical activity and was sometimes profuse in men, but unusual and rare in women. Shedding from the skin is increased by friction from clothes and is more predominant from the skin of the perineal area. These workers proposed the use of bacteria-proof underpants, e.g. closely woven Ventile material. Screening to identify staff for whom *the* pants might be useful was deemed difficult!

Normal cotton clothing frequently worn in the operating room does little to prevent the passage of bacteria on the skin scales as the diameter of the holes at the interstices of the cloth is normally greater than 80 μm and much interest has been shown in the use of a complete coverall system made from a disposable non-woven fabric (9). This concept is considered to be important in diminishing airborne bacteria as a major source of infection in total joint replacement operations (10).

Extensive work by Whyte *et al.* (11) compared the bacterial dispersion rate of people wearing operating-room clothing made from several types of polyester fabric with conventional cotton clothing, total-body exhaust gowns and disposable clothing.

Fabrics studied

1. *Cotton fabric*: The total body exhaust (TBE) gowns were made from a tightly woven cotton fabric known as Ventile L34.
2. *Disposable non-woven fabric*: Sontara fabric known as Fabric '450'.
3. *Polyester fabrics*: Selguard types T85382, T85895, T-303.

All these fabrics incorporated anti-static grids or strips.

The polyester clothing was demonstrated to be much superior to conventional cotton clothing and at least as good as the TBE gowns and disposable gowns. Other factors, such as fabric pore size, air permeability, particle removal efficiency, and wet strike through were also measured. The polyester fabrics were tested in the laboratory and whilst 'in use' in theatres and were quite well accepted, although not considered quite as comfortable as cotton. The use of a double layer of polyester fabric was successful in preventing penetration of blood or fluid through the area of the gown protected.

These fabrics can be easily washed and they can be autoclaved between 50 to 100 times before functional deterioration occurs. The ability to *resist penetration* of moist contamination poses further constraints as it is likely that under wet conditions it is the individual bacterial cells that penetrate; more closely woven and waterproof fabric would seem to be necessary. Closs and Tierney (12) found that 36 per cent of 243 operations produced blood soak-through of gowns. Disposable plastic aprons were never worn under linen gowns and the feedback from the surgeons on completion of the study suggested extreme discomfort occurred due to sweating when wearing plastic aprons. Other factors such as economy, safety, particularly electrostatic safety, and aesthetic appeal have to be considered.

A variety of materials are now available:

1. *Ventiles*—tightly woven cottons whose fibres swell when wet, preventing the further passage of water.
2. *Disposable fabrics*—all non-woven in cellulose, e.g. Protek theatre wear.
3. *Cellulose plus man made fibre*—60 per cent Terylene, 40 per cent cellulose, e.g. Fabric '450'.
4. *Man-made fibre*—high-density spunbounded polythene, e.g. Tyvek.

Some non-woven fabrics incorporate a plastic film bonded to them for extra water repellancy. This is either a double layer or with the PTFE film sandwiched between two layers of woven fabric, e.g. Gore-tex.

The effectiveness of any fabric is reduced or completely lost by poor *design* in the finished garment (7). This is probably due to escape of contamination around openings at the neck, waist, wrist, and ankles as with the standard pyjama style jacket and trousers. Improved designs have blocked these exits without detriment to user comfort.

Moylan *et al.* (13) have demonstrated the beneficial effects on surgical wound infection rates of commercially available disposable gown and drape systems. In a 21-month study involving 2 181 clean and clean contaminated general surgical procedures the overall infection rate was reduced from 6.5 per cent to 2.83 per cent, with substantial cost savings.

Because over 90 per cent of body bacterial emissions come from below the neck, the body exhaust system worn with the walk-in Howorth–Solihull gowns, developed specially for this application not only captures, contains and removes the body emissions of the surgical team which would otherwise be transported on, and disseminated by, their warm body convection currents into the ultra clean air zone, but it also keeps them cool and refreshed so fatigue is reduced.

Gloves

Using gloves during surgery serves two purposes: to protect the surgeon from contamination by blood and exudate from the patient and the patient from transfer of micro-organisms from the surgeon's hands. Wearing rubber gloves obviously reduces the risk of contaminating the operation but minute holes do develop during surgery thus emphasizing that they are not an entirely reliable barrier against contamination of wounds. Devenish and Miles (14) in 1939 found minute holes in 20 per cent of gloves through which bacteria could escape. Church and Sanderson (15) using a dye watertightness test demonstrated punctures in 11.5 per cent of 130 surgical gloves used in one operating theatre on four successive days of operating. Of more importance is the collaborative report which describes eight patients who developed hepatitis B after major gynaecological surgery performed by a surgeon who was a carrier of HB antigen (16). Often, the wearer of the glove is unaware of the fact that the glove has been punctured. Other workers have explored the feasibility of wearing two pairs of gloves and conclude that double gloving does confer some protection with the puncture rate falling from 11 per cent of outer gloves to 2 per cent of inner gloves (17). Surgical staff will have to balance the enhanced safety of introducing a second barrier between themselves and the patients against possible discomfort or reduced sensitivity and dexterity.

More recently, Dalgleish and Malkovsky (18) have examined a wide variety of surgical gloves for the ability to prevent transmission of the human immunodeficiency virus (HIV). Six types of gloves (e.g. Featherlite, starch-free Biogel II E. B. 12, starch-free Biogel s961/1, Regent Sensor, Regent Dispo) withstood severe compression tests and also exhibited direct antiviral properties. No penetration of HIV through the intact glove was detected. However, new, unused gloves have existing holes prior to use emphasizing the fact that the manufacturing process of surgeon's gloves is complicated and demanding. Both inter-lot variation and lot-to-lot variations of the frequency of gloves with pin-holes were found in one study (19).

Gloves should be used once and discarded. They should not be washed or disinfected between use as these manoeuvres may cause subsequent deterioration. During a laboratory assessment of the antimicrobial effectiveness of glove washing and re-use in dental surgical practice 17 per cent of the gloves showed evidence of micropuncture after five sequential inoculations and washings (20).

Masks

Micro-organisms are constantly being shed from exposed skin and from mucous membranes so masks, drapes, hoods, and gowns are used as barriers to decrease shedding into the air and to prevent wound contamination. These barriers are most effective when their pore size is so small that they do not allow passage of bacteria, even during use and when wet. Nowadays face-masks are worn for many and varied procedures but their use is seriously being questioned. During quiet talking and breathing there is little or no expulsion of bacteria-laden particles (21). The practice of wearing masks became important as a vital barrier in the prevention of spread of *Streptococcus pyogenes* in obstetric surgery in the 1940s but recent evidence suggests that this is no longer necessary (22).

An efficient mask must be capable of arresting low momentum droplets which contaminate the front of the operator's gown and his/her sterile gloves and subsequently to the wound. There are few reports of the effect of mask-wearing on infection rates in patients. Ayliffe *et al.* (23) found no evidence of transfer of *Staph. aureus* from staff to patients in an isolation unit with positive pressure ventilation where masks were not worn, other than on the hands of the nurses. In one recent study, staff stopped wearing masks during vaginal delivery and the incidence of puerperal infection in 1750 consecutive cases (3.6 per cent) was the same as in the previous 1750 cases when masks had been worn (22). In a randomized prospective, but unpublished, study in Belfast more than 8000 surgical operations were reviewed after half of the operations were conducted by surgeons not wearing masks. Preliminary results suggest that there was no difference between the two groups. However, the patients studied under-went general surgical operations, e.g. large bowel surgery and not implant surgery of any kind. This may suggest that for certain types of surgery, face masks may *not* be beneficial.

When it is agreed that masks should be worn, e.g. in implant surgery, a high efficiency filtration rate mask should be worn by all members of staff scrubbed and assisting at the operating table; this includes the anaesthetists. It is questionable whether masks are necessary for other members of staff not assisting at the table, e.g. circulating nurses, operating departmental assistants whilst routine general surgery is in progress. There is no need for staff to wear masks in other parts of the theatre complex, e.g. in corridors, patient transfer zones, or sister's office.

A fresh mask must be worn for each operation and care used when the mask is discarded. Manipulation of the mask during use will simply contaminate the outside with skin commensals including staphylococci.

When first introduced masks were made of several layers of gauze or linen and were *re-used* after they had been sterilized. The masks were improved when a piece of paper or cellophane was inserted between the linen layers to provide an impervious barrier. In the last few years these types have been replaced by disposable theatre masks made out of synthetic fibres which are more tolerable. Some, with fibreglass inserts, which were very efficient filters caused facial eruptions and were replaced with filters made of polyester (e.g. Bard Vigilon, Deseret — no glass, White Knight — no glass) or polypropylene (3M 1818 and Filtron) (24). Paper masks have no place in operating theatres as they become wet within a very few minutes and lose their barrier qualities. In addition they do not fit the face or nose well enough to prevent lateral dispersal of large droplets.

The efficiency of masks in use has been tested under a variety of in use situations and with a variety of tests (25). Differences have been found in the efficiencies of similar masks. The fact that some masks prove uniformally good is understandable, but it is difficult to explain a variation between 36.8 per cent and 98.4 per cent for the same mask.

Spectacle wearers often suffer from fogging, i.e. escape of breath in the vicinity of spectacle lenses. Surgical anti-fog masks have a flexible noseband which helps the mask to conform to facial contours and yet retains a very high efficiency of filtration.

Eye-protection

Masks and protective eyewear or face shields should be worn during procedures that are likely to generate droplets of blood or other body fluids to prevent exposure of mucous membranes of the mouth, nose, and eyes. A variety of anti-fog goggles, wrap around spectacles and face shields are now available which are efficient, easy to wear and pleasant in appearance. They are lightweight, adjustable and do not obstruct vision. An educational programme is necessary to introduce surgeons to these new barriers.

Hair/beard cover

All members of staff entering the theatre area must wear their hair in a neat style. Long hair should be tied back in such a way that when the head is bent forward hair does not fall forward, occlude vision, or at worst fall into a surgical wound. Hair must be completely covered by a close-fitting cap made of synthetic material. Once the head cover is in place it must not be adjusted or manipulated as this facilitates the dispersal of many bacteria-carrying particles. Beards should be fully covered by a mask and a hood of the balaclava type which is tied securely at the neck.

Footwear

There is little evidence to show that the floor plays a significant role in the spread of infection in hospital and expensive efforts to minimize bacterial contamination of feet are unnecessary. Nevertheless, it is probably rational to keep contamination of floors of operating theatres to a minimum by routine mopping with hot water and detergent (see later). Operating room staff should wear clean, comfortable, antislip and antistatic shoes. Plastic overshoes are commonly worn by visitors but are an expensive luxury. Putting on overshoes can be potentially hazardous; cross-infection has been reported in an intensive therapy unit due to hand-contamination from the floor when putting on the overshoes. If there is a constant risk of spillage, e.g. in genitourinary surgery, then ankle length antistatic boots can be worn. These boots should conform to British Standard BS5451 which allows static electricity in the body to leak away rather than being transmitted to a patient in the form of an electrostatic shock.

A variety of styles of shoes and clogs are available which allows choice with style. They should fit snugly and must not be allowed to produce a bellows effect. If sufficient shoes or half wellingtons are not available then freshly laundered socks can be provided to act as hygienic inserts.

Preparation of the patient

Cultures from post-operative wound infections often suggest that organisms are transferred from other areas of the patient to the operative site (endogenous transfer) despite the use of antiseptics at this site. This led Swedish workers to consider whether whole-body disinfection would be beneficial (26). The results of these studies suggested that infection rates may be reduced by whole-body disinfection. The pre-operative programme is as follows

1. *Pre-operative day*—Whole-body disinfection with four per cent chlorhexidine detergent soap before changing to hospital clothes.
2. *Pre-operative evening*—Whole-body disinfection with chlorhexidine before retiring to a clean bed.
3. *Operative day*—Whole-body (top to toe) disinfection before changing to operation dress.

The effect of pre-operative whole-body washing with chlorhexidine detergent on the incidence of post-operative wound infection was assessed in a placebo-controlled trial of 1989 patients (27). Patients bathed or showered with 4 per cent w/v chlorhexidine ('Hibiscrub'), placebo, or conventional bar soap on two occasions in the 24 h before operation. The overall infection rate for patients treated with chlorhexidine was 9 per cent, 12.8 per cent with the bar soap, and 11.7 per cent in the placebo groups; in the 'clean' surgery group, infections were 7.2 per cent, 10.2 per cent and 10 per cent respectively. The *Staph. aureus* infection rate in the 'clean' group was 3 per cent for chlorhexidine and 6 per cent for bar soap.

This obvious improvement in infection rates has *not* been demonstrated by other workers. For example, Ayliffe *et al.* (28) found that a single pre-operative bath with 'Hibiscrub' did not influence the infection rate in more than 5000 patients. Further studies by the European Working Party on Control of Hospital Infections (29) in a prospective, randomized, double-blind placebo controlled study of 2813 patients could not demonstrate a reduction in the incidence of infection of clean wounds. These findings are in contrast to the results of the study by Hayek *et al.* (27) whose trial design is criticized.

Given that it is undesirable to spread organisms around the body (possibly by bathing) and that *Staph. aureus* is an important pathogen within the resident microflora, logic would suggest that measures which reduce the skin microflora would decrease infection rates. Cruse and Foord (30), in a 10-year prospective study of more than 62 000 surgical operations, found that the infection rate for clean wounds in patients who did not shower before operation was 2.3 per cent whereas those who showered using a hexachlorophane-detergent preparation had an infection rate of 1.3 per cent. It may be that following two or more 'top to toe' showers with an appropriate (e.g. Hibiscrub) skin antiseptic, followed by an all over rub of body oil, that skin dispersion of staphylococci will be reduced enough to effect wound infection rates. All signs of skin infection in the patient should be pre-treated or covered with waterproof dressings.

Pre-operative shaving

Hair adjacent to the operative site is often removed to prevent the wound from becoming contaminated with hair during the operation. However, the method of hair removal can injure the skin and such injury may increase the risk of infection by promoting increased skin colonization with bacteria (30). Using clippers or a depilatory cream to remove hair seems to cause less skin injury. Cruse and Foord in 1973 (31) found the infection rate was 2.3 per cent in patients who were shaved, but only 1.7 per cent when they were not shaved and had only their pubic hair clipped. In patients who had neither shaving nor clipping the infection rate was 0.9 per cent. Depilatory cream is less traumatic and gives equally effective low rates of infection.

If hair removal is necessary, doing it immediately before the operation may reduce the risk of infection. Gone are the days when a patient is shaved from head to toe for a hair-lip repair!

Pre-operative screening

Pre-operative screening of nasal or pre-sternal swabs is commonly performed on cardiac surgical wards to identify patients carrying *Staph. aureus*, particularly methicillin resistant strains which might be responsible for subsequent sternal wound infection or prosthetic valve endocarditis (32). In practice pre-operative isolation of *Staph. aureus* has rarely, if ever altered pre-operative management and the commonest potential pathogen *Staph. epidermidis* was often disregarded. The cost of processing pre-operative samples can only be justified if the source of an operative infection would be identified as endogenous, and selective prophylaxis altered accordingly. In a study of 314 patients undergoing cardiac surgery Ridgway *et al.* were unable to demonstrate the value of pre-operative screening cultures and considered the exercise not to be cost effective (33). Likewise the ritual of pre-operative screening for carriage of *Streptococcus pyogenes* in gynaecological patients has lapsed. In general, the mere presence of potentially pathogenic micro-organisms is not commensurate with subsequent infections.

Transport of the patient

A design of operating suites has been recommended in which the 'Sterile' zone, including the operating and sterilizing rooms is approached through a clean zone, where theatre clothes are worn. The clean zone is approached through a protective zone where the staff change into theatre clothes, footwear, etc. (34). Between the protective and clean zones in some operating suites a transfer zone is provided, where patients are transferred from the ward trolleys to 'clean' theatre trolleys; this arrangement is thought to have some value in protecting the aseptic zone against contamination from trolleys. Ayliffe *et al.* in 1969 studied the effect of transfer areas on the clean zones in operating suites (35). They were unable to demonstrate any beneficial effect of a transfer zone on the state of cleanliness and bacterial contamination of the clean zone. They felt that it was hard to justify the inclusion of a transfer area for trolleys in the theatre suite. Transfer to the theatre table in the anaesthetic room could be arranged without a special transfer area.

Elaborate and expensive systems do exist involving complex longitudinal transfer trolleys or systems involving mechanical equipment resembling fork lift trucks!

Trolleys are exposed to some degree of contamination during the journeys to and from the wards and should be generally cleaned at least after each day's use and after use for an infected patient. The risk from trolley wheels is very low. Recent work by Lewis *et al.* confirm that using one trolley did not significantly influence the bacterial counts in the theatre and anaesthetic room (36).

Passing the trolley wheels over a sticky (peel off) mat in the transfer area may remove dirt from them but their bacteriological value is doubtful, and the cost scarcely justifies their use.

Drapes

The patient drape is used to isolate the wound site from the patient's own skin bacteria. Whilst cotton drapes are still in constant use it has been known for at least 30 years that when wet they are totally unsuitable in preventing bacterial contamination. Early work by Cruse and Foord in 1973 (31) determined that adhesive plastic skin drapes were *not* associated with a reduction in wound infection. With the usual cloth drapes, the infection rate was 1.5 per cent (186 of 11 893); with plastic drapes, 2.4 per cent (140 of 5714). Whilst these figures are impressive more recent work has confirmed this still to be the case (37). The use of incisional adhesive plastic drapes remains controversial and no convincing demonstration of any anti-infective effect seems to exist.

Theatre cleaning

Much effort is expended on the cleaning of operating theatres. Walls, floors, and furniture are often cleaned after operating sessions and sometimes between operations. Early work by Froud *et al.* in 1966 (38), following extensive environmental testing, confirmed that only horizontal, upward-facing surfaces were heavily contaminated by particles settling from the air. Walls were only slightly contaminated and ceilings even less. The walls and ceilings of the corridor, which were cleaned only twice a year, were not more contaminated than those of theatres which were cleaned twice a week. The floors of the theatres readily became contaminated after cleaning, partly by contact with footwear and partly by the settling of bacteria from the air.

It is generally accepted in the UK to use detergent and water for hospital cleaning rather than chemical disinfectants (39). Disinfectants are reserved for special situations such as the terminal cleaning of isolation rooms and after spillage of infected body fluids.

Cleaning between cases

Air is only one of several possible sources of micro-organisms, others include endogenous and person-to-person spread. All equipment in close contact with breaks in the skin or mucous membranes, or introduced into a sterile body area, should be sterile. These items, e.g. instruments, suture materials are replaced between patients and can be supplied as re-usable items from the TSSU or as single-use items supplied from an industrial irradiation plant. Other items such as large ventilators or anaesthetic machines not in direct contact with the patient can be wiped down with a disposable cloth or sponge using warm water and detergent. If necessary, i.e. after direct contamination, this can be followed by drying with a large, alcohol impregnated, wipe.

The clean up period between patients may be of the order of 20 min which, with an air change of 20 to 30 times per hour, will provide five to six air changes during this period. Bacterial contamination is directly proportional to the number of staff in the operating room and to the degree of activity. Floors should be wet mopped using freshly laundered stay flat mops, fresh hot water, and a general purpose detergent. Walls only need to be spot cleaned with water and detergent if obviously splashed. The idle practice of staff leaning against the walls must be avoided as this is the only way that operative hands can be contaminated from the walls.

Whilst it is prudent to schedule contaminated and dirty cases to the end of the list this is not always practicable since *all* the cases may be contaminated/dirty, e.g. colorectal surgery. There is no evidence to suggest that there is an increased risk of infection when a clean operation follows a dirty case. Nevertheless, implant surgery is often scheduled for a designated theatre as a matter of operational policy. There is no need to set aside a 'dirty' theatre for specific cases. Except for implant surgery the vast majority of wound infection is caused by endogenous bacteria which are best controlled by relevant chemoprophylaxis.

Great attention must be paid to the type and care of cleaning materials. Most floor-cleaning equipment readily becomes contaminated and, unless there is expert supervision of both the cleaner and the materials, major contamination can occur. All spray cleaned items need to be carefully decontaminated at the end of each day and stored in a dry condition. A recent survey (40) revealed that hospital detergent cleaning fluids, while in use, frequently contain large numbers of bacteria, especially Gram-negative bacilli. Therefore it is probable that during cleaning Gram-negative and other bacteria are being redistributed in the patients' environment.

It is imperative that good cleaning techniques are employed and are supervised according to advice from the Infection Control Committee, and in accordance with the local Disinfection Policy.

Cleaning after dirty cases

Modern theatre design and the use of high quality finishing materials allows frequent washing without causing damage. During the course of a routine large bowel operation it is unlikely that the walls of the operating theatre will become visibly contaminated. Pus or faecal material under pressure, however, may discharge beyond the confines of the operating table and will have to be dealt with.

Without good theatre discipline operating theatres tend to become cluttered with unnecessary items of large equipment. The fewer items brought into the theatre the fewer will need to be cleaned. Horizontal surfaces must be reduced to the absolute minimum. This should leave the large operating lamp and the floor. Walls need only be cleaned once a week and ceilings once a month. If the surfaces are coated with a hard gloss finish (humidity and temperature tolerable) they need only be washed often enough to look clean since dingy surroundings tend to undermine the morale of members of staff.

Disinfectants play an important part in the emergency decontamination of blood and body spills (see later). In UK hospitals, phenolic-and chlorine-releasing disinfectants are recommended by the PHLS and the DHSS (41) because they are relatively economic as well as effective. In the past there has been a tendency to use phenolics rather than hypochlorites since they are less inactivated by organic soiling, but, with increasing concern over transmission of viruses, hypochlorites may now be preferred because of their superior activity against a broad spectrum of viruses.

For bacterial contamination of the floor and walls the phenolics, clearsol 1 per cent and stericol 2 per cent can be used as a terminal disinfectant, i.e. when the mess has been cleaned up. Personnel should use gloves, eye protection, a plastic disposable apron and disposable cloth/paper towels. For light contamination, surfaces can be disinfected with sodium dichloroisocyanurate (NaDCC) at 2500 p.p.m. of available chlorine or sodium hypochlorite (NaOCL) at 2500 p.p.m.; contamination by blood spillages will be dealt with later.

Extensive sampling of the inanimate environment, in the absence of an identifiable problem with nosocomial infection is not cost-effective and is not required after dirty cases as a means to determine the efficacy of the cleaning procedure.

Environmental contamination

Gross spillages

If blood is spilled—either from a container or as a result of an operative procedure—the spillage should be dealt with as soon as possible. The spilled blood should be covered completely, either by sodium dichloroisocyanurate (NaDCC) granules or by disposable towels which are then treated with 10 000 p.p.m. sodium hypochlorite solution (NaOCL).

Before treating a major spill, staff should don impervious gloves and a plastic apron. If there is any danger of further splashing then protective eye wear must be used. Such spillages must be covered for 5 to 10 min with disinfectant or with paper towels soaked in disinfectant. Once all the liquid blood has been absorbed, the granule mass can be scooped up and placed in a plastic waste bag marked for incineration. Any remaining traces of blood–granule mixture should be removed with paper towels soaked in NaDCC or NaOCL at 10 000 p.p.m.

Hypochlorite, which may deteriorate on storage, is known to be adversely affected by organic matter but the recommended concentration presents a considerable over-allowance although recent work casts some doubt on this (42). For treatment of blood spills, chlorine-releasing compounds NaDCC granule formulation, which produce higher available chlorine concentrations and contain spilled material, offer an effective alternative.

Unfortunately, hypochlorite releasing compounds are corrosive to metals and bleach fabrics. Freshly activated 2 per cent alkaline glutaraldehyde is active against Hepatitis B and HIV viruses and is non-corrosive to metals. However, glutaraldehyde is an irritant and has sensitizing properties and must be handled with great care. It is expensive and because of its great propensity to cause skin sensitization it must not be splashed about. Further guidance on protection against infection with HIV and Hepatitis viruses has now been published (43).

If blood is spilled on to drapes, theatre gowns etc these are discarded into appropriately coded laundry bags to be regarded as infected linen and washed accordingly (HC(87)30). If single-use disposable linen and gowns are used these are disposed of by incineration.

Sharps disposal

The most common and important method of transmission of blood borne viruses (e.g. HBV and HIV) to health care personnel is by the direct percutaneous inoculation of infected blood by needle or other sharp instrument. The surgical aspects of AIDS will be considered in Chapter 33 but care in the disposal of sharps will lessen environmental contamination. There is no evidence of transmission of HBV by inhalation of droplets, nevertheless a safe system of counting gauze swabs must minimize environmental splashing.

Surgical or other single use gloves can not protect workers from sharps injuries. Wearing two sets of gloves with glutaraldehyde cream between does not lessen the risk of inoculation. Other staff must not be put at risk by careless disposal of sharps and all workers must be reminded of their responsibilities under the Safety at Work Act.

Current advice is not to resheath used needles *unless* there is a safe means available. Local safety policies must dictate which method of disposal is used. All disposable sharps must be promptly placed in a secure puncture-resistant bin/box suitable for incineration. The Department of Health has a specification for sharps containers and a British Standard is in preparation. When syringes containing arterial blood are to be sent to the laboratory, needles must be removed and blind hubs attached to the syringes. Intravascular guidewires, broken glass, and glass slides must be disposed of as sharps. General rubbish and broken bottles must not go into sharps boxes. Sharps boxes must carry 'Danger of Infection' (Biohazard) markings.

Suction disposal

Many episodes of infection have been related to the use of clinical suction apparatus (44). These may arise from misuse of equipment or from design limitations, i.e. lack of specific safety devices to prevent contamination and spread of bacteria to the environment. Most suction apparatus incorporates in-line air filters situated between the collecting vessel and suction source. Without these the suction lines, pumps and discharge readily become contaminated with Gram-negative bacilli. Inappropriate handling of such contaminated equipment facilitates direct transmission of many moisture loving organisms. In addition devices need to be incorporated to prevent overflow of fluid and the generation of froth. There is a risk of contamination when the collecting vessels are removed for emptying. Aerosols may pass through the apparatus and be emitted to the environment in the exhaust air with the potential for widespread cross-infection. Blenkharn in 1988 examined a variety of devices to prevent airborne infection from clinical suction apparatus (45).

Collecting vessels may be single use, e.g. Receptal, or multiple use, consisting of glass or polypropylene. Glass is heavy and is prone to fracture either during the emptying, cleaning, drying or autoclaving procedures. Care must be taken not to allow the contents of the jar to exceed two-thirds full. Antifoam additives may help in the prevention of foam and froth within the collecting vessel, e.g. foamtrol. There is no advantage in adding disinfectants to the bottle when in use as they are often ineffective. When the bottles are not in use they should be decontaminated and stored dry. The single use sterile catheter must not be connected or the container seal broken until put into use.

In free-standing units a filter (BS4199 Part I, 1967) for electrically driven apparatus should be fitted between the collection bottle and the pump; the filter should not be in the outlet to the atmosphere, because the pump may become clogged with coagulated protein if not protected by a filter.

Extreme care should be taken when these collecting vessels are emptied. Free standing units can be electrically disconnected and wheeled to the sluice. The vessel is dismantled and gently lifted and poured carefully down a low-level sluice. The vessel is then rinsed out with warm detergent. They can then be dried in a drying cabinet at 80 °C for about 10 min. Alternatively the vessels can be capped and transported in purpose designed cardboard containers back to the Hospital Sterile and Decontamination Unit (HSDU) where they are emptied, machine washed and heat disinfected. There is no need to sterilize them as heat at 80 °C for 10 min will readily kill vegetative bacteria remaining on the surface of a clean glass vessel.

References

1. Working Party (1972). Ventilation in operation suites. Report of a joint working party. Medical Research Council and DHSS.
2. Lidwell, O.M., Lowbury, E.J.L., Whyte, W., Blowers, R., Stanley, S.J., and Lowe, D. (1983). Airborne contamination of wounds in joint replacement operations: the relationship to sepsis rates. *J. Hosp. Infect.*, **4**, 111–31.
3. Charnley, J. (1964). A clean air operating enclosure. *Br. J. Surg.*, **51**, 202–5.
4. Lidwell, O.M., Lowbury, E.J.L., Whyte, W., Blowers, R., Stanley, S.J., and Lowe, D. (1982). The effect of ultra-clean air in operating rooms on deep sepsis in the joint after total hip or knee replacement: a randomised study. *Br. Med. J.*, **285**, 10–4.
5. Meers, P.D. (1983). Ventilation in operating rooms. *Br. Med. J.*, **286**, 244–5.
6. Clark, R.P., Reed, P.J., Seal, D.V., and Stephenson, M.L. (1985). Ventilation conditions and air-borne bacteria and particles in operating theatres: proposed safe economies. *J. Hyg. (Camb.)*, **95**, 325–35.
7. Mitchell, N.J., Evans, D.S., and Kerr, A. (1978). Reduction of skin bacteria in theatre air with comfortable, non-woven, disposable clothing for operating theatre staff. *Br. Med. J.*, **1**, 696–8.
8. Hill, J., Howell, A., and Blowers, R. (1974). Effect of clothing on dispersal of *Staphylococcus aureus* by males and females. *Lancet*, **ii**, 1131–3.
9. Whyte, W., Bouley, P.V., Hamblen, D.L., Fisher, W.D., and Kelly, I.G. (1983). A bacteriologically occlusive clothing system for use in the operating room. *J. Bone Joint Surg. (Br)*, **65**. 502–6.
10. Lidwell, O.M., Elson, R.A., Lowbury, E.J.L., *et al.* (1987). Ultraclean air and antibiotics for prevention of post-operative infection. *Acta. Ortho. Scand.*, **58**, 4–13.
11. Whyte, W., Hamblen, D.L., Kelly, I.G., Hambraeus, A., and Laurell, G. (1990). An investigation of occlusive polyester surgical clothing. *J. Hosp. Infect.*, **15**, 363–74.
12. Closs, S.J. and Tierney, A.J. (1990). Theatre gowns: a survey of the extent of user protection. *J. Hosp. Infect.*, **15**, 375–8.
13. Moylan, J.A., Fitzpatrick, K.T., and Davenport, K.E. (1987). Reducing wound infections. Improved gown and drape barrier performance. *Arch. Surg.*, **122**. 152–7.
14. Devenish, E.A. and Miles, A.A. (1939). *Lancet*, **i**, 1088–94.
15. Church, J. and Sanderson, P. (1980). Surgical glove punctures. *J. Hosp. Infect.*, **1**, 84.
16. Collaborative Study. (1980). Acute hepatitis B associated with gynaecological surgery. *Lancet*, **i**, 1–6.
17. Matta, H., Thompson, A.M., and Rainey, J.B. (1988). Does wearing two pairs of gloves protect operating theatre staff from skin contamination? *Br. Med. J.*, **297**, 597–8.
18. Dalgleish, A.G. and Malkovsky, M. (1988). Surgical gloves as a mechanical barrier against human immuno-deficiency viruses. *Br. J. Surg.*, **75**, 171–2.
19. Paulssen, J., Eidem, T., and Kristiansen, R. (1988). Perforations in surgeon's gloves. *J. Hosp. Infect.*, **11**, 82–5.
20. Bagg, J., Jenkins, S., and Barker, G.R. (1990). A laboratory assessment of the antimicrobial effectiveness of glove washing and re-use in dental practice. *J. Hosp. Infect.*, **15**, 73–82.
21. Shooter, R.A., Smith, M.A., and Hunter, C.J.W. (1959). A study of surgical masks. *Br. J. Surg.*, **47**, 246–9.
22. Turner, M.J., Crowley, P., and MacDonald, D. (1984). The unmasking of delivery room routine. *J. Obstet. Gynaecol.*, **4**, 188–90.
23. Ayliffe, G.A., Babb, J.R., Taylor, L., and Wise, R. (1979). A unit for source and protective isolation in a general hospital. *Br. Med. J.*, **2**, 461–5.
24. Rogers, K.B. (1981). Face masks: which, when, where and why? *J. Hosp. Infect.*, **2**, 1–4.
25. Quesnel, L.B. (1975). The efficiency of surgical masks of varying design and composition. *Br. J. Surg.*, **62**, 936–40.
26. Brandberg, A. and Andersson, I. (1981). Pre-operative whole body disinfection by shower bath with chlorhexidine soap: effect on transmission of bacteria from skin flora. In *Skin micro-*

biology: relevance to clinical infection (ed. H. I. Maibach and R. Aly), pp. 92–9. Springer-Verlag, New York.

27. Hayek, L. J., Emerson, J. M., and Gardner, A. M. N. (1987). A placebo controlled trial of the effect of two pre-operative baths *or* showers with chlorhexidine detergent on post operative wound infection rates. *J. Hosp. Infect.*, **10**, 165–72.
28. Ayliffe, G. A. J., Noy, M. F., Babb, J. R., Davies, J. G., and Jackson, J. (1983). A comparison of pre-operative bathing with chlorhexidine-detergent and non-medicated soap in the prevention of wound infection. *J. Hosp. Infect.*, **4**, 237–44.
29. Rotter, M. L., Larsen, S. O., Cooke, E. M., *et al.* (1988). A comparison of the effects of pre-operative whole-body bathing with detergent alone and with detergent containing chlorhexidine gluconate on the frequency of wound infections after clean surgery. The European Working Party on Control of Hospital Infections (EWPCHIN). *J. Hosp. Infect.*, **11**, 310–20.
30. Cruse, P. J. E. and Foord, R. (1980). The epidemiology of wound infection. A 10-year prospective study of 62 939 wounds. *Surg. Clin. North Am.*, **60**, 27–40.
31. Cruse, P. J. E. and Foord, R. (1973). A five-year prospective study of 23 649 surgical wounds. *Arch. Surg.*, **107**, 206–9.
32. Keighley, M. R. B. and Burdon, D. W. (1979). Cardiovascular surgery. In *Antimicrobial prophylaxis in surgery*, Chapter 8, p. 136. Pitman Medical, Tunbridge Wells.
33. Ridgway, G. L., Wilson, A. P. R., and Kelsey, M. C. (1990). Pre-operative screening cultures in the identification of staphylococci causing wound and valvular infections in cardiac surgery. *J. Hosp. Infect.*, **15**, 55–63.
34. Medical Research Council. (1962). Design and ventilation of operating-room suites for control of infection and comfort. *Lancet*, **ii**, 945–51.
35. Ayliffe, G. A. J., Babb, J. R., Collins, B. J., and Lowbury, E. J. L. (1969). Transfer areas and clean zones in operating suites. *J. Hyg. Camb.*, **67**, 417–25.
36. Lewis, D. A., Weymont, G., Nokes, G. M., *et al.* (1990). A bacteriological study of the effect on the environment of using a one-or-two-trolley system in theatre. *J. Hosp. Infect.*, **15**, 35–53.
37. Cordtz, T., Schouenborg, L., Laursen, K., *et al.* (1989). The effect of incisional plastic drapes and redisinfection of operation site on wound infection following caesarean section. *J. Hosp. Infect.*, **13**, 267–72.
38. Froud, P. J., Alder, V. G., and Gillespie, W. A. (1966). Contaminated areas in operating theatres. *Lancet*, **ii**, 961–63.
39. Lowbury, E. J. L., Ayliffe, G. A. J., Geddes, A. M., and Williams, J. D. (1981). *Control of hospital infection — a practical handbook*. Chapman & Hall, London.
40. Werry, C., Lawrence, J. M., and Sanderson, P. J. (1988). Contamination of detergent cleaning solutions during hospital cleaning. *J. Hosp. Infect.*, **11**, 44–9.
41. Ayliffe, G. A. J., Coates, D., and Hoffman, P. N. (1984). *Chemical disinfectants in hospitals*. PHLS, London.
42. Bloomfield, S. F. and Miller, E. A. (1989). A comparison of hypochlorite and phenolic disinfectants for disinfection of clean and soiled surfaces and blood spillages. *J. Hosp. Infect.*, **13**, 231–9.
43. Expert Advisory Group on AIDS. (1990). Guidance for Clinical Health Care Workers: Protection against Infection with HIV and Hepatitis Viruses DHSS. HMSO, London.
44. Blenkharn, J. I. and Hughes, V. M. (1982). Suction apparatus and hospital infection due to multiply-resistant *Klebsiella aerogenes*. *J. Hosp. Infect.*, **3**, 173–8.
45. Blenkharn, J. I. (1988). Safety devices to prevent airborne infection from clinical suction apparatus. *J. Hosp. Infect.*, **12**, 109–15.

3

Surgical factors influencing infection

DAVID J. LEAPER

Introduction

We now assume that a low incidence of infection will follow surgery, particularly elective and clean surgery, and it is easy to forget the pioneer work (much of it based on trial and error) which has led to this satisfactory state of affairs. The precise ritual of operative surgery is now entrenched for all time, some of it based on hard scientific evidence and controlled clinical trials, some based on common sense, some still purely anecdotal. This chapter covers the surgical factors which may influence the development of post-operative infection which must not be overlooked or replaced by a blind faith in antimicrobial prophylaxis. In contaminated surgery it is less likely that surgical factors are so important in the determination of post-operative infection and there is no doubt that antimicrobials have significantly changed surgical practice. Equally the importance of the adequacy of pre-operative nutrition and the patient's host defence must be recognized. Many environmental factors during the pre-and post-operative stay on the ward and in the operating theatre have been highlighted by careful audit and surveillance (1). The recognition that a prolonged pre-operative stay can allow nosocomial acquisition of resistant organisms (such as multiple resistant coagulase negative staphylococci, so important in prosthetic surgery) serves as an example. These factors are covered in other chapters.

Many of the surgical factors which influence the incidence of post-operative infection are not easily measured. However, there is no doubt that some are surgeon-related variables (2). It is surely obvious that the surgeon who practices Halstedian gentleness with tissues, with anatomical skill and accurate placement of sutures and apposition, will enjoy the best results. Attention to haemostasis and reduction of dead space is not so easily quantified. An incision made with a scalpel is less likely to be infected than one made with diathermy (3);

bleeding vessels in the wound edge which are tied, rather than diathermied, leave less devitalized tissue to become infected (4). The use of bipolar diathermy reduces the amount of coagulation as it is more accurate but is not universally accepted. However, diathermy allows the operation to be performed more quickly and reduces blood loss, helping to maintain optimal perfusion which lessens the risk of infection. None of these exemplifying factors has been prospectively studied in contaminated surgery where wound infection is directly related to the number and pathogenicity of endogenous organisms introduced to the wound (see Chapter 5). Therefore the bulk of this chapter relates to the minimalization of infection in clean, elective surgery.

Normal skin bacteria and control

The significance of the skin bacteria may be regarded as controversial (5). They comprise commensals (or residents), transients, and pathogens. The commensals include aerobic and anaerobic bacteria such as the propionibacteria (diphtheroids and coryneforms) and *Staphylococcus epidermidis*. This latter coagulase-negative organism, formerly titled *Staph. albus*, is a potential pathogen in prosthetic surgery particularly where nosocomial acquisition of the multiple resistant form (MRCNS) is a well recognized hazard. The transient organisms, not usually found in skin, include *Staph. aureus* (and hospital-acquired methicillin resistant forms—MRSA) and coliforms which have greater infective potential. Other pathogens which can temporarily contaminate skin include *Streptococcus pyogenes*, bacteroides, clostridia (as spores), and candida as well as *Staph. aureus* and coliforms. They are the cause of endogenous infection after clean surgery, and are particularly associated with contamination of skin caused by shaving or poor pre-operative hygiene. Resident organisms occur in highest numbers in the groin, axillae, and on the feet. The external nares may harbour *Staph. aureus* and the fauces *Strep. pyogenes*.

The size of an inoculum of organisms which will cause a wound infection is 1×10^6 organisms/g tissue (6) but it is unusual for this figure to be reached in clean surgery where infection is more likely to be related to other factors. The bacterial population of normal skin in healthy patients is controlled by the dryness of skin, the low pH, desquamation, and by a high salt content (7). Lipids in the skin have antimicrobial properties, as do secretions from other specialized epithelia which also clear bacteria by macrophages and by ciliary action (8). In addition, interbacterial competition further reduces bacterial counts (9).

The effectiveness of pre-operative skin preparation to reduce skin bacteria to as low a count as possible depends largely on the effectiveness of the sampling technique used (10). Techniques which use swab or plate harvesting do not recover as many bacteria as biopsies. Sampling cannot differentiate antimicrobial inhibition from the microbicidal effects of skin preparation.

Pre-operative skin preparation

Shaving

By tradition patients are shaved before surgery, presumably for aesthetic reasons but also to allow post-operative dressing changes to be made more easily. It is now well recognized that shaving brushes can harbour organisms and that the risk of infection increases the longer the time between shaving and surgery (3). It is not clear why we do not shave patients immediately before surgery or resort to depilatory creams. Clumsily shaved skin, often caused by the patients themselves performing an unsupervised shave the night before surgery, damages the deeper layers of skin causing bleeding or wound exudate which acts as a medium for bacterial growth and risks exogenous as well as endogenous contamination. However, once the skin is divided it has been shown that a scalpel change is unnecessary (unless the blade is blunt) (11).

Depilation

Hair removal could be avoided in many operations but, when infection by skin organisms is a hazard, should be effected by shaving immediately pre-operatively or by a depilatory cream. In clean surgery the incidence of wound infection can be reduced from 2 to 5 per cent (following shaving) to less than 1 per cent using a depilatory cream (3, 12).

General hygiene

Patients with open skin infections should not have surgery unless there is an overwhelming indication. Simple hygienic measures and social washing are required and should be supervised by nursing staff and monitored by an infection control officer (if such exists). Clean theatre clothing should allow easy access for surgery. The use of total body washes (13) can disperse organisms (14) but total body antiseptic washes have been used in some centres where the incidence of wound infection has been halved (15).

Skin preparation and antiseptics

Skin preparation

The antiseptics used most popularly for preparing the patients skin immediately prior to surgery are alcoholic chlorhexidine (0.5 per cent) (Hibiscrub) (16) or alcoholic 10 per cent povidone –iodine (1 per cent available iodine) (Betadine) (17). One application of either solution reduces skin flora by 80 to 95 per cent. Commensal organisms on the skin can be almost eliminated and the skin can be rendered almost sterile by repeated use of aqueous chlorhexidine (see surgical scrub). However prolonged, repeated use disturbs this low level of equlibrium by releasing organisms from the deeper layers of skin which cannot be reached by the action of antiseptics (18, 19).

Surgical scrub

Almost complete sterility of the hands can be achieved using a 5-minute handwash with aqueous 4 per cent chlorhexidine or aqueous 7.5 per cent (w/v) povidone–iodine, including 2 minute spent with a brush on the nails alone. Only a 2 to 3 minute hand-wash is required between cases (without further brushing) and the antiseptic continues to exert its effect after gloves are donned.

Surgical scrubbing has been a ritual for over 100 years following acceptance of the Semmelweis doctrine using chlorinated lime, and Lister's phenol. Prolonged washing has been advocated for over 50 years (20) but only damages skin with the attendant risk of the emergence of organisms from deeper layers of skin, particularly when the whole forearm is brushed. The use of an alcoholic iodine solution, chlorhexidine, or povidone iodine, after the surgical scrub but just before gloving may improve effectiveness and prolong the action of the antiseptic under gloves during surgery, but this is not a widespread practice.

Social hand-washing and minor procedures

It is accepted that medical and nursing attendants should wash their hands between patients during ward rounds, particularly after inspecting wounds, but as any infection control officer knows this is almost impossible to police. Social handwashing with soap and water, and adequate drying of the skin, is sufficient for minor procedures such as placement of an intravenous drip cannula but this is not adequate for the placement of central venous lines. Isopropyl alcohol (70 per cent) wipes are sufficient to sterilize patient skin rapidly. Chlorhexidine and povidone–iodine may be used but soap is cheaper and a quaternary ammonium compound such as cetrimide (Savlon) has a useful detergent action for cleaning as well as being antimicrobial, but is not so effective (21). Disposable towels for hand drying are ideal but unpopular.

Other uses of antiseptics in surgical practice

Antiseptics are used not only for skin preparation and surgical scrub but also in the management of open wounds healing by secondary intention, and as prophylactic agents during surgery to prevent post-operative infection (17). Table 3.1 lists the antiseptics commonly used in surgical practice. It should be remembered that all antiseptics are rapidly inactivated after contact with body fluids, necrotic material or pus (22). Other antiseptics, such as glutaraldehyde and the phenols, are used for instrument and surface disinfection and should not be used on tissues. There are some which are used for specialized treatments, such as silver sulphadiazine in treatment of burns. Other agents claimed to have antiseptic properties, such as hydrogen peroxide, have no substantiated use.

Antiseptics in open wounds healing by secondary intention

Surgeons may be faced with infection and breakdown of sutured wounds, or have to deal with wounds electively left open to granulate such as an excised pilonidal sinus, chronic leg ulcers (venous, arterial or diabetic) or even pressure (decubitus) sores. Recognized antiseptics have been used since the days of Semmelweis and Lister as topical antimicrobial agents in a rather unquestioned way, and before then non-recognized antiseptics have been used anecdotally for millenia. In 1919 Fleming asserted that an antiseptic must be an effective antimicrobial without toxic side-effects (23). There is no evidence that successful healing necessarily requires a sterile wound surface and, in fact, the contrary could be the case (24). Compelling experimental evidence has shown that antiseptics, particularly hypochlorites, are toxic to healing tissue and that they might be unnecessary (25–27). Hypochlorites act as desloughing agents probably by killing the surface layer of granulation tissue to enable separation of adherent necrotic

Table 3.1. Classification of antiseptics commonly used in general surgical pratice.

Name	Presentation	Uses	Comments
Chlorhexidine (Hibiscrub)	Alcoholic 0.5% Aqueous 4% (biguanide)	Skin preparation Skin preparation. Surgical scrub In dilute solutions in open wounds	Has cumulative effect. Effective against Gram-positive organisms and relatively stable in presence of pus and body fluids.
Povidone–iodine (Betadine)	Alcoholic 10% Aqueous 7.5%	Skin preparation Skin preparation. Surgical scrub In dilute solutions in open wounds	Safe fast acting broad spectrum. Some sporidical activity. Antifungal. Iodine is not free but combined with polyvinylpyrrolidone (povidone).
Cetrimide (Savlon)	Aqueous	Hand-washing Instrument and surface cleaning	*Pseudomonas* spp. may grow in stored contaminated solutions. Ammonium compounds have good detergent action (surface active agent).
Alcohols	70% ethyl, isopropyl	Skin preparation	
Hypochlorites	Aqueous preparations (Eusol, Milton, Chloramine T)	Instrument and surface cleaning. (Debriding agent in open wounds?)	Should be reserved for use as disinfectant.
Hexachlorophane	Aqueous bisphenol	Skin preparation Hand-washing	Has action against Gram-negative organisms.

slough. Mechanical excision is probably quicker and less damaging. Dilute aqueous solutions of chlorhexidine and povidone iodine may act as antimicrobials and reduce odour, but do not appear to be so toxic. In addition, the cytotoxic effect of antiseptics may be useful as an adjunct to the operative treatment of cancer (28, 29). The use of antiseptics in open wound care may be largely replaced by the range of dressings now available (see later in this chapter).

Antiseptics used as intra-operative prophylactic agents

Lister successfully used phenol as an intra-operative agent to prevent infection after surgery for compound limb fractures but the evidence that antiseptics are useful during modern surgical procedures is controversial. To have any chance of success they must surely be used before tissues are contaminated in the decisive period after wounding (30). Despite early encouraging reports of intra-operative wound lavage with antiseptics (31, 32) success has not been repeated by other workers (33–35). This controversy is similar to the use of topical antimicrobial lavage with tetracycline which has also been shown to reduce wound infections in contaminated surgical procedures (36) but bears further investigation by prospective controlled comparative and blinded clinical trials. Without any definite evidence that topical antiseptics and antimicrobials cause harm to tissues at operation, their use must remain the individual surgeons choice although it is quite obvious that copious lavage with an antimicrobial can reduce bacterial contamination.

Intra-operative surgically-related factors

Gloves

Gloves were originally devised to protect the hands of operating theatre staff when toxic antiseptics were being used. They are now part of the aseptic ritual, but whether any breaks in the technique of donning gloves, or intra-operative glove damage, directly relates to post-operative infection in general surgery is not clear. In prosthetic surgery it is logical that contamination from gloves is important and that breaks in gloving routine or intra-operative damage must be avoided. Similarly, during surgery on patients with transmissible diseases great care must be taken to avoid operator trauma and damaged gloves. Nevertheless, holes appear in gloves during surgery in up to 50 per cent of operations. The incidence can be minimized by a scrupulous 'no touch' technique but this is difficult to perfect in practice. Electronic circuitry can be devised to activate an alarm buzzer when gloves are perforated (and can be changed) but has not gained much acceptance (37).

Wound incise drapes

Thin sheet, transparent polymeric incise drapes were introduced 30 years ago (38, 39). Most are made of polyurethane with one adhesive side and they have also been used extensively as dressings over primarily sutured wounds and open wounds healing by secondary intention. When used as incise drapes they can cover the whole operative field and adhere to surrounding disposable or reusable linen drapes, thereby avoiding the need for towel clips. Incise drapes are particularly useful in isolating an abdominal stoma or infected focus from a freshly made wound but there is no evidence that their use reduces post-operative wound infection (40, 42). Antiseptic impregnation of incise drapes, with povidone–iodine, has been shown to reduce the skin bacterial count but not to prevent an increase in bacteria colonizing the wound during an operation (43). In clean general surgical operations it is unlikely that any effect on wound infection would be seen, and the use of incise drapes is unnecessary, but they may be of use in prosthetic implant surgery.

Wound guards

The use of a polymeric sheet placed over the wound edge, with an attached ring in the peritoneum to hold it in place, does reduce bacterial contamination of the wound edge during open viscus surgery (44). However, as with incise drapes the theoretical corollary of a reduction in the incidence of wound infection, has not been proven. (45, 48). The use of wound guards in general surgery should be viewed with scepticism.

Drains

There are several theoretical reasons to use drains after surgical procedures. They would seem to be common sense but in reality have little real proven value. It is classical surgical teaching to minimize dead space, particularly in the wound. This can be achieved by anatomical layered closure but the increased number of sutures introduces more foreign body material and risks devascularization of tissue and increased infection. Alternatively, a drain may help to reduce dead space and prevent the collection of blood, exudate or other body fluid which acts as a culture medium. However, there is doubt that dead space needs to be avoided (49) or that drains effectively reduce dead space and lessen the risk of infection (50, 51). Despite this it is not easy to dissuade surgeons from the use of drains where there is a potential dead space or an oozing wound with potential infection.

There are two types of drain available for wound drainage: the open type, where secondary infection may easily track into the wound; and the closed suction type, where reflux of potentially infected material is prevented, but these are liable to block as the surrounding tissues occlude the drain holes (52). Closed system suction drains are preferable but introduce a foreign body reaction which may enhance infection and stimulate collagenolysis (53, 54).

Wound closure

There is a multiplicity of techniques and materials for closing wounds. Any technique should avoid tension and there is no definite need to avoid dead space, although haemostasis is important. The hypoxia at the wound edge is the stimulus, through released chemoattractants, to macrophage function which in turn directs fibroblastic activity and angiogenesis in the healing wound (55, 56). There is biochemical evidence that a dynamic collagenolytic zone exists around a healing wound and if sutures are placed within this zone they are at risk of cutting out (57). Infection widens this zone and the chance of wound failure is minimized by the use of the least amount of the least reactive, monofilament, and usually synthetic polymer suture.

Local factors in wound closure, other than technique, which reduce the risk of infection are adequate attention to debridement of foreign bodies or contamination, and avoidance of excessive trauma. Tied bleeding vessels make a wound less prone to infection than diathermy haemostasis (4). The maintainance of optimal tissue perfusion during surgery and in the early post-operative period when wound healing begins is probably the single most important determinant of the success of healing and avoidance of wound infection. Perfusion, measured as tissue oxygen tension, is a useful and accurate parameter for monitoring this (58–61).

Sutures

The function of wound closure techniques is to hold wound edges together until healing is complete. In some instances sutures may be required to hold a wound together without great strength (in bowel anastomosis), but to ensure a leak proof apposition, or with great strength (in abdominal wall aponeurotic muscle layer closure). It takes up to six months to reach the full tensile strength in the latter situation and even when complete this is only three-quarters of pre-wound strength (62). Once healing is complete the sutures are relatively unimportant but if an absorbable suture is used then its integrity must persist until wound tensile strength has reached an appropriate level. The use of catgut alone in the abdominal wall serves as an example: it is associated with an unacceptable rate of wound breakdown and should not be used for this purpose. In some situations a prolonged suture life is necessary. In vascular surgery, non-biodegradable monofilament sutures (such as polypropylene) are required to prevent anastomotic separation or aneurysm formation.

Table 3.2. Modern sutures and recommendations for their use.

Suture type	Example (Trade name)	Presentation	Comments
Natural—absorbable	Plain catgut Chromic catgut	Monofilament twist collagen Monofilament twist collagen chromicisation delays absorption	Highly irritant in tissues. May predispose to infection in contaminated wounds. Useless in deep wound closure (abdominal wall) with high suture failure rate and infection. Still popular for bowel anastomosis and ties. 21-day catgut can disrupt within a few days in infected wounds.
Non-absorbable	Silk (silicone coat)	Twist or braid for best handling and knotting.	Biodegradeable and irritant. No use for long term security. Should not be used in contaminated wounds. Braids risk capillarity and may increase infection.
	Cotton, linen	Braided	Used for tying ligatures—being replaced by modern polymeric absorbables.
	Stainless steel wire	Monofilament	Used for strength, closing abdominal and chest wounds, with low infective risk but difficult to tie. Safe in contaminated wounds.
Synthetic—absorbable (All polymers)	Polyglycolic acid (Dexon) Polyglactin (Vicryl) Polydioxanone (PDS) Polyglyconate (Maxon)	Braided with final coat for handling and knotting. Braided Monofilament Monofilament	Replacing catgut as resorption rates are predictable and irritative effect in tissues is lessened. Some (PDS) have long life tissue integrity and may be used for wound deep layers and skin closure. Shorter life sutures may relate to wound irritation but subcuticular sutures do not require removal. Braids ideal for ligature ties.
Non-absorbables	Polyamide (Nylon, Nuralon) Polyester (Dacron) Polypropylene (Prolene) Polyethylene Polybutester (Novafil) Polytetrafluoroethylene (PTFE)	Extruded polymers as mono-filaments or braids which may be coated for easier handling and knotting.	Nylon is briodegradeable and should not be used in vascular surgery where Prolene, Polybutester or PTFE monofilaments should be used. As monofilaments they may be used for wound closure with low infection rates. No irritation in tissues unless knots become infected by contamination. Subcuticular sutures require removal. These give the best cosmetic results in skin because of no irritation (if braids not used) and very fine sutures have high tensile strength. Braided forms used for deep tissue apposition (hernia repair) with low infection rates.

However, sutures are foreign bodies. They can potentiate infection, particularly in the presence of contamination, and have a necrotizing effect if tied too tightly, again adding to the risk of infection. Their use for closure of dead space is probably unwarranted (49, 63).

The foreign body effect of sutures can be minimized by the use of monofilament, non-absorbable materials which have high tensile strength, as well as by techniques which use as little material as possible without an unnecessarily large diameter of suture (continuous fine sutures use less material than interrupted). Natural suture materials, particularly the absorbable catgut group, have a pronounced tissue reaction and, together with any devitalized or ischaemic tissue, render the wound liable to infection with a much lower inoculum (64). The irritative effect of catgut in tissues is almost matched by that of other natural, but so called non-absorbable sutures, such as silk, linen, or cotton. They are biodegradeable and, as well as potentiating infection, they are irritating to the tissues, (particularly if braided, when capillarity is enhanced) and have their tensile strength reduced by infection (65-68). The suture abscesses seen in skin after the use of silk reflect these features. The herring-bone scars which result are not acceptable. Knots left deep in the tissues have the same effect and knots with several throws, even using monofilament, non-absorbable materials, may act as a nidus for persistent infection. Knot and suture sinuses are unusual following adequate antibiotic prophylaxis but knots can be kept to a minimum by using loops or continuous techniques. A classification of modern sutures and recommendations for their use is shown in Table 3.2. Most suture materials are swaged on to their needles and are therefore atraumatic as they are passed through tissues. The lessened tissue damage reduces the infective risk, particularly when a fine suture can be used such as the monofilament non-absorbable polymers which have a high tensile strength. In bowel and other tissues, where atraumatic technique is required, round bodied needles may be used whereas in tough tissues, such as skin, cutting needles are required. Skin can safely be closed after clean surgery without wound infection using polymeric absorbables or non-absorbables (69). Continuous closure can be undertaken after contamination providing antibiotic prophylaxis or treatment is adequate (70, 71). Subcuticular techniques give the best cosmetic results.

Tissue adhesives

The use of cyanoacrylates to close wound edges is attractive but wound edges need to be dry with near perfect haemostasis. They are expensive with no clear advantage and have not gained widespread use.

Skin clips

The use of clips (and tapes) is time honoured and has been related to low rates of wound infection (72). Modern inserting devices are expensive. They do save time (73, 74) but it has been reported that results are bettered with the use of tapes (75, 76).

Skin tapes

Sutures may be replaced by skin tapes within a few days of surgery and give very good cosmetic results with no hatching and fine white scar lines. They promote healing biology by spreading the tensile strength evenly along the whole length of the wound, and are related to low wound infection rates (77, 78). Tapes may be impossible to apply at the end of an operation if haemostasis is not adequate and may be difficult to remove when healing is complete. The use of an adhesive polyurethane dressing acts in a similar fashion and adhesion may be facilitated by skin drying agents.

Wound closure and foreign bodies

The foreign body effect of sutures, particularly natural, non-absorbable braids such as silk, has already been discussed. Severely contaminated wounds can be left open to heal by secondary intention or submitted to delayed primary or secondary suture. Open wounds do not become infected (75, 79), yet even in the presence of severe contamination, with adequate mechanical irrigation and appropriate antibiotic therapy, primary closure is safe (36, 71). Contamination and devitalisation are common to military wounds and require specialised care. (See Chapter 18.) In essence, because of foreign bodies (particularly clothing and soil) and devitalization a much smaller inoculum of organisms can lead to wound infection requiring techniques of fasciotomy and debridement (80, 81).

Dressings

The ideal dressing does not exist but some notable advances have been made in the last 20 to 30 years which overshadow the Paré aphorism: '*je le pensay*, *Dieu le guarist*' (I dress the wound, God heals it). Whether dressings are necessary after primary wound suture has still to be answered but there is no doubt that the moist wound environment afforded by appropriate dressings does improve epithelialization and granulation tissue formation (82, 83). Dressings can retain heat and the antimicrobial effect of wound exudate (84–86). However, a wound that is kept open and allowed to dry develops a coagulum which resists secondary infection even if scab formation may delay epithelialization by a few hours or days. A useful compromise might be the use of polymeric adhesive sheet dressings which act as a tape closure, maintain the moist environment and wound exudates, and prevent over-zealous wound cleansing and dressing changes which risk secondary infection. These dressings are leak proof so that 'strike through' is not an infection risk and excessive exudate can be aspirated through the dressing. Thick absorbent dressings do risk skin maceration and once exudate reaches the dressing surface bacteria may easily migrate from the exterior to the wound surface (strike through).

Dressings are equally important for wounds healing by secondary intention whether these are dehisced, infected wounds or chronic skin ulcers (which are often referred for surgical care). The requirements for an ideal surgical dressing are shown in Table 3.3, modified from another source (87).

Table 3.3. The ideal surgical dressing.

Absorbent and able to remove excess exudate.
Maintain moist environment, aid own tissues to debride necrotic material and promote healing.
Prevent trauma to underlying healing granulate tissue or to prevent shed of foreign particles into the wound.
Be leakproof and prevent 'strike through' and secondary infection.
Maintain temperature and gaseous exchange.
Allow simple dressing changes, easy application and removal, and be pain free.
Be odourless, cosmetically acceptable, and comfortable.
Be inexpensive

There is a plethora of dressings now available ranging from those with an historical background and indications for their use (and are surprisingly still popular) to modern polymeric materials which have been tailor-made for their function. There are very few scientifically acceptable trials which show any clear advantages and the surgical practitioner may, in effect, choose which dressing he or she wishes. Table 3.4 gives an indication of the range of dressings and some of their individual functions (24, 88). The use of antiseptic impregnated dressings confers no obvious advantage as sterility of an open wound surface is not a prerequisite for healing. The moist wound healing environment may be inappropriate in ischaemic or diabetic ulcers where maceration may lead to invasive infection which needs systemic antibiotic therapy based on organisms harvested by microbiological culture. A wound which yields pathogens but shows no clinical evidence of infection does not warrant antibiotic therapy, either topically or systemically. The risk of allergy or emergence of resistant organisms and cross-infection precludes the use of empiric therapy (89). Healing by secondary intention does not require the ulcer or wound surface to be sterile (90) and the aphorism of 'treat the patient, not the microbiology swab' holds true. There is no definite evidence that the prolonged use of any surgical dressing for surgical debridement is justified. It is far more logical to debride necrotic tissue with a scalpel, scissors, or by irrigation (with or without a general anaesthetic) but chlorinated solutions are certainly best avoided once the wound is clean (91).

Conclusions

We have entered an era of surgery where post-operative infection, particularly after elective, clean operations, is at its lowest. It is not a time for complacency. We must not forget

Table 3.4. Surgical dressings.

Type	Name (Example)	Indications and comments
Debriding agents	Benoxyl—benzoic acid Aserbine—benzoic and salacyclic acid Variclene—lactic acid	Used only in necrotic sloughing skin ulcers. Provide acidic environment. Claimed to enhance healing with debriding action.
Enzymatic agents	Varidase—streptokinase/streptodornase	Activate fibrinolysis and liquify pus on chronic skin ulcers.
Bead dressings	Debrisan Lodosorb Other paste dressings	Remove bacteria and excess moisture by capillary action in deep granulating wounds. Antimicrobials may be added but with questionable topical benefit.
Polymeric films	Op-site Bioclusive	Primary adhesive transparent dressings for sutured wounds or donor sites.
Foams	Silastic (elastomer) Lyofoam	Elastomeric dressing can be shaped to fit deep cavities and granulating wounds. Absorbent and non adherent.
Hydrogels	Geliperm Scherisorb	Maintain moist environment. Polymers can absorbe exudate, or antiseptics (but adding antiseptics is of doubtful benefit). Semi-permeable, allow gas exchange.
Hydrocolloids	Comfeel Granuflex	Complete occlusion. Promote epithelialisation and granulation tissue. Maintain moisture without gaseous exchange across them.
Fibrous polymers	Kaltostat Sorbsan	Absorptive alginate dressings. Derived from natural (sea weed) source. Like polymeric hydrocolloids and hydrogels can pack deep wounds.
Biological membranes	Porcine skin, amnion	Used for superficial chronic skin ulcers. No proven advantage.
Simple miscellaneous	Gauzes. Viscose/cotton with non adherent coating. (Melolin)	Simple absorptive dressings only used as secondary dressings to absorb exudate.
	Tulles. Non adherent paraffin impregnation. Paste bandages. Coal tar zinc additives	Added antimicrobials probably confer no benefit. Added charcoal absorbents may reduce swelling. Relatively cheap but of questionable effectiveness.

the pioneer surgery, however anecdotal, which has led to modern theatre technique. Those time-honoured rituals should be obeyed and kept in force until there is hard evidence that they may be safely abandoned. We should continue to perfect surgical technique and not rely on prophylaxis with increasingly broad-spectrum antibiotics. Equally, our interest and advancement of knowledge in tissue physiology and perfusion, host defences, nutrition, and bacterial invasion must continue.

References

1. Report Ad Hoc Committee on Trauma. (1964). Division Medical Sciences. National Academy of Sciences—National Research Council. *Ann. Surg.*, **160** (suppl.), 1–192.
2. Russell, R.C.G. (1987). Surgical Technique. *Br. J. Surg.*, **74**, 763–4.
3. Cruse, P.J.E., and Foord, R. (1980). The epidemiology of wound infection. A 10 year prospective study of 62 939 wounds. *Surg. Clin. North Am.*, **60**, 27–40.
4. Arnot, R.S., Evans, M., and Pollock, A.V. (1975). The influence of two methods of haemostasis on the rate of wound sepsis: a random controlled trial of ligature and diathermy. *Br. J. Surg.*, **62**, 655.
5. Selwyn, S. and Ellis, H. (1972). Skin bacteria and skin disinfection reconsidered. *Br. Med. J.*, **i**, 136–40.
6. Roettinger, W., Edgerton, M.T., Kurtz, L.D., Prusak, M., and Edlich, R.F. (1973). Role of inoculation site as a determinant of infection in soft tissue wounds. *Am. J. Surg.*, **126**, 354–8.
7. Selwyn, S. (1980). Skin preparation, the surgical scrub and related rituals. In *Controversies in surgical sepsis* (ed. S. Karran). Praeger Scientific, Eastbourne, UK. pp. 23–32.
8. Aly, R., Maibach, H.I., Rahman, R., Shinefield, H.R., and Mandel, A.D. (1975). Correlation of human in vivo and in vitro cutaneous antimicrobial factors. *J. Infect. Dis.*, **131**, 579–3.
9. Selwyn, S. (1980). Microbial interactions and antibiosis. In *Skin microbiology: relevance to clinical infection* (ed. H.I. Maibach and R. Aly). Springer-Verlag, New York.
10. Selwyn, S., Anderson, I.S., and Rogers, T.R. (1979). Quantitative studies on the decontamination of skin and mucous membranes in relation to immunodeficient patients. In *Clinical and experimental gnotobiotics* (ed. T.M. Fliedner), pp. 281–4. Gustav Fischer, Stuttgart.
11. Jacobs, H.B. (1974). Skin knife-deep knife: The ritual and practice of skin incisions. *Ann. Surg.*, **179**, 102–4.
12. Seropian, R. and Reynolds, B.M. (1971). Wound infections after pre-operative depilatory versus razor preparation. *Am. J. Surg.*, **121**, 251–4.
13. Ayliffe, G.A.J., Noy, M.F., Babb, J.R., Davies, J.G., and Jackson, J. (1983). A comparison of pre-operative bathing with chlorhexidine detergent and non-medicated soap in the prevention of wound infection. *J. Hosp. Infect.*, **4**, 237–44.
14. Speers, R., Bernard, H., O'Grady, F., and Shooter, R.A. (1965). Increased dispersal of skin bacteria into the air after shower-baths. *Lancet*, **i**, 478–80.
15. Brandberg, A. and Anderson, I. (1981). In *Skin microbiology: relevance to clinical infection* (ed. H. Maibach and R. Aly). Springer-Verlag, New York, pp. 92–96, 98–102.
16. Ojajarvi, J. (1976). An evaluation of antiseptics used for hand disinfection in wards. *J. Hygiene*, **76**, 75–82.
17. Proceedings of the III World Congress on Antiseptics. (1985). *J. Hosp. Infect.*, **6**, Suppl A.
18. Lilly, H.A. and Lowbury, E.J.L. (1971). Disinfection of the skin: an assessment of some new preparations. *Br. Med. J.*, **3**, 674–7.
19. Lilly, H.A., Lowbury, E.J.L., and Wilkins, M.D. (1979). Limits to progressive reduction of resident skin bacteria by disinfection. *J. Clin. Path.*, **32**, 382–5.
20. Price, P.B. (1938). The bacteriology of normal skin: a new quantitative test applied to a study of the bacterial flora and the disinfectant action of mechanical cleansing. *J. Infect. Dis.*, **63**, 301–18.
21. Sanford, J.P. (1970). Disinfectants that don't. *Ann. Intern. Med.*, **72**, 282–3.
22. Russell, A.D., Hugo, W.B., and Ayliffe, G.A.J. (1982). *Principles and practice of disinfection, preservation and sterilisation.* Blackwell Scientific Publications, Oxford.
23. Fleming, A. (1919). The action of chemical and physiological antiseptics in a septic wound. *Br. J. Surg.*, **7**, 99–129.
24. Anon. (1991). Local applications to wounds. *Drug Ther. Bull.* (In press.)
25. Brennan, S.S. and Leaper, D.J. (1985). The effect of antiseptics on the healing wound: a study using the rabbit ear chamber. *Br. J. Surg.*, **72**, 780–2.
26. Leaper, D.J. and Simpson, R.A. (1986). Antiseptics and healing. *J. Antimicrob. Chemother.*, **17**, 135–7.
27. Lucarotti, M.E., Morgan, A.P., and Leaper, D.J. (1990). The effect on antiseptics and the moist environment on ulcer healing; an experimental and biochemical study. *Phlebology*, **5**, 173–79.
28. Umbleby, H.C. and Williamson, R.C.N. (1984). The efficacy of agents employed to prevent anastomotic recurrence in colorectal carcinoma. *Ann. R. Coll. Surg. Engl.*, **66**, 192–4.
29. Lucarotti, M.E., White, J., Deas, J., Silver, I.A., and Leaper, D.J. (1990). Antiseptic toxicity to breast carcinoma in tissue culture—an adjuvant to conservative therapy? *Ann. R. Coll. Surg. Engl.*, **72**, 388–92.
30. Burke, J.F. (1961). The effective period of preventing antibiotic action in experimental incisions and dermal lesions. *Surgery*, **50**, 161–8.
31. Gilmore, O.J.A. (1977). A reappraisal of the use of antiseptics in surgical practice. *Ann. R. Coll. Surg. Engl.*, **59**, 93–103.
32. Stokes, E.J., Howard, E., Peters, J.L., Hackworth, C.A., Milne, S.E., and Witherow, R.O. (1977). A comparison of antibiotic and antiseptic prophylaxis of wound infection in acute abdominal surgery. *World J. Surg.*, **1**, 777–82.
33. Crosfil, M., Hall, R., and London, D. (1969). The use of chlorhexidine antisepsis in contaminated surgical wounds. *Br. J. Surg.*, **56**, 906–8.
34. Pollock, A.V. and Evans, M. (1975). Povidone iodine for the control of surgical wound infection: a controlled trial against topical Cephaloridine. *Br. J. Surg.*, **62**, 292–4.
35. Galland, R.B., Saunders, J.H., Moslen, J.G., and Darrell, J.H. (1977). Prevention of wound infection in abdominal operations by perioperative antibiotics or povidone iodine. *Lancet*, **ii**, 1043–5.
36. Krukowski, Z.H. and Matheson, N.A. (1988). 10 year computerised audit of infection after general surgery. *Br. J. Surg.*, **75**, 857–61.
37. Hamer, A.J. (1987). Electronic device for the detection of breaches in asepsis during surgical procedures. *Br. J. Surg.* **74**, 1038–9.
38. Artz, C.P., Conn, J.H., and Howard, H.S. (1960). Protection of the surgical wound with a new plastic film. *J. Am. Med. Assoc.*, **174**, 1865–8.
39. Page, W.G. (1960). A new transparent plastic surgical drape. *Am. J. Surg.*, **100**, 590–2.
40. Paskin, D.L. and Lerner, H.J. (1969). A prospective study of wound infections. *Am. Surg.*, **35**, 627–9.

41. Lilly, H. A., London, P. S., Lowbury, E. J. L., and Porter, M.F. (1970). Effects of adhesive drapes on contamination of operation wounds. *Lancet*, **ii**, 431–2.
42. Jackson, D. W., Pollock, A. V., and Tindall, D. S. (1971). The value of a plastic adhesive drape in the prevention of wound infection. *Br. J. Surg.*, **58**, 340–2.
43. Lewis, D., Leaper, D. J., and Speller, D. C. E. (1984). Prevention of bacterial colonisation of wounds at operation: comparison of iodine impregnated (Ioban) drapes with conventional methods. *J. Hosp. Infect.*, **5**, 431–7.
44. Raahave, D. (1976). Effect of plastic skin and wound drapes on the density of bacteria in operation wounds. *Br. J. Surg.*, **63**, 421–6.
45. Harrower, H. W. (1968). Isolation of incisions into body cavities. *Am. J. Surg.*, **116**, 824–6.
46. Maxwell, J. G., Ford, C. R., Pederson, D. E., and Richards, R. C. (1969). Abdominal wound infections and plastic drape protectors. *Am. J. Surg.*, **118**, 844–8.
47. Alexander-Williams, J., Oates, G. D., Brown, P. P., Burdon, D. W., McCall, J., Hutchison, A. G., and Leers, L. J. (1972). Abdominal wound infections and plastic wound guards. *Br. J. Surg.*, **59**, 142–6.
48. Psaila, J. V., Wheeler, M. H., and Crosby, D. L. (1977). The role of plastic wound drapes in the prevention of wound infection following abdominal surgery. *Br. J. Surg.*, **64**, 729–32.
49. Ferguson, D. J. (1968). Clinical application of experimental relations between technique and wound infection. *Surgery*, **63**, 377–81.
50. Alexander, J. W., Korelitz, J., and Alexander, N. S. (1976). Prevention of wound infection. A case for closed suction drainage to remove wound fluids deficient in opsonic proteins. *Am. J. Surg.*, **132**, 59–63.
51. Bartolo, D. C. C., Andrews, H., Virjee, J., and Leaper, D. J. (1985). A comparative clinical and ultrasonic trial of the new Reliavac drain after cholecystectomy. *J. R. Coll. Surg. Edinb.*, **30**, 358–9.
52. Harland, R. N. L. and Irving, M. H. (1988). Surgical drains. *Surgery*, **1**, 1360–2.
53. Hawley, P. R. (1969). The aetiology of colonic anastomotic leaks with special reference to the role of collagenase. MS thesis, University of London.
54. Magee, C., Rodeheaver, G. T., and Golden, G. T. (1976). Potentiation of wound infection by surgical drains. *Am. J. Surg.*, **131**, 547–9.
55. Silver, I. A. (1969). The measurement of oxygen tension in healing tissue. *Prog. Resp. Res.*, **3**, 124–35.
56. Hunt, T. K., and Halliday, B. (1980). Inflammation in wounds: from laudable pus to primary repair and beyond. In *Wound healing and wound infection: theory and surgical practice* (ed. T. K. Hunt). Appleton-Century-Crofts, New York.
57. Adamson, R. J., Musco, F., and Enquist, I. F. (1966). The chemical dimensions of a healing incision. *Surg. Gynecol. Obstet.*, **123**, 515–21.
58. Gottrup, F., Firmin, R., Hunt, T. K., and Mathes, S. J. (1984). The dynamic properties of tissue oxygen in healing flaps. *Surgery*, **95**, 527–36.
59. Jonsson, K., Jensen, J. A., Goodson, W. H., West, J. M., and Hunt, T. K. (1987). Assessment of perfusion in post-operative patients using tissue oxygen measurements. *Br. J. Surg.*, **74**, 263–7.
60. Lancaster, J. F. and Leaper, D. J. (1988). Tissue oxygen measurements and sepsis scoring. *Surg. Res. Comm.*, **3** (Suppl 1), 50.
61. Gote, H., Raahave, D., and Baech, J. (1990). Tissue oximetry as a possible predictor of lethal complications after emergency intestinal surgery. *Surg. Res. Comm.*, **7**, 243–9.
62. Douglas, D. M. (1952). The healing of aponeurotic incisions. *Br. J. Surg.*, **40**, 79–84.
63. De Holl, D., Rodeheaver, G., Edgerton, M. T., and Edlich, R. F. (1974). Potentiation of infection by suture closure of dead space. *Am. J. Surg.*, **127**, 716–20.
64. Howe, C. W. (1966). Experimental studies on determinants of wound infection. *Surg. Gynecol. Obstet.*, **123**, 507–14.
65. Posthlethwait, R. W., Willigan, D. A., and Ulin, A. W. (1975). Human tissue reaction to sutures. *Ann. Surg.*, **181**, 144–50.
66. Bucknall, T. E., (1981). Abdominal wound closure: choice of suture. *J. R. Soc. Med.*, **74**, 580–5.
67. Bucknall, T. E., Teare, L., and Ellis, H. (1983). The choice of a suture to close abdominal fascia. *Eur. Surg. Res.*, **15**, 59–66.
68. Capperauld, I. and Bucknall, T. E. (1984). Sutures and dressings. In *Wound healing for surgeons* (ed. T. E. Bucknall and H. Ellis). Baillière Tindall, Eastbourne, UK.
69. Leaper, D. J. and Benson, C. E. (1985). A controlled trial of polypropylene or polydioxanone sutures for subcuticular skin closue after inguinal surgery. *J. R. Coll. Surg. Edinb.*, **30**, 234–6.
70. Foster, G. E., Hardy, E. G., and Hardcastle, J. D. (1977). Subcuticular suturing after appendicectomy. *Lancet*, **i**, 1128–9.
71. Leaper, D. J., Kennedy, R. H., Sutton, A., Johnson, E., and Roberts, N. (1987). Treatment of acute bacterial peritonitis: a trial of imipenem against ampicillin–metronidazole–gentamicin. *Scand. J. Infect. Dis.*, **52**, 7–10.
72. Stillman, R. M., Marino, C. A., and Seligman, S. J. (1984). Skin staples in potentially contaminated wounds. *Arch. Surg.*, **119**, 821–2.
73. Stephens, F. O., Hunt, T. K., and Dunphy, J. E. (1971). Studies of traditional methods of care on the tensile strength of skin wounds in rats. *Am. J. Surg.*, **122**, 78–80.
74. Harrison, I. D., Williams, D. F., and Cuschieri, A. (1975). The effects of metal clips on the tensile properties of healing skin wounds. *Br. J. Surg.*, **62**, 945–9.
75. Edlich, R. F., Rodeheaver, G., and Kuphal, J. (1974). Techniques of closure: contaminated wounds. *Ann. Emerg. Med.*, **3**, 375–82.
76. Johnson, A., Rodeheaver, G. T., Durand, L. S., Edgerton, M. T., and Edlich, R. F. (1981). Automatic disposable stapling devices for wound closure. *Ann. Emerg. Med.*, **10**, 631–5.
77. Forrester, J. C. (1980). Collagen morphology in normal and wound tissue. In *Wound healing and wound infection: theory and surgical practice* (ed. T. K. Hunt), Chapter 10. Appleton-Century-Crofts, New York.
78. Forrester, J. C. (1980). Sutures and wound repair. In *Wound Healing and wound infection: theory and surgical practice* (ed. T. K. Hunt), Chapter 15. Appleton-Century-Crofts, New York.
79. Edlich, R. F., Rogers, W., Kasper, G., Kaufman, D., Tsung, M. S., and Wangensteen, O. H. (1969). Studies in the management of the contaminated wound. *Am. J. Surg.*, **117**, 323–9.
80. Rodeheaver, G. T., Pettry, D., Turnbull, V., Edgerton, M. T., and Edlich, R. F. (1974). Identification of the wound infection–potentiating factors in soil. *Am. J. Surg.*, **128**, 8–12.
81. Cooper, G. T. and Ryan, J. M. (1990). Interaction of penetrating missiles with tissues: some common misapprehensions and implications for wound management. *Br. J. Surg.*, **177**, 606–10.
82. Winter, G. (1972). Epidermal regeneration studies in the domestic pig. In *Epidermal wound healings* (ed. H. I. Maibach and D. T. Rovee). Year Book Medical Publishers, Chicago.
83. Brennan, S. S., Foster, M. E., and Leaper, D. J. (1984). A study of microangiogenesis in wounds healing by secondary intention. *Microcirc. Endothelium Lymphatics*, **1**, 657–69.
84. Hohn, D. C., Ponce, B., Burton, R. W., and Hunt, T. K. (1977).

Antimicrobial systems of the surgical wound. *Am. J. Surg.*, **133**, 597–603.
85. Buchan, I. A., Andrews, J. D., and Lang, S. M. (1981). Laboratory investigation of the composition and properties of pig skin wound exudate under Op site. *Burns*, **8**, 39–46.
86. Leaper, D. J., Brennan, S. S., Simpson, R. A., and Foster, M. E. (1984). Experimental infection and hydrogel dressings. *J. Hosp. Infect.*, **5** (suppl. A), 69–73.
87. Turner, T. D. (1986). Recent advances in wound management products. In *Advances in wound management* (ed. T. D. Turner, R. J. Schmidt, and K. G. Harding), pp. 3–6. Wiley, Chichester.
88. Anon. (1986). Dressings for ulcers. *Drug. Ther. Bull.*, **24**, 9–12.
89. Kim, J. H., and Gallis, H. A. (1989). Observations on spiraling empiricism: its causes, allure and perils, with particular reference to antibiotic therapy. *Am. J. Med.*, **87**, 201–6.
90. Leaper, D. J. (1986). Antiseptics and their effect on healing tissue. *Nursing Times*, **82**, 45–57.
91. Morgan, D. A. (1989). Chlorinated solutions: E (useful) or (e) useless?. *Pharm. J.*, **257**, 219–20.

4

Surgical infection and altered host defence mechanisms

JEAN I. TCHERVENKOV and JONATHAN L. MEAKINS

Introduction

Despite many recent advances in the field of surgery and medicine, and better antibiotics, bacterial sepsis remains one of the leading causes of morbidity and mortality in surgical patients. In recent times more complex surgery is performed on an increasingly aging population. With the advent of intensive care units, sicker patients are treated more aggressively and life-threatening sepsis in such specialized units with associated organ failure may be as high as 30 per cent (1). The great epidemics of past centuries are now well controlled through massive immunization programmes, better hygiene, and better nutrition. The early enthusiasm with the use of antibiotics has been replaced with the realization that, although they are powerful and important adjuncts in treatment of infections, they are not the ultimate answer.

If further progress is to be made in the control of morbidity and mortality from infection, the biology and pathophysiology of the septic process must be understood to make a rational, systematic approach to treatment modalities. Recently, this approach to sepsis has permitted surgeons to identify better the 'immunocompromised host' and knowledge of host defence abnormalities in surgical patients will enable us to develop new and rational therapeutic approaches in the near future.

Determinants of infection

The determinants of infection can be divided, for simplicity's sake, into three major components: (1) the micro-organism producing the infection; (2) the environment (local factors) in which the infection is produced; (3) the host defence mechanisms. There is a continuous, dynamic interaction among these factors that represents the state of homeostasis, i.e. a balanced interaction between the three determinants.

The opposite situation, where all the determinants are altered, can be seen in the patients treated in the surgical intensive care unit (SICU). Here, the patient is greatly threatened by sepsis, exposure to many pathogenic, antibiotic resistant organisms, in the setting of environmental (local defences) alterations (catheters, drains, open wounds) and altered host defences. If we could identify the specific determinants contributing to an infection and put a weight value on each, an equation of susceptibility to infection would result.

The first two determinants of infection, the environment and bacteria, have been extensively investigated. Short of creating the 'sterile' environment in surgery, which is impossible for all practical considerations, the principles of antisepsis and asepsis are essentially unchanged since the great discoveries of the late 1800s to early 1900s. In the case of bacteria, we have learned that even the rational use of antibiotics, although proven helpful, is just a partial solution. Often the rational or irrational use of broad-spectrum antibiotics may induce an ecological vacuum in the host's normal bacterial flora that is soon replaced by opportunistic and more virulent pathogens and in an immunocompromised host this effect is often detrimental to clinical outcome. At present, surgeons and internists approach sepsis mainly through the first two determinants of infection: the bacteria and the environment. Only recently has there been a resurgent interest in the third determinant 'host defence mechanisms'. The work of Sir Ashley Miles and J.F. Burke (2–4) defined the 'early decisive period of antimicrobial action', i.e. host defence, during which bacterial infection may become established. The host is the determining factor. More recently the work of Dinarello (5, 6) has expanded this concept by his description of the 'acute phase response'. This response is a non-specific host defence mechanism of mammals to microbial infection, injury, and inflammatory disease, and includes dramatic changes in metabolic, haematologic and immunologic states. This process results in the identification of 'the invader' as foreign and its localization and eradication before it disseminates throughout the host. This concept is important in understanding the process of sepsis and eventual outcome in the immunocompromised patient.

Technological advances in the last thirty years have permitted the identification of suppressed host defences in relation to the surgical patient (7). However, these tests often require special expertise to perform and to interpret. A simple test or formula, not handicapped by such premises, capable of identifying those at risk of sepsis would be of paramount benefit in the fight against infection.

Host defences to infection

Traditionally, and for simplicity, host defences to sepsis can be subdivided into the humoral response, non-specific immunity (phagocytic cell response), specific immunity (cell-mediated response), and complement. The division of host defences into these categories, although useful in their understanding, may be more of historical significance stemming from early immunological research, rather than reflecting the real host response to sepsis. Recent evidence suggests that their interdependence is more intricate than initially suspected (8, 9).

This interdependence is reflected in the host's inflammatory response to sepsis, alternatively referred as the acute-phase response (8, 9). Alteration or suppression of a normal acute phase response by various disease states may be the key process by which infections become established in the surgical patient.

Humoral immunity

Humoral immunity describes the immune process responsible for the production of immunoglobulins (Fig. 4.1). Since the discovery in the early 1940s by Tisehus and Kabat that the gamma globulin fraction of protein contained most of the serum antibody function, five different classes of immunoglobulins have been identified in man. These are IgG, IgM, IgA, IgE, and IgD. Immunoglobulins or antibodies are highly specialized glycoprotein molecules that bind to foreign antigens in a highly specific manner, can resist proteolysis and autodigestion and bind to phagocytic cell membrane, making them highly valuable in host defence.

The most abundant and widely distributed immunoglobulin is IgG. It is present both intravascularly and interstitially, crosses the placenta, activates complement and its half-life is 23 days. It is immunogenic against most infectious agents including bacteria. Receptors for the Fc portion of the IgG molecule exist on monocytes, polymorphonuclear leucocytes (PMNs), reticulo-endothelial cells, and certain lymphocytes.

IgA is the second most abundant immunoglobulin and is found almost exclusively in the external secretory system of man (i.e. respiratory tract, GI tract, reproductive system etc.). Receptors for IgA are found on lymphocytes, PMNs and monocytes. The IgA molecules are synthesized as monomers, but are secreted from plasma cells as dimers linked by a 'J' chain. The significance of this is not certain. Its primary function is to prevent attachment of bacteria to mucosal surfaces.

IgM is the largest of all known immunoglobulins and because of this is mostly restricted to the intravascular compartment. It is a highly efficient agglutinator of particulate antigen such as bacteria and is a potent inducer of the complement cascade. IgM is thought to be the first antibody

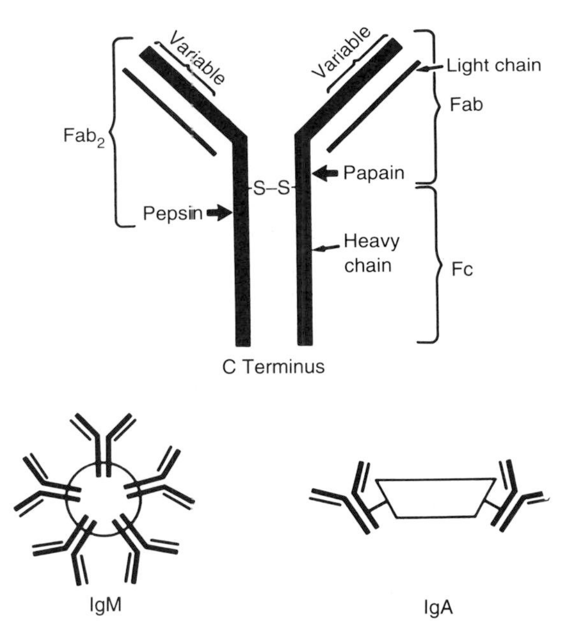

Fig. 4.1. The basic structure of the immunoglobulin molecule. The IgM pentamere and IgA dimere are specialized macromolecules composed of single immunoglobulin molecules joined by disulfide bonds or a secretory structure.

elaborated during antigenic challenge and peaks within a few days, but declines following IgG production.

IgD is the most recently discovered immunoglobulin to have a role in host defences. It is mostly found on the surface of lymphocytes and may act as a surface receptor for the initiation of the immune response.

IgE is present in serum only in trace amount and has the ability to attach to skin and initiate the allergic reaction. It is a secretory immunoglobulin and like IgA is mostly found in the lining of the respiratory and GI tracts. Deficiency of IgE and IgA have been found in patients susceptible to nosocomial infections (10).

Antibodies are produced by B-lymphocytes in response to 'exposure' by an antigen and are very unique to that antigen. This property is known as 'specificity' and is determined by the primary amino acid sequence of the antibody molecule. The initiation and antibody formation in response to antigen is a complex process that involves the interaction of antigen, macrophage, T-lymphocytes and B-lymphocytes (11).

Complement

The complement system is an important part of the body's immune system. Originally, the term complement was used to describe an auxillary factor in the serum that was not heat-inactivated and acted upon an antibody-coated cell causing its destruction. Today we know the complement system involves 20 or more different protein molecules circulating in their inactive forms in serum and, when activated, take part in an intricate amplificatory cascade system that plays an important role in host defence. These proteins are synthesized mostly by the liver, but have also been isolated from lymphocytes, macrophages and cells of the reticulo-endothelial system (12).

There are two pathways of the complement cascade. The classical pathway is activated by antigen–antibody complexes

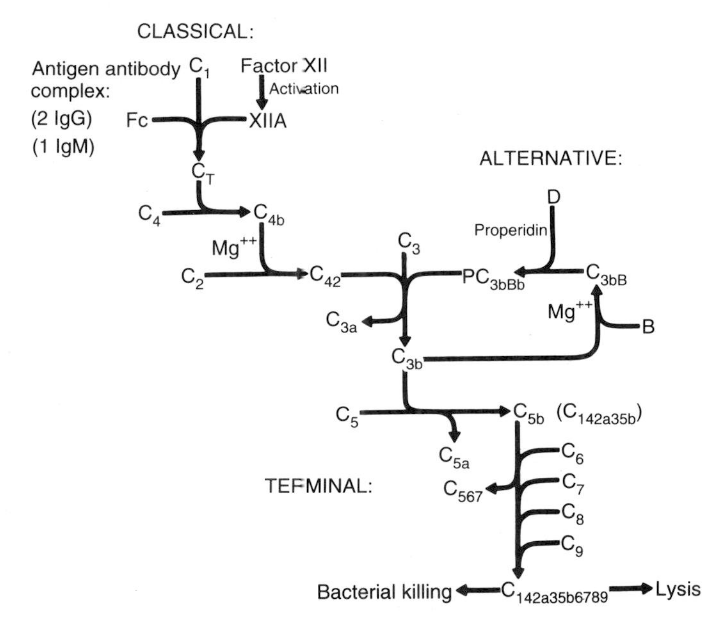

Fig. 4.2. The complement cascade system showing the classical and alternate pathways.

Table 4.1. Biological effects of some complement cascade products.

Substance	Activity
C3a	Smooth muscle contraction Increased vascular permability Degranulation of mast cells and basophils Platelet aggregation
C4a	Opsonization and facilitation of phagocytosis Smooth muscle contraction Increased vascular permeability
C5a	Chemotaxis of neutrophils, monocytes, basophils, eosinophils Degranulation of mast cells and basophils Aggregation of platelets Increased macrophage secretion of interleukin-1 Release of hydrolytic enzymes from neutrophils
C5a-des-arg	Chemotaxis of neutrophils Release of hydrolytic enzymes from neutrophils

and the alternate pathway activated by a variety of stimulants including bacterial lipopolysaccharide (Fig. 4.2).

The complement system cascade generates biological products important to inflammation and host defence (Table 4.1). Both the classical and alternate complement pathways can be further subdivided into the initiation phase, the amplification phase, and the membrane attack phase (Fig. 4.2).

Central to both complement cascades is the cleavage of C3 into Ca3 and C3b. C3b under the influence of factor B, a zymogen-like plasma protein, is involved in a complex positive feedback mechanism that results in a fast consumption of C3 and the generation of more C3a and C3b. C3a acts as an anaphylatoxin while C3b acts as a catalyst for the cleavage of C5 into C5a and C5b. C5b further reacts with C6, C7, C8, and C9 and forms the membrane attack complex (MAC) that causes cell lysis and death. C3b and C5b are important opsonins that greatly facilitate phagocytosis of bacteria by PMNs. C5a is formed in serum or plasma and is rapidly, and irreversibly, converted to C5a des-arg (12, 13). This protein looses its spasmogenic activity, but retains its chemotactic and degranulating activity on neutrophils. Chemotactic response to C5a has been exhibited by PMN's monocytes, basophils, eosinophils, and macrophages (14). More recently, C5a receptors were found on macrophages and C5a was shown to induce Interleukin-1 production by macrophages (15, 16). Interleukin-1 (IL-1), or leucocytic pyrogen, is a macrophage-secreted monokine produced in response to bacterial invasion and is a potent chemotactic agent for inflammatory cells including PMNs (8, 17).

Non-specific immune responses

All living organisms must maintain homeostasis in order to survive in the face of a changing environment. Both the human body and animals respond in a remarkably similar fashion in the face of altered homeostasis. This non-specific response to 'foreign' substances such as bacteria invading the host has been recently described and called the acute-phase reaction (8). This reaction is mediated by the host and results in the identification of the 'invader' before it has a chance to disseminate throughout the host. Bacteria and bacterial by-products are the most potent known inducers of the acute-phase response (8, 9).

It appears now that the monocyte-macrophage cell is the pivotal cell to the acute phase response. The monocyte-macrophage and its secretory products or family of products, known as interleukin-1 (IL-1), appear to be the primary mediators of host defence to infection. Rather than being the primary mediator, IL-1 is thought to be the highlight of many host reactions of the acute-phase response and may act directly or in concert with other host substances or hormones in the body (8, 9).

Circulating blood monocytes, the interstitial macrophages of the reticulo-endothelial system, lung, peritoneum, bone marrow, and dendritic cells such as the keratinocytes and Langerhan's cells all produce substantial quantities of IL-1 in response to bacteria and other antigen (8). Their strategic location in the human body at the interface of the host and its environment make them ideal 'watchtowers'.

Phagocytic cells are thought to be the most important in host defences against bacteria. These cells are capable of ingesting particles and other substances and represent the host's initial encounter with bacteria. The two most important phagocytic cells are the polymorphonuclear leucocyte (PMN) and the monocyte-macrophage.

Neutrophils (PMNs)

Neutrophils (PMNs) arise in the bone marrow from a common ancestral cell. Their precursors, in order of increasing maturity, are myeloblasts, promyelocytes, metamyelocytes, and band cells. The PMN represents the end cell of myeloid differentiation and cannot divide further. There is a large storage of PMNs in the bone marrow that can be mobilized when needed to replenish circulating PMNs when infection or other disturbance in homeostasis occurs. Once the PMN enters the circulation, it remains for only a short time (about 12 h) before entering the tissues. There it remains for two or three days before completing its life span. PMN delivery to a site of infection is mediated by substances known as chemoattractants. Under their influence, the circulating PMN adheres to the walls of small vessels and exits to the interstitial tissues. There it moves in a unidirectional manner along an increasing gradient of chemoattractant towards a site of microbial contamination. This property, chemotaxis, can be measured experimentally *in vitro* and *in vivo* and is a useful method of determining PMN function (18–23). Many substances are chemotactic *in vitro* and some like C5a, IL-1 and bacterial cell wall products play a role *in vivo* (14, 23–26). However, the kinetics of these reactions are yet undefined and are currently under study. Antibodies and C3b greatly enhance phagocytosis of bacteria by PMNs and receptors for them have been demonstrated on PMNs (27).

Monocytes

The circulating monocyte is part of the mononuclear phagocytic cell system (MPS) (28, 29) also known as the reticulo-endothelial system (RES), which is distributed throughout the body. These cells are present in the interstitial tissues of the lung (30), peritoneum (31), synovium, the liver (Kupffer cells), spleen, bone marrow, and lymph nodes (32). Other cells having macrophage like properties are the keratinocytes, Langerhan's cells, corneal epithelial cells, gingival exudate cells, astrocyte glial cells, and renal mesangial cells (8, 24, 32).

The monocyte originates in the bone marrow from a stem cell and matures from a monoblast to a promonocyte to a monocyte. It can move into tissues where it differentiates further into tissue macrophages. These cells remove and destroy bacteria, damaged tissue cells, neoplastic cells, and various other macromolecules such as antigen–antibody complexes. The monocyte-macrophage, however, is more than a non-specific phagocyte. In the last decade, immunologists working with the mononuclear phagocyte have recognized its critical role in antigen 'recognition' and 'processing' (32, 34). It 'presents' antigen to competent T-lymphocytes and also secretes soluble products necessary for T-lymphocyte activation. Originally, this product was called lymphocyte activating factor (LAF) (35, 36), but as its function became elucidated, it was more recently renamed interleukin-1 which also refers to B cell-activating factor (BAF), endogenous pyrogen (EP), and helper peak-1 factor (8, 37).

The initial macrophage antigen reaction achieves a twofold purpose. The association of antigen and macrophage results in yet undetermined cellular changes that spell out a foreign substance to the host. This is a non-specific reaction and results in the activation of macrophages and production of IL-1 or other monokines. This results in the attraction of T-lymphocytes to the site of antigen and sets an immune response in action.

The acute-phase response is characterized clinically by fever, net nitrogen catabolism, hypoglycaemia, aminoacidaemia, proteinuria, hypozincaemia, and increased synthesis in hepatic acute-phase proteins. These include fibrinogen, C-reactive protein, serum amyloid A protein, haptoglobin, ceruloplasmin, a-macroglobulin, and complement components. There is also an increased release in the circulation and an increased synthesis of PMNs by the bone marrow (8). Fever, as defined by a rise of the hypothalamic thermostat centre, is the most prominent component of the acute phase response (8, 38). Fever has been associated with increased antibody production in relation to an increased T-cell function (T-helper subset) (39) increased phagocystosis and bacteriocidal capacity by PMNs and decreased bacterial survival (8, 40). IL-1 production and activity is also increased at febrile temperatures (41). These effects of fever are thought to be beneficial in increasing host survival from sepsis. Animal studies support this concept (8, 41).

Although not yet fully understood or characterized , the acute-phase response is thought to result from the antigen–macrophage interaction and IL-1 production. At present, however, it is known that antigen phagocytosis is not required (43, 44). Bacteria and endotoxin are the most potent known inducers of IL-1 production (8, 45, 46, 43), not all stimulators of macrophages results in the IL-1 production (2) and antigen antibody complexes and C5a are also very potent inducers of

IL-1 production by macrophages (8, 16, 17, 47). The above interactions help in the identification process of self versus non-self by the host.

Some aspects of the acute-phase response occur within hours after the onset of infection. These are fever, neutrophilia, nitrogen catabolism, and muscle protein degradation. Others, such as synthesis of acute-phase reactants begin soon after infection, but take several days to evolve (8).

The local effects of antigen–macrophage interaction and IL-1 production set in motion the 'signals' for the host to deliver the effector cells, (the neutropils and monocytes), to the site of infection. This must be accomplished quickly in order to 'localize' the infectious agent.

Specific immune response

Specific immunity refers to a process of immune response that results in products (cells or proteins) capable of reacting to antigens in a specific manner.

The two processes involved in antibacterial host resistance are humoral immunity and antibody production, and cell-mediated immunity and the production of specifically sensitized T-lymphocytes. The delayed-type hypersensitivity (DTH) reaction is the prototype of cell-mediated immunity. Classically, the DTH reaction is a specific cutaneous response to a specific antigen reintroduced cutaneously into a pre-sensitized host. However, more recent experiments on specific immunity have demonstrated a remarkable similarity between the induction (afferent arc) of the humoral and DTH immune responses to an antigen in an immunologically naïve host. Evidence suggests that many naturally occurring antigens, including bacterial products, can stimulate both the production of specific antibody and a DTH response (11, 48).

Delayed-type hypersensitivity reaction

Delayed type hypersensitivity reaction is the chemical type of cell mediated immunity (CMI) and describes an *in vivo* test used to assess CMI. The test is performed by injecting antigens intradermally and measuring the resultant skin induration at 24, 48, and 72 h. Most DTH reactions are maximal at 48 h, but some may peak at 24 h, others at 72 h.

Although first observed by Jenner in 1798 with the 'vaccinia' injections and later observed by Koch in 1890 while working with guinea-pigs infected with the tubercle bacilli, the term 'delayed-type hypersensitivity' was first used in 1921 by Zinsser (49). He described an erythematous indurated skin reaction following an intracutaneous challenge with a bacterial antigen in a previously 'sensitized' patient. In 1942 Chase and Landsteiner established that the DTH response required sensitized lymphocytes (50, 51).

The 'afferent arc' of the DTH response refers to a sequence of cellular events in response to an 'antigen' never encountered before by the host. This process, also referred to as 'sensitization', involves the interaction between T-lymphocytes and the antigen in association with histocompatibility or 'self-recognition' antigens on the surface of a macrophage or a dendritic cell (42, 52, 57).

Following initial antigen–macrophage interaction production of IL-1 by these macrophages is stimulated and T-lymphocytes are attracted in a non-specific manner to the site of antigen. The majority of these T-cells are of the 'helper' subset and are 'activated' by IL-1 and macrophage contact to produce lymphokine of which the principle one is called IL-2. Interleukin-2 and IL-1 together are thought to induce T-cell transformation into 'T-memory cells'. The DTH response to infections of the same antigen subsequently rests on these memory T-cells. The degree of specificity observed in antigen recognition by T-memory lymphocytes is only equalled by the specificity seen in B-lymphocyte antibody production. Evidence suggests that receptors on T-lymphocytes, B lymphocytes, and macrophages, capable of reacting to the same antigen, are all coded by the same variable region on a gene (11, 54).

Phagocytes (PMNs and circulating monocytes), are also recruited by monokines, lymphokines, and other substances elaborated in the initial phase of a DTH reaction (52, 54). At present, their function remains largely unknown but they are thought to act non-specifically in removing the foreign antigen. Thus, the sensitization phase of a DTH response is an interaction between T-cells, macrophages, monokines (IL-1), lymphokines (IL-2 and others), involved in a positive feedback mechanism that results in specific T-memory cell production capable of reacting to the same antigen subsequently. If unchecked, however, this reaction can consume large numbers of macrophages, PMNs' and lymphocytes. Evidence suggests that the same processes that elaborate the production of T-memory 'helper-subtype' lymphocytes also results in the production of T-memory 'suppressor-subtype' lymphocytes. T-suppressor lymphocytes regulate T-helper and B-lymphocyte functions and thus moderate both cell-mediated and humoural immunity (11, 52, 54, 55). This process of sensitization to an antigen is usually complete within two to three weeks.

Upon 'recall' antigen reinjection at a later date, the same process is repeated but is tremendously accelerated and amplified under the influence of T-memory lymphocytes. This is known as the efferent arc and is commonly referred to as the DTH reaction seen cutaneously following the injection of 'recall antigen'. Less than 1 per cent of the resultant cell infiltrate in a DTH response comprises specifically sensitized lymphocytes (T-memory cells). The majority are PMNs, macrophages, non-specific T-lymphocytes and the occasional basophil and plasma cell (52). Platt *et al.* (55) found that larger infiltrates of PMNs and basophils in a DTH reaction were associated with a more intense central necrosis and dermal reaction. Degranulation of PMNs and basophils releases vasoactive amines that induce local vasodilatation. Proteins leak and activation of the clotting system results in the deposition of fibrin, trapping large amounts of protein and fluid which assumes the consistency of a gel.

It is this local deposition of fibrin gel and not the actual infiltration of leucocytes that is responsible for the induration that is felt clinically in a DTH reaction. Indirectly, however, the deposition of this fibrin gel reflects the normal delivery and function of leukocytes and the normal function of the clotting cascade. The function of this fibrin gel deposition locally is thought to restrict the spread of bacteria or the diffusion of soluble antigen, thus localizing foreign substances. Even though the DTH reaction is described as a specific immune response the participation of the non-specific 'inflammatory' immune response is essential in its final clinical manifestation (52–54, 56). The induration measured at 24 or 48 h in a DTH reaction reflects a normal specific or cell-mediated immune response, a normal non-specific or phagocytic immune response, and a normal clotting system cascade.

The immunology of wound healing

The repair, or 'healing', of injured vertebrate tissues is a complex interaction of molecular cascade and feedback systems, and cellular processes (57, 58). For simplicity the process can be divided into three distinct but well-integrated stages: inflammation; migration and proliferation of connective tissue cells and blood vessels; and deposition of new connective tissue matrix. The ability of vertebrates to repair injured tissue is vital to the maintenance of homeostasis and ultimate survival. Repair of injured tissues is limited by the speed of the slowest biochemical process. Minor injuries are easily and quickly repaired. Following a major injury, as in large burns or multiple trauma victims, the repair mechanisms are taxed heavily and the rate of repair may be dangerously slow. This results is a life-threatening situation.

The initial signals following injury within the first hours seem to arise from the coagulation process itself. The complement and coagulation cascades are activated post injury and platelets migrate to the wound. Fibrin, fibrin-split products, C5a, elastin peptides, F-met peptides, monokines, and platelets have all been shown to play a significant role in chemotaxis of PMNs, monocytes, and lymphocytes and the subsequent steps in repair (59, 60). Basically, cells that arrive early into wounds produce 'factors' that recruit cell types which arrive later in the process of wound healing. Neutrophils reach the wound early in the first hours and kill bacteria that may contaminate the wound. However, they contribute nothing to wound healing and repair (60).

It has been shown that platelets, the inflammatory response and macrophages are absolutely *essential* in the normal healing process of wounds (59–61). Early post injury, the platelets, and fibrin-split products are the initiators and essential directors of healing and repair until the macrophages arrive (62). Platelets have been shown to secrete an important, and perhaps the most important, chemoattractant for connective tissue cells, the platelet-derived growth factor (PDGF) (60, 63, 64). In addition, lymphokines and fibronectin are also important chemoattractants for fibrocytes (65). Fibronectin also stimulates chemotaxis for endothelial cells (66, 67). Serious impairment of the early inflammatory response in a wound severely reduces healing of that wound (61). Wound healing can occur without the presence of granulocytes and lymphocytes, but the macrophage is essential in tissue repair processes (62). The macrophages probably take over from the platelets and fibrin as the major directors of repair a few days after injury and continue directorship until healing is complete. Macrophages secrete macrophage-derived growth factor (MDGF) that stimulates mitosis in fibroblasts (68). In addition, they secrete wound angiogenesis factor (WAF) in response to tissue hypoxia (61). Fibroblasts and capillary endothelial cells in culture, multiply best at a pO_2 of 40 mmHg. Lactate and hypoxia also greatly stimulate macrophages to secrete WAF and cause fibroblasts to induce collagen synthesizing enzymes (69).

Within three days after injury fibroblasts proliferate and, supported by new vessels, become the dominant element of a healing wound. After one week in a primary healing wound, a collagenous 'glue' is actively secreted among the pre-existing large collagen fibres and a rich capillary network spans the wound. Open wounds heal similarly, however, because they are open granulation tissue forms. Open wounds 'close' and heal more slowly and with greater expenditure of physiological resources as epithelial structures creep from the edges, obeying the same signals that modulate fibroblasts. Granulation tissue is very sensitive to hypoxia and vasoconstriction. Any form of sustained shock induces granulation tissue necrosis and predisposes open wounds to bacterial infection.

Throughout the repair process inflammatory cells and fibroblasts lyse and remodel collagen which fibroblasts synthesize and deposit new collagen fibres. This forms a stronger, more flexible and elastic scar.

How do wounds 'decide' to stop healing? For the most part, it is still a mystery, however, Knighton *et al.* (70) and Hunt (60) may have answered this question. Using rabbit ear chambers, they have studied healing in response to high and low pO_2. They have observed that at hypoxic levels the macrophage secretes WAF and MDGF in high quantities. As the wound becomes better vascularized, the pO_2 increases and the macrophage secrets less WAF and MDGF. Furthermore, hyperbaric oxygen has been shown to be beneficial for rapid healing of burn wounds (22, 59). Using hyperbaric oxygen on burn wounds, Ketchum *et al.* (70) have noticed an increase in wound capillary density. Presumably hyperbaric oxygen allows for the rapid growth and survival of granulation tissues which require a higher pO_2 and yet does not increase the interstitial pO_2 of deep wound tissues where macrophages continue their production of angiogenesis factor undisturbed by high pO_2. Knighton *et al.* have shown that when macrophages are exposed to air a pO_2 of 150 mmHg no angiogenesis factor was produced. However, the same macrophages produced massive levels of angiogenesis factor when cultured at a pO_2 of 15 mmHg or less (71).

Thus it appears that wound healing is a self regulating process centred around the macrophages. As wounds get better vascularized and oxygenated, and as lactic acid is cleared, the macrophages stop further production of WAF and MDGF. This in turn stops the support mechanism for further fibrocyte mitosis and production of collagen.

Alteration of host defence in surgical patients

Intuitively, the clinical surgeon knows from experience that the incidence of sepsis is increased when managing patients who are elderly, traumatized, uraemic, suffering from cancer, malnourished, and those with severe pancreatitis or haemorrhagic shock. However, such bedside assessment of a particular patient is unreliable and often guesswork. The question of how to identify the surgical patient with altered host defences is important in order to implement better therapeutic modalities in an organized and rational manner. It would allow us to understand the physiological alterations in immune function and to assist in the development of specific therapy based on defined abnormalities. A simple and reproducible clinical test or formula that can identify the patient at risk and quantify his immune dysfunction at any phase of his illness would be invaluable.

The approach initiated by MacLean *et al.* (72) to this problem was prompted by the study of a 13-year-old boy seen at the Royal Victoria Hospital (Montreal, Canada) two months after an appendicectomy for perforation and generalized peritonitis. At that time the patient had a high output intestinal fistula, intra-abdominal abscesses requiring drainage, septicaemia, respiratory failure, and malnutrition. Despite repeated laparotomies for drainage of an abscess, total parenteral nutrition of 3000 calories per day, a miriad of antibiotics and other efforts of modern surgery, he eventually died five months later of sepsis. Blood cultures before his demise grew *Staphylococcus aureus*, *Streptococcus faecalis*, *Staph. epidermidis* and *Candida albicans*. The patient's inability to localize and control infection prompted the study of his immune response. He had normal levels of immunoglobulins, but failed to respond to recall DTH antigens (mumps, purified protein derivative (PPD), trichophyton, varidase, and candida). He also accepted a skin graft without a sign of rejection for up to 44 days and had a serum inhibitor of the mixed lymphocyte culture (MLC) response of his own lymphocytes to allogeneic lymphocytes.

In a subsequent pilot study in 50 pre-operative and 55 ICU patients the same recall antigens were used to identify patients at risk of sepsis. Anergy was defined as no response $\geqslant$ 5 mm to any of the five antigens; relative anergy as a single response. The DTH response was measured at 24 and 48 h following the intradermal injection of 0.1 cc of the 5 antigens in the arm of the patient. In the case of an elliptical induration, the mean of the two diameters was recorded. Anergic and relatively anergic patients had a significant higher incidence of sepsis and septic-related morbidity than reactive patients. In subsequent studies, regardless of the patient population studied (pre-operative, post-operative, intensive care, trauma, general surgical, or non-operative surgical, cancer, and GI bleeding), the presence of altered DTH response to recall antigens identified a patient population at increased risk to ordinary Gram-negative and Gram-positive bacteria.

Host defence parameters have now been studied in association with sepsis related morbidity and mortality in 2202 surgical patients admitted to the general wards or the surgical intensive care unit (SICU) of the Royal Victoria Hospital (73). Host defence measurements included DTH response, circulating leucocyte counts and haemoglobin levels, neutrophil adherence, chemotaxis, phagocytic and bactericidal functions, circulating serum albumin, serum globulin, serum immunoglobulin, and complement levels. Major sepsis was defined as the presence of a positive blood culture, an abscess identified at laparotomy, or autopsy, or confirmed by needle aspiration under ultrasound or computerized tomography guidance. Minor sepsis was defined as wound infection, pneumonia, urinary tract infection, cellulitis or other soft tissue infections.

Table 4.2. Clinical outcome in all patients based on admission skin-test response.

Skin-test Response	No.	Sepsis no. (%)*	Death no. (%)†
Reactive	1373	113 (8)	54 (4)
Relatively anergic	306	65 (21)	45 (15)
Anergic	523	175 (33)	161 (31)

*x2 = 186.3, 2 d.f., $p < 0.0001$. †x2 = 265.1, 2 d.f., $p < 0.0001$.

All 2202 patients (1211 men and 991 women) underwent skin testing. Haematologic assays were done on the majority of patients except for phagocytosis and bactericidal assays (done on 152 patients) and immunoglobulin data (done on 302 patients). Based on DTH skin testing, done on admission to hospital (Table 4.2), the rate of sepsis was 8 per cent (113/1373) in the reactive group, 21 per cent (65/306) in the relatively anergic group, and 33 per cent (175/523) in the anergic group. The anergic patients showed an increased susceptibility of developing bacterial sepsis and a decreased ability to handle major sepsis. Of the 175 anergic patients who developed major sepsis in hospital 92 (53 per cent) died. In contrast, only 25 (23 per cent) of 113 reactive patients with major sepsis died from their infection. Seriously ill patients admitted to the SICU had the same strong association between a decreased DTH response and major sepsis and sepsis related mortality (Table 4.3).

Pre-operative skin testing in patients (n = 1184, Table 4.4) who were matched for operative time, operative trauma, and type of surgery, also showed the same distribution of major sepsis and sepsis-related mortality. Skin test reactivity was not

Table 4.3. Clinical outcome in 553 patients in the intensive care unit based on skin test response on entry to the unit.

Skin-test Response	No.	Sepsis no. (%)*	Death no. (%)†
Reactive	175	58 (33)	25 (14)
Relatively anergic	110	45 (41)	29 (26)
Anergic	268	128 (48)	101 (38)

*x2 = 9.3, 2 d.f., $p < 0.0094$. †x2 = 28.9, 2 d.f., $p < 0.0001$.

Table 4.4. Clinical outcome in patients first skin tested pre-operatively, based on pre-operative response.

Skin-test Response	No.	Sepsis no. (%)*	Death no. (%)†
Reactive	876	66 (8)	36 (4)
Relatively anergic	131	21 (16)	16 (12)
Anergic	177	54 (31)	47 (27)

*x2 = 76.5, 2 d.f., $p < 0.0001$. †x2 = 99.7, 2 d.f., $p < 0.0001$.

a fixed phenomenon but could change during the course of a patients' hospital stay. Fifty per cent of the reactive patients who underwent grade four surgery were anergic when tested on day 3 post-operation. The majority recovered their DTH response by day 7. However, in this group of patients that were reactive pre-operation and became anergic on day 3 post-operation (Grade 4 surgery), 5 per cent remained anergic one week post-operation. Those patients that did not recover DTH reactivity had a similar rate of sepsis and sepsis related mortality as those who were anergic pre-operation (i.e. 32 per cent). Such changes in DTH reactivity showed a strong association with the development of sepsis and sepsis-related death. In the 98 patients who were reactive pre-operation on admission but deteriorated to a non-reactive status during hospitalization sepsis developed in 43 (44 per cent) and 39 (40 per cent) died. In contrast 326 patients who were anergic on admission recovered their DTH response during hospitalization and of these 81 (20 per cent) developed major sepsis and only 23 (7 per cent) died from sepsis.

Sequential DTH skin testing was done on 465 patients during hospitalization (Table 4.5). Skin testing ranged from 2 to 31 weekly determinations (mean 5.3 ± 0.4 tests). This demonstrated that patients who maintained reactivity throughout their hospital stay had a much lower incidence of major sepsis and sepsis related death compared with those who became, and remained, anergic during hospitalization.

Table 4.5. Sequential skin-test response and clinical outcome in patients with the same skin-test response throughout the hospital stay.

Skin-test Response	No.	Sepsis no. (%)	Death no. (%)
Reactive	295	35 (12)	6 (12)
Relatively anergic	35	15 (50)	6 (20)
Anergic	140	59 (42)	78 (56)

Christou (73), has shown a more meaningful way of expressing the DTH response. Rather than expressing the DTH response as three fixed arbitrary classifications of reactive, relatively anergic, and anergic, it was expressed as the DTH score. The DTH score was defined as the sum of the diameters of the skin-test reactions to all five antigens (i.e. mumps, PPD, varidase, candida, and trichophyton). A bivariate logarithmic regression was done using the percentage of patients within a particular DTH score range who had sepsis as the dependent variable and the DTH score as the independent variable. A 4 mm range was independently used. There was a strong correlation between the DTH score (x) and sepsis development (y) thus $y = 35.1 - 7.5x$, $r = -0.95$ (Fig. 4.3). The DTH skin response in surgical patients indicates a transient, acquired immunodeficiency consisting of abnormalities at many levels of the immune response.

In addition to DTH response, other immunological parameters were studied on normal and anergic patients. Abnormalities in neutrophil function, as reflected by decreased *in vitro* chemotaxis, decreased phagocytosis, and bacteriocidal killing assays, and by cell adherence, have been demonstrated in the anergic and relatively anergic patients (74, 75).

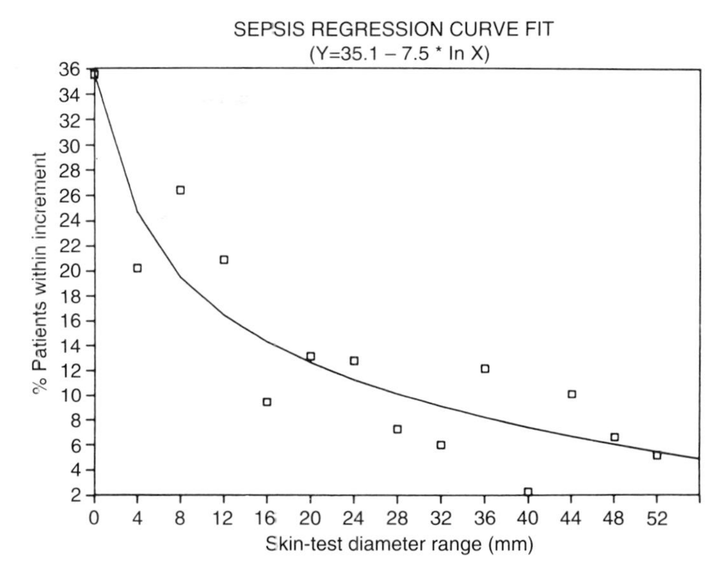

Fig. 4.3. Sepsis regression curve fit delayed type hypersensitivity (DTH) score (mm) and sepsis rate in 2202 surgical patients assessed by DTH response on entry into study

Using the technique of Zigmund and Hirsh *in vitro* neutrophil chemotaxis was decreased in the anergic patients (90.4 ± 2.9 u) when compared with laboratory controls (128.1 ± 2.4 u), reactive patients (123.3 ± 3.1 u), or relatively anergic patients (103.7 ± 2.0 u). Neutrophil adherence to nylon fibre was increased in the anergic and relatively anergic patients (85.0 ± 7.0 per cent and 84.3 ± 7.9 per cent) compared with laboratory controls or reactive patients (71.5 ± 3.8 per cent and 72.5 ± 13.1 per cent). There was a direct correlation between increased adherence and decreased chemotaxis. Patients demonstrating decreased neutrophil chemotaxis (less than 115 ± 1.0 u) and anergy had a rate of sepsis of 66 per cent and mortality of 37 per cent compared with no sepsis or mortality in those patients with normal DTH response and normal PMN chemotaxis. Recovery of the DTH response was accompanied by recovery of neutrophil chemotaxis (73, 74, 76).

Serum inhibitors of PMN chemotaxis have been isolated. Two such inhibitors have been implicated, one with a molecular weight of 110 kilodaltons, and the other with a molecular weight of 310 kilodaltons (1). Other studies support these findings (75, 77, 78). This has been studied much more extensively in the burn patient. Ninnemann *et al.* (79) have identified in burn patients a serum component that has immunosuppressive properties against lymphocytes and neutrophils. This serum component has a molecular weight between 1000 and 5000 daltons; contains a protein, carbohydrate and lipid component; has a structure that is heat stable, pH stable and unaffected by treatment with trypsin, proteinase K, DNase, and RNase; and has a non-cytotoxic immunosuppressive mode of action. It appears that the suppressive activity is dependent upon a prostaglandin portion of this low molecular weight complex.

Bactericidal activity has also been shown to be suppressed in the anergic or burn patient (80–82). *In vivo* delivery of leucocytes to an inflammatory focus was tested in the anergic patients using the Sykes–Moore skin window chambers placed over an epithelial abrasion of the forearm according to the method described by Rebuck and Crowley (21, 83). Patients with a decreased DTH response and PMN chemotaxis had a reduced leucocyte delivery in the chambers. The fluid from the chambers of patients with a decreased DTH response also had less chemoattraction capability to PMN's when tested *in vitro*. A similar study done on patients following grade three and four surgery showed a similar decrease in leucocyte delivery to skin windows on the second post-operative day and a return to normal by day 7 (84). This finding paralleled the DTH skin test response but not the *in vitro* PMN chemotaxis showing that *in vitro* PMN chemotaxis does not reflect the *in vivo* situation in anergic patients.

Cell-mediated immunity and the DTH response, which is classically thought to reflect cell-mediated immunity and lymphocyte function, have been extensively studied in normal and anergic patients. The *in vitro* lymphocyte response as tested by mixed lymphocyte cultures (MLC), lymphocyte proliferation to PPD, and the ability of *in vitro* activated lymphocytes to elicit a skin reaction when reinjected intradermally was assessed in 43 anergic surgical patients (85). A normal MLC response was present in over 80 per cent of the patients and 24 (56 per cent) had a positive proliferation to PPD. The cells or the supernatant of MLC's from patients with positive *in vitro* response to PPD were reinjected subcutaneously back into the patients. A normal skin response was present in 79 per cent of patients with a normal *in vitro* response to PPD, but only 20 per cent of patients with a negative *in vitro* response to PPD had a normal skin test response following either injection of cells or MLC supernatent from patients with a positive *in vitro* response to PPD. These findings suggest that *in vivo* block of lymphocyte activation may be at the source of immunosuppression in the anergic patients.

Humoral immunity was also assessed in surgical patients using specific immunoglobulin production to tetanus toxoid (86, 87) and to pneumococcal polysaccharide (88). *In vivo* and *in vitro* measurement of specific antitetanus IgG production was done on day 14 (day of maximal response) after immunization. In the anergic group of patients the antibody response was significantly reduced compared with reactive patients or laboratory control. In contrast, total immunoglobulin production was increased in the anergic group compared with reactive controls, showing that the mechanisms of specific humoral immune response to antigen is most affected.

Classically tetanus toxoid, a protein antigen, is thought to be T-lymphocyte dependent. However, most common bacterial antigens are not protein but polysaccharide molecules. For this reason antibody response to a 23 valent penumococcal polysaccharide (Pneumovax) vaccine was tested in reactive, anergic, and laboratory control patients. Both *in vitro* and *in vivo* response was tested. Total specific antipneumovax IgG, IgA, IgM *in vivo* production was the same in all three groups of patients and there was good correlation between *in vivo* and *in vitro* specific antibody response. Because many common bacterial antigens are not protein but polysaccharides, this finding raises the possibility of active immunization of the anergic surgical patients with bacterial vaccines. Further work is necessary in this field, both in identifying pathogens commonly found in the immunocompromised host and assessing the ability of inducing active immunization against these pathogens. This form of therapy may prove useful and inexpensive in the septic, anergic patient.

In anergic surgical patients the DTH response to keyhole limpet haemocyanin (KLH), a protein antigen, was restored by injecting it together with lymphokines prepared from mixed lymphocyte cultures of reactive laboratory controls (90). *In vitro* lymphocyte proliferation of anergic patients was also increased by the use of lymphokines together with the KLH antigen but not by KLH alone. In an animal model of lethal acute bacterial peritonitis, the use of mixed lymphocyte culture supernatants (i.e. lymphokines/monokines) significantly increased early survival from 0 per cent to 56 per cent (90). These data support the theory that anergy in surgical patients, perhaps amongst other things, is a failure at the macrophage-T-lymphocyte interaction after antigen recognition and lack of, or reduced production or inhibition of, lymphokine/monokine activity. This results in the subsequent failure to recruit non-specific leucocytes such as PMNs and monocytes and a failure to amplify the immune response. Serum opsonic activity, important for bacterial phagocytosis and killing by neutrophils, has been shown to be suppressed in patients with a decreased DTH response (92). In a group of trauma patients, this serum opsonization defect was important only in those with associated neutrophil abnormalities (92–94).

Trauma

There appears to be an innate immunosuppression following any form of injury (95, 96). Immunosuppression post trauma correlates with the magnitude of injury, appears early post trauma, and affects all aspects of immunity. Burn trauma is the most severe form of trauma, causing profound alterations of immune function and as such is the prototype when studying surgical immunodeficiency (97, 98).

Decreased systemic and local host defences in the presence of an abnormal environment, the burn wound, predisposes these patients to sepsis. In addition, local factors in an SICU, such as invasive monitoring, therapeutic devices, or loss of protective airway mechanisms while patients are intubated, further predispose the injured or burn victim to sepsis. The burn injury or trauma may be the 'tipping' factor superimposed on other pre-morbid conditions such as age, malignancy, malnutrition, or medications predisposing the patient to sepsis. When considering immunosuppression following burn, or other forms of trauma, the healing process forms an intricate part of the whole process of survival. Factors that promote or influence the healing process may also be immunosupressive allowing sepsis to take root and progress. The host is caught in a dichotomy between healing or bacterial sepsis.

The determinants of infection in burn injury, namely host defences and an abnormal environment, are severely altered. In addition, local factors present in the SICU environment such as invasive monitoring and therapeutic devices, and antibiotic resistant bacteria further tip the balance in favour of bacterial sepsis.

Suppression of cell-mediated immunity post-burn injury has long been recognized (99). A decrease in the number of T-cells (100, 101) and a reversal in the ratio of the helper–inducer to suppressor subtypes have been reported in both human and animal studies (102, 103). Using monoclonal antibodies as cell markers, an increase in the T-suppressor to T-helper cell ratio was identified soon after burn trauma. It was maximum at one week and returned to normal two weeks' post-burn. Persistently elevated T-suppressor to T-helper ratios beyond two weeks' post-injury correlated closely with septic mortality.

There is increasing evidence in the literature that T-suppressor lymphocytes may be induced by inhibitory or suppressive monocyte–macrophage type cells (104, 105). These cells appear to be particularly attracted by degraded fragments of connective tissue present at sites of injury, and secrete monokines similar to IL-1 that stimulate macrophages and inhibit other leucocytes, including T-lymphocytes and neutrophils (8, 105). More recently IL-1 has been implicated in the generation of concanavalin A-induced T suppressor cells (106). Kupper *et al.* (107) have isolated from burn wound blister fluid a molecule with the same molecular weight and function as IL-1 and Wood *et al.* (108) have found that serum IL-1 increases immediately after burn injury. These findings can explain the acute phase-like response seen after burn trauma (i.e. fever, negative nitrogen balance, and muscle wasting). However, a direct cause and effect between IL-1 and the activation of T-suppressor cells has not been found.

Serum inhibitory factors, linked to endotoxin, prostaglandin E, interferon, and cutaneous burn toxin, have been identified in burn patients using gel chromatography (95, 109, 110). However, Wolfe *et al.* (111) has shown that serum immunosuppressive activity following burn trauma does not correlate with prostaglandin E_2, cortisol, or endotoxin. The same group has put forward the concept that burn-induced circulatory suppressor factors are products of suppressor cells (112). They have evidence that the suppressive material is an alpha-globulin associated polypeptide.

Suppressor T-cells and macrophages from animal and human source have been shown to secrete protein suppressor factors that non-specifically inhibit cell-mediated immune response *in vitro* (113–115). Suppressor T-cells, when cultured with prostaglandin E_2, release two such factors. Suppressor T-cells also produce a glycoprotein called soluble immune response suppressor (SIRS) (114, 116). In response to SIRS suppressor macrophages produce a non-antigen specific suppressor factor (116). Their importance in the overall immunosuppressor post-burn injury is not yet established.

Early post-burn host defence depression has also been associated with increased prostaglandin and thromboxane secretion (117). Increased production of prostaglandin E and F, and thromboxane B_2 by monocytes from burned patients has been demonstrated (118–120). Other important sources of these compounds may be stimulated platelets and neutrophils (121). In burned patients reduced mixed lymphocyte response and the appearance of suppressor T-cell activity is associated with increased prostaglandin E synthesis by monocytes (122). Prostaglandin E_2 was shown to activate suppressor T-cells directly (133, 123) and also by reducing the antigen-presenting capability of macrophages (124). Prostaglandins F and E_2 are potent inhibitors of the expression of Ia antigens on macrophages. Expression of these antigens on the cell wall of macrophages is essential to their function as antigen presenting cells and the initiation of the immune response (125). It is thought that reduced antigen presentation by macrophages results in the interaction of T-cells with soluble rather than membrane bound antigen, favouring activation of T-suppressor lymphocytes (126, 127).

Thromboxane B_2 and certain prostaglandins have also been shown to inhibit complement production by monocytes (128). Thromboxane A_2, which has been shown to be elevated post burn injury (129), has also been shown to increase platelet aggregation (130). Jacob *et al.* (131) have shown that, by using ibuprofen, complement-mediated *in vitro* aggregation of neutrophils can be inhibited. He postulated that ibuprofen exerted its protective effect by inhibiting the metabolism of arachidonic acid in the neutrophil, thus reducing prostaglandin and thromboxane synthesis. Decreased PMN chemotaxis and increased PMN nylon fibre adherence is evident in anergic surgical patients post-trauma and sepsis (76, 77). However, no available data at present has established cause and effect between neutrophil function and arachidonic acid metabolite activity in anergic surgical patients or post-burn injury. Latter *et al.* (132) showed increased survival post 30 per cent burn injury with indomethacin in an animal model. Serum prostaglandin levels in the animals given indomethacin was lower.

Humoral immunity is also altered post-trauma. Serum levels of immunoglobulins were shown to drop post-burn with a nadir from two to five days (133, 134). In burn patients, low IgG levels were found in those who died of sepsis (100). In an animal model, generation of antibody-forming cells was decreased on days 3 to 8 post-burn injury (135). This was corrected by adding T-lymphocytes and macrophages from uninjured animals, suggesting that trauma and burns affect humoural immunity by affecting T-lymphocytes and macrophages rather than B-lymphocytes. Trauma patients have reduced anti-tetanus toxoid IgG production and this correlated with the presence of cutaneous anergy. This was confirmed in an animal model using 30 per cent scald burn (Nohr 1986; unpublished material).

Trauma and surgery appear to be associated with decreased levels of complement factors and serum opsonic activity (138, 139). Activation of the complement cascade appears early post-burn injury and trauma, and results in increased complement by-products. These investigators have found that the alternate pathway is preferentially inhibited when the classical pathway is activated, resulting in consumptive opsinopathy. Activated complement factors facilitate fibronectin depletion reducing serum opsonic activity and thereby impede reticuloendothelial system clearance and phagocytic activity of PMNs and monocytes (117, 140). Complement activation, in particular C3a, activates suppressor T-cells *in vitro* (141), but does not inhibit *in vivo* antibody response (142), suggesting that its activity may be limited to the microenvironment. In a burn animal model, activation of the alternate complement pathway was associated with increased mortality (143). However, it is not clear how all this relates to infection control following burn injury or trauma in humans (117).

Trauma, surgery, and burns result in a graded suppression of PMN function. Alexander and Wixson (135) were among the first to report dysfunction of bacterial killing by PMNs from burn victims. This dysfunction correlated with the appearance of life-threatening sepsis (92). Since then others have reported suppressed *in vitro* PMN chemotaxis, phagocytosis, degranulation, and bacterial killing post-burn trauma (145–149). *In vitro* PMN chemotaxis is suppressed following trauma and correlated with the DTH response, the severity of injury, and the rate of sepsis (76). Others report suppression of PMN chemotaxis, phagocytosis, killing and opsonic capacity after major surgery (150–152). The *in vivo* delivery of technecium-99 colloid (^{99}Tc) labelled phagocytes to a DTH reaction and a bacterial abscess is decreased soon after burn injury in an animal model (152). This, however, appears not to be due to an intrinsic phagocytic cell abnormality but to the 'burn or trauma milieu' effect on phagocytes (Fig. 4.4 and 4.5). Cell delivery of phagocytes from 30 per cent burned rats radiolabelled with ^{99}Tc and reinjected into non-burned rats was normal. This suggests that in the *in vivo* situation, increased PMN inhibitor production (79, 95, 96) or decreased PMN chemoattractants (137–139), may be responsible for decreased PMN delivery to a septic focus. These defects in PMN function and activity may be the most important factors in sepsis post-trauma.

Cell-mediators, important in humoural immunity, cell-mediated immunity, and non-specific inflammation, have recently been shown to be affected post-injury. Wood *et al.* (108) studied IL-1 and IL-2 levels in 23 burned patients and found that IL-2 levels were reduced and IL-1 levels were increased immediately (48 h) post-burn trauma. There was a reduction of T-helper lymphocytes in the peripheral circulation, but this did not correlate with serum IL-2, suggesting that cell function rather than absolute numbers is more important

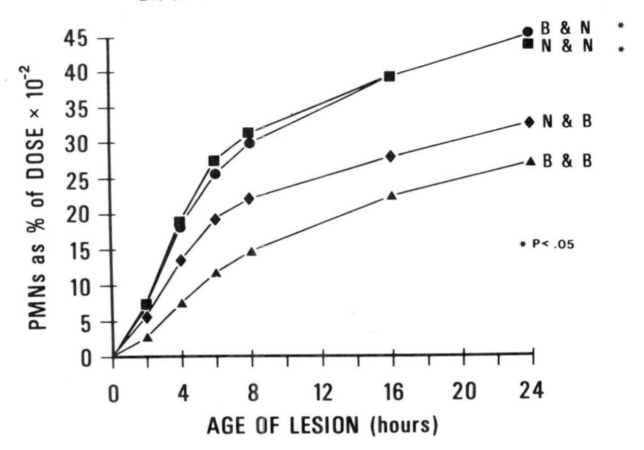

Fig. 4.4. Influx into a bacterial (*Staph. aureus*) abscess of ^{99}Tc-labelled phagocytes from burned or sham burned rats injected into burned or sham burned rats. When reinjected into normal (sham burned) rats labelled phagocytes from burned rats influx normally into a bacterial abscess.

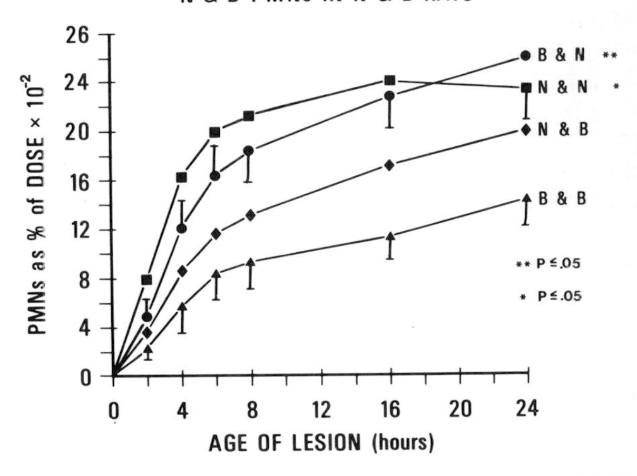

Fig. 4.5. Influx into a DTH reaction (to KLH) of ^{99}Tchn-labelled phagocytes from burned or sham burned rats injected into burned or sham burned rats. A similar cell influx pattern as in the bacterial abscess is apparent.

in immunosuppression post injury. Septic patients and patients with greater per cent burns showed a lower IL-2 production. Patients with lower than 30 per cent burns, or non-septic patients, returned to normal IL-2 production by day 10 post-burn. Those with greater than 30 per cent burns or sepsis did not recover IL-2 production throughout their hospitalization. Interleukin-1 production returned to normal after one week post-burn. This study confirms the profound suppression of T-helper lymphocyte function and alteration of macrophage function seen in animal studies post-burn. Further studies in this area should shed light into immunosuppressor mechanisms post trauma.

In summary, bury injury, trauma, and surgical trauma in the form of major surgical procedures, result in profound transient immunosuppression predisposing the host to sepsis. Alteration of T-lymphocyte, macrophage, DTH, humoral immunity, PMN function have been identified. Immunosuppression occurs immediately post injury, recovers with healing (10–14 days) and has a nadir ranging from 2 to 7 days. It preceeds sepsis, and is persistent in those patients that eventually suffer from sepsis and septic death. Serum inhibitors, some with characteristics of prostaglandins, others with characteristics of IL-1 like properties, still others not yet characterized have been identified. These have a profound effect on T-lymphocytes (both T-helper and suppressor cells), PMNs, and macrophages. Teleologically, this inhibition post-injury may be a normal response related to the 'healing processes' and the prevention of acute immune reaction of host to self-denatured proteins. The host is, therefore, caught in a dichotomy between healing and sepsis, in the midst of breached defences.

Malnutrition

Malnutrition frequently accompanies underlying illnesses such as cancer, obesity, inflammatory bowel disease, peptic ulcer disease, chronic and acute pancreatitis, chronic infections, and trauma victims. In the obese and the elderly, malnutrition is particularly insidious and may be more than a simple lack of caloric or protein intake. Deficiencies in important vitamins, minerals and rare divalent cations may be present. In particular zinc, copper, vitamins B_6 and A, folate, biotin, thiamin, and riboflavin are all important to the normal function of leukocytes and the immune response (153–157). In surgical patients and in particular trauma, burn, or septic patients the acute phase response puts a tremendous demand on the patients' metabolism. Unlike the Third World malnourished children, from whom most of the data on malnutrition and sepsis was collected, surgical patients that are septic have a tremendously accelerated metabolic response, and simple extrapolation of data between the two groups is difficult. Nevertheless, there are innate immune function abnormalities related to malnutrition.

Obesity is a form of malnutrition and these patients have a higher incidence of wound sepsis. Local factors such as blood supply and wound ischemia have been extensively investigated and no doubt account for the increased wound sepsis. However, recent evidence in obese mice or adolescents and adults show neutrophil and lymphocyte dysfunction (158, 159).

Zinc deficiency is associated with reduced cell-mediated immune function (153). However, following bacterial sepsis, trauma, and cancer there is a state of hypozincaemia and hypoferraemia (8). These changes are part of the acute phase response and are mediated by IL-1. Bacteria are known to require zinc and iron for rapid growth and metabolism (160, 161). Zinc is part of DNA polymerase and transcriptase of bacteria. Low blood or tissue iron levels severely limits bacterial growth at febrile temperatures (39°C) (8). However, it is not certain whether hypoferraemia and hypozincaemia at the onset of sepsis represents host adaptability to bacterial infection or merely consumption by an increased immune metabolism.

Copper is another divalent cation that is part of superoxide dismutase and cytochrome-c oxidase (162, 163). Infants with inherited copper deficiency and adults with acquired copper deficiency suffer recurrent bacterial sepsis (8). Following bacterial sepsis IL-1 induces hepatic synthesis of ceruloplasmin and increases serum copper levels. However, high levels of these cations, especially zinc and copper are immunosuppressive, particularly on T-lymphocytes (64).

Simple malnutrition can be classified as marasmus (primarily protein and total caloric deprivation) or kwashiokor (protein and visceral protein depletion). Anthropometric measurements of malnutrition include height, weight, midarm circumference, triceps skin fold, and creatinine to height index. Serum albumin, transferrin, or total lymphocytes have also been used to assess nutritional status. However, in an acutely ill patient these are not reliable. Dynamic nutritional assessment uses the rate of weight loss, nitrogen balance, and body composition analysis, such as the isotope dilution techniques (Nae/Ke). Pure kwashiorkor or marasmus is not the usual presentation of surgical patients. Nearly 40 per cent of the surgical patients over the age of 70 years old have some form of protein malnutrition.

Immune deficiencies present in protein malnutrition include suppression of cell-mediated immunity, the afferent and efferent arcs of the DTH response, bactericidal function of PMNs, and humoral immunity (155, 164). In the rat and in humans, protein deprivation results in atrophy of the thymus, spleen, and tonsillar lymph nodes. Histological examination of lymph nodes reveals reduced cellularity of the germinal and T-cell paracortical areas, the latter more severely (136). Lymphopenia and anergy are present in many malnourished patients. Although there is a significant statistical relationship between DTH skin test response and nutritional state, because of wide variability DTH does not accurately assess nutritional status. Persistence of the anergic state in the presence of adequate nutritional therapy in surgical patients normally signifies persistance of the underlying illness or sepsis (136, 165). In an animal model protein deprivation resulted in anergy, as assessed by the DTH response to keyhole limpet haemocyanin (KLH) (166). Survival from bacterial peritonitis challenge in this model was best assessed by the DTH response (anergy) rather than by the nutritional status of the animals.

Malnutrition affects cell-mediated immunity more adversely in children than in adults (155, 167, 168). Mitogen response of T-lymphocytes has been shown to decrease in malnourished children, adults, guinea pigs, and dogs. T-cell subpopulations were studied and reduction of T-helper cells and their receptors to antigen has been reported (136, 164).

Humoral immunity is also affected, but the changes are more complex. Polyclonal hyperimmunoglobulinaemia exists with protein malnutrition but there is also a reduction of IgG response to T-cell dependent antigens. As in the trauma patients, antibody response (IgG) to immunization with antigen is mostly due to abnormal T-helper cell function (8, 155). B-cell function appears quite resistant to malnutrition. B-lymphocytes from protein-malnourished patients produced normal plaques when incubated with T-lymphocytes from well-nourished controls, but lost this activity when incubated with T-lymphocytes from protein-malnourished patients (136, 155). Nohr *et al.* assessed humoral immunity in an animal model of acute nutritional deprivation (169) and long-term protein deprivation (170). In the acute nutritional deprivation model, all food was withheld from rats for 72 h, and the animals were re-fed for seven days. The IgG response to tetanus toxoid (TT) and the DTH skin test response to KLH were assessed. The average weight loss was 15 per cent in the acutely starved rats. Both the DTH response and anti-TT response were down following acute starvation and failed to return to normal with re-feeding despite a return to normal weight of the rats. It appears that the adverse effect of acute starvation on the immune system outlasts simple weight recovery with refeeding. Even though simple extrapolation from this animal study into humans is not entirely correct, the surgeon should nevertheless be aware that perioperative nutritional depriviation may be an important contributing factor to acquired immune deficiency post-operatively. This may be especially true in some patients when one considers the additive effect of acute nutritional deprivation, surgical trauma, and the pre-morbid state of the patient.

The long-term protein deprivation model consisted of feeding the rats a 2 per cent protein diet for eight weeks and refeeding them with normal diet for four weeks. Again there was a progressive decrease of the DTH response and anti-TT response and this correlated directly to the degree of malnutrition and weight loss. The DTH response also correlated directly with the antibody response.

Polymorphonuclear function, such as chemotaxis and bactericidal activity, is depressed in protein malnutrition, but phagocytosis is normal (136, 155, 171). Following acute protein deprivation alveolar macrophage phagocytosis is depressed in rats but bactericidal capacity is normal (172). Depression of phagocytosis persists despite re-feeding back to normal weight. *In vivo* phagocytic cell delivery to a DTH skin test response and a cutaneous bacterial abscess were assessed post-protein-deprivation in an animal model (173). There was a progressive delay and reduced delivery of total number of phagocytic cells in the early hours (first 8 h) of the DTH response and bacterial skin abscess following protein deprivation up to ten weeks. Cell delivery returned quickly back to normal with refeeding.

In the malnourished host the best immune response to antigenic challenge, both humoral and cell-mediated, appears soon after refeeding, usually in the first four days (136, 174). This may be an important therapeutic consideration especially for active immunization with bacterial vaccines.

Sepsis

In the surgical patient bacterial infections are of most significance. Viral and parasitic infections are much less frequent and fungal infections are significant only in the severely immunosuppressed. The impact of sepsis on host defences are hard to assess in surgical patients in the presence of other associated factors. In addition, the systemic effect on the host is not the same for all infections and is influenced by the nature of the organism, the route of infection and the premorbid state of the host. Recently, a general consensus has developed amongst researchers which states that the systemic response to sepsis is not only secondary to a direct effect of bacteria on the host but is also due to the host's response to that micro-organism.

There are three manifestations of bacterial sepsis: the acute, the chronic, and the toxigenic. To the surgeon the acute type is most important. Such infections are caused by nosocomial Gram-positive and Gram-negative bacteria. Bacterial sepsis is characterized by fever, chills, obtunded mental status, and a general feeling of malaise. In the very old or immunocompromised patient a change in mental status or general well-being may be the only 'clue' to a septic process. Sepsis is accompanied by immunologic, haemotologic, and metabolic changes. This process is termed the acute-phase response, and is mediated by the host in response to an invading micro-organism. It mobilizes 'host resources' in an attempt to 'localize', control, and if possible erradicate bacteria that have breached mechanical defences. It is a dose-graded response; bacteria and bacterial products such as endotoxins are the most potent inducers. Central to this response is the macrophage and its equivalent cell in the skin, interstitial tissues, lung, and the reticuloendothelial system. These cells secrete IL-1 when induced by bacteria and its products.

During sepsis there is a rapid shift in metabolism toward the production of acute-phase reactants and an associated body protein catabolism to provide the energy and amino-acid building blocks required (8, 175–177). The body stores of protein most affected are initially the skeletal muscle and albumin, and subsequently systemic organ proteins. The object of the acute phase response is to recruit and deliver immunologically competent leukocytes and associated humoral factors and at the same time mobilize the hosts metabolic processes important to immune cell function in order to localize the invading micro-organisms. Failure to eradicate the invaders results in the ongoing stimulation of the acute phase response and continued illness as witnessed in a patient with an undrained intra-abdominal abscess. Failure to localize the invading micro-organisms results in their dissemination and continued stimulation of the acute phase response, dissemination of stimulated leucocytes, and self-mutilation of the host. Continued metabolic catabolism and indiscriminate release of proteases and oxygen intermediates by stimulated PMNs becomes a vicious cycle that leads ultimately to progressive organ failure and death (178, 179).

With the advent of potent antibiotics against Gram-positive bacteria, Gram-negative sepsis emerged in the 1960s as the major threat to patient survival and focused attention on septic shock and its haemodynamic manifestations (180). With advances in haemodynamic monitoring and support the metabolic and immunologic alteration in bacterial sepsis became the focus of our attention (181). Even though multiple organ failure (MOF) has been described over 15 years ago, Bane (182) and Fry *et al.* (183) were the first to establish its lethality and correlation with disseminated sepsis. By the late 1970s, MOF had replaced septic shock as the manifestation of systemic infection. Many patients with MOF had intra-abdominal infections, often occult, and MOF came to be regarded as an indication for laparotomy (184, 185). However, laparotomy performed to find an infectious focus was negative in many patients. In 1980, the authors described a group of patients who clinically behaved as septic patients (fever, leucocytosis, organ dysfunction) yet had persistently negative cultures (186). Norton has reported a similar experience (187). There is growing evidence to suggest that in these patients on maximum antibiotic therapy, appropriate surgical intervention, and diligent physiological and haemodynamic support, the 'motor' of the MOF syndrome is the GI tract and its vast source of bacteria.

Clinically, the GI tract function is profoundly altered following sepsis. The mucosa of the GI tract, in concert with the gut associated lymphoid tissues, provides an effective barrier to the entry of micro-organisms and endotoxin. Multiple factors, including the tight junctions between epithelial cells, specific epithelial IgA antibody, and local cell-mediated immunity, support this barrier function (193, 194). In addition, the bulk of the reticuloendothelial system and more than 70 per cent of the total macrophage number, the liver and lungs are attached in series to the GI tract. The Kupffer cell and the alveolar macrophage are extremely efficient filters of particulate matter originating from the GI tract. Kupffer cell blockade in an animal model of haemorrhagic shock is associated with subsequent systemic bacteraemia (188), and mechanical obstruction of the bile ducts reduces hepatic phagocytosis with a concomitant increase in pulmonary localization of viable *E. coli* (189). There was a decreased DTH response following Kupffer cell activation with bacteria injected through the portal vein and ablation of Kupffer cells restored DTH response (190).

Changes in intestinal flora, under the influence of a wide use of antibiotics, coupled with impairment of the normal barrier function of the GI tract, allow the bowel to serve as a reservoir of pathogens that enter systemic circulation and fuel the ongoing sepsis (191) Keller *et al.* (192) have shown Kupffer cells are capable of secreting a monokine similar to IL-1 in response to endotoxin and can modulate *in vitro* hepatocyte–protein synthesis. Thus, a potential role for this cell population in the pathogenesis of both the metabolic and immunologic aberrations of MOF is suggested. In the persistent septic state associated with MOF, aberrations of the GI tract are evident: bacterial flora are altered both qualitatively and quantitatively: the intestinal mucosa is altered both morphologically and functionally, and bacterial translocation probably occurs: reticuloendothelial function is suppressed and mediates altered hepatocyte function: systemic immunity is continually suppressed. It is as if someone forgot to turn the engine off. Perhaps in some of these patients that are in an overdrive state of their immune response with the result being MOF, we should be approaching the question from the opposite end. As in any physiological response there is an initiation phase, the process itself, and a termination phase. The questions we should be asking ourselves, perhaps, are what terminates the acute phase response and initiates healing post-sepsis? Does the patient with MOF and sepsis have a protracted acute-phase response and is there failure to initiate 'healing' and termination of the process?

The effect of sepsis on host defences is variable depending at what phase of the process we intervene. In early sepsis, there is, generally, immunopotentiation followed quickly by immunosuppression. This is reflected by decreased DTH response, decreased levels of complement and opsonization, and a decreased PMN chemotaxis (136). Many of the immunologic findings described previously as the acute phase response can be attributed to IL-1 activity.

In an animal model, Bohnen *et al.* (193) demonstrated a reduced DTH response to KLH following septic peritonitis. The DTH skin test response predicted mortality from intraperitoneal sepsis in this model when assessed at the time of bacterial intraperitoneal innoculation. Reactive animals had less intraperitoneal abscesses and a lower mortality compared with anergic animals. Also, a higher bacterial innoculum was associated with a higher rate of anergy. Humoral immunity is also affected by sepsis but most studies are not conclusive. There is a direct relationship between survival and the titre of specific IgG against infecting organisms in Gram-negative sepsis (194, 195).

Immunotherapy and support of immune function

Maintenance of physiology

Correction of the underlying causes of altered chemotaxis and normal physiological processes is the basis of good surgical care and immunotherapy. There is no 'magic bullet' that can be given to the surgical immunocompromised patient in order to restore normal physiology and normal immune function. Minimizing and quickly correcting altered physiologic states such as hypovolaemia, hypoxaemia, hypoventilation, inadequate tissue perfusion, and altered acid–base balance, can all be regarded as immunotherapy (1, 2). Adherence to good surgical principles to minimize tissue trauma, bacterial contamination, tissue ischaemia, and creating a favourable milieu for the healing process are also important aspects of host defence. At the present time there are three therapeutic approaches to anergic patients with sepsis: surgery and restoration of normal physiology with careful respiratory and haemodynamic support, nutritional support, antibiotherapy and immunopotentiation.

Surgery

Drainage of an abscess, resection of perforated or ischaemic bowel, or excision of a septic focus have long been recognized as the most useful treatment for many septic complications. Today it is becoming clearer that these procedures are also physiologically sound. Following surgical intervention for a septic focus, there is restoration of normal physiologic and immunologic status such as return of pre-morbid DTH skin test, neutrophil function, and lymphocyte function (1, 196). Other beneficial interventions are control of haemorrhagic shock, resection of carcinoma, and resection of necrotic or thermally injured tissue (1, 197, 198). Aggressive and timely surgical intervention in the immunocompromised septic patient is physiologically sound. In the context of the 'acute-phase response' and sepsis, removal of the bacterial bond restores the balance in favour of the patient. This is followed by a recovery phase conducive to healing.

Nutritional supplementation

Cellular and biochemical bodily functions require a constant source of energy. Three basic nutritional substances provide this source of energy: carbohydrate, protein, and fat. Sepsis and trauma are associated with an increased metabolic rate and are not simple cases of undernourishment that easily respond to simple nutritional supplementation (8, 171, 199). Trauma and sepsis are associated with an accelerated rate of certain biochemical reactions, and the acute-phase response requires new protein synthesis and building blocks to maintain immunocompetence. Catabolism, protein loss, and negative nitrogen balance are part of this shift in protein synthesis and metabolism. The healthy individual has some nutritional reserves in the form of fat and muscle. A shift in metabolism is, therefore, essential and is a normal physiological response to sepsis or trauma. These sources are finite, however, and eventually other causes such as visceral proteins are mobilized. If there is ongoing sepsis, and food is not supplied exogenously, catabolism continues and multiple organ failure and death follow (175). This process usually takes seven to ten days. Early and aggressive nutritional support is, therefore, essential. In the purely malnourished, non-septic, non-injured host, nutritional therapy restores skin test response, humoral immunity, and PMN function (164, 170, 173, 175). However, the anergy or immunosuppression following sepsis, trauma, or major surgery is not completely restored by nutritional supplementation (200–202). This suggests intrinsic suppressive processes, which does not preclude supportive nutritional therapy.

The choice of nutritional support, total parenteral nutrition or enteral nutrition is controversial. Often the choice is made for us as in severe sepsis, or certain surgical patients, the bowel cannot be effectively used for nutritional support. Preliminary data appears to favour enteral feeding (200), although benefits for both have been claimed and there is no real conclusive data favouring one or the other. The usefulness of various combinations of TPN solutions is also under investigation. Initial studies have presented equivocal results (203).

Immunomodulators

Agents designed as immunomodulators of host defence against bacteria are divided into those from biological sources and those synthetically derived. Biological agents can be further subdivided as endogenous or exogenous. Endogenous biological agents are usually derived from the patient himself but may be from other mammalian sources. An example of this is passive immunization. Exogenous biological agents are derived from viral, bacterial, or fungal sources and often lead to active immunization.

Biological response modifiers may also be classified according to their mechanism of action. These agents may act by (a) removing suppressor factors, (b) replenishing stores of endogenous host defence factors, (c) restoring deficient mechanisms to normal, or (d) hyperstimulating already normal host defence mechanisms. Immunomodulators may have specific or non-specific reactions to antigen. Specific action is usually seen in biologically derived immunomodulators while synthetically derived immunomodulators tend to act in a more non-specific way. History tells us that the use of antigen-specific biologically derived materials, such as vaccines or antisera, have had the most success therapeutically.

Tissue or cell products that have been used in animal models as positive immunomodulators include thymic extracts such as thymopictin or TP5 (204, 205). T-cell function and DTH response were improved in man and survival in a burned septic animal model was also improved. Replacement therapy with isolated mature neutrophils in patients with severe neutropenia and sepsis has shown some promise. However, problems with cell source, isolation, short shelf-life, allo-immunization, and the presence of neutrophil inhibitors in the anergic surgical patients may obviate its therapeutic usefulness (203). Perhaps the greatest use of leucocyte replacement therapy lies in bone marrow harvesting in cancer patients before massive chemotherapy with subsequent marrow autotransplantation.

Active and passive immunization have been most successful therapeutically in bacterial or viral infections. Their use has been mostly as prophylaxis. It is thought that in the anergic state vaccination or active immunization may not be practical against bacteria. However, recent work by Nohr *et al.* (88) has demonstrated that anergic surgical patients can still mount a good humoral response when injected with a pneumococcal (polysaccharide) vaccine. There appears to be substantial cross-reactivity between bacterial serotypes. Many bacterial species exhibit the same surface antigens, and active immunization with one can induce protection against another. For example, cross-reactivity between pneumococcal vaccine serotypes and several *E. coli* and *Klebsiella* species has been described (206). In an animal model pneumococcal vaccination protected against lethal injections of *E. coli* and *Klebsiella*.

It remains to be determined whether active immunization to other bacteria can induce adequate antibody levels and whether adequate antibody response makes a difference in overall survival in the anergic septic surgical patient with progressive multiple organ failure. Vaccination is still of value prophylactically in those patients susceptible to certain bacterial infections. Examples are *Pneumovax* or *Pseudomonas* polyvalent vaccine in patients undergoing splenectomy or in burn victims, respectively (207).

For reasons stated above, passive immunization may be of greater benefit to anergic surgical patients. The recent discovery of monoclonal antibodies raised against specific bacterial cell-wall antigens may prove useful in sepsis. Dunn and Ferguson (208) used monoclonal antibodies raised against core glyoproteins of *E. coli* and showed protective value in animals with bacterial peritonitis with these bacteria (208, 209). In future, genetic recombinant technology will permit the production of large quantities of monoclonal antibodies. Some clinical studies are presently under way. Alternatively the use of polyclonal human antibodies recovered from immunized individuals may also be of value. Screening blood from blood bank donors has shown the presence of high titres of anti-bacterial antibodies (210). Plasma from such subjects could be used as a source for the large-scale production of antibacterial antibodies that could be used to treat surgical anergic patients with sepsis.

Recent advancement in the knowledge of the function and preparation of mixed lymphocyte culture supernatants, lymphokines, and monokines has opened another potential avenue for the treatment of septic anergic patients. However, further animal and human studies are necessary.

Adjuvents are substances that cause non-specific stimulation of the immune system. Most are bacterial products. Some include BCG, muramyl dipeptide (MDP), *Corynebacterium parvum*, and zymosan. BCG increases antibody response; MDP enhances T-helper cell function and improves local infection control and survival after bacteraemia in mice (211–213); *C. parvum* increased survival to bacterial challenge in a rodent model (214). However, most of the benefit is seen when innoculation is done at least one week prior to bacterial infection and the benefit during overwhelming sepsis is probably minimal (214).

Synthetic drugs have also been investigated for potential immunomodulator effect. Levamisole hydrochloride and lithium carbonate have been shown to improve neutrophil function and the DTH response (203). Levamisole was tested in anergic pre-operative patients. Neutrophil chemotaxis and DTH improved, sepsis was significantly reduced, however, the overall mortality rate, although lower, was not reduced significantly (196). However, the number of patients used was small and further studies are necessary, perhaps using a combination of immunomodulators.

Summary

Immunomodulators, however, whether effective in improving immune function or survival, do not absolve the surgeon of the responsibility to provide sound surgical therapy. The benefit of these agents, or new treatment modalities, can only be adequately assessed in the face of optimal, presumably established, surgical care and antibiotherapy. The surgeon should recognize that immunotherapy is not a substitute but only adjuvent to the adherence of basic surgical principles.

References

1. Meakins, J. L. (1981). Clinical importance of host resistance to infection in surgical patients. *Adv. Surg.*, **15**, 225–55.
2. Miles, A. A., Miles, E. M., and Burke, J. F. (1957). The value and duration of diffuse reactions of the skin to the primary lodgement of bacteria. *Br. J. Exp. Pathol.*, **38**, 79.
3. Miles, A. A. (1980). The inflammatory response in relation to local infection. *Surg. Clin. North Am.*, **60**, 93.
4. Burke, J. F. (1961). The effective period of preventive antibiotic action in experimental incisions and dermal lesions. *Surgery*, **50**, 161.
5. Dinarello, C. A. and Wolff, S. M. (1982). Molecular basis of fever in humans. *Am J. Med.*, **72**, 799.
6. Atkins, E. (1984). Fever: the old and the new. *J. Infect. Dis.*, **149**, 339.
7. Howard, R. J. (1982). Prospects for the control of host defenses. *Surgery*, **92**, 138.
8. Dinarello, C. A. (1984). Interleukin-1. *Rev. Infect. Dis.*, **6**, 51–95.
9. Dinarello, C. A. (1984). Interleukin-1 and the pathogenesis of the acute-phase response. *N. Engl. J. Med.*, **311**, 1413.
10. Chipps, B. E., Talamo, R. C., and Binbelstein, J. A. (1978). IgA deficiency, recurrent pneumonias and bronchiectasis. *Chest*, **73**, 519.
11. Herscowitz, H. B. (1985). Immunophysiology: Cell function and cellular interactions in antibody formation. In *Immunology* III (ed. J.A. Bellanti), Vol 7, p. 117. W. B. Saunders Co., Philadephia.
12. Kunkel, S. H., Ward, P. A., Caporale, L. H., and Vogel, C. W. (1985). The complement system. In *Immunology* III (ed. J. A. Bellanti), Vol 6, p. 106. W. B. Saunders Co., Philadephia.
13. Fernandez, H. N., Henson, P. M., Otain, A., *et al.* (1978). Chemotactic response to human C3a and C5a anaphylatoxins: evaluation of C3a and C5a leukotaxis *in vitro* conditions. *J. Immunol.*, **120**, 109.
14. Hugil, Te. (1981). The structural basis for anaphylatoxins and chemotactic functions of C3a, C4a and C5a CRC. *Crit. Rev. Immunol.*, **1**, 321.
15. Chenoweth, D. E., Goodman, M. G., and Weigle, W. O. (1982). Demonstration of a specific receptor for human C5a anaphylatoxin on murine macrophages. *J. Exp. Med.*, **156**, 68.
16. Goodman M. E., Chenoweth, D. E., and Weigle, W. O. (1982). Induction of Interleukin-1 secretion and enhancement of humoral immunity by binding of human C5a to macrophage surface C5a receptors. *J. Exp. Med.*, **156**, 912.
17. Sander, D. L., Mounessa N. L., Katz, Sl. *et al.* (1984). Chemotactic cytokines: The role of leukocytic pyrogen and epidermal cell derived thymocyte activity factor (ETAF) for polymorphonuclear leukocytes. *J. Immunol.*, **132**, 828.
18. Boyden, S. (1962). The chemotactic effect of mixtures of antibody and antigen on polymorphonuclear leukocytes, *J. Exp. Med.* 1962; **115**, 453.
19. Zigmond, S. H. and Hirsh, J. G. (1973). Leukocyte locomotion and chemotaxis; new methods for evaluation and demonstration of a cell-derived chemotactic factor. *J. Exp. Med.*, **137**, 367.
20. Nelson, R. D., Quie P. G., and Simmons, R. L. (1975). Chemotaxis under agarose: a new and simple method for measuring chemotaxis and spontaneous migration of human polymorphonuclear leukocytes and monocytes. *J. Immunol.*, **115**, 1650.
21. Rebuck, J. W. and Crowley, J. H. (1955). A method of studying leukocytic functions *in vivo*. *Ann. NY Acad. Sci.*, **59**, 757.
22. Otani, A., and Hugli, T. E. (1977). Leukocyte chemotaxis: A new *in vivo* testing technique. *Inflammation*, **2**, 67.
23. Goldberg, B. S., Weston, W. L., Kohler, P. F. *et al.* (1979). Transcutaneous leukocyte migration *in vivo*: cellular kinetics, platelets and C5a dependent activity. *J. Invest. Dermatol.*, **72**, 248.
24. Luger, T. A., Charon, J. A., Colot, M. *et al.* (1983). Chemotactic properties of partially purified human epidermal cell-derived thymocyte activating factor (ETAF) for polymorphonuclear and mononuclear cells. *J. Immunol.*, **131**, 816.
25. Issehutz, A. C. and Movat, H. Z. (1980). The *in vivo* quantitation and kinetics of rabbit neutrophil leukocyte accumulation in the skin in response to chemotactic agents and Escherichia coli. *Lab. Invest.*, **42**, 310.
26. Cololitz, I. G. and Movat, H. Z. (1984). Kinetics of neutrophil accumulation in acute inflammatory lesions induced by chemotoxins and chemotoxinogens. *J. Immunol.*, **133**, 2169.
27. Porter, R. R. (1981). Interactions of complement components with antibody – antigen aggregates and cell surfaces. *Immunol. Today.*, **2**, 143.
28. Atkins, E. Bodel, P., and Francis, L. (1967). Release of an endogenous pyrogen *in vitro* from rabbit mononuclear cells. *J. Exp. Med.*, **126**, 357.
29. Dinarello, C. A., Bodel, P. T., and Atkins E. (1968). The role of the liver in the production of fever and in pyrogenic tolerance. *Trans. Assoc. Am. Physicians*, **81**, 334.
30. Simon, P. L. and Willoughby, W. F. (1981). The role of subcellular factors in pulmonary immune function: physicochemical characterization of two distinct species of lymphocyte-activating factor produced by rabbit alveolar macrophages. *J. Immunol.*, **126**, 1534.
31. Murphy, P. A., Simon, P. L., and Willoughby, W. F. (1980). Endogenous pyrogens made by rabbit peritoneal exudate cells are identical with lymphocyte-activating factors made by rabbit alveolar macrophages. *J. Immunol.*, **124**, 2498.
32. Lee, K. C., Wong, M., and McIntyre, D. (1981). Characterization of macrophage subpopulations responsive to activation by endotoxin and lymphokines. *J. Immunol.*, **126**, 2474.
33. Rosenthal, A. S. (1980). Regulation of the immune response-role of the macrophage. *N. Engl. J. Med.*, **303**, 1153–6.
34. Unanue, E. R. (1978). The regulation of lymphocyte functions by the macrophage. Immunol Rev 1978, **40**, 227–55.
35. Gery, I., Gershon, R. K., and Wahsman, B. H. (1972). Potentiation of the T-lymphocyte response to mitogens. I. The responding cell. *J. Exp. Med.*, **136**, 128–42.
36. Grezy, I. and Wahsman, B. H. (1972). Potentiation of the T-lymphocyte response to mitogens II. The cellular source of potentiating mediator(s). *J. Exp. Med.*, **136**, 143–55.
37. Aarden, L. A., Bumner, T. K., Cerottini J-C *et al.* (1979). Revised nomenclature for antigen-non-specific T cell prolifera-

tion and helper factors. (Letter). *J. Immunol.* 1979; **123.**, 2928–9.
38. Dinarello, C.A. and Wolff, S.M. (1982). Exogenous pyrogens. In *Pyretics and antipyretics* (ed. A.S. Milton), p. 73. Springer-Verlag, Berlin.
39. Janpel, H.D., Duff, G W., Gershon, R.K. *et al.* (1983). Fever and immunoregulation. III. Hypothermia augments the primary *in vitro* humoral immune response, *J. Exp. Med.* **157**, 1229.
40. Van Oss, C.S., Absolom, D.R., Moore, L.L. *et al.* (1980). Effect of temperature on the chemotaxis, phagocytic engulfment, digestion and O_2 consumption of human polymorphonuclear leukocytes. *J. Reticuloendothel. Soc.*, **27**, 561.
41. Duff, G.W. and Durum, S.K. (1983). The pyrogenic and nitrogenic actions of Interleukin-1 are related. *Nature*, **304**, 449.
42. Kluger, M.T., Ringler, D.H., and Anver, M.R. (1975). Fever and survival. *Science* 1975; 188: 166.
43. Buttler, T., Spagmedo, P.J., Goldsmith, G.H. *et al.* (1982). Interaction of Borrelia spirochetes with human mononuclear leukocytes causes production of leukocytic pyrogen and thromboplastin. *J. Lab. Clin. Med.*, **99**, 709.
44. Bodel, P. (1976). Colchicine stimulation of pyrogen production by human blood leukocytes. *J. Exp. Med.*, **143**, 1015.
45. Etin, R.J., Wolff, S.M., McAdam, K.P.W.J. *et al.* (1981). Properties of reference *Escherichia coli* endotoxin and its phthalylated derivatives in humans. *J. Infect. Dis.*, **144**, 329.
46. Ikejima, T., Dinarello, C.A., Gill, M.D. *et al.* (1983). Toxic shock (TS) strains of staphilococcus aureus are potent inducers of human leukocytic pyrogen (LP) and lymphocyte activating factor (LAF). *Clin. Res.*, **31**, 496A.
47. Duff, G.W., Gekowski, K.M., and Atkons, E. (1982). Endogenous pyrogen production stimulated by immune complexes. *Clin. Res.*, **30**, 364A.
48. Milon, G., Marchal, G., Seman, M. *et al.* (1983). Is the delayed-type hypersensitivity observed after a low dose of antigen mediated by helper T-cells? *J. Immunol.*, **130**, 1103.
50. Chase M.V. (1945). Cellular transfer of cutaneous hypersensitivity to tuberculin. *Proc. Soc. Exp. Biol. Med.*, **59** 134.
51. Landsteiner, K. and Chase M.W. (1942). Experiments on transfer of cutaneous sensitivity of simple chemical components. *Proc. Soc. Exp. Biol Med.*, 49–688.
52. Razzaque-Ahmed, A. and Blose, D.A. (1983). Delayed-type hypersensitivity skin testing. A review. *Arch. Dermatol.*, **119**, 934.
53. Woody, J.N., Bellanti, J.A., and Sell, K.W. (1985). Immunogenetics. In *Immunology* III (ed. J.A. Bellanti), Vol. 3, p. 54. W.B. Saunders Co., Philadelphia.
54. Platt, J.L., Grant, B.W., Eddy, A.A. *et al.* (1983). Immune cell populations in cutaneous delayed-type hypersensitivity. *J. Exp. Med.*, **158**, 1227.
55. Asano, Y. and Hodes, R.J. T cell regulation of B cell activation: Antigen-specific and antigen-nonspecific supressor pathways are mediated by distinct T cell subpopulations. *J. Immunol.*, **30**, 1061.
56. Bellanti, J.A. and Rocklin, R.E. (1985). Cell-mediated immune reactions. In *Immunology* III (ed. J.A. Bellanti), p. 176. W.B. Saunders Co, Philadelphia.
57. Ross, R. (1969). Wound healing *Sci. Am.*, **220**, 40.
58. Howes, R.M. and Hoopes, J.E. (1977). Current concepts in wound healing. *Clin. Plast. Surg.*, **2**, 173–9.
59. Hunt, T.K. (1984) Can repair processes be stimulated by modulators (cell growth factors, angiogenic factors, etc.) without adversely affecting normal processes? *J. Trauma.*, **24**, 39–49.
60. Grotendwist G.R. (1984). Can collagen metabolism be controlled? *J. Trauma*, **24**, 49.
61. Hunt, T.K., Andrews, W.S., Halliday, B., *et al.* (1981). Coagulation and macrophage stimulation of angiogenesis and wound healing. In *The surgical wound* (ed. P. Dimen and G. Hlock-Smith), pp. 1–18. Lea & Febiger, Philadelphia.
62. Ross, R. (1980). Inflammation, cellular proliferation, and formation of connective tissue in wound healing. In *Wound healing and wound infection* (ed. T.K. Hunt), pp. 1–10. Theory and surgical practice. Appleton-Century-Crofts, New York.
63. Seppa, H.E., Grotendwist, G.R., Seppa, S., *et al.* (1982). Platelet derived growth factor is a chemoattractant for fibroblasts. *J. Cell. Biol.*, **92**, 584–8.
64. Grotendwist, G.R., Chang, T., Seppa, H.E.J., *et al.* (1982). Platelet-derived growth factor is a chemoattractant for vascular smooth muscle cells. *J. Cell. Physiol.*, **113**, 261–6.
65. Bowezsox, J.C. and Sogente, N. (1982). Chemotactic response of endothelial cells in response to fibronectin. *Cancer Res.*, **42**, 2547–51.
66. Bauda, M.J., Knighton, D.R., Hunt, T.W., and Werb, Z. (1982). Isolation of a nonmitogenic angiogenesis factor from wound fluid. *Proc. Natl. Acad. Sci., USA*, **79**, 7773–7.
67. Schilling, J.A., Joel, W., and Shuelyey, H.M. (1959). Wound healing: a comparative study of the histochemical changes in granulation tissue contained in stainless steel wire mesh and polyvinyl sponge cylinders. *Surgery*, **46**, 702–10.
68. Martin, B.M., Ginbrane, M.A., Unanue, E.R., *et al.* (1981). Macrophage derived growth factor: Production by cultured human mononuclear blood cells. *Fed. Proc.*, **40**, 335.
69. Langness, U. and Udentfrienld, S. (1973). Collagen hydroxiplase activity and anaerobic metabolism. In *Biology of fibroblast* (ed. E. Krilonen and J. Pikkarainen), pp. 373–8. Academic Press, London.
70. Ketchum, S.A. III, Thomas, A.N., and Hall, AD. (1970). Angiogenic studies of the effects of hyperbaric oxygen on burn wound revascularization. In *Proceedings of the Fourth International Congress on Hyperbaric Medicine* (ed. J. Wode and T. Iwa), pp. 388–94. Williams and Wilkins, Baltimore.
71. Knighton, D.R., Silver, I.A., and Hunt, T.K. (1981). Regulation of wound healing angiogenesis—effect of oxygen gradients and inspired oxygen concentration. *Surgery*, **90**, 262–70.
72. MacLean, L.D., Meakins, J.L., Taguchi, K. *et al.* Host resistance in sepsis and trauma. *Ann. Surg.*, **182**, 207.
73. Christou, N.V. (1985). Host defense mechanisms in surgical patients: a correlative study of the delayed hypersensitivity skin-test response, granulocyte function and sepsis. *Can. J. Surg.*, **28**, 39.
74. Christou, N.V., Meakins, J.L. (1984). Neutrophil function in anergic surgical patients. *Arch. Surg.*, **190**, 557.
75. Buffone, V., Meakins, J.L., and Christou, N.V. (1984). Neutrophil function in surgical patients. *Arch. Surg.*, **119**, 39.
76. Meakins, J.L., Pletsch, J.B., Bubenick, O. *et al.* (1977). Delayed hypersensitivity: Indicator of acquired failure of host defenses in sepsis and trauma. *Ann. Surg.*, **186**, 241.
77. Christou, N.V., Meakins, J.L., and MacLean, L.D. (1981). The predictive role of delayed hyper-sensitivity in preoperative patients. *Surg. Gynecol. Obstet.*, **152**, 297.
78. Van Epps, E.D., Palmer, D.L., and Williams, R.C. (1974). Characterization of serum inhibitors of neutrophil chemotaxis associated with anergy. *J. Immunol.*, **113**f. 189.
79. Ninnemann, J.L. and Ozkan, A.N. (1985). Definition of a burn-injury induced immunosuppressive serum component. *J. Trauma*, **25**, 113.
80. Christou, N.V. and Meakins, J.L. (1982). Phagocytic and bactericidal functions of polymorphonuclear neutrophils from anergic surgical patients. *Can. J. Surg.*, **25**, 444.

81. Alexander, J. W. Emerging concepts in control of clinical infection. *Surgery*, **75**, 934.
82. Alexander, J. W., Ogle, C. K., Stinnett, J. D., and MacMillan, B. G. (1978). A sequential prospective analysis of immunologic abnormalities and infection following severe thermal injury. *Ann. Surg.*, **188**, 809.
83. Superina, R. A., Christou, N. V., and Meakins, J. L. (1984). Failure of neutrophil delivery into skin windows in anergic patients. *Surg. Forum*, **35**, 113.
84. Morris, J. S., Buffone, V., Meakins, J. L. *et al.* (1984). *In vivo* polymorphonuclear neutrophil (PMN) delivery to skin windows, *in vitro* PMN chemotaxis, and their relation to serum chemoattraction. *Surg. Forum*, **35**, 113.
85. Rode, H. N., Christou, N. V., Bubenick, O. *et al.* (1982). Lymphocyte function in anergic patients. *Clin. Exp. Immunol.*, **47**, 155.
86. Nohr, C. W., Christou, N. V., Broadhead, M., Meakins, J. L. (1983). Failure of humoral immunity in surgical patients. *Surg. Forum.*, **34**, 127.
87. Nohr, C. W., Christou, N. V., Rode, H., Gordon, J., and Meakins J. L. (1984). *In vivo* and *in vitro* humoral immunity in surgical patients. *Ann. Surg.*, **200**, 373.
88. Nohr, C. W., Latter, D. A., Meakins, J. L., and Christou, N. V. (1986) *In vivo* and *in vitro* humoral immunity in surgical patients: Antibody response to pneumococcal polysaccharide. *Surgery*, **100**, 229.
89. Puyana, J. C., Rode, H. N., and Meakins, J. L. *et al.* (1986). Restoration of primary immune response in anergic surgical patients by lymphokines. *Surg. Forum*, **37**, 103.
90. McPhee, M. J., Zakaluzny, I., Marshall J., *et al.*, (1986). Mixed lymphocyte culture supernatants provide effective immunotherapy for acute peritonitis in immunosuppressed rats. *Surg. Forum*, **37**, 105.
91. Van Dijk, W. C., Verburgh, H. A., Van Rijswjik, R. E. N., *et al.* (1982). Neutrophil function, serum opsonic activity and delayed hypersensitivity in surgical patients. *Surgery*, **92**, 21.
92. Alexander, J. W., Ogle, C. K., Stinnett, J. D., *et al.* (1978). A sequential, prospective analysis of immunologic abnormalities and infection following severe thermal injury. *Ann. Surg.*, **188**, 809.
93. Alexander, J. W., Stinnett, J. D., Ogle, C. K., *et al.* (1979). A comparison of immunologic profiles and their influence on bacteremia in surgical patients with a high risk of infection. *Surgery*, **86**, 94.
94. Bjornson, A. B. and Alexander, J. W. (1974). Alterations of serum opsonins in patients with severe thermal injury. *J. Lab. Clin. Med.*, **83**, 372.
95. Ninnemann, J. L. (1982). Immunologic defenses against infection: alterations following thermal injuries. *J Bone Care Rehab*, **3**, 355.
96. Lundy, J. and Ford, C. M. (1983). Surgery, trauma and immune suppression. Evolving the mechanism. *Ann. Surg.*, **197**, 434.
97. Alexander, J. W. and Moncrief, J. A. (1966). Alterations of the immune response following severe thermal injury. *Arch. Surg.*, **93**, 75.
98. Gelfand, J. A. (1984). Infections in burn patients: A paradigm for cutaneous infection in the patient at risk. *Am. J. Med.*, **72**, 158.
99. Ninnemann, J. L., Fisher, J. C., and Frank, H. A. (1978). Prolonged survival of human skin allografts following thermal injury. *Transplantation*, **25**, 69.
100. Ischizawa, S., Sabai, H., Sarlese, H. E. *et al.* (1978). Effect of thymosis on T-lymphocyte functions in patients with acute thermal burns. *J. Trauma.*, **18**, 48.
101. Bauer, A. R., McNeil, C., Teewtelman *et al.* (1978). The depression of T-lymphocytes after trauma. *Am. J. Surgery.*, **136**, 674.
102. Antonacci, A. C., Good, R. A., and Gupta, S. (1982). T-cell subpopulations following thermal injury. *Surg. Gynecol. Obstet.*, **155**, 1.
103. McIrvine, A. J., O'Mahony, J. B., Saporoschetz, I., *et al.* (1982). Depressed immune response in burn patients: Use of monoclonal antibodies and functional assays to define the role of suppressor cells. *Ann. Surg.*, **196**, 297.
104. Holt, P. G., Warner, L. T., and Mayrhofer, G. (1981). Macrophages as effectors of T suppression: T-lymphocyte dependent macrophage-mediated suppression of mitogen induced blastogenesis in the rat. *Cell Immunol.*, **63**, 57.
105. Henson, P. M. (1985). Mechanisms of tissue injury produced by immunologic. In *Immunology* III (ed. J. A. Bellanti), p. 218. W. B. Saunders Co, Philadelphia.
106. Beer, D. J., Dinarello, C. A., Rosenwasser, L. J., *et al.* Human monocyte-derived soluble product(s) has an accessary function in the generation of histamine and concanavalent induced suppressor T cells. *J. Clin. Invest.*, **70**, 393.
107. Kupper, T. S., Deitch, E. A., Baher, C. C., and Wong, W. (1986). The human burn wound as a primary source of Interleukin-1 activity. *Surgery*, **100**, 409.
108. Wood, J. J., Rodrich, M. L., O'Mahony, J. B., *et al.* (1984). Inadequate Interleukin-2 production: a fundamental immunological deficiency in patients with major burns. *Ann. Surg.*, **200**, 311.
109. Ninnemann, J. L., Condie, J. T., Davis, S. E., *et al.* (1982). Isolation of immunosuppressive serum components following thermal injury. *J. Trauma*, **22**, 837.
110. McCloughlin, G. A., Wu, A. V., Saporoschetz, I., *et al.* (1979). Correlation between anergy and a circulatory immunosuppressive factor following major surgical trauma. *Ann. Surg.*, **190**, 297.
111. Wolfe, J. H. N., Wu, A. V. O., O'Connor, N. E., *et al.* (1982). Anergy, immunosuppressive serum and impaired lymphocyte blastogenesis in burn patients. *Arch. Surgery.*, **117**, 1266.
112. Constantian, M. B. (1978). Association of sepsis with an immunosuppressive polypeptide in the serum of burn patients. *Ann. Surg.*, **188**, 209.
113. Rogers, T. J., Nowowickjski, I., and Webb, D. R. (1980). Partial characterization of a prostoglandin-induced suppressor factor. *Cell Immunol.*, **50**, 82.
114. Tadakuma, T. and Pierce, C. W. (1976). Site of action of a soluble immune response suppressor (SIRS) produced by concanavalin-A activated spleen cells. *J. Immunol.*, **117**, 967.
115. Pierce, C. W. and Kapp, J. A. (1980). Activities of non-specific and specific suppressor T-cell factors in immune responses. *Agents Actions* (Suppl), **7**, 126.
116. Anne, T. M. and Pierce, C. W. (1981). Mechanisms of action of macrophage-derived suppressor factor produced by soluble immune response suppressor-treated macrophages. *J. Immunol.*, **127**, 368.
117. Bjornson, A. B. and Bjornson, H. S. (1984). Theoretical interrelationships among immunologic and hematologic sequelae of thermal injury. *Rev. Inf. Dis.*, **6**, 704.
118. Antonacci, A. C., Calvano, S. E., Reaves, L. E., *et al.* (1984). Autologous and allogenic mixed-lymphocyte responses following thermal injury in man: the immunomodulatory effects of Interleukin-1, Interleukin-2, and a prostaglandin inhibitor, WY-18251. *Clin. Immunol. Immunopathol.*, **30**, 304.
119. Shires, G. T. and Dineen, P. (1982). Sepsis following burns, trauma and intra-abdominal infections. *Arch. Intern. Med.*, **142**, 2012.
120. Kuehl, F. A. Jr. and Egan, R. W. (1980). Prostaglandins, arachidonic acid, and inflammation. *Science*, **210**, 9.

121. Weksler, B.B. and Goldstein, I.M. (1980). Prostaglandins: Interactions with platelets and polymorphonuclear leukocytes in hemostasis and inflammation. *Am. J. Med.*, **68**, 419.
122. Miller, C.L. (1983). Monitoring of lymphocyte function. In Abstracts of the 40th International Burn Research Conference, San Antonio, Texas, January 1983.
123. Webb, D.R. and Nowowiejski, I. (1978). Mitogen-induced changes in lymphocyte prostaglandin levels: a signal for the induction of suppressor cell activity. *Cell Immunol.*, **41**, 72.
124. Snyder, D.S., Beller, D.I., and Unanue, E.R. (1982). Prostaglandins modulate macrophage lc expression. *Nature*, **299**, 163.
125. Unanue, E.R. (1981). The regulatory role of macrophages in antigenic stimulation. Part two: symbiotic relationship between lymphocytes and macrophages. *Adv. Immunol.*, **31**, 1.
126. Ischizaha, K. Adachi, T. (1976). Generation of specific helper cells and suppressor cells *in vitro* for the IgE and IgG antibody responses. *J. Immunol.*, **117**, 40.
127. Pierce, C.W. and Kapp, J.A. (1978), Antigen-specific suppressor T-cell activity in genetically restricted immune spleen cells. *J. Exp. Med.*, **148**, 1271.
128. Lappin, D.F. and Whaley, K. (1982). Prostaglandins and prostaglandin synthetase inhibitors regulate synthesis of complement components by human monocytes. *Clin. Exp. Immunol.*, **49**, 623.
129. Herndon, D.N., Abston, S., and Stein, M.D. (1984). Increased thromboxane B_2 levels in the plasma of burned and septic burned patients. *Surg. Gynecol. Obstet.*, **159**, 210.
130. Weksler, B.B. and Goldstein, I.M. (1980). Prostaglandins: interactions with platelets and polymorphonuclear leukocytes in hemostasis and inflammation. *Am. J. Med.*, **68**, 419.
131. Jacob, H.S., Moldow, C.F., Flynn, P.J., *et al.* (1982). Therapeutic ramifications of the interaction of complement, granulocytes, and platelets in the production of acute lung injury. *Ann. NY Acad. Sci.*, 384–489.
132. Latter, D.A., Tchervenkov, J.I., Nohr, C.W., and Christou, N.V. (1987). The effect of indomethacin on burn-induced immunosuppression. *J. Surg. Res.*, **43**, 246–52.
133. Shorr, R.M., Ezshler, W.B., and Gramelli, R.L. (1984). Immunoglobulin production in burned patients. *J. Trauma.*, **24**, 319.
134. Miller, C.L. and Trunkey, D.D. (1977). Thermal injury: defects in immune response induction. *J. Surg. Res.*, **22**, 621.
135. Alexander, J.W. and Wixson, D. (1970). Neutrophil dysfunction and sepsis in burn injury. *Surg. Gynecol Obstet.*, **131**, 431.
136. Meakins, J.L. and Nohr, C.W. (1983). Assessment of immunologic responsiveness. In *Nutrition and metabolism in the surgical patient* (ed, J.R. Kirkpatrick), p. 107. Futura Publishing, New York.
137. Lanser, M.E. and Saba, T.M. (1982). Opsonic fibronectin deficiency and sepsis, cause or effect? *Ann. Surg.*, **195**, 340.
138. Bjornson, A.B., Altemeier, W.A., and Bjornson, H.S. (1980). Complement, opsonins, and the immune response to bacterial infection in burned patients. *Ann. Surg.*, **191**, 323.
139. Gelfand, J.A., Donelan, M., and Burke, J.F. (1983). Preferential activation and depletion of the alternative complement pathway by burn injury. *Ann. Surg.*, **198**, 58.
140. Hautanen, A. and Keshi-Oja, J. (1983). Interaction of fibronectin with complement component C3. *Scand. J. Immunol.*, **17**, 225.
141. Charriant, C., Senik, A., Kolf, J.P. *et al.* (1982). Inhibition of *in vitro* natural killer activity by the third component of complement: role for the C3a fragment. *Proc. Natl. Acad. Sci. USA*, **79**, 6003.
142. Morgan, E.L., Weigle, W.O., and Hyeli, T.E. (1982). Anaphylatoxin mediated regulation of the immune response. I. C3a mediated suppression of human and murine humoral immune responses. *J. Exp. Med*, **155**, 1412.
143. Gelfand, J.A., Denelan M., and Hawiger, A. (1982). Alternative complement pathway activation increases mortality in a model of burn injury in mice. *J. Clin. Invest.*, **70**, 1170.
144. Grogan, J.B., (1976). Altered neutrophil phagocytic function in burn patients. *J. Trauma*, **16**, 734.
145. Deitch, E.A., Gelder, F., and McDonald, J.C. (1982). Prognostic significance of abnormal neutrophil chemotaxis after thermal injury. *J. Trauma.*, **22**, 199.
146. Warden, G.D., Mason, A.D., and Pruitt, B.A. (1974). Evaluation of leukocyte chemotaxis *in vitro* in thermally injured patients. *J. Clin. Invest.*, **54**, 1001.
147. McManus, A.T. (1983). Examination of neutrophil function in a rat model of decreased host resistance following burn trauma. *Rev. Infect. Dis.*, **5**, 5898.
148. Christou, N.V., McLean A.P.H., and Meakins, J.L. (1980). Host defense in blunt trauma: Interrelationships of kinetics of anergy and depressed neutrophil function, nutritional status, and sepsis. *J. Trauma*, **20**, 833.
149. Alexander, J.W. and Meakins, J.L. (1972). A physiological basis for the development of opportunistic infections in man. *Ann. Surg.*, **176**, 273.
150. Alexander, J.W. and Fisher, M.W. (1974). Immunization against pseudomonas in infection after thermal injury. *J. Inf. Dis.*, **130**, 152.
151. Allen, R.C. and Pruitt, B.A. (1982). Humoral-phagocyte axis of immune defense in burn patients–chemoluminogenic probing. *Arch. Surg.*, **117**, 133.
152. Tchervenkov, J.I., Latter, D.A., Psychogios J, *et al.* (1986). Decreased phagocytic cell delivery to inflammatory lesions is due to the host 'trauma environment' not to intrinsic cellular defects. *Surg. Forum*, **37**, 90–2.
153. Allen, J.I., Kay, N.E., and McClain, C.J. (1981). Severe zinc deficiency in humans: Association with reversible t-lymphocyte dysfunction. *Ann. Intern. Med.*, **95**, 154.
154. Axelrod, A.E. (1971)., Immune processes in vitamin deficiency states. *Am. J. Clin. Nutr.*, **24**, 265.
155. Chandra, R.K. (1980). Cell-mediated immunity in nutritional inbalance. *Fed. Proc.*, **39**, 3088.
156. Good, R.A., West, A., and Fernandes, G. (1980). Nutritional modulation of immune responses. *Fed. Proc.*, **39**, 3098.
157. Cannon, P.R., Wissler, R.W., Woolridge Beditt EL: (1944). The relationship of protein deficiency to surgical infection. *Ann. Surg.*, **170**, 514.
158. Chandra, R.K. and Au, B. (1980). Spleen hemolytic plaque-forming cell response and generation of cytotoxic cells in genetically obese (S57B1/6J ob/ob) mice. *Int. Arch. Allergy Appl. Immunol.*, **62**, 94.
159. Chandra, R.K. and Kutty, K.M. (1980). Immunocompetence in obesity. *Acta Paediatr. Scand.*, **69**, 25.
160. Bullen, J.J. (1981). The significance of iron in infection. *Rev. Inf. Dis.*, **3**, 1127.
161. Sugarman, B. (1983). Zinc and infection. *Rev. Infect. Dis.* **5**, 137.
162. Prolusko, J.R. and Lukascwycz, O.A. (1981). Copper deficiency suppresses the immune response in mice. *Science*, **213**, 559.
163. Newerne, P.M., Hunt, C.E. and Young, V.R. (1968). The role of diet and the reticuloendothelial system in the response of rats to Salmonella typhimirium infection. *Br. J. Exp. Pathol.*, **49**, 559.
164. Chandra, R.K. (1988). Nutrition, immunity, and infection: Present knowledge and future directions. *Lancet* 1983, **1**, 688.
165. Forse, R.A., Christou, N.V., Meakins, J.L., *et al.* (1981).

Reliability of skin testing as a measure of nutritional state. *Arch. Surg.*, **116**, 1284.
166. Ing. A.F.M., Meakins, J.L., McLean, A.P.H., *et al.* (1982). Determinants of susceptibility to sepsis and mortality: malnutrition *vs* anergy. *J. Surg. Res.*, **32**, 249.
167. Bistrian, B.R., Sherman, M., Blackburn, G.L., *et al.* (1977). Cellular immunity in adult marasmus. *Arch. Intern. Med.*, **137**, 1408.
168. Law, D.K., Dudrick, S.J., and Abdou, N.I. (1973). Immunocompetence of patients with protein-calorie malnutrition: The effects of nutrition repletion. *Ann. Intern. Med.*, **79**, 545.
169. Nohr, C.W., Tchervenkov, J.I., Meakins, J.L., and Christou, N.V. (1985). Malnutrition and humoral immunity: Short-term acute nutritional deprivation. *Surgery*, **98**, 769.
170. Nohr, C.W., Tchervenkov, J.I., Meakins, J.L., and Christou, N.V. (1986). Malnutrition and humoral immunity: Long-term protein deprivation. *J. Surg. Res.*, **40**, 432.
171. Dionigi, R., Zonta, A., Dominioni, L., *et al.* (1976). The effects of total parenteral nutritional on immunodepression due to malnutrition. *Ann. Surg.*, **185**, 467.
172. Shennib, H., Chier, C.R., Mulder, D.S., and Lough, J.O. (1984). Depression and delayed recovery of alveolar macrophage function during starvation and refeeding. *Surg. Gynecol. Obstet.*, **158**, 535.
173. Tchervenkov, J.I., Latter, D.A., Psychogios, J. *et al.* (1988). *In vivo* phagocytic cell delivery to inflammatory lesions in long-term protein deprivation. *Surgery*, **103**, 463–89.
174. Law, D.K., Dudrick, S.J., and Abdon, N.I. (1974). The effect of dietary protein depletion on immunocompetence: The importance of nutritional repletion prior to immunologic induction. *Ann. Surg.*, **179**, 168.
175. Baracos, V., Rodemann, H.P., Dinarello, C.A., *et al.* (1983). Stimulation of muscle protein degradation and prostaglandin E_2 release by leukocyte pyrogen (Interleukin 1). A mechanism for the increased degradation of muscle proteins during fever. *N. Engl. J. Med.*, **308**, 553.
176. Clowes, G.H.A., George, B.C., Ville, C.A., *et al.* (1983). Muscle proteolysis induced by a circulating peptide on patients with sepsis or trauma. *N. Engl. J. Med.*, **308**, 545.
177. Newman, J.J., Goodwin, C.W., Mason, A.D., *et al.*, (1984). Altered protein metabolism in diaphragms from thermally injured rats. *J. Surg. Res.*, **36**, 177.
178. Baggiolini, M., Bretz, U., Dewald, B. *et al.* (1978). The polymorphonuclear leukocyte. *Agents Actions*, **8**, 3.
179. Fantone, J.C. and Ward, P.A. (1982). Role of oxygen-derived free radicals and metabolites in leukocyte-dependent inflammatory reactions. *Am. J. Pathol.*, **107**, 397.
180. Altemeier, W.A., Tood, J.C., and Inge, W.W. (1967). Gram-negative septicemia: a growing threat. *Ann. Surg.*, **166**, 530.
181. MacLean, L.D., Mulligan, W.G., McLean, A.P.H., *et al.* (1967). Patterns of septic shock in man: A detailed study in 56 patients. *Ann. Surg.*, **166**, 543.
182. Baue, A.E. (1975). Multiple, progressive or sequential systems failure: A syndrome of the 1970's. *Arch. Surg.*, **110**, 779.
183. Fry, D.E., Pearlstein, L., Fulton, R.L., *et al.* (1980). Multiple system organ failure: the role of uncontrolled infection. *Arch. Surg.*, **115**, 136.
184. Polk, H.C., Shields, C.L. (1977). Remote organ failure: A valid sign of occult intra-abdominal infection. *Surgery*, **81**, 310.
185. Meakins, J.L. (1979). Occult signs of sepsis. *Can. J. Surg.*, **22**, 505.
186. Meakins, J.L., Wicklund, B., Forse, R.A., *et al.* (1980). The surgical intensive care unit: current concepts in infection. *Surg. Clin. North. Am.*, **60**, 117.
187. Norton, L.W. (1985). Does drainage of intra-abdominal pus reverse multiple organ failure? *Am. J. Surg.*, **149**, 347.
188. Purdy, B.J., Spencer, R.C., and Dudley, H.A.F. (1977). Hepatic reticuloendothelial protection against bacteremia in experimental hemorrhagic shock. *Surgery*, **81**, 193.
189. Katz, S., Grosfield, J.L., Gross, K., *et al.* (1984). Impaired bacterial clearance and trapping in obstructive jaundice. *Ann. Surg.*, **199**, 14.
190. Marshall, J.C., Lee, C., Meakins, J.L., *et al.* (1987). Kupffer cell modulation of the systemic immune response. *Arch. Surg.*, **122**, 191.
191. Carrico, C.J., Meakins, J.L., Marshall, J.C., Fry, D., Maier, R.V. (1986). Multiple-organ failure syndrome: the gastrointestinal tract: The 'Motor' of MOF. Panel discussion SIS 1985. *Arch. Surg.*, **121**, 196.
192. Keller, G.A., West, M.A., Hartly, J.T., *et al.* (1985). Modulation of hepatocyte protein synthesis by endotoxin-activated Kupffer cells: III. Evidence for a role of a monokine similar to but not identical with interleukin-1. *Ann. Surg.*, **201**, 436.
193. Bohnen, J.M., Christou, N.V., Chiasson, L., *et al.* (1984). Anergy secondary to sepsis in rats. *Arch. Surg.*, **114**, 117.
194. Clumek, N., Delespesse, G., and Butzler, J.P. (1980). Humoral immunity and circulating immune complexes in gram-negative bacteremia and septic shock. In *Bacterial endotoxins and host response* (ed. M.K. Agarwal), p. 79. Elsevier–North Holland Biomedical Press, Amsterdam.
195. Zinner, S.H., McCabe, W.R. (1976). Effects of IgM and IgG antibody in patients with bacteremia due to gram-negative-bacilli. *J. Infect. Dis.*, **133**, 37.
196. Meakins, J.L., Christou, N.V., Shizgal, H.M., *et al.* (1979). Therapeutic approaches to anergy in surgical patients: Surgery and levamisol. *Ann. Surg.*, **190**, 286.
197. Tompkins, R.G., Burke, J.F., Schoenfeld, D.A., *et al.* (1986). Prompt eschar excision: a treatment system contributing to reduced burn mortality. A statistical evaluation of burn care at the Massachusetts General Hospital (1974–1984). *Ann. Surg.*, **204**, 272.
198. Stratta, R.J., Soffle, J.E., Ninnemann, J.L., *et al.* (1985). The effect of surgical excision and grafting procedures on postburn lymphocyte suppression. *J. Trauma.*, **25**, 46.
199. Tayek, J.A. and Blackburn, G.L. (1984). Goals of nutritional support in acute infections. *Am. J. Med.*, **76**, 81.
200. Alexander, J.W. (1986). Nutrition and infection: new perspectives for an old problem. *Arch. Surg.*, **121**, 966.
201. O'Mahony, J.B., McIrvine, A.J., Palder, S., *et al.* (1984). The effect of short term post-operative intravenous feeding upon cell-mediated immunity and serum suppressive activity in well nourished patients. *Surg. Gynecol. Obstet.*, **159**, 27.
202. Christou, N.V., Superina, R., Broadhead, M., *et al.*, (1982). Post-operative depression of host resistance determinants and effects of peripheral protein sparing therapy. *Surgery*, **92**, 786.
203. Sax, H.C., Talamini, M.A., and Fisher, J.E. (1986). Clinical use of branched chain amino acids in liver disease, sepsis, trauma, and burns. *Arch. Surg.*, **121**, 358.
204. Gorshi, A., Korrzak-Kowalslea, G., Nowacyzk, M., *et al.* (1982). Thymosin: An immunomodulator of antibody production in man. *Immunology*, **47**, 497.
205. Hess, M.L. and Manson, N.H. (1983). The paradox of steroid therapy: inhibition of oxygen free radicals. *Circ. Shock*, **10**, 1.
206. Young, L.S., Martin, W.J., Meyer, R.D., *et al.* (1977). 15 Gram-negative rod bacteremia: Microbiologic, immunologic and therapeutic considerations. *Ann. Intern. Med.*, **86**, 456.
207. Jones, R.J., Roe, E.A., and Gupta, J.L. (1980). Controlled trials of pseudomonas immunoglobulin and vaccine in burn patients. *Lancet*, **2**, 1263.

208. Dunn, D.L. and Ferguson, R.M. (1982). Immunotherapy of gram-negative bacterial sepsis: Enhanced survival in a guinea pig model by use of rabbit antiserum to *Escherichia coli* J5. *Surgery*, **92**, 212.
209. Dunn, D.L., Mack, P.A., Candie, R.M., *et al.* (1984). Anti-core endotoxin $F(ab)_2$ horse immunoglobulin fragments protect against the lethal effects of gram-negative bacterial sepsis. *Surgery*, **96**, 440.
210. Gaffin, S.L., Badsha, N., Brock-Utne, J.G., *et al.* (1982). An ELISA procedure for detecting human anti-endotoxin antibodies in serum. *Ann. Clin. Biochem.*, **19**, 191.
211. Peters, L.C., Hanna, M.G., Gutterman, J.V., *et al.* (1974). Modulation of the immune response of guinea pigs by repeated BCG scarification. *Proc. Soc. Exp. Biol. Med.*, **147**, 344.
212. Sugimoto, M., Germain, R.N., Chediel, and Benacerz, B. Enhancement of carrier-specific helper T cell function by the synthetic adjuvant, *N*-acetyl muramyl-L-alanyl-D-isoglutamine (MDP). *J. Immunol.*, **120**, 980.
213. Polk, H.C., Calhoun, J.H., Blanchard, J.P., *et al.* (1981). Nonspecific enhancement of host defenses against infection: Experimental evidence of a new order of efficacy and safety. *Surgery*, **90**, 376.
214. Calhoun, K., Trachtenberg, L., Hart, K., and Polk, H.C. (1979). Corynebacterium parvum: Immunomodulation in local bacterial infections. *Surgery*, **87.**, 52.
215. Nohr. C.W. and Meakins, J.L. (1985). Biological response modifiers. In *Surgical infections in intensive care units* (ed. J.L. Meakins). Churchill Livingstone, London.

5

Wound contamination and post-operative infection

DENNIS RAAHAVE

'Every operation in surgery is an experiment in bacteriology'.
Lord Moynihan, 1920 (1).

Introduction

Post-operative wound infection can be disastrous; it involves suffering for the patient, a risk to other patients, and extra costs because of the need for more operations, blood, antibiotics, nursing, and prolonged hospitalization. Over the last few decades many factors have been identified which contribute to the risk of post-operative wound infection (2–7). Common risk factors are the type and duration of surgery, the age of the patient and the host defence capability, but bacterial contamination of the operative field is probably the most important.

Bacterial contamination

Type of operation

It has become apparent that the risk of post-operative infection is closely related to the type of operation performed (3–4, 7–9). Entry into viscera which contain bacteria always involves a high risk, even with antibiotic prophylaxis. Ever since the National Research Council study of the effects of ultraviolet irradiation on wound infections (2), which showed that ultraviolet light was not protective, wounds have been classified as clean, potentially contaminated, contaminated or dirty, depending on the degree of bacterial contamination (10–14) (see Chapter 1).

Clean wounds

These are uninfected operative wounds in which no inflammation is encountered, and the respiratory, alimentary or genitourinary tracts are not entered.

Potentially contaminated wounds

These are operative wounds in which the respiratory, alimentary or genitourinary tracts are entered under controlled conditions (no significant spillage).

Contaminated wounds

These include operative wounds where acute inflammation (without pus) is encountered, or where there is gross spillage from a hollow viscus.

Dirty wounds

These are operative wounds in the presence of pus or a perforated viscus.

In a study of 62 939 wounds (4) the infection rate of clean wounds was 1.5 per cent, of potentially contaminated wounds 9 per cent, of contaminated wounds 20 per cent and of dirty wounds 43 per cent. These rates have declined during the 1980s, now being 7–8 per cent for potentially contaminated wounds, 11–12 per cent for contaminated and 23–27 per cent for dirty wounds. The clean infection rate still remains between 1–2 per cent (7, 15).

Wound contamination

Contamination of the wound during operation has been difficult to prove, a majority of bacteriology swabs being without growth, both after incision and before closure of the wound (16, 17). Some studies have indicated the presence of wound bacteria, both in clean operations (wound washings) (18) and in contaminated operations, where swabs have been taken from the peritoneal cavity at operation, the rectus sheath and the subcutaneous tissue, have given positive findings on some occasions (19). In a previous study, a culture from the subcutaneous fat after fascial closure was suggested as the best predictor of the organisms likely to be responsible for the post-operative infection (20).

Measuring contamination

Different types of wounds — for example, the open (traumatic) wound, the burn wound, a skin graft bed or the operative incision, represent different problems in sampling for quantitative bacteriological culture. Swabs have been used widely but are inadequate to indicate the true degree of contamination (21–23). While burn and traumatic wounds have been sampled by impression gauze (24) or by homogenized tissue samples (25), these methods have, apparently, not been used for operation wounds. More recent, quantitative sampling of such wounds has also been done by irrigation procedures and membrane filter contact techniques (11, 26, 27). Clearly there was a need for a quantitative method to measure the degree of contamination, and not just the manifest infection.

For more than a decade Raahave *et al.* (15, 28–30) have attempted to determine the numbers of aerobic and anaerobic bacteria responsible for intra-operative wound contamination. The ultimate aim of these studies was to correlate the degree of wound contamination with the wound classification (clinical category), and with the subsequent occurence of post-operative wound infection. First, therefore, the use of velvet pads (Fig. 5.1) was evaluated in an experimental laboratory model, simulating intra-operative sampling of *Staphylococcus epidermidis, Escherichia coli*, and *Bacteroides fragilis* (29, 31, 32), since these organisms are important pathogens in post-operative wound infections. This, so-called velvet pad rinse technique, yielded quantitatively high recoveries of the test bacteria (Fig. 5.2). The method has been further tested and validated by others (27, 33).

Second, four types of wounds were sampled during operation: the clean wound, the potentially contaminated wound,

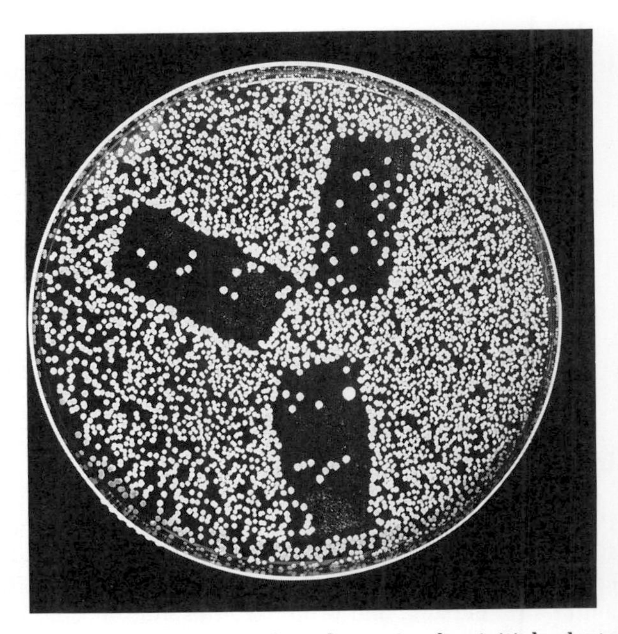

Fig. 5.2. Residual colonies of test bacteria after initial velvet pad sampling and subsequent incubation.

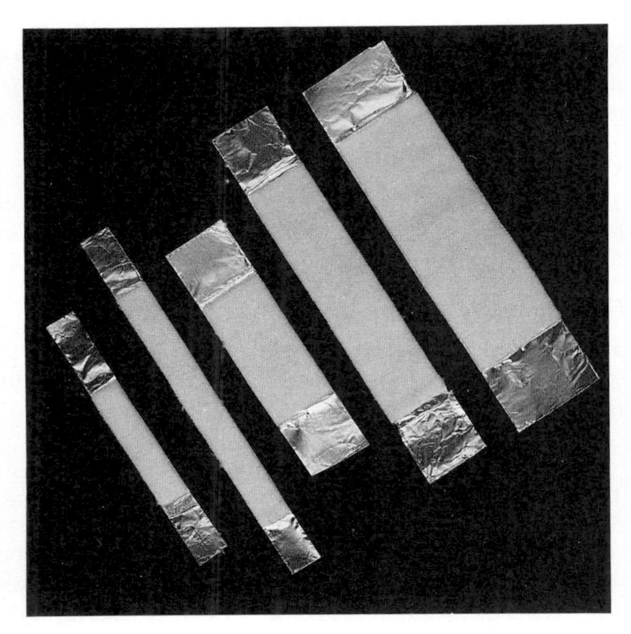

Fig. 5.1. Different sizes of sterile velvet pads, suitable for wound sampling.

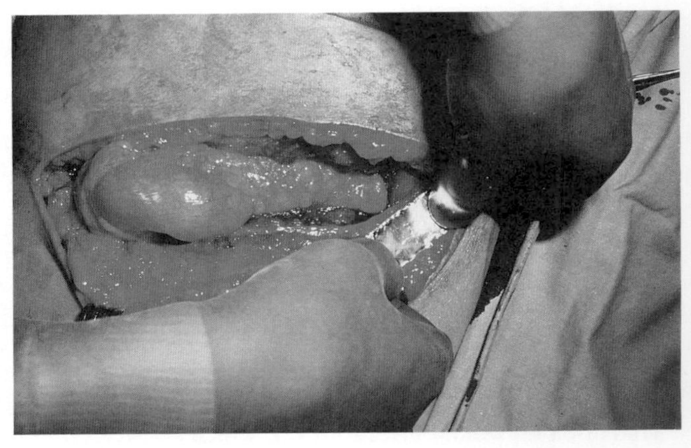

Fig. 5.3. Velvet pad sampling of bacteria before closure of contaminated operated wound. (See plate section.)

Plate Section

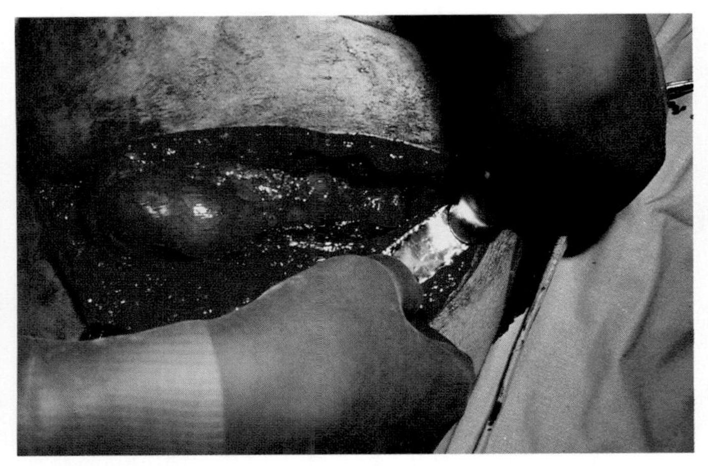

Fig. 5.3. Velvet pad sampling of bacteria before closure of contaminated operated wound.

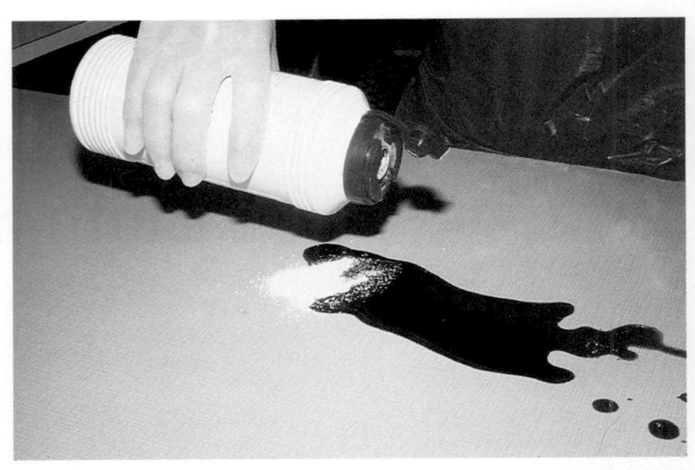

Fig. 6.2. Using chlorine-releasing powders or granules (NaDCC) to remove small blood spillages.

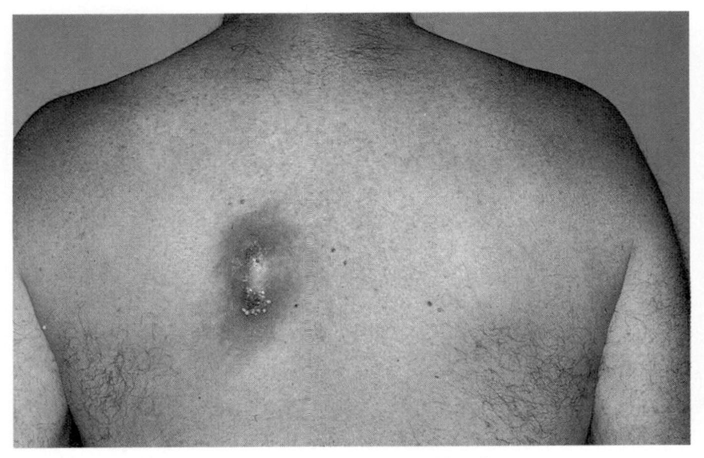

Fig. 15.1. An infected sebaceous cyst of back.

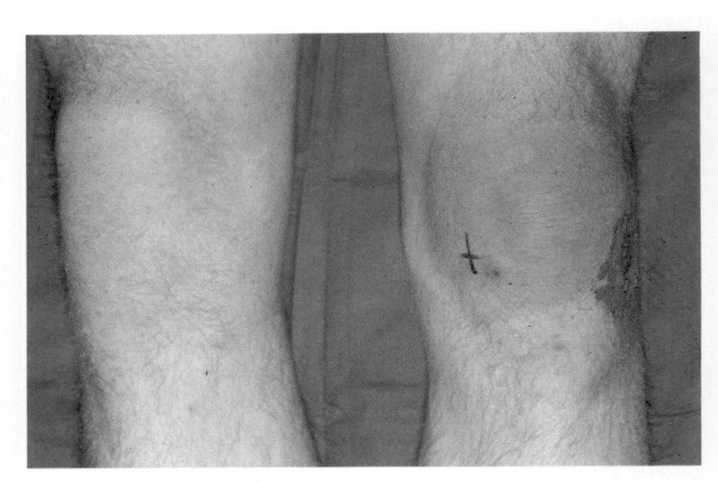

Fig. 15.2. An infected pre-patellar bursa.

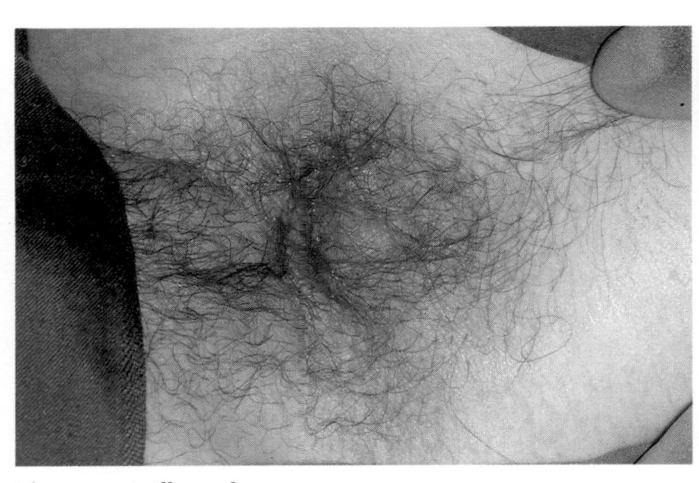

Fig. 15.3. Axillary abscess.

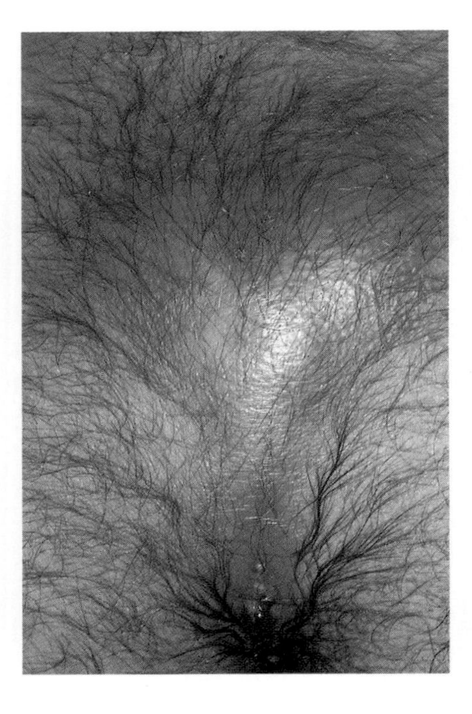

Fig. 15.4. Pilonidal abscess of natal cleft.

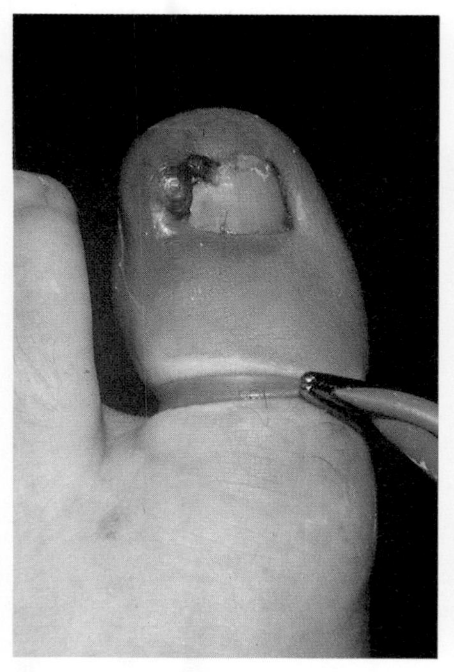

Fig. 15.5. Infected ingrowing toe nail.

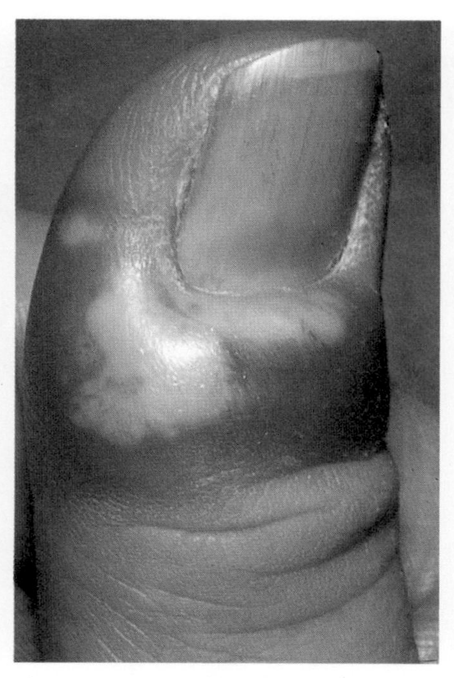

Fig. 15.6. Paronychia of the thumb.

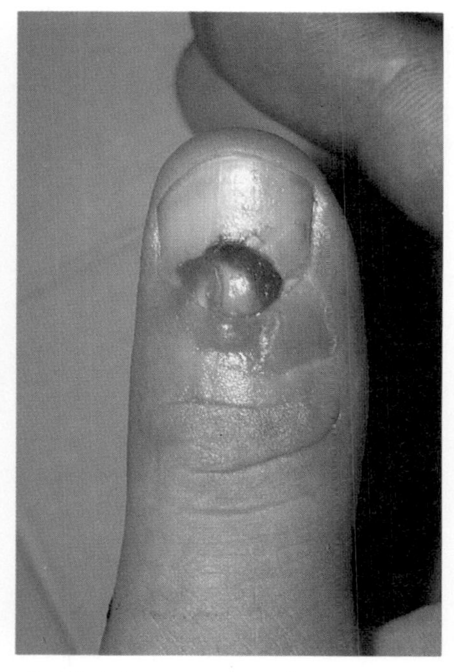

Fig. 15.7. Pyogenic granuloma.

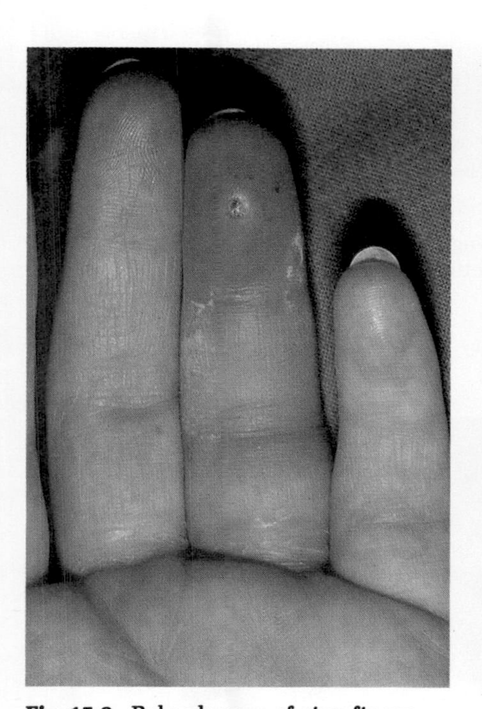

Fig. 15.8. Pulp abscess of ring finger.

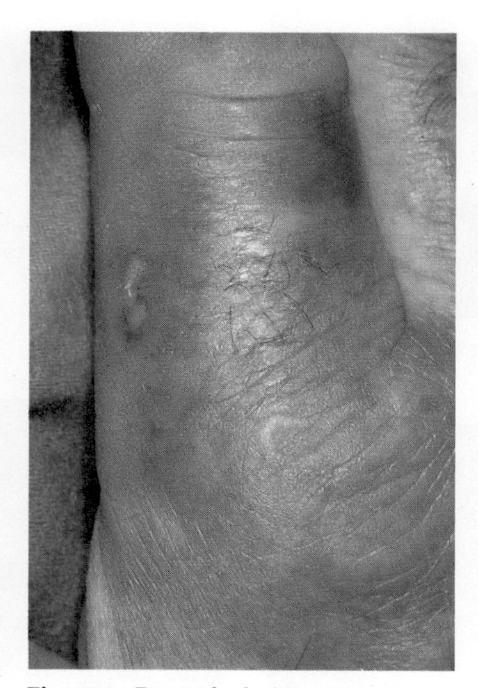

Fig. 15.9. Einsipaloid of Rosenbach.

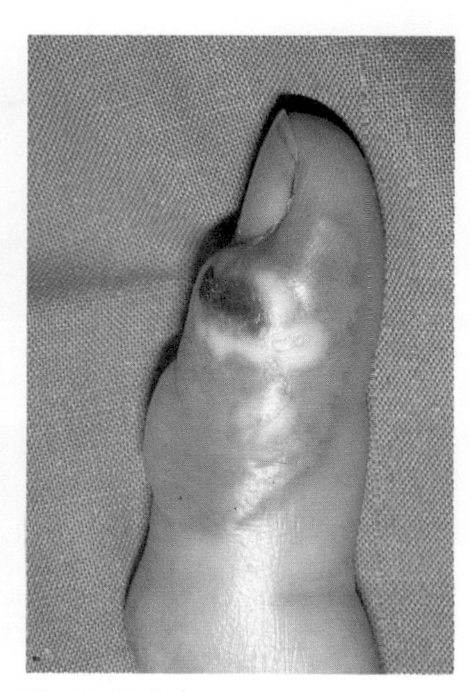

Fig. 15.10. Orf.

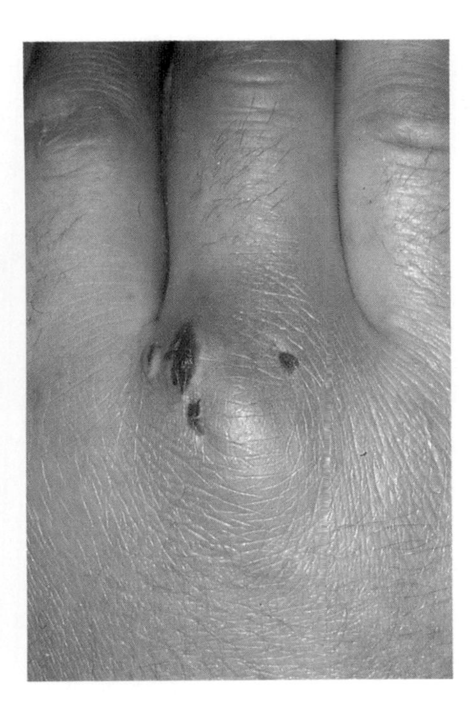

Fig. 15.11. Teeth marks over MCP joint.

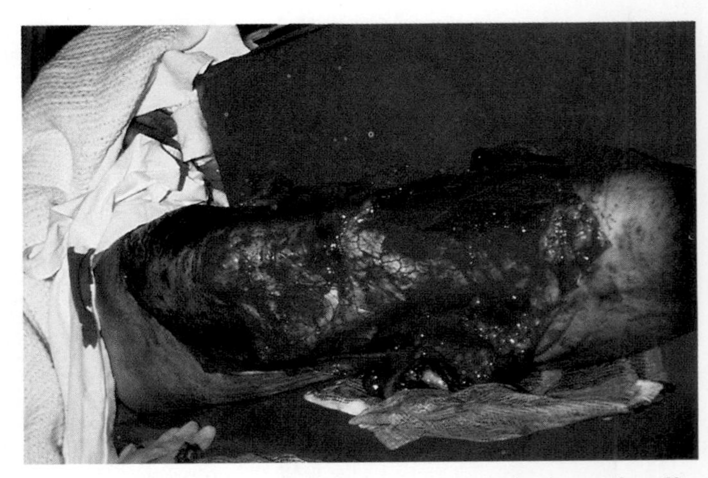

Fig. 16.1. An open fracture of the leg as a result of a road traffic accident.

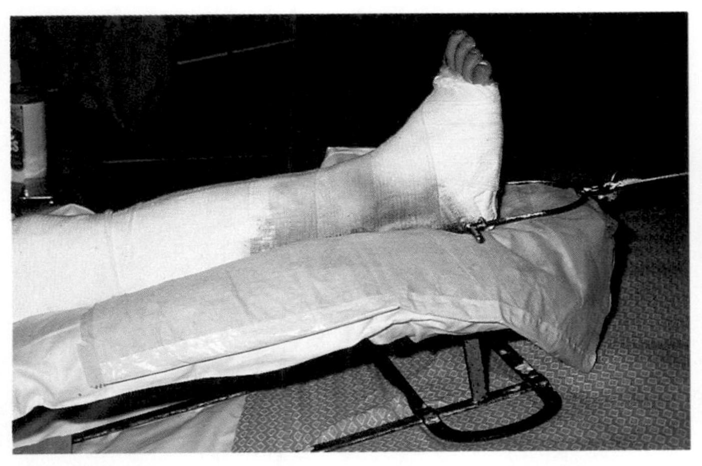

Fig. 16.2. Traction and plaster for a distal open tibial fracture.

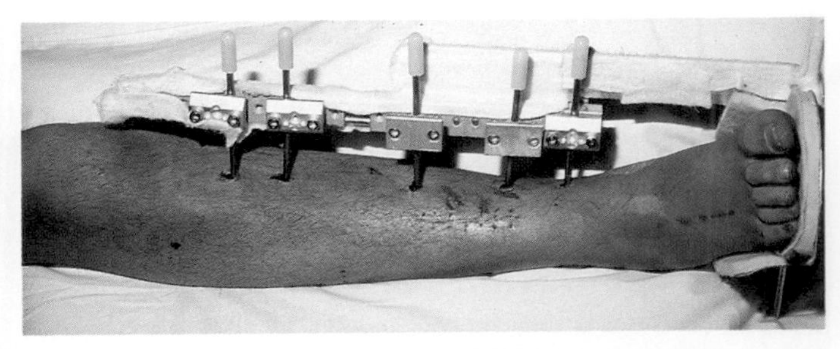

Fig. 16.3. Sukhtian–Hughes external fixation, single bar system, for an open tibial fracture.

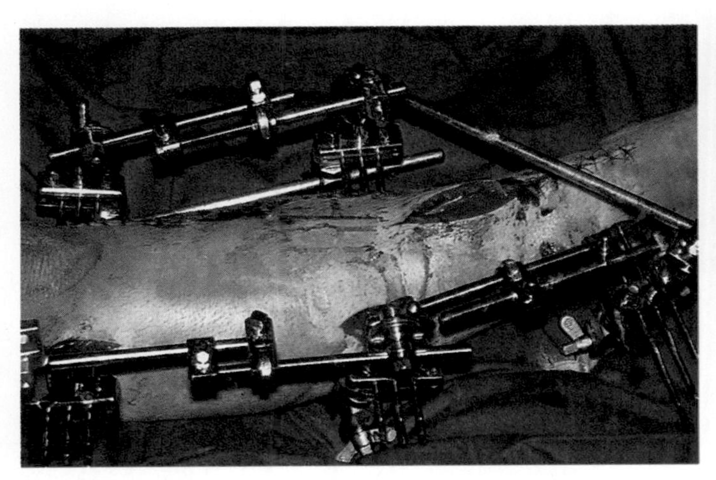

Fig. 16.4. Hoffman external frame for an open tibial fracture.

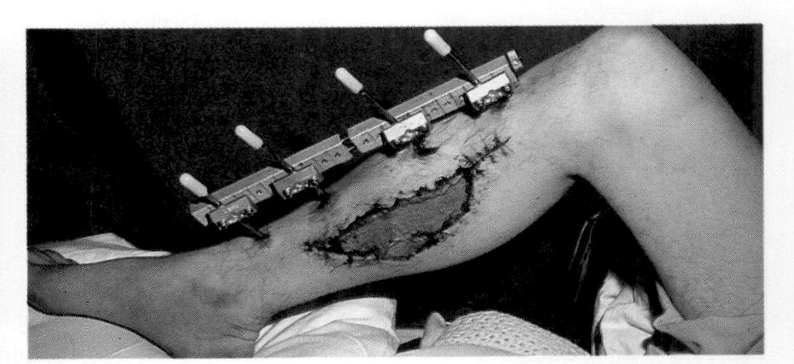

Fig. 16.5. Split skin graft for an open fracture. There is a Sukhtian–Hughes external fixation system in place.

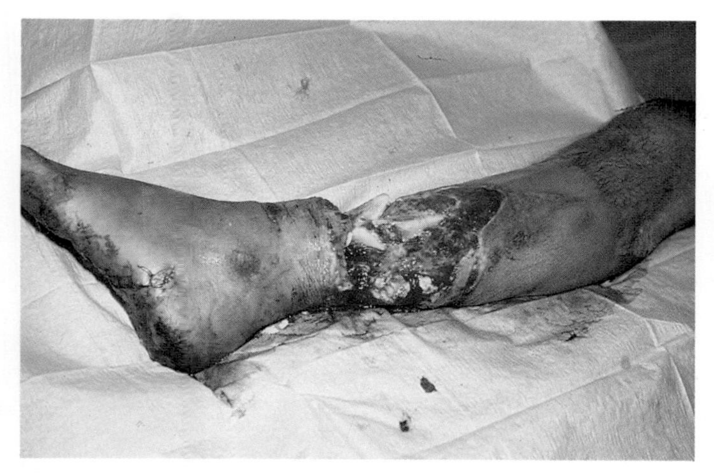

Fig. 16.6. Infected non-union of the tibia.

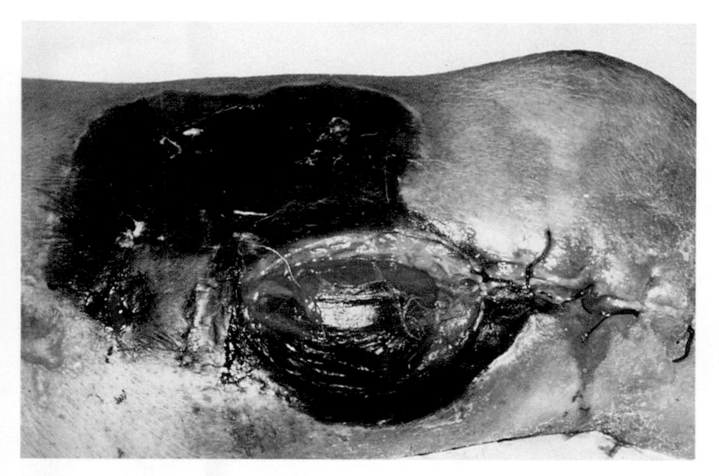

Fig. 18.1. Gas gangrene of the leg demonstrating blanched oedematous skin, purple discoloration, haemorrhagic bullae, frank necrosis, and an extending margin of erythema. Tight skin sutures and brown watery discharge are also shown.

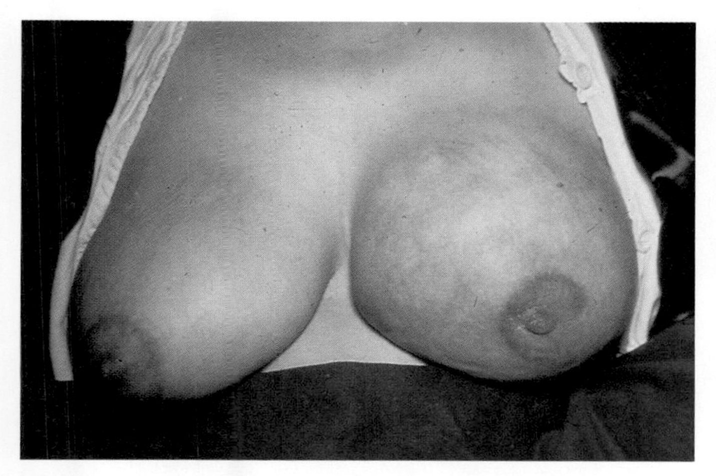

Fig. 22.2. Puerperal mastitis of the left breast. Note the erythema and oedema and obvious signs of inflammation in the left breast, particularly medially.

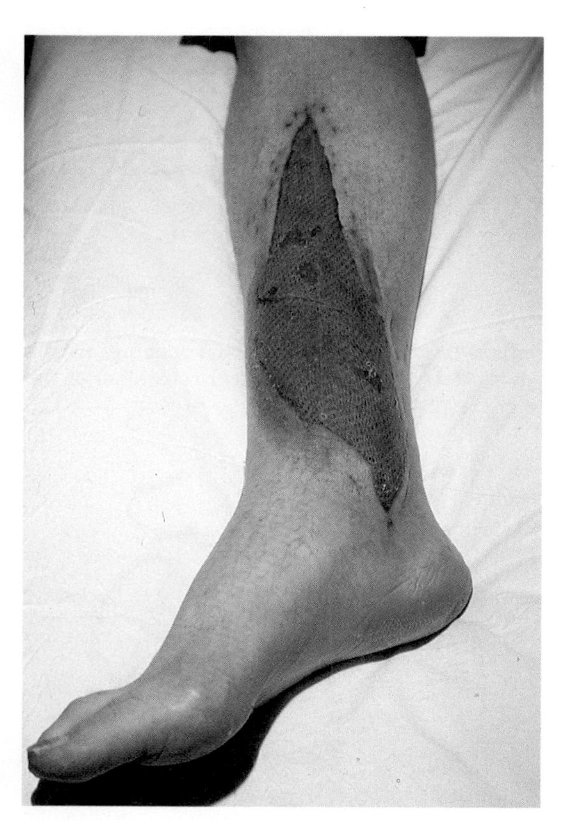

Fig. 16.7. A myocutaneous flap for a distal tibial fracture.

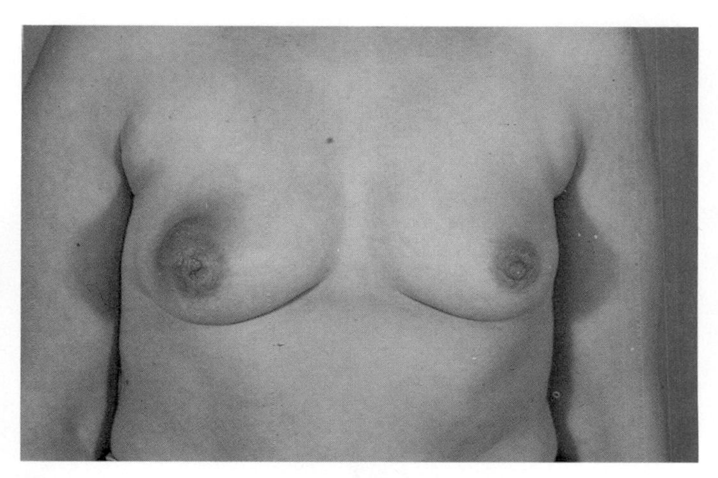

Fig. 22.4. Periareolar abscess of the right breast associated with periductal mastitis. The right nipple is retracted towards the site of infection and an obvious abscess is evident pointing at the areolar margin.

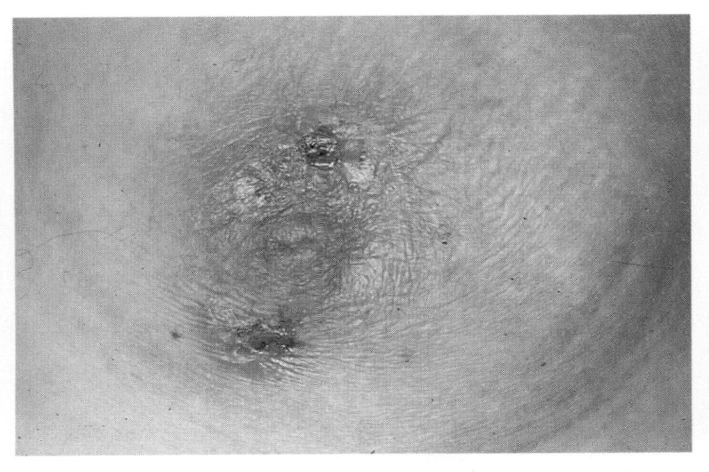

Fig. 22.6. Mammillary fistula with two external openings from a single diseased duct. Note the slit-like central retraction of the nipple at the site of the diseased duct.

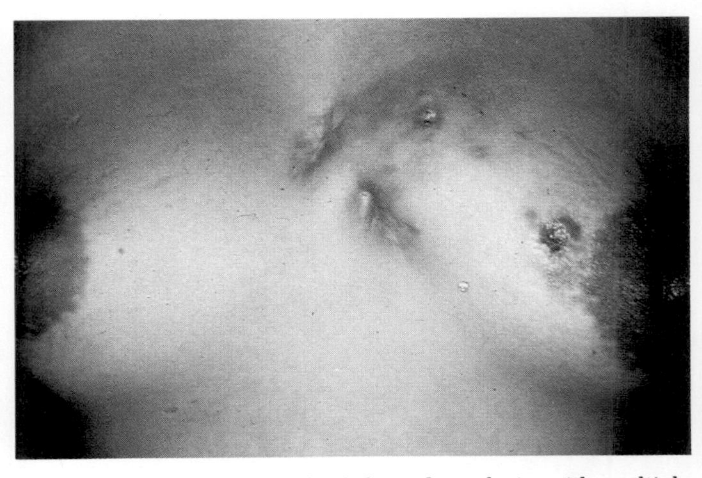

Fig. 22.8. Left breast involved by tuberculosis with multiple sinuses.

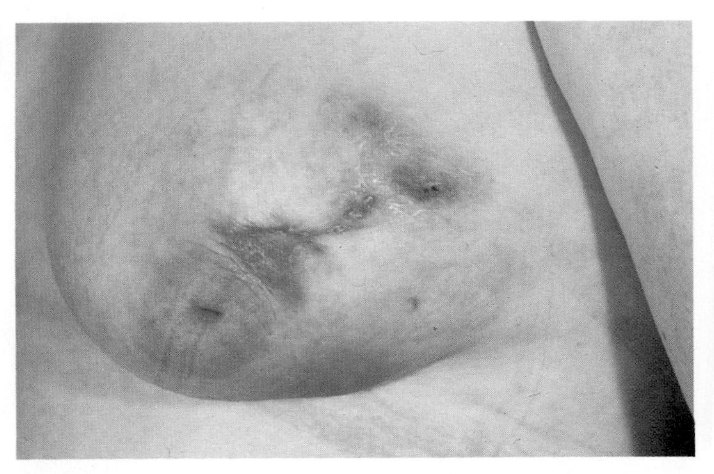

Fig. 22.9. Left breast affected by granulomatous lobular mastitis with evidence of multiple scars, sinuses and nipple retraction.

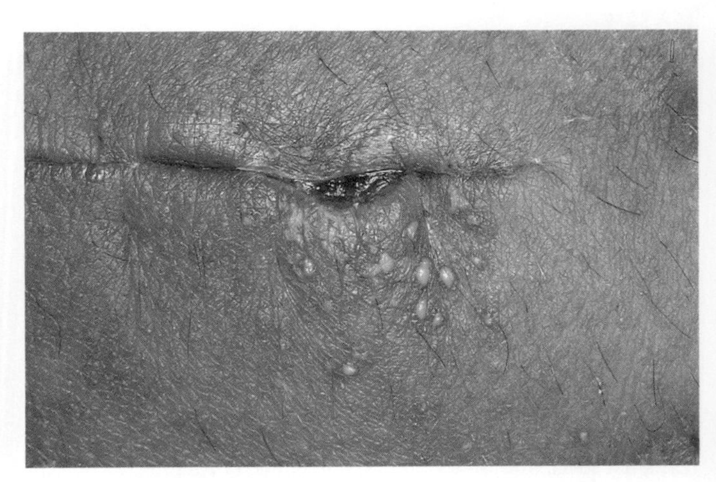

Fig. 23.1. Superficial skin infection.

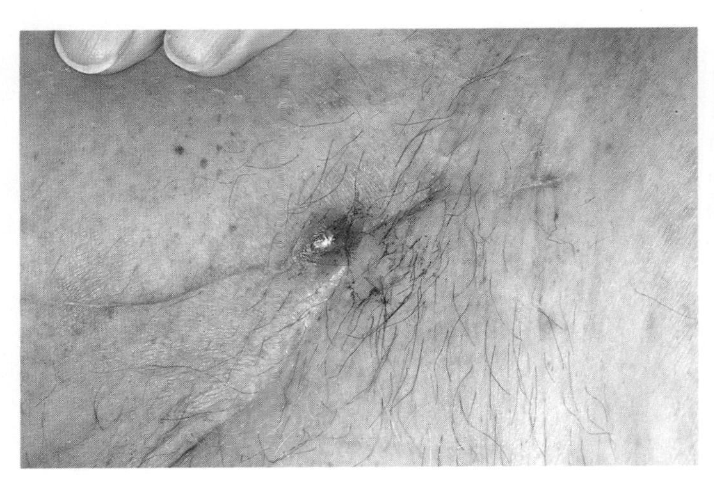

Fig. 23.2. Infection of subcutaneous tissues.

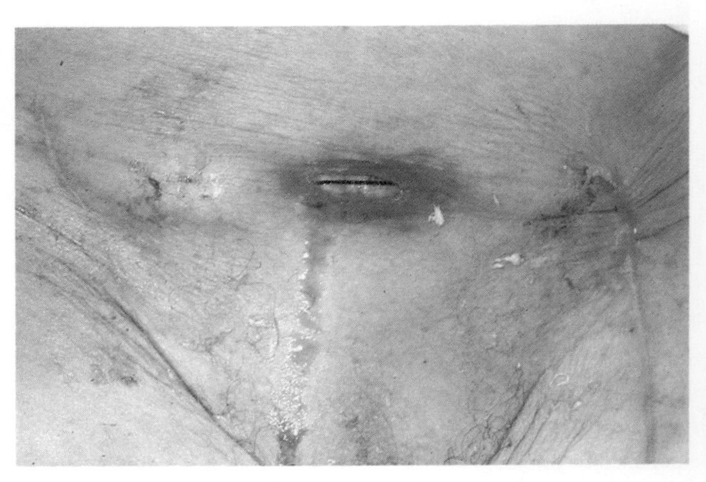

Fig. 23.3. Graft exposed in the wound.

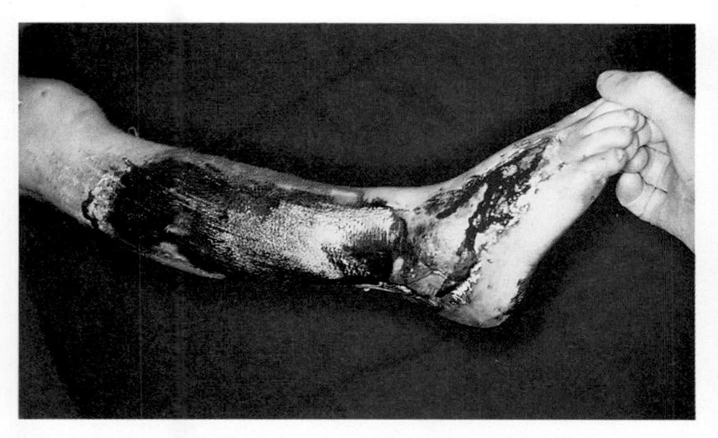

Fig. 25.1. Result following incorrect treatment by primary suture of an extensive degloving injury. The devitalized flap has necrosed and become infected.

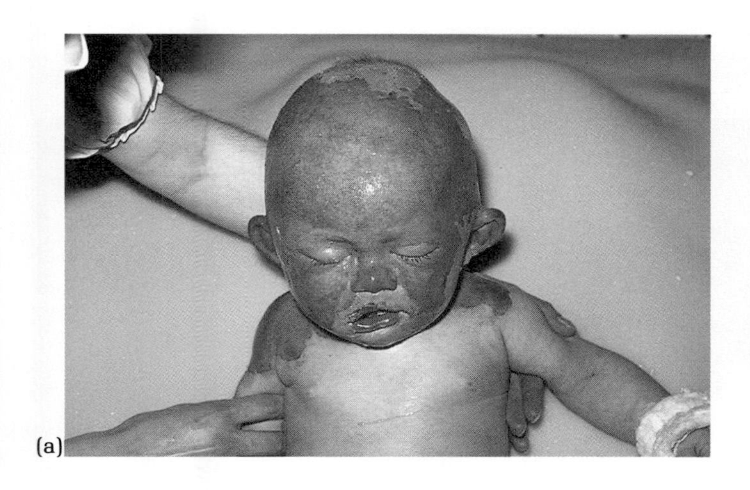

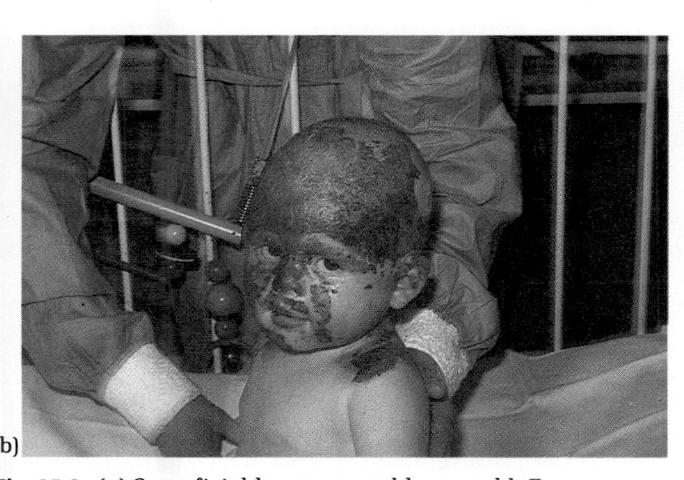

Fig. 25.2. (a) Superficial burns caused by a scald. Exposure treatment is ideal for burns of the face; (b) Result eight days later. The scabs separated easily after a bath.

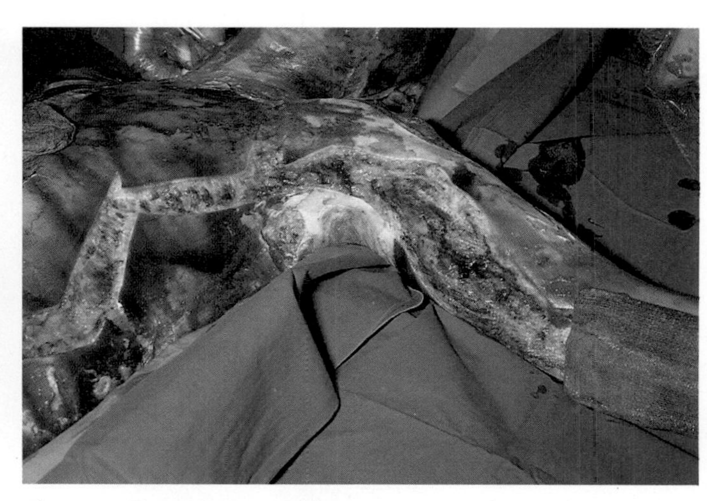

Fig. 25.3. Escarotomy used for emergency release of constricting escar in a circumferential flame burn of trunk and arm. Incision down to viable tissue increases the risk of infection and a Flamazine gauze dressing has been used.

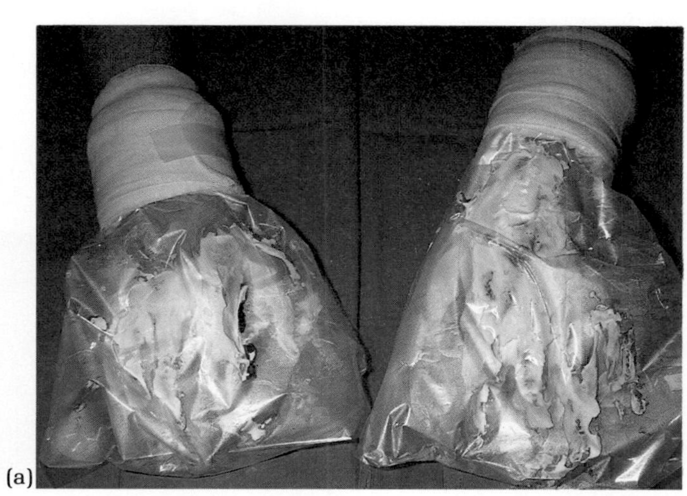

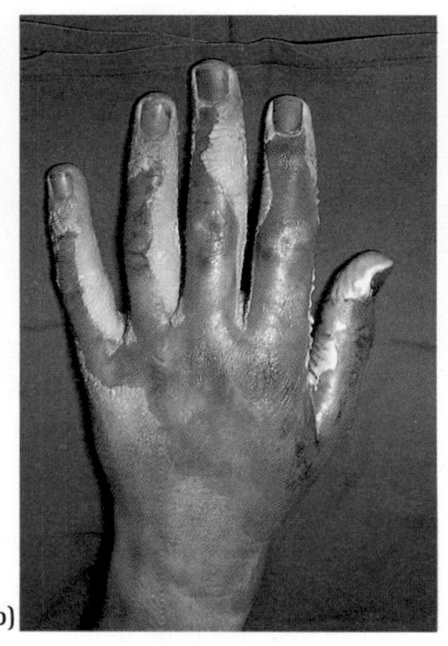

Fig. 25.4. (a) Polythene bags used for bilateral hand burns. The burn is smeared with Flamazine cream and the bag is changed daily; (b) Left hand completely healed at eight days.

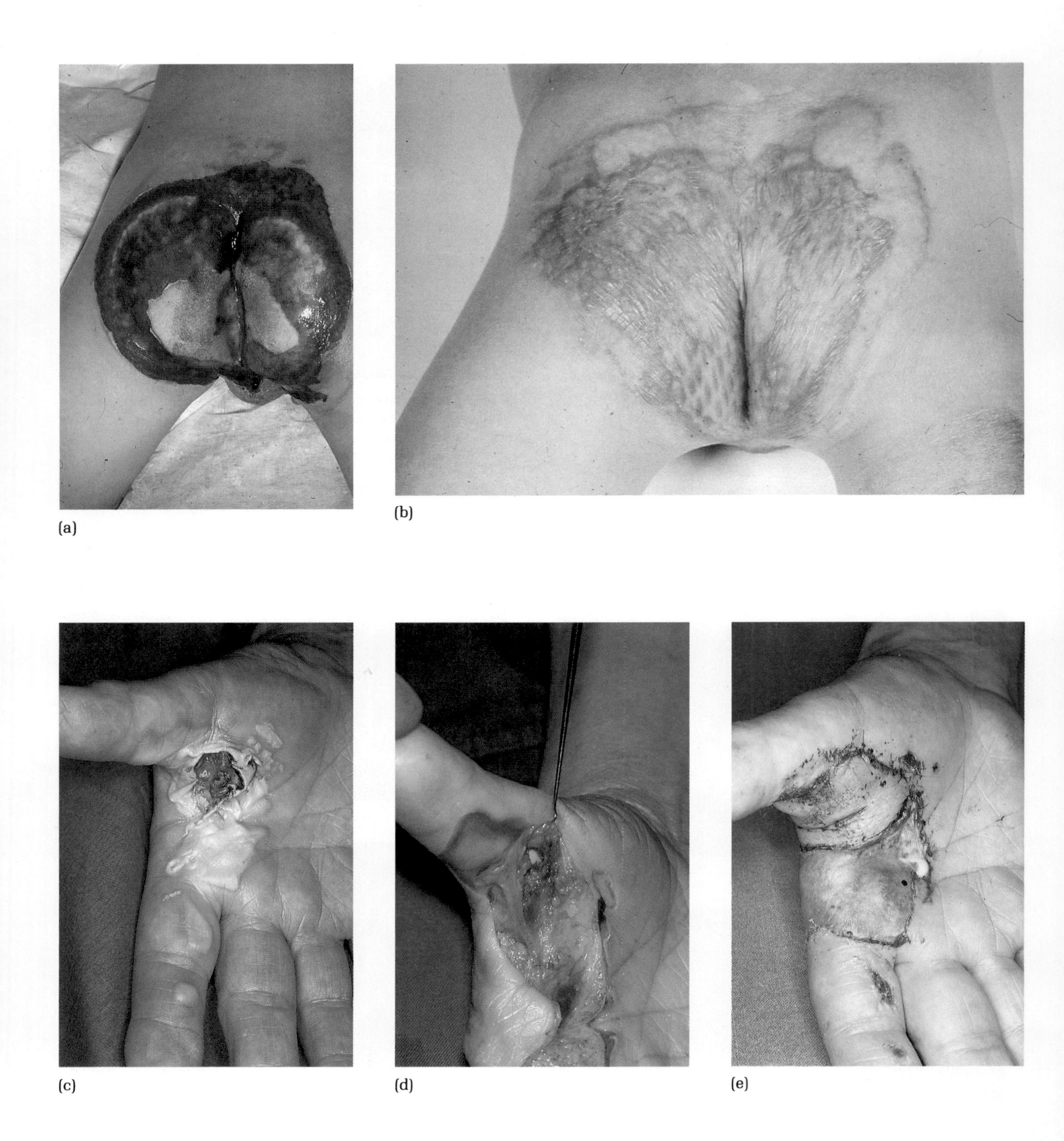

(a) (b) (c) (d) (e)

Fig. 25.5. Early excision of burns: (a) Deep burn of perineum treated by exposure for 48 h followed by excision and grafting. Mesh grafts were used to encourage take in a potentially contaminated area. Rapid healing took place; (b) Result at three months; (c) Deep electrical burn of the thumb; (d) Early excision and flap repair is essential to prevent infection. The metacarpo-phalangeal joint has been opened; (e) Local flap repair to the area of exposed joint and tendon, split skin graft to the area with a good vascular bed. The healed wound one week later.

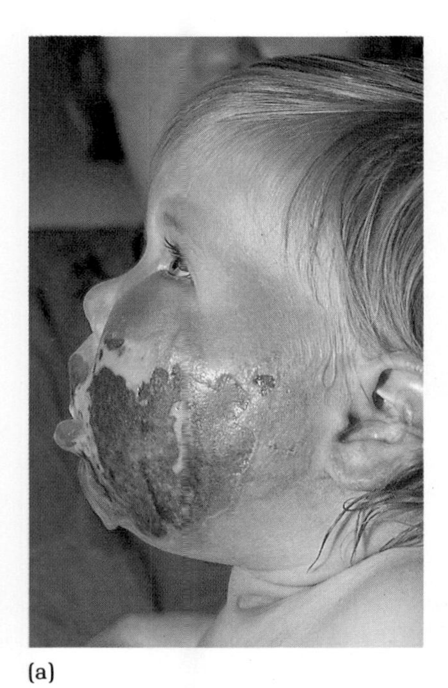

(a)

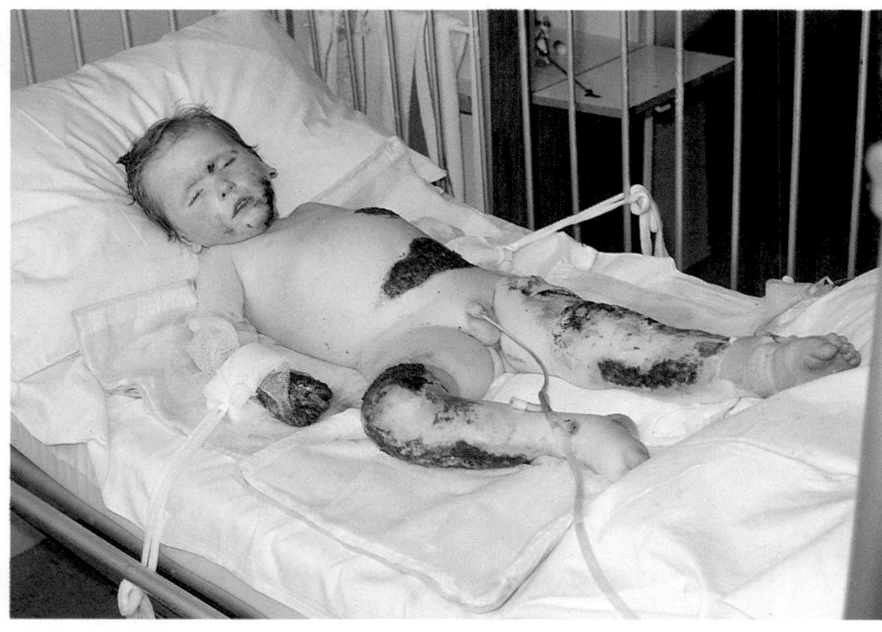

(c)

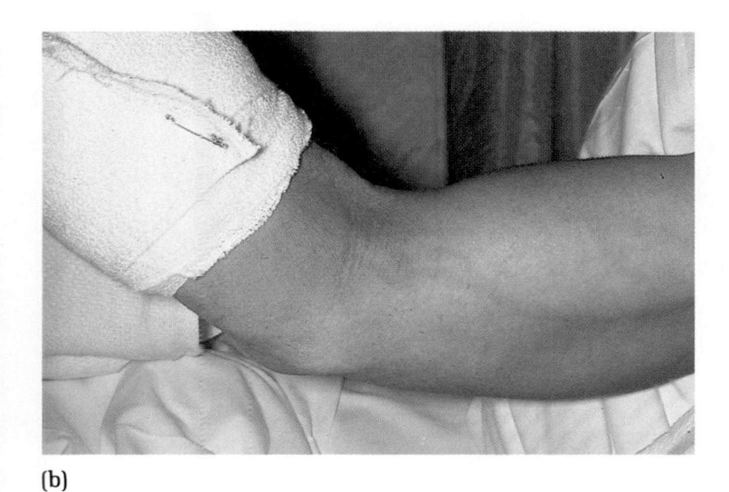

(b)

Fig. 25.6. Infected burns: (a) *Streptococcus pyogenes* infection in a 4-day-old contact burn. Note the surrounding erythema and the weeping exudate; (b) Erythema beyond the edge of this dressed burn and lymphangitis is diagnostic of infection; (c) Severe systemic infection in a child with flame burns. Blood culture grew *Pseudomonas aeruginosa*—as suggested by the green discoloration on the burn. The right hip is flexed and abducted and a joint aspirate grew *Staph. aureus*.

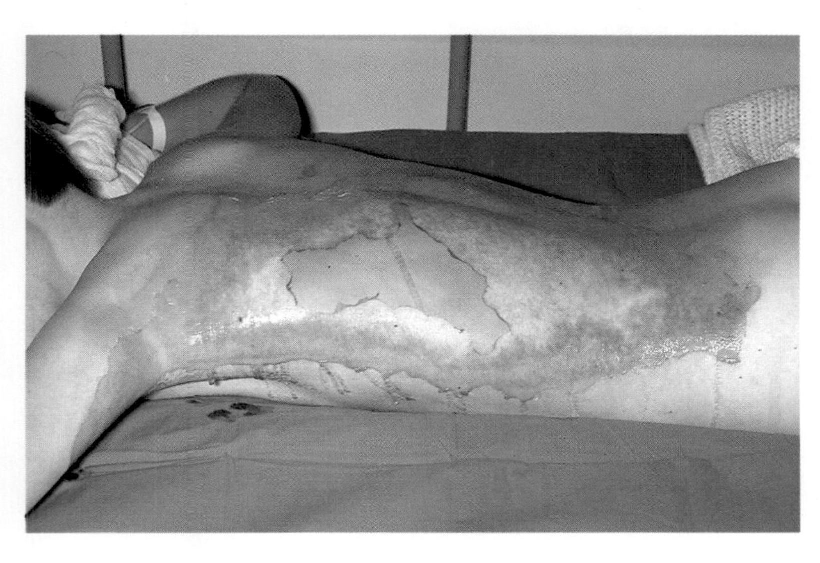

Fig. 25.7. The erythema at the edge of this flame burn signifies a superficial burn at the edge of a deeper burn, not infection.

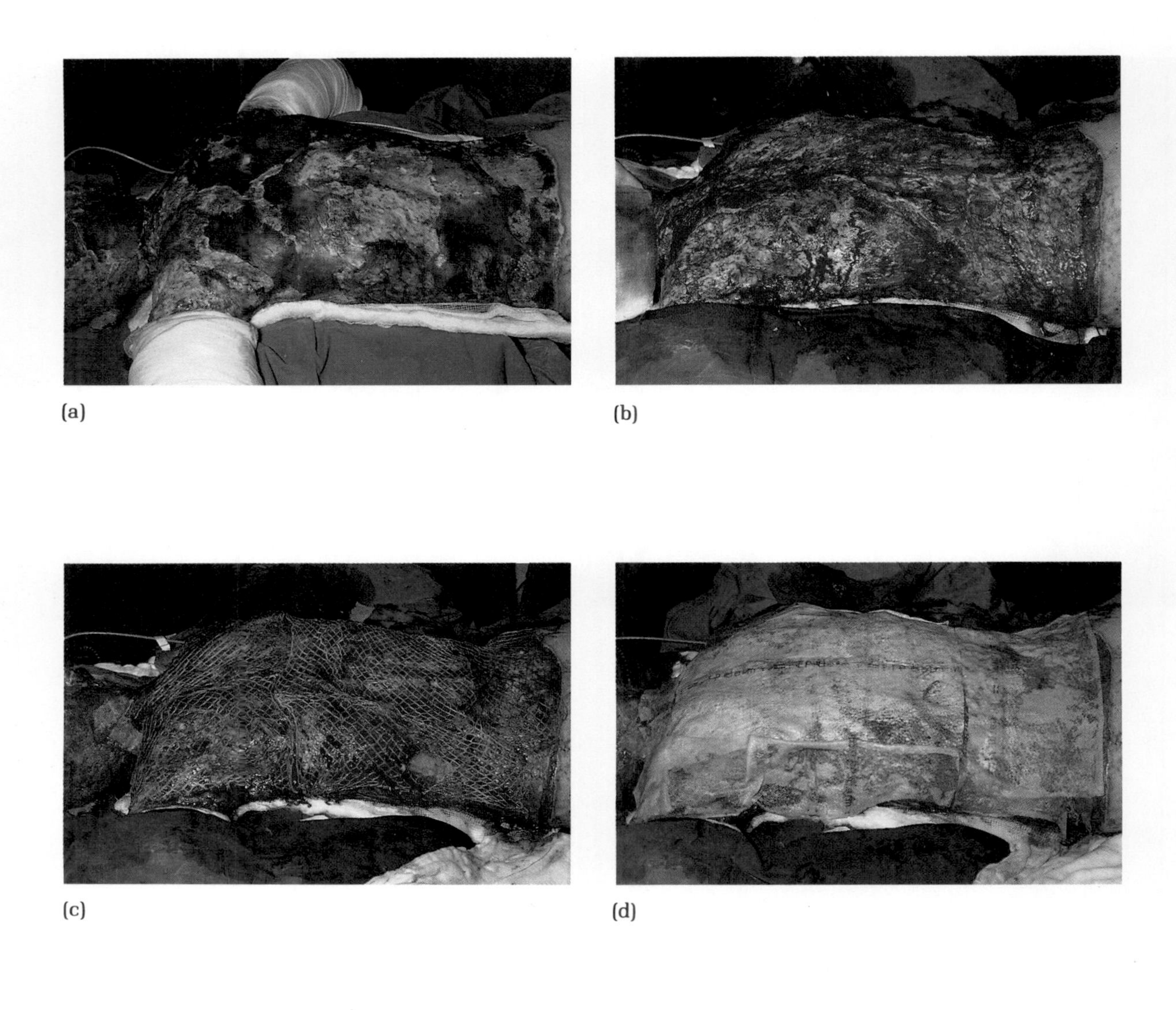

(a) (b) (c) (d)

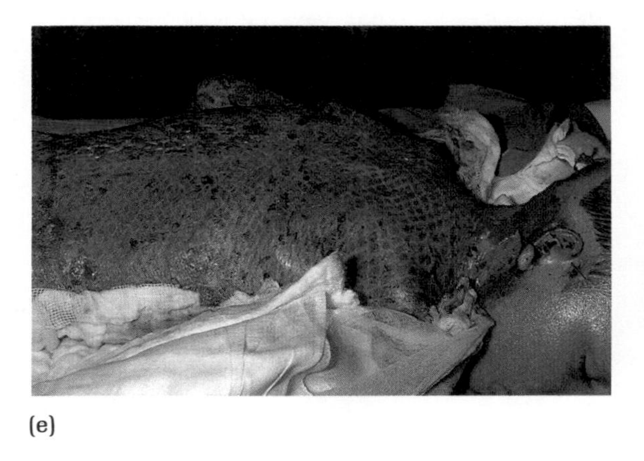

(e)

Fig. 25.8. Excision and grafting of a 60 per cent flame burn: (a) The slough on the back is still present two weeks after injury. The patient has been lying on a bed of Flamazine on a convential dressing while the burn of the front was excised and grafted; (b) There is no infection present but systemic antibiotic is essential during surgical debridement as a bacteraemia is inevitable; (c) Expanded mesh grafts are applied to the burn; (d) A layer of lyophilized pig skin is applied under the dressing to prevent dessication of the bed while the mesh heals; (e) Good take of the grafts three weeks later despite the patient having to lie on them for part of the time.

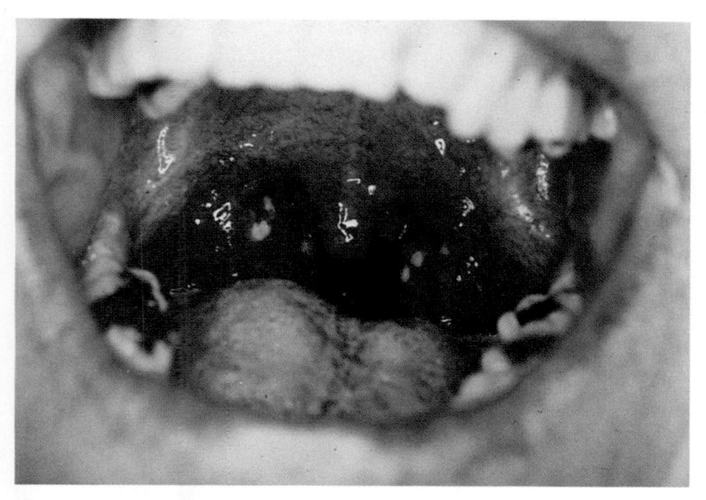

Fig. 27.6. Acute follicular tonsillitis.

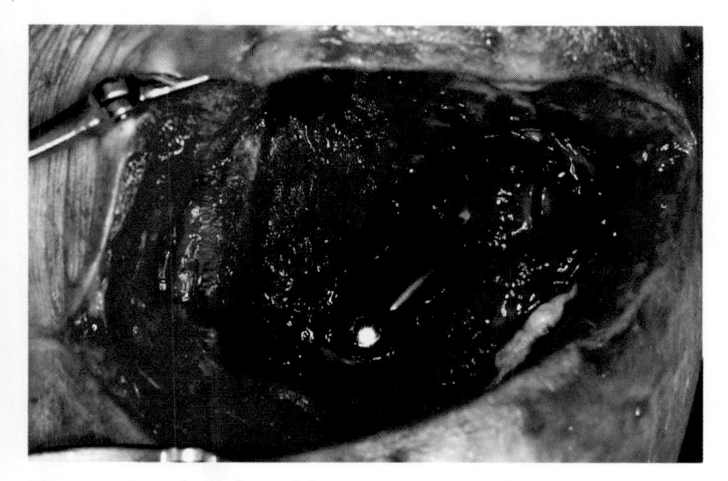

Fig. 30.2 In infected total hip replacement showing pus at the operation site.

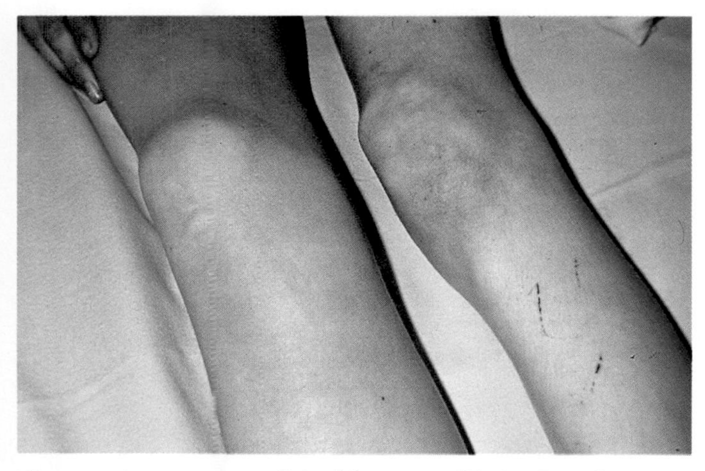

Fig. 30.5 Acute osteomyelitis of the upper tibia in a boy of 10 years of age.

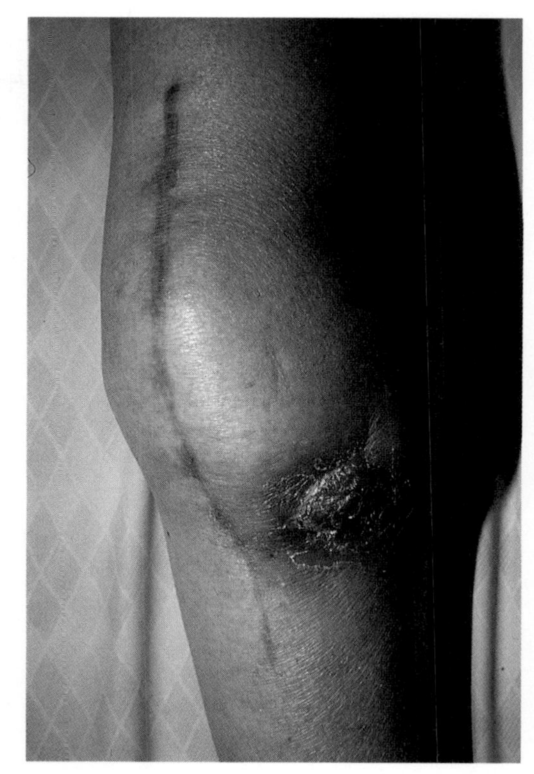

Fig. 30.1 An infected total knee replacement.

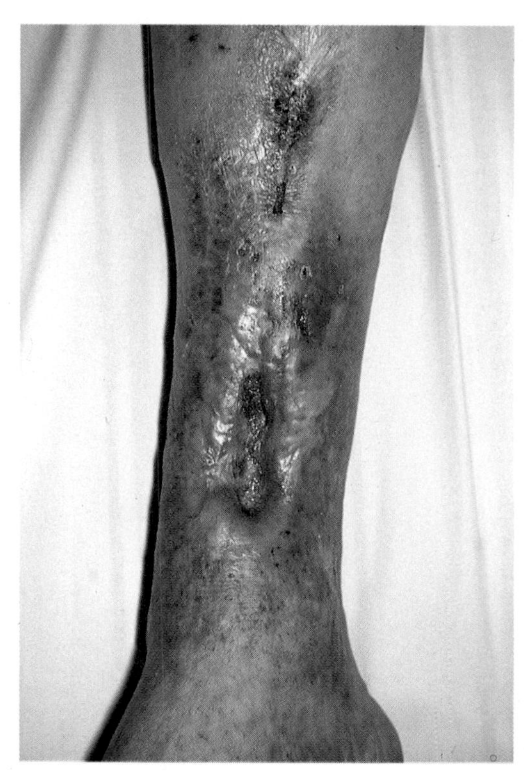

Fig. 30.7 Chronic osteomyelitis of the tibia.

the contaminated wound and the dirty wound, by use of pads of cotton velveteen, backed by aluminium foil, extending at both ends so that the pads could be handled without touching the velvet surface. All samples were taken under aseptic conditions (Fig. 5.3). After sampling, each velvet pad was placed in a sterile Erlenmeyer flask with sterile saline or peptone water. The flasks were flushed with carbon dioxide and sealed, and transported to the laboratory. In the laboratory, the flask with its contents was agitated in a shaker for 10 min. Blood agar plates and lactose bromethymol blue plates were inoculated aerobically and anaerobically with aliquots from wound samples, using an aerobic cabinet. Further identification was by morphology, Gram's stain, fermentation and biochemical tests. After incubation the number of colony-forming units (cfu) were counted and estimated for each sample.

Contamination level

A few investigators have attempted to estimate the level of contamination of operation wounds. Using a wound irrigation technique, Bartlett *et al.* found an average of 10^{2-3} anaerobic and aerobic bacteria per millilitre (11), while Scheibel *et al.* reported a range of zero to 10^5 cfu per millilitre (34).

The author's studies demonstrated, for the first time, a fully quantitative measure of aerobic and anaerobic bacterial contamination in surgical procedures covering the spectrum from clean to dirty operations (15, 30, 35–37). The degree of contamination was expressed as the density of bacteria in the wound, i.e. colony forming units per unit area (cfu/cm^{-2}).

The level of aerobic and anaerobic contamination (upper confidence limit 95 per cent) was for clean wounds 2.2 cfu/cm^{-2}, for potentially contaminated wounds 2.4×10^1 cfu/cm^{-2}, for contaminated wounds 1.1×10^3 cfu/cm^{-2}, and for dirty wounds 3.7×10^3 cfu/cm^{-2}.

These studies (15) also demonstrated that the bacterial density during operation could be correlated with the clinical category of the operative wounds, i.e. clean, potentially contaminated, contaminated or dirty. This implies that classifying wounds by degree of clinically judged contamination rests on a sound quantitative bacteriological basis, and confirms the criteria used for the wound categories.

The frequencies of isolation of aerobic and anaerobic species from wounds showed that aerobic Gram-positive cocci, anaerobic peptococcus species and pepto-streptococcus species and propionebacterium species, were isolated with the same frequency from all wounds irrespective of category. *E. coli*, other Gram-negative bacilli and *Bacteroides* species were isolated with significantly increasing frequencies in potentially contaminated, contaminated and dirty wounds. Following these investigations, others have used the pad method for wound sampling, most often semiquantitatively (38–40).

Although the bacterial densities measured only mirror, and this imperfectly, the contamination at the given stage of operation, it may be inferred that operation wounds harbour both aerobic and anaerobic commensals after incision, the so-called 'background' contamination present in conventional operating theatres. However, when bacteria-containing viscera are opened or inflammatory processes are already present, the wound is also challenged by this new flora.

Post-operative wound infection

An infected wound is usually defined as a wound with a collection of pus that empties spontaneously or after incision (41) (see Chapter 9). In 85 per cent of cases this happens within the first 14 days post-operatively (7), although late wound infections can occur up to 30 years after surgery (42). Infection is the ultimate result of a process, which starts immediately after wounding (incision). Here, bacteria from various sources contaminate the surgical wound, which is frequently an entrance to one of the body cavities.

Infective dose of bacteria

In clean operations, wound infections are ten times more common if bacterial cultures are positive (operation wound washings) than if they are negative (18). In colorectal surgery, when swabs were taken at operation from the peritoneal cavity, rectus sheath, and subcutaneous tissue, giving positive findings on some occasions, a close correlation was found between tissue contamination and the incidence of wound infection (19).

A few investigators have sought to determine the number of bacteria necessary to create a clinical wound infection (with pus). Robson found a value of 10^5 bacteria per gram of tissue was the critical count for successful reclosure of surgical wounds without sepsis (25). In experimental studies, it required 10^6 cocci to produce pus in volunteers (43), but as few as 15 organisms have been shown to be sufficient to cause septic lesions (44). The author has shown that the bacterial density in a wound showed a high correlation with the wound category (15), and also that there was a significant rise in the median values of intra-operative bacterial densities for wounds which later developed infection (30).

A few studies have tried to determine a threshold for infection of the operative wound (34, 45). Earlier, Bartlett *et al.* (11) irrigated surgical wounds with Ringer's lactate solution at the time of closure. They obtained wound irrigation specimens and determined which bacteria were present. However, they were unable to predict subsequent wound infection on this basis. More recently, however, the author (15, 30) has demonstrated a high correlation between the density of aerobic and anaerobic bacteria during surgery, and post-operative wound infection. The exponential curve found presenting as a dose–response curve (Fig. 5.4), appears to represent a true biological relationship between the densities of wound bacterial contamination and the occurrence of wound infection. This confirms the original experimental work by Morris *et al.* (46), using a guinea-pig skin-bacterial injection model.

In the author's human 'experimental' model the *median* infective dose of aerobic and anaerobic bacteria together was found to be 4.6×10^5 cfu $\times$ cm^{-2} wound (30). This model also allows a reliable prediction of wound infection on the basis of contamination during operation, not merely the identification of patients at risk on the basis of parietal swab cultures (47).

In recent studies by Pollock *et al.* (47) and Raahave *et al.* (15, 30), culture of purulent discharge from patients with wound infection showed the same species patterns of aerobic and

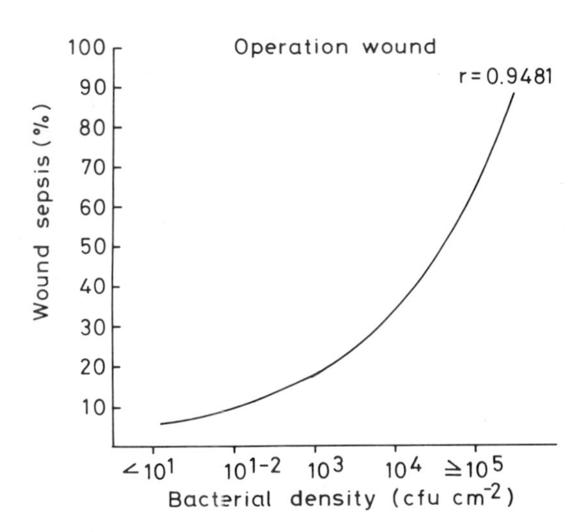

Fig. 5.4. Correlation between pre-closure bacterial densities (aerobic and anaerobic) in operation wound and post-surgical wound infection

anaerobic bacteria as for those organisms isolated during operation. This was earlier not the case, probably because of inadequate sampling methods.

It is widely recognized today that both aerobic and anaerobic organisms are implicated in many wound infections (11, 30, 47, 48). Although there has been a dramatic decline in the incidence of post-operative wound infection after contaminated operations, where there has been proper administration of antibiotics (12–14), *E. coli* and *Bacteroides fragilis* are still the dominating micro-organisms isolated (15, 30, 47). This is consistent with the animal studies by Onderdonk *et al.* (49) and by Kelly (50), who confirmed that both organisms contribute equally and synergistically to abscess formation. In these models, however, *E. coli* predominates in the first stage of infection, while *B. fragilis* seems to be the important pathogen in the abscess formation (51). The finding of *E. coli* and *B. fragilis* with the same high frequency on the appendix, in the peritoneal exudate and in the wound points to the inflamed viscera as the original source (30).

In addition, the route of wound contaminants could be lymphatic- or blood-borne (52–54). Although wound sampling was not done, it has been shown clearly that there is a good correlation between air contamination and the post-operative infection rate (55).

Non-bacterial factors

As has been shown, post-operative wound infections are initiated primarily during operation as a result of the presence of bacteria, the patient being the main source of this (endogenous) contamination. However, sites of low, or even zero, bacterial density were close to sites with a high density in the operation wound, (36). The infective dose was also significantly different for each wound category—clean, potentially contaminated, and dirty wounds. This seems to show that factors other than the degree of the bacterial contamination influence the outcome (15).

The dose–response relationship demonstrated (Fig. 5.4) also points to infection as being a quantitative expression of the relationship between the bacteria and local and systemic host defences. The presence of bacteria at wound closure interferes with the chronological sequence of inflammation, fibroplasia, and connective tissue formation in the healing wound (56). Polymorphonuclear neutrophils are attracted to the area of complement activation, migrate through the capillary walls, are activated, and engulf opsonized bacteria into phagosomes, killing them both by an oxygen-dependent mechanism and by anaerobic processes. Superoxide, hydrogen peroxide and hydroxyl ions are generated from molecular oxygen and are microbicidal. Thus, elimination of bacteria from experimental wounds is impared under hypoxic conditions (57). Wound hypoxia has been demonstrated by tissue oximetry to be fairly common in post-operative patients (58, 59), also as a result of tissue hypoperfusion (60). Very recently, low tissue oxygen tensions within the first 24 h post-operatively predicted death after intestinal emergency operations (61).

In brief, phagocytosis of contaminating and invading bacteria triggers a series of metabolic changes that result in a 15 to 20 fold increase in oxygen consumption over basal rates (62). A serious side-effect is the damage to wound tissues by oxygen-free radicals. Once all the bacteria have been dealt with, the process of inflammation and repair will continue. From this it would seem obvious that non-traumatizing surgery is desirable, to avoid creating necrotic tissue and to reduce the likelihood of a haematoma in the wound. A haematoma or necrotic tissue will act as a culture medium, enhancing bacterial infection, inhibiting phagocytosis and producing an anaerobic environment (63).

The presence of a silk suture was earlier shown to decrease dramatically the number of staphylococci necessary to form a pustule in human volunteers (43). Nowadays, biomaterials are used widely within different fields of surgery, and have the common feature that a much smaller inoculum is needed to create an infection (64).

Surgical expertise

To the clinical surgeon, operating is a technical skill acquired during training and developed by experience: most surgeons recognize that technical difficulties apparent at the time of operation may have an important influence on the outcome. The surgical literature is almost silent about the complication and infection rates for different surgeons. However, some surgeons seem to encounter complications more often than others (4).

Thus, in-hospital mortality for patients with malignant obstruction of the large bowel, primarily resected by surgeons under training, was almost double that of equivalent cases treated by consultants (65). In contrast, surgical seniority had no impact on mortality in primary, elective resection (65). Similar trends have been reported in other areas of surgical practice, where the risk of wound infection was closely related to the technical expertise of the surgeon (66). These patterns were seen especially in contaminated operations, in comparison with clean operations. In a wound surveillance study, there was a significant difference between the post-operative infection rates for the surgeons performing general surgery, while this was not the case for orthopaedic surgeons (7).

It seems quite apparent, then, that wound contamination, and thus control of it, is an essential factor in operating. Of course, no surgeon will condone overt spillage of the contents of a hollow viscus which he is incising or excising. Good, careful operative technique also involves the use of instruments, clamps, suction and swabbing. In many contaminated and dirty cases it will be a clear advantage to set up a 'dirty zone' where heavily contaminated equipment can be placed (67). In so doing, bacterial-containing organs should not be touched by the surgeon's or assistant's fingers, to avoid the spread of bacteria to the entire field, including the wound.

Advances in medical technology have provided sterile barrier materials of plastic which are impervious to bacteria. Bacteriological studies of laparotomy wounds have shown that a plastic wound drape considerably reduces the density of exogenous and in particular endogenous bacteria (68).

Alternatively the incised peritoneum can be pulled up through the wound and sutured to the wound edges, whereby the peritoneum acts as a combined mechanical and biological barrier against contaminating bacteria. If there are no bacteria in the wound, surgical skill becomes less important. On the other hand a safe surgical technique is mandatory to control wound contamination. Much effort has been and is still being exerted to lower wound contamination while operating. 'Bacteriological thinking' will add considerably to an uncomplicated post-operative course for the patient.

Wound contamination control

Wound infection *per se* has previously been the accepted measure of contamination, because means of measuring wound contamination were inexact. However, as host immunity and tissue resistance intervene between contamination and infection, the magnitude of contamination would appear to be a better index of the many efforts exerted to lower wound contamination. These include sterile barriers, surgical scrub, skin disinfection and the use of antibiotics (69).

Quantitative assessment of contamination of the wound by velvet pad sampling (15, 28–33, 38, 39, 68) could be used to determine the effectiveness of the new regimen introduced. Until now, it has also been claimed that surgical technique cannot be measured. As outlined, however, handling of bacteria-containing viscera can now be ascribed a value by determining the resultant number of bacteria in the wound. In addition, physiological wound parameters, i.e. tissue oxygen, can also be measured (61). Over the past two decades the use of prophylactic antibiotics has considerably reduced the incidence of post-operative infective complications. Most regimens now rely on the presence of an adequate concentration of an effective antibiotic in the wound at the time of parietal contamination, with the aim of controlling it (12–14, 70).

Other control precautions

Scientific studies only mirror the real clinical world, and this imperfectly, and here continuous surveillance has been necessary. By this means, total infection rates have decreased significantly with time (4, 7, 71). However, it is not unambiguously clear how this has been achieved. The improvement could lie in a better patient preparation, in better operative technique and support, and in improved post-operative care. A better outcome for the patient, i.e. avoiding infection, is synonymous with quality improvement. Undoubtedly, continuous registration of risk factors, operations performed and post-operative course and outcome, will be a future demand for guarantee of quality. Whether surgeons' personal wound infection rates should be reported or not, with the aim of controlling infection, is debatable. Studies detailed here (7, 65, 66) show significant differences between individual surgeons' rates according to the classification of the surgical wound. It has been argued that comparisons between colleagues at the same institution should also include an adjustment for surgical procedure and severity of patient illness (72). Even so, surgeon-specific infection rates would have no meaning in most hospitals, because of the small numbers of operations (72).

Conclusions

Post-operative wound infection is the end result of many factors, only one of which is the presence of bacteria in the operative field.

The risk of post-surgical infection is closely related to the type of operation performed. All operation wounds harbour bacteria shortly after incision. The flora isolated at this stage are both aerobic and anaerobic commensals, constituting 'background contamination' in conventional operating theatres. However, when bacteria-containing viscera are opened, the bacterial densities increase significantly prior to wound closure. The majority of contaminating bacteria reach the surfaces of the wound from an endogenous source by contact in the widest sense, also with gloves and instruments as vectors (Fig. 5.5). Sites of low bacterial density are close to sites of high density.

There is a consistent correlation between the density of bacteria during operation and wound classification, i.e. clean, potentially contaminated, contaminated, and dirty wounds. Also, there is a high correlation between the density of bacteria prior to closure and post-operative wound infection.

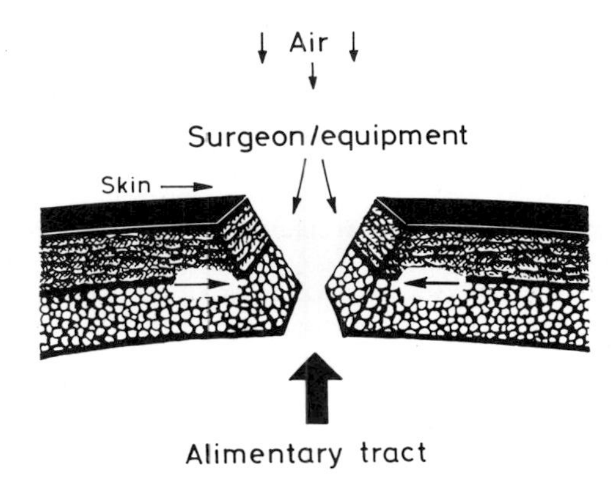

Fig. 5.5. Wound contamination with bacteria from different sources.

The median infective dose of aerobic and anaerobic bacteria is 4.6×10^5 cfu/cm^{-2} in the operative wound. However, the patient could fail to mount an adequate defence against invading organisms (i.e. hypoxia, severity of illness, coexisting diseases, immunodepression), and a smaller inoculum could then be of clinical relevance.

The present technique of velvet pad sampling of bacteria has been elaborated to include anaerobic and aerobic bacteria, and seems to be preferable, where a quantitative measurement of intra-operative contamination is needed.

The surgeon, incising the skin and deeper tissue layers, breaks natural barriers and opens up tissue planes which are primarily sterile. If there are no bacteria in the wound, surgical skill seems to be less important. Bacterial contamination of the operation wound follows consistent patterns, depending mostly on the type of operation. This permits the surgeon to predict the amount and type of contaminating bacteria, allowing him to take adequate measures to prevent and combat parietal contamination. The surgeon should be able to control wound contamination from a bacteria-containing viscus safely throughout the operation, quite apart from the use of antisepsis and sterile barriers. It is surgical technique which distinguishes good and bad surgeons. As part of quality assurance, continuous wound surveillance and reporting of infection rates seem mandatory.

It should now be axiomatic that reducing bacterial contamination reduces infection and that the surgeon's skill in controlling contamination is crucial.

References

1. Moynihan, B. J. A. (1920). The ritual of a surgical operation. *Br. J. Surg.*, **8**, 27–35.
2. National Academy of Sciences. (1964). Ad hoc Committee of the Committee on Trauma: Post-operative wound infections: the influence of ultraviolet irradiation of the operating room and of various other factors. *Ann. Surg.*, **160**, (Suppl 2), 1–92.
3. Davidson, A. I. G., Clark, C., and Smith, G. (1971). Post-operative wound infection: A computer analysis. *Br. J. Surg.*, **58**, 333–7.
4. Cruse, P. J. E. and Foord, R. (1980). The epidemiology of wound infection: A ten-year prospective study of 62 939 wounds. *Surg. Clin. North Am.*, **60**, 27–40.
5. Haley, R. W., Culver, D. H., Morgan, W. M., White, J. W., Emori, T. G., and Hocton, T. M. (1985). Identifying patients at high risk of surgical wound infection. A simple multivariate index of patient susceptibility and wound contamination. *Am. J. Epidemiol.*, **121**, 206–15.
6. Christou, N. V., Nohr, C. W., and Meakins, J. L. (1987). Assessing operative site infection in surgical patients. *Arch. Surg.*, **122**, 165–9.
7. Bremmelgaard, A., Raahave, D., Beier-Holgersen, R., Pedersen, J. V., Andersen, S., and Sørensen, A. I. (1989). Computer-aided surveillance of surgical infections and identification of risk factors. *J. Hosp. Infect.*, **13**, 1–18.
8. Jepsen, O. B., Larsen, O. S., and Thomsen, V. F. (1969). Post-operative wound sepsis in general surgery. II. An assessment of factors influencing the frequency of wound sepsis. *Acta Chir. Scand.*, (Suppl 396), 80–90.
9. Broete, L., Gillquist, J., and Tärnvik, A. (1976). Wound infections in general surgery. Wound contamination, rates of infection and some consequences. *Acta Chir. Scand.*, **142**, 99–106.
10. Matheson, D. M., Arabi, Y., Baxter-Smith, D., *et al.* (1978). Randomized multicentre trial of oral bowel preparation and antimicrobials for elective colorectal operations. *Br. J. Surg.*, **65**, 597–600.
11. Bartlett, J. G., Gordon, R. E., Gorbach, S. L., *et al.* (1978). Impact of oral antibiotic regimen on colonic flora, wound irrigation cultures and bacteriology of septic complications. *Ann. Surg.*, **188**, 249–54.
12. Baum, M. L., Anish, D. S., Chalmers, T. C., *et al.* (1981). A survey of clinical trials of antibiotic prophylaxis in colon surgery: Evidence against further use of no-treatment controls. *N. Engl. J. Med.*, **305**, 795–9.
13. Guglielmo, B. J., Hohn, D. C., Koo, P. J., Hunt, T. K., Sweet, R. L., and Conte, J. E. (1983). Antibiotic prophylaxis in surgical procedures. *Arch. Surg.*, **118**, 943–55.
14. Raahave, D., Hesselfeldt, P., and Pedersen, T. B. (1988). Cefotaxime i.v. versus oral neomycin–erythromycin for prophylaxis of infections after colorectal operations. *World J. Surg.*, **12**, 369–73.
15. Raahave, D. and Friis-Møller, A. (1989). Measuring operative wound contamination predicts post-operative wound infection. *Surg. Res. Comm.*, **5**, 31–9.
16. Jepsen, O. B. (1972). Post-operative wound sepsis in general surgery. VI. The occurrence of infecting staphylococci. *Acta Chir. Scand.*, **138**, 335–41.
17. Wilson, B. D., Surgalla, M. J., and Yates, J. W. (1974). Aerobic and anaerobic surgical wound contamination in patients with cancer. *Surg. Gynecol. Obstet.*, **139**, 329–32.
18. Dillon, M. L., Postlethwait, R. W., and Bowling, K. A. (1969). Operative wound cultures and wound infections: A study of 342 patients. *Ann. Surg.*, **170**, 1029–34.
19. Hughes, E. S. R. (1967). Asepsis in large bowel surgery. *Med. J. Aust.*, **2**, 663–6.
20. Polk, H. C. (1973). Post-operative wound infection: Prediction of some responsible organisms. *Am. J. Surg.*, **126**, 592–4.
21. Peach, S. and Hayek, L. (1974). The isolation of anaerobic bacteria from wound swabs. *J. Clin. Pathol.*, **27**, 578–82.
22. Kelly, M. and Warren, R. E. (1978). The value of an operative wound swab sent in transport medium in the prediction of later clinical wound infection: a controlled clinical and bacteriological evaluation. *Br. J. Surg.*, **65**, 81–8.
23. Nyström, P. O. (1978). The microbiological swab sampler—a quantitative experimental investigation. *Acta Pathol. Microbiol. Scand. B*, **86**, 361–7.
24. Brentano, L. and Gravens, D. L. (1967). A method for the quantitation of bacteria in burn wounds. *Appl. Microbiol.* **15**, 670–1.
25. Robson, M. C., Shaw, R. C., and Heggers, J. P. (1970). The reclosure of post-operative incisional abscesses based on bacterial quantification of the wound. *Ann. Surg.*, **171**, 279–82.
26. Lilly, H. A., Lowbury, E. J. L., London, P. S., and Porter, M. F. (1970). Effects of adhesive drapes on contamination of operation wounds. *Lancet*, **ii**, 431–2.
27. Craythorn, J. M., Barbour, A. G., Matsen, J. M. *et al.* (1980). Membrane filter contact technique for bacteriological sampling of moist surfaces. *J. Clin. Microbiol.*, **12**, 250–5.
28. Raahave, D. (1979). Bacterial densities in operation wounds (Thesis). Copenhagen, University of Copenhagen, Denmark. p. 84.
29. Raahave, D. and Friis-Møller, A. (1982). Velvet pad surface sampling of aerobic and anaerobic bacteria: An *in vitro* laboratory model. *J. Clin. Pathol.*, **35**, 1356–60.
30. Raahave, D., Friis-Møller, A., Bjerre-Jepsen, K., Knudsen, J. T., and Rasmussen, L. B. (1986). The infective dose of aerobic and

anaerobic bacteria in post-operative wound sepsis. *Arch. Surg.*, **121**, 924–9.
31. Raahave, D. (1975). Experimental evaluation of the velvet pad rinse technique as a microbiological sampling method. *Acta Pathol. Microbiol. Scand. B*, **83**, 416–24.
32. Raahave, D. (1975). New technique for quantitative bacteriological sampling of wounds by velvet pads: Clinical sampling trial. *J. Clin. Microbiol.*, **2**, 277–80.
33. Benediktsdóttir, E. and Hambraeus, A, (1983). Isolation of anaerobic and aerobic bacteria from clean surgical wounds: An experimental and clinical study. *J. Hosp. Infect.*, **4**, 141–8.
34. Scheibel, J.H. Nielsen, M.L., and Wamberg, T. (1978). Septic complications in colorectal surgery after 24 hours versus 60 hours of pre-operative antibiotic bowel preparation. *Acta Chir. Scand.*, **144**, 527–32.
35. Raahave, D. (1974). Bacterial density in operation wounds. *Acta Chir. Scand.*, **140**, 585–93.
36. Raahave, D. (1976). Bacterial density in laparotomy wounds during gastrointestinal operations. *Scand. J. Gastroenterol.*, **11** (suppl. 37), 135–42.
37. Raahave, D, Friis-Møller, A., Bülow, S., Jakobsen, B.H., Knudsen, J.B., and Nilsson, T. (1986). Whole bowel irrigation: A bacteriologic assessment. *Infections in Surgery.*, **5**, 12–8.
38. Nyström, P.-O. (1979). Contamination with enterobacteria and post-operative wound infection after appendectomy. *Acta Chir. Scand.*, **145**, 411–3.
39. Møller-Petersen, J., Højbjerg, T., Jensen, K.M.E., *et al.* (1982). Contamination of urological wounds by aerobic bacteria. *Scand. J. Urol. Nephrol.*, **16**, 109–14.
40. Benediktsdóttir, E. and Kolstad, K. (1984). Non-spore-forming anaerobic bacteria in clean surgical wounds—air and skin contamination. *J. Hosp. Infect.*, **5**, 38–49.
41. Ljungquist, U. (1964). Wound sepsis after clean operations. *Lancet*, **i**, 1095–7.
42. Krogh, J., Jess, P., Raahave, D., and Göte, H. (1989). Sene post-operative sårinfektioner. *Ugeskr. Læger*, **151**, 100–1.
43. Elek, S.D. and Conen, P.E. (1957). The virulence of *Staphylococcus pyogenes* for man. A study of the problem of wound infection. *Br. J Exp. Pathol.*, **38**, 573–86.
44. Foster, W.D. and Hutt, M.S.R. (1960). Experimental staphylococcal infections in man. *Lancet*, **ii**, 1373–6.
45. Törnquist, A., Ekelund, G., Forsgren, A., *et al.* (1981). Single dose doxycycline prophylaxis and perioperative bacteriological culture in elective colorectal surgery. *Br. J. Surg.*, **68**, 565–8.
46. Morris, P.J., Barnes, B.A., and Burke, J.F. (1966). The nature of the 'irreducible minimum' rate of incisional sepsis. *Arch. Surg.*, **92**, 367–70.
47. Pollock, A.V. and Evans, M. (1987). Microbiologic prediction of abdominal surgical wound infection. *Arch. Surg.*, **122**, 33–7.
48. Raahave, D., Hesselfeldt, P., Pedersen, T.B., Zachariassen, A., Kann, D., and Hansen, O.H. (1989). No effect of topical ampicillin prophylaxis in operations upon the colon or rectum. *Surg. Gynecol. Obstet.*, **168**, 112–4.
49. Onderdonk, A.B., Bartlett, J.G., Louie, T., *et al.* (1976). Microbial synergy in experimental intra-abdominal abscess. *Infect. Immun.*, **13**, 22–6.
50. Kelly, M.J. (1980). Wound infection: A controlled clinical and experimental demonstration of synergy between aerobic (*Escherichia coli*) and anaerobic (*Bacteroides fragilis*), bacteria. *Ann. R. Coll. Surg. Engl.*, **62**, 52–9.
51. Bartlett, J.G. and Gorbach, S.L. (1979). An animal model of intra-abdominal sepsis. *Scand. J. Infect. Dis.*, **191** (Suppl).: 26.
52. Eade, M.N. and Brooke, B.N. (1969). Portal bacteraemia in cases of ulcerative colitis submitted to colectomy. *Lancet*, **i**, 1008–9.
53. Burton, R.C. (1972). Gram-negative bacteraemia in colonic and rectal surgery. *Med. J. Aust.*, **1**, 367–9.
54. Orth, H.D., Gierhake, F.W., Zimmermann, K., Hoffmann, K., and Ruscher, I. (1972). Intraoperative bakteriämien in der Abdominal-chirurgie. *Langenbecks Arch. Chir.*, **330**, 307–15.
55. Lidwell, O.M., Lowbury, E.J.L., Whyte, W., Blowers, R., Stanley, S.J., and Lowe, D. (1983). Airborne contamination of wounds in joint replacement operations: the relationship to sepsis rates. *J. Hosp. Infect.*, **4**, 111–31.
56. Hunt, T.K., Knighton, D.R., Thakral, K.K., Andrews, W., Michaeli, D. (1984). Cellular control of repair. In *Soft and hard tissue repair* (ed. T.K. Hunt, R.B. Heppenstall, E. Pines, D. Rovee), pp. 3–19. Praeger Scientific, New York.
57. Hohn, D.C., Mackay, R., Halliday, B., *et al.* (1976). Effect of O_2 tensions on microbicidal function of leukocytes in wounds and *in vitro*. *Surg. Forum*, **27**, 18–20.
58. Chang, N., Goodson, W.H., Gottrup, F. and Hunt, T.K. (1983). Direct measurement of wound and tissue oxygen tension in post-operative patients. *Ann. Surg.*, **197**, 470–8.
59. Gottrup, F., Firmin, R., Chang, N., Goodson, W.H., and Hunt, T.K. (1983). Continuous direct tissue oxygen tension measurement by a new method using an implantable silastic tonometer and oxygen polarography. *Am. J. Surg.*, **46**, 399–403.
60. Jönsson, K., Jensen, J.A., Goodson, W.H., West, J.M., and Hunt, T.K. (1987). Assessment of perfusion in post-operative patients using tissue oxygen measurements. *Br. J. Surg.*, **74**, 263–7.
61. Göte, H., Raahave, D., and Bæch, J. (1990). Tissue oximetry as possible predictor of lethal complications after emergency intestinal surgery. *Surg. Res. Comm.*, **7**, 243–9.
62. Knighton, D.R., Halliday, B.H., and Hunt, T.K. (1984). Oxygen as an antibiotic. *Arch. Surg.*, **119**, 199–204.
63. Robson, M.C. and Heggers, J.P. (1984). Quantitative bacteriology and inflammatory mediators in soft tissue. In *Soft and hard tissue repair* (ed. T.K. Hunt, R.B. Heppenstall, E. Pines, and D. Rovee), pp. 483–507. Praeger Scientific, New York.
64. Wadström, T., Eliason, I., Holder, I., and Ljungh, Å. (ed.). (1990). *Pathogenesis of wound and biomaterial-associated infections*. Springer-Verlag, London.
65. Phillips, R.K.S., Hittinger, R., Fry, J.S., and Fielding, L.P. (1985). Malignant large bowel obstruction. *Br. J. Surg.*, **72**, 296–302.
66. Karran, S.J., Hunt, M.de la, Townend, I., *et al.* (1985). Prevention of infection in high risk biliary operations. *Antibiot. Chemother.*, **33**, 59–72.
67. Frankel, A. and Kark, A.E. (1969). Assisting at operations. In *Pye's surgical handicraft* (ed. J. Kyle), pp. 145–69. John Wright, Bristol.
68. Raahave, D. (1976). Effect of plastic skin and wound drapes on the density of bacteria in operation wounds. *Br. J. Surg.*, **63**, 421–6.
69. Maki, D.G. (1976). Lister revisited: Surgical antisepsis and asepsis. *N. Engl. J. Med.*, **294**, 1286–7.
70. Raahave, D. (1975). Penicillin concentrations in abdominal operation wounds after intravenous administration. *Scand. J. Gastroenterol.*, **10**, 551–5.
71. Mead, P.B., Pories, S.E., Hall, P., Vacek, P.M., Davis, J.H., and Gamelli, R.L. (1986). Decreasing the incidence of surgical wound infections. *Arch. Surg.*, **121**, 458–61.
72. Scheckler, W.E. (1988). Surgeon-specific wound infection rates—A potential dangerous and misleading strategy. *Infect. Control Hosp. Epidemiol.*, **9**, 145–7.

6

The action of disinfectants and antiseptics and their role in surgical practice

JOHN R. BABB

Introduction

Cleaning, disinfection, and sterilization are all processes which remove or destroy micro-organisms present on instruments, environmental surfaces, and the skin. Which of these processes is used will depend on the risks associated with the use of the item, the target micro-organisms, nature of the surface and its ability to withstand the decontamination process.

Sterilization

If the item penetrates intact skin or mucous membranes, enters sterile body cavities or is in contact with a breach in the skin or mucous membranes, a sterilization process is required. This will ensure that all micro-organisms are destroyed including the more tolerant pathogenic species such as Clostridial spores and slow viruses.

The most widely used method of sterilization is autoclaving. This process is extremely reliable, safe, and comparatively inexpensive. Unfortunately, there are some items that will not tolerate the pressure fluctuations and high temperatures used in this process, i.e. 100 to 200 kPa and either 121 °C (unwrapped instruments) or 134 °C (porous loads) and a chemical process is required for these. A few hospitals have Sterile Service Departments (SSDs) that are equipped with ethylene oxide or sub-atmospheric steam and formaldehyde sterilizers. These processes, although suitable for heat sensitive items, are lengthy, require microbiological monitoring and involve the use of toxic substances and expensive equipment. Items sterilized using ethylene oxide also require lengthy aeration before re-use. Consequently, these processes are unsuitable for many heat sensitive instruments, particularly those which are required promptly for re-use. For these a sporicidal disinfectant, or sterilant, is required (1).

Disinfection

Disinfection is also a process which removes or destroys micro-organisms but does not usually include bacterial spores and slow viruses. It is normally utilized for making used instruments and equipment free from infection risk and safe to handle. It is used for non-invasive items that are in contact with mucous membranes, diseased or damaged skin and body fluids, e.g. gastrointestinal endoscopes, respiratory equipment, and spillage. As with sterilization, heat is the preferred method. Items may be immersed in boiling water for 10 min, disinfected at 73 °C using sub-atmospheric steam, pasteurized at temperatures between 65 °C and 100 °C or processed using one of the many washer disinfectors that are currently available. Washer disinfectors are particularly useful for anaesthetic circuits and respiratory equipment which do not require a sporicidal process and that would be damaged by repeated autoclaving. Washer disinfectors are also useful for processing dirty surgical instruments which, if not handled carefully, may be hazardous to theatre and SSD staff. If the use of hot water or steam is impractical, disinfectants should be used (1).

Cleaning

Cleaning is also a method of decontamination and is an essential prerequisite or component of all sterilization and disinfection processes. Cleaning will remove large numbers of micro-organisms and the organic material on which they thrive. It will also remove material which may inactivate or prevent the penetration of a disinfectant, hot water, or steam. Cleaning and drying alone will usually suffice for those items which are either remote from the patient or in contact with intact healthy skin, e.g. walls, floors, furniture, and sphygmomanometer cuffs.

The classification of items and surfaces in relation to risk, with examples and process options, is shown in Table 6.1. Following the use of one or more of these options it is important to ensure that the item does not become recontaminated with potential pathogens before re-use. Sterilized items should be suitably contained or wrapped to prevent environmental contamination. The usual methods are double wraps of paper

Table 6.1. Classification of items and surfaces in relation to risk.

Risk category	Method of decontamination	Process options	Examples of items/surfaces
High risk In contact with a break in the skin or mucous membrane or introduced into a sterile body area (if sterilization is not practical high level disinfection may be adequate).	Cleaning and sterilization	**Heat tolerant** Autoclave Hot air oven **Heat sensitive** Single use Ethylene oxide Low temperature steam and formaldehyde Sporicidal disinfectants e.g. glutaraldehyde	Surgical instruments, laparoscopes arthroscopes, cardiac catheters implants, infusions, injections, needles, syringes, swabs, surgical dressings, sutures.
Intermediate risk In contact with intact mucous membranes, body fluids, or contaminated with particularly virulent or readily transmissible organisms, or if the item is to be used on highly susceptible patients or sites.	Cleaning and disinfection (or sterilization)	All the above and **Heat tolerant** Boiling Pasteurization Low temp. steam washer disinfectors **Heat sensitive** disinfectants, e.g. glutaraldehyde, Chlorine releasing agents, alcohol, clear soluble phenolics	Respiratory and anaesthetic equipment, GI endoscopes, bronchoscopes, thermometers, vaginal speculae, body fluid spillage, dirty instruments prior to reprocessing, bed pans.
Low risk In contact with normal and intact skin.	Cleaning usually adequate disinfection if known infection risk	Manual cleaning with detergent. Automated cleaning/disinfection Disinfectants.	Trolley tops, operating table, wash-bowls, lavatory seats, baths, wash hand basins, bedding, patient supports.
Minimal risk Remote, not in direct contact with patients or immediate surroundings. Unlikely to be contaminated with a significant number of pathogens or be transferred to a susceptible site.	Cleaning alone	Manual or automated cleaning, damp dusting, wet mopping, dust attractant mops, vacuum cleaners.	Floors, walls, furniture, ceilings, drains.

or linen, or specifically designed containers. Processed items should be stored dry, with packaging intact and free from dust. Surfaces that have been cleaned and disinfected should be left dry to discourage subsequent microbial proliferation.

It is the responsibility of all hospital staff, and more especially those working in operating theatres, to minimize the risk of transmission of infection on the skin and inanimate surfaces. Cleaning, disinfection, and sterilization are all methods by which potentially pathogenic micro-organisms are removed or destroyed so preventing them from reaching a susceptible site, e.g. a surgical wound, in sufficient numbers to initiate an infection. The selection and use of disinfectants in surgical practice for the skin, environmental surfaces and heat labile items will be discussed here.

Disinfection policy

A disinfectant is a chemical compound which can destroy micro-organisms and an antiseptic is a non-toxic disinfectant which can be safely applied to the skin or living tissues. Some disinfectants, e.g. glutaraldehyde and the chlorine-releasing agents can, under certain conditions, kill bacterial spores as well as viruses and vegetative bacteria. These are described as sterilants or cold sterilizing solutions.

Those persons responsible for producing and implementing a disinfection policy are the members of the Infection Control Committee and Team. This would normally include those familiar with the properties and use of disinfectants such as the Microbiologist, Pharmacist, Infection Control Doctor, and Nurse. Discussions on the selection of disinfectants should also include representatives of the users, e.g. surgeons, physicians, nurses, technicians, and operating department assistants.

The Infection Control Committee may produce their own policy or, as is most likely, adopt the recommendations of reference laboratories, professional societies or the Department of Health. Factors taken into account when producing a disinfectant policy include the nature of the items or surfaces to be processed, the range of antimicrobial activity required, contact time, stability, inactivation, cost, and corrosiveness. Micro-organisms vary in their susceptibility to disinfectants: Gram-positive bacteria are comparatively sensitive, Gram-negative bacilli less sensitive, tubercle bacilli relatively resistant and spores highly resistant. Viruses vary according to their structures. Enveloped or lipophilic viruses, e.g. Herpes simplex and HIV, are more susceptible than the non-enveloped or hydrophilic viruses, e.g. the enteroviruses, but, with the exception of the slow viruses, these are more readily destroyed than mycobacteria and bacterial spores. The properties of several widely used disinfectants are shown in Table 6.2.

Policies should include disinfectants for heat-sensitive instruments and equipment, spillage, the skin, and mucous membranes. It is usual to include in the policy the method of application, health and safety data, and at least one alternative for each of the purposes listed.

Disinfectants: heat-sensitive instruments and equipment

Most surgical instruments and invasive items are either heat tolerant or single use. There are, however, a few items, e.g. endoscopes, tonometers, cryosurgical probes, and transducers which are not. Broad spectrum, non-damaging disinfectants are required for these.

Aldehydes

Glutaraldehyde (2 per cent) is probably the most widely used instrument disinfectant. It is an alkylating agent and is effective against bacteria, including mycobacteria, spores, viruses, and fungi (2). It is non-corrosive and will not damage rubber, lens cements, and plastics. It is therefore compatible with flexible fibreoptic endoscopes (3) and many other complex heat-sensitive instruments. Unfortunately, aldehydes are toxic, irritant and allergenic (4) and have therefore become a prime

Table 6.2. Properties of principal disinfectants.

	Disinfectants	Antimicrobial activity: Vegetative bacteria	Mycobacteria	Spores	Enveloped viruses	Non-enveloped viruses	Corrosive/ damaging	Toxic/ irritant	Inactivation by organic matter
Spillage and environment	chlorine releasing agents 1000–10 000 p.p.m. available Cl_2	+++	++	++	+++	++	Yes	Yes	Yes
	Clear soluble phenolics 0.6–2%	+++	+++	–	+	–	slight	Yes	No
Heat sensitive equipment and instruments	2% glutaraldehyde and other aldehydes	+++	++ (Slow)	++ (Slow)	+++	+++	No	Yes	No
	60–80% alcohol (ethanol & isopropanol)	+++	++	–	++	+	slight	No	Yes
Skin and mucous membrane	Chlorhexidine 0.5–4%	++	–	–	+	–		No	
	povidone iodine 7–10%	++	+	+	++	+		No	
	60–80% alcohol	++	++	–	++	+		No	

+++ Excellent activity ++ Good activity + Some activity – Little or no activity objective for assessment for Control of Substances Hazardous to Health (COSHH) (5). When using glutaraldehyde and other aldehyde containing disinfectants, gloves and a plastic apron should always be worn in addition to eye-protection if splashing is likely. Immersion and storage tanks should be covered, the disinfectant stored away from sources of heat and preferably used away from busy areas. Fume cupboards or local exhaust ventilation should be installed to remove toxic vapour in endoscopy units or theatres where large quantities of aldehydes are used (6). The current short-term occupational exposure limit (10 min reference period) is 0.2 p.p.m. (0.7 mg m^{-3}) (7) but it is likely that this requirement will become more stringent.

Immersion times vary depending upon the nature of the aldehyde, its concentration, the type of contamination and the time available for processing. If 2 per cent activated alkaline glutaraldehyde is used, vegetative bacteria (2) and most viruses (8), including HIV, (9, 10), are destroyed in under 4 min. Longer immersion times of 10 to 30 min are usually recommended for HBV (11), 60 min for tubercle bacilli (12) and other mycobacteria (13), and 3 h for bacterial spores (14). If lower concentrations are used, e.g. to reduce irritancy, longer immersion times will be required (15).

Cleaning prior to disinfection is essential as glutaraldehyde is a fixative. Cleaning is particularly important with narrow lumen instruments, biopsy forceps, and cytology brushes. Channel blockages are expensive to clear and a misdiagnosis could be made if dirty biopsy forceps or cytology brushes are used (16).

All items should be thoroughly rinsed after disinfection to remove toxic residues. The rinse water rapidly becomes contaminated with glutaraldehyde and should be changed frequently. Potable water is usually sufficient for items in contact with intact mucous membranes but, if the microbiological quality of water is poor, the patient is immunocompromised or the item is invasive, sterile water should be used. Some patients have been misdiagnosed as having mycobacterial infections following bronchoscopy because rinse water was contaminated with acid-fast bacilli (17, 18). There is also a risk of infection in the compromised host with water-borne organisms such as *Pseudomonas aeruginosa* (19) and legionella.

The most widely used aldehydes are the two per cent activated alkaline glutaraldehydes ('Cidex', 'Asep', 'Totacide 28'). Once activated these become more effective but unstable and should be used within the 14 to 28 days specified by the manufacturer (14). The period of re-use, (within this 14 to 28 days), will depend on the cleanliness of the item and the number and size of instruments processed. Organic material, detergent and water from the cleansing process will be transferred to the disinfectant so reducing its potency. Stable acid glutaraldehydes are available for the small volume, or occasional user, but these are less effective and longer immersion times may have to be used.

Other aldehydes, or mixtures, such as 10 per cent succine dialdehyde and formaldehyde (Gigasept) and 2 per cent glutaraldehyde with 7 per cent phenate, ('Sporicidin') are also effective and may be used as alternatives (15, 20).

Alcohol (60 to 90 per cent ethanol or isopropanol)

Alcohol is an alternative instrument disinfectant but it will not destroy bacterial spores and some viruses. It has the advantage that it works rapidly and evaporates, leaving surfaces dry. Provided items have been thoroughly cleaned, alcohol will destroy vegetative bacteria, including mycobacteria (21), fungi, HIV (9, 10), HBV (22, 23), and most viruses. It is therefore particularly useful for the rapid disinfection of dropped instruments, ampoules, razors, laryngoscopes, thermometers, and endoscopes. Alcohol wipes are available which may be used to clean and disinfect electrical equipment and large items unsuitable for immersion, e.g. radiographic equipment and trolley tops. Isopropanol (60 to 80 per cent) is normally preferred as a bactericide, but 70 to 90 per cent ethanol is more effective as a virucidal agent (8, 24). The addition of antiseptics such as chlorhexidine are of benefit for skin disinfection but are not necessary for instruments and environmental surfaces, and may leave sticky residues. Rubber swells, plastics may be hardened and epoxy lens cements may be weakened by frequent or prolonged contact with alcohol. Immersion times should, therefore, be limited to 10 min or, in the case of flexible fibre-optic endoscopes, to 4 min. Alcohol is flammable and care should be taken to avoid sources of ignition, especially when using naked flames or diathermy.

Other agents

Quaternary Ammonium Compounds (QACs), are used in some hospitals, particularly where aldehyde sterilization is a problem, for between patient cleaning and disinfection of flexible GI endoscopes (3, 20). They are good cleansing agents, are non-corrosive and non-irritant. Unfortunately, they are ineffective against spores and tubercle bacilli and have little or no virucidal activity. They should, therefore, only be used where the risks of transmission of infection are low or providing their use is followed by a more effective agent such as alcohol.

Iodophors were formerly used for the disinfection of flexible fibreoptic endoscopes. They are non-irritant, bactericidal, virucidal, and tuberculocidal but *in vitro* tests have proved disappointing. Povidone–iodine is too thick to pass readily down the channels of endoscopes and sticks to lenses (8).

Stabilized hydrogen peroxide 3 to 6 per cent, is used to disinfect hydrophilic (soft) contact lenses and tonometers (25) (see later). Nebulized hydrogen peroxide, or formaldehyde vapour has also been used to disinfect ventilators but these are now largely protected by filters and incorporate the use of disposable or heat tolerant circuits. A synergistic sporicidal effect has been observed with a mixture of hydrogen peroxide and peracetic acid but these agents are corrosive and are not generally recommended at the present time.

Infective agents that may require unique recommendations are the slow viruses such as that of Creutzfeld–Jakob disease. The agent has been transmitted very rarely by corneal transplantation, human growth hormone, and brain electrodes. Particular care is necessary when handling items contaminated with brain tissue, CSF, and blood from such patients or if the diagnosis is suspected. Slow viruses are particularly tolerant and steam sterilization for 18 min at 134 °C or 121 °C for 1 h, or immersion in 1 N sodium hydroxide or a chlorine-releasing agent (> 5000 p.p.m. av. Cl_2) for 1 h is recommended for those items that cannot be destroyed by incineration (26).

Endoscopes

The flexible fibre-optic endoscopes currently available will not tolerate temperatures in excess of 60 °C and consequently cannot be disinfected or sterilized using hot water or steam. Some rigid endoscopes are now autoclavable, and these are preferred, but most will tolerate boiling water and sub-atmospheric steam at 73 °C (with or without formaldehyde). Ethylene oxide, although effective and non-damaging, is a lengthy process and is available in comparatively few hospitals. Immersion in a suitable, non-damaging, and effective disinfectant is, therefore, the only practical solution in most hospitals (27).

The decontamination procedure selected should relate to the risks associated with the investigation, e.g. is the procedure invasive, has the patient a known immune deficiency or communicable disease? The disinfectant chosen should be effective against patient associated transmissible organisms, e.g. *Salmonella* spp, *Mycobacterium tuberculosis*, Hepatitis B and HIV as well as the opportunistic pathogens, e.g. *Ps. aeruginosa* and the Gram-negative bacilli, which thrive in the moist narrow channels and valves of the endoscope between periods of use (28). The relatively high cost of these instruments, and the personal preference of the user, often means few endoscopes are available for routine use. It is, therefore, essential to adopt a rapid but effective method of decontamination between patients if a busy session is to be completed in a reasonable time (Fig. 6.1). A more thorough technique, which includes longer exposure times, is recommended where the risk of transmission of infection is particularly great, e.g. before endoscopic retrograde cholangiopancreatography (ERCP) and at the beginning and end of a days list (29). Decontamination should include the cleaning and disinfection of all channels (suction, biopsy, air, and water) the insertion tube, telescope, trochar, water bottle, and all support equipment. Accessible channels, valve ports, and external surfaces should be cleaned with a detergent and a soft brush. The insertion tube, telescope and trochar should be wiped with a gauze swab or paper wipe to remove adherent organic soil. If an automated washer/disinfector is not available, a syringe and tubing should be used to irrigate all accessible channels.

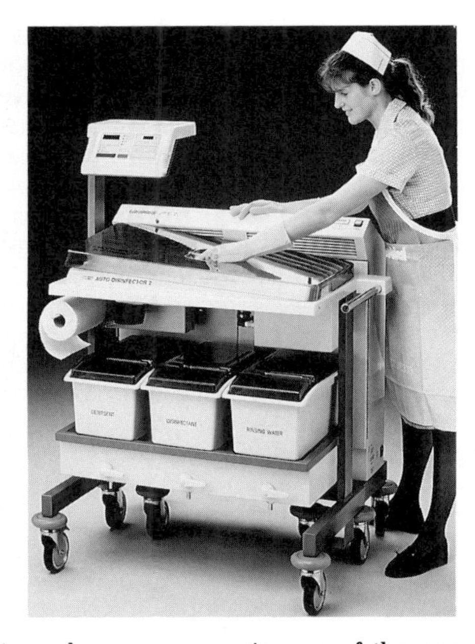

Fig. 6.1. An endoscopy nurse using one of the many automatic washer disinfectors for flexible fibreoptic endoscopes. Suitable clothing and exhaust ventilation should be provided if aldehydes are used. (Photo: Courtesy of KeyMed Limited.)

Two per cent glutaraldehyde or 10 per cent succine dialdehyde is recommended for disinfection as these disinfectants exhibit a wide range of antimicrobial activity and are non-damaging. The current immersion times (29, 30) are shown in Table 6.3. Although it is currently recommended that, for cold sterilization, endoscopes (e.g. laparoscopes, arthroscopes, and cystoscopes) are immersed in glutaraldehyde for 3 h, this is rarely practical. It is unlikely that chemically tolerant pathogenic spores will be present in large numbers after thorough cleaning. Immersion in 2 per cent glutaraldehyde for at least 10 minutes is recommended if mycobacterial infections are not suspected. It is essential that, if items are immersed in glutaraldehyde, they are thoroughly cleaned first and rinsed afterwards. Cleaning with a QAC, such as Dettol ED, followed by disinfection with 60 to 80 per cent alcohol, has been recommended as an alternative to glutaraldehyde for gastrointestinal endoscopes if irritancy or sensitization is considered a major problem and the risks of patients acquiring communicable diseases is low (29). However, this combination is less effective and 2 per cent glutaraldehyde is still preferred. If alcohol is used, care should be taken to avoid lengthy immersions as these may damage lens cements. One leading manufacturer, (Olympus) does not recommend immersion in alcohol in excess of 4 min. Rinsing is not necessary after immersion as alcohol evaporates. Alcohol is particularly useful for rinsing bronchoscopes and invasive instruments when sterile water is not available or the microbiological quality of the tap water cannot be assured (30).

Table 6.3. Endoscopes.

UK immersion times for 2 per cent glutaraldehyde		
Endoscope	**Recommendation**	**References**
All endoscopes	30 min HBV and HIV	11
	1 h *Mycobacterium tuberculosis*	12, 29, 30
	3 h Cold sterilization	14
Gastrointestinal endoscopes	4 min between patients	
	20 min beginning and end of list	
	1 h after symptomatic AIDS patient	29
	1 h *Mycobacterium tuberculosis*	
Bronchoscopes	20 min between patients	
	1 h beginning and end of list	
	1 h known or suspected mycobacterial infection	30

Alternative agents such as the peroxygen compounds and peracetic acid are currently under investigation as less irritant alternatives to glutaraldehyde, but it is too early to endorse their use without further study. Thorough cleaning should, however, greatly reduce the need for disinfection.

Several machines are now available which automatically clean and disinfect the channels and surfaces of fibrescopes (27, 31, 32). These machines are effective and studies have shown that they offer a more reliable decontamination process than has hitherto been achieved manually. Should a machine be purchased it should be effective, convenient, non-damaging, and sufficiently adaptable to accommodate the range of instruments used. Enclosed tanks and covered trays will reduce the risk of splashing and exposure to the disinfectant. Machines should be programmable or have a disinfectant hold facility which enables the user to select a suitable contact period. All channel irrigation is important and so is a terminal rinse. Water and detergent tanks and all circuitry, if not automatically decontaminated during the cycle, should be cleaned and disinfected before each session. If this is not done equipment associated infections with atypical mycobacteria and Gram-negative bacilli, e.g. *Ps. aeruginosa* and legionella, are likely.

In recent years, a range of immersible flexible fibrescopes has been introduced. These can be totally immersed should disinfection of the control box and light-guide connector prove necessary. They also have removable valves which allow access to all channels. A leak detector and all channel irrigation device are available for these instruments. These are easy to use and extremely effective.

The selection of a safe and effective decontamination procedure will reduce the likelihood of infection, staff sensitization, channel blockages, and the deterioration of an expensive item of equipment (27). It is recommended that, before changing your disinfectant policy, the opinions of the manufacturers and the professional organisations are sought. Suitable courses on user maintenance and decontamination are available and can be arranged with the manufacturers or Endoscopy Nurses Association.

Disinfectants: spillage and the environment

The routine disinfection of theatre floors, walls, and other environmental surfaces remote from the patient is wasteful and unnecessary as floors and horizontal surfaces in occupied areas rapidly become recontaminated after cleaning and disinfection (33). However, disinfectants are required to protect staff whilst removing potentially infectious material such as spilt blood and other body fluids. It may also be necessary to disinfect surfaces in contact with infected patients or dirty instruments e.g. the operating table, patient supports, trolley tops, sinks, and dirty instrument containers. Micro-organisms do not thrive on clean dry surfaces and those dispersed by the theatre occupants, are removed by the theatre ventilation or, once settled, are difficult to redisperse provided appropriate cleaning techniques such as damp dusting and wet mopping, are used.

Most of the more effective environmental disinfectants, e.g. chlorine-releasing agents and phenolics, damage surfaces and are irritant to the user. Gloves and a plastic apron should be worn and eye protection if splashing is likely.

Chlorine-releasing agents

The disinfectants most suitable for environmental surfaces, particularly if blood is present, are the chlorine-releasing agents. They are available in liquid form as sodium hypochlorite or bleach and as tablets, powders or granules which contain sodium dichloroisocyanurate (NaDCC) (34–36). These agents exhibit a broad spectrum of antimicrobial activity and are particularly effective as virucides (8, 10, 22–24). They are fast acting and comparatively inexpensive. The concentration used will be dependent on the amount of organic matter present, the nature of the contamination, and the type of surface. Chlorine-releasing agents are readily inactivated by organic material, damage rubber, and are corrosive to metals (14, 37). They are therefore largely unsuitable for surgical instruments.

Once prepared at in-use concentrations the chlorine-releasing agents are unstable and should be used immediately. For the removal of spilt blood and other body fluids at least 10 000 p.p.m. av. Cl_2 is recommended to accommodate the organic load (38). Lower concentrations of 200 to 1000 p.p.m. av. Cl_2 are suitable for precleaned surfaces, theatre furniture and cleaning equipment. Solutions of sodium dichloroisocyanurate (NaDCC), have a lower pH and are less stable but are more effective than equivalent concentrations of sodium hypochlorite. They are also less corrosive and more convenient to use (37). Detergents and cream cleansers are normally suitable for sluices, sinks, and wash-hand basins but should a disinfectant be required, a non-abrasive chlorine-releasing agent may be used. Chlorine-releasing agents are incompatible with cationic detergents and should not be mixed with acids as this may lead to the rapid release of chlorine.

NaDCC formulations are supplied as powders or granules and these can be applied directly to small blood spills (e.g. less than 30 ml) (36) (Fig. 6.2). Once the spillage is absorbed, residues can be removed with a paper towel or disposable cloth and a second moist cloth used to clean the surface. For larger spills, on floors, furniture, and other surfaces, a solution

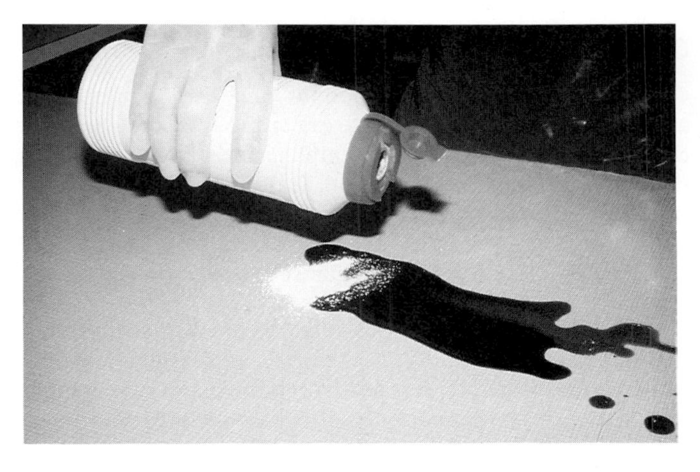

Fig. 6.2. Using chlorine-releasing powders or granules (NaDCC) to remove small blood spillages. (See plate section.)

should be prepared by either dissolving one or more tablets in an appropriate amount of cold water or by preparing a suitable dilution of bleach. This solution may be applied either with a cloth or mop and bucket. A fresh solution of 1000 p.p.m. av. Cl_2 should be used to disinfect cleaning equipment. Once prepared, solutions are comparatively unstable and should be used either immediately or within 24 h. Dry, undissolved tablets and powders are stable for years.

Although primarily intended for environmental surfaces, chlorine-releasing agents are also used, at low concentrations, for disinfecting tonometer prisms (39) (500 p.p.m. av. Cl_2 for 5 min) and for some respiratory, dialysis, and catering equipment. If damage to the surface is likely, items should be thoroughly cleaned first, a low concentration of chlorine used (i.e. less than 1000 p.p.m. av. Cl_2) and the surface washed afterwards to remove the corrosive agent.

Clear soluble phenolics

At one time phenolics (Clearsol, Stericol, Izal) played a prominent role in environmental disinfection. Unfortunately, recent studies have shown them to be poor virucidal agents (8, 24) and with the current focus on the transmission of HIV and HBV, the chlorine-releasing agents are now more popular.

Clear soluble phenolics are highly effective against non-sporing bacteria, including tubercle bacilli and fungi (40, 21). They are inexpensive, stable at in-use concentrations, are not readily inactivated by organic material (41), and usually contain a compatible detergent. They are therefore used to remove faeces, urine, sputum, and other spillage provided an effective virucide is not required. Many clear soluble phenolics contain corrosion inhibitors and have been used to disinfect sigmoidoscopes and post mortem instruments but heat, glutaraldehyde, or alcohol would seem more appropriate. Phenolics have also been used for bed pans, urinals, wash bowls, suction bottles and receivers, especially where no means of heat treatment is available. Phenolics are not recommended for the routine treatment of mattress covers and supports as they damage plastic and rubber, thus increasing permeability (42). Chlorine-releasing agents or, if the spillage is small, alcohol wipes would be most suitable.

Other agents

Quaternary ammonium compounds and ampholytic agents are used primarily in catering areas but may also be used for cleaning non-critical environmental surfaces in the operating theatre, e.g. walls, floors, and furniture. They are 'user friendly' and have some detergent properties but are unsuitable for spillage because of their inactivation and poor spectrum of activity. They are ineffective against spores, tubercle bacilli, and most viruses (24).

Formaldehyde has occasionally been used to disinfect rooms, including operating theatres, and bulky items of medical equipment (1). It is a slow sporicide and is only effective on clean exposed surfaces. It is extremely irritant to the eyes, skin, and respiratory mucosa and should not therefore be used unless it can be safely contained and discharged. The effectiveness of formaldehyde in reducing the numbers of micro-organisms in the air and on surfaces has not been demonstrated and several disadvantages are associated with this technique, e.g. disinfection is not accompanied by cleaning, or possible inhalation of toxic residues. A more effective technique would be to ventilate the room and clean and disinfect the surfaces.

Disinfectants: skin and mucous membranes

Many different types of micro-organisms exist on the skin (43). These include the resident flora, which largely consist of Gram-positive cocci such as *Staphylococcus epidermidis*, micrococci and diphtheroids, and transient bacteria which may be deposited on the skin as a result of contact with patients, or their immediate environment. The transient flora do not thrive on the skin and can substantially be removed by a thorough wash with soap and water. Although most transient micro-organisms survive for only a limited period on the skin, some may last several days. These have been described as temporary residents. They include bacterial spores, *Staph. aureus*, *Acinetobacter* sp., *Candida albicans*, and some strains of *Klebsiella aerogenes*.

The resident skin flora are far more difficult to remove and, if a substantial reduction is necessary, an antiseptic will be required. Most resident skin micro-organisms are not highly virulent and are rarely implicated in outbreaks of hospital acquired infection. The majority of the resident micro-organisms are found in the superficial skin layers but approximately 10 to 20 per cent inhabit deep epidermal layers. Large numbers of micro-organisms are also found as residents of mucous membranes, i.e. mouth, nose, and vagina.

The numbers of transient or resident micro-organisms present on the skin and mucous membranes can substantially be reduced by cleaning with soap or detergent and water or by the application of non-irritant skin disinfectants (antiseptics) such as chlorhexidine, povidone–iodine, or alcohol (44). Antiseptics are of value in reducing the numbers of endogenous micro-organisms present on the skin or mucous membranes prior to surgery or other invasive procedures, e.g. during the insertion of a catheter and, to remove or destroy micro-organisms present on the hands of surgeons, nurses, and other hospital staff (45–47). Ideally the skin should be sterilized, or free from all micro-organisms, prior to an invasive procedure. This is, however, impractical without destroying or severely damaging the skin. Cleaning and disinfection is therefore more appropriate. Antiseptics may also occasionally be used to treat carriers or dispersers of particularly resistant, virulent, or communicable strains, e.g. Methicillin-resistant *Staph. aureus* (MRSA) (48).

Hand washing and disinfection

Hand washing and disinfection has repeatedly been described as the most important infection-control procedure (49, 50). Studies have shown high rates of hand carriage of pathogenic species during outbreaks. Also, in one study, 30 per cent of nurses in a large district general hospital were found to be carrying *Staph. aureus* and Gram-negative bacilli on their hands

(46). Neither of these organisms is commonly found as part of the normal resident skin flora but frequently occur as pathogens. Counts were, on occasions, as high as 10^7 with a median count of 10^3 to 10^4. In a much larger study, Cruse and Foord initially indicated that the risk of post-operative wound infection increased threefold during clean surgery if the surgeon's gloves became punctured during the operation (51) but, in the continuation of this study, no longer see this effect. (See Chapter 1.) In spite of the fears of acquiring infection with blood-borne viruses, the incidence of surgical glove punctures is high. In a recent study of general surgery, gloves became punctured during 34.5 per cent of all operations with an overall incidence of single-glove puncture of 12.7 per cent (52). Much higher incidences of glove perforation have been detected in cardiothoracic surgery. Punctures are primarily due to contact with sharp instruments, bone splinters, needles, or to the use of inferior gloves. It would therefore appear logical to adopt a highly effective hand-washing/disinfection technique before donning surgical gloves. This will minimize the risk of micro-organisms passing through holes or tears and the likelihood of surface contamination whilst donning the glove.

In most hospital wards and departments, hand-cleansing with bar or liquid soap or detergent will remove most, if not all, of the transient skin flora (46). It is, however, important that a thorough technique is used (53). This should include the fingertips, thumb, and other contact sites which are often missed (54). Antiseptic formulations are occasionally recommended for ward (hygienic) hand-wash. They are slightly more effective than soap and water in removing the transient flora and may exhibit a cumulative or persistent effect. They are therefore more suitable for use when nursing immunocompromised patients or during outbreaks of infection. The agents most commonly used are those containing alcohol, chlorhexidine, or povidone–iodine. Hexachlorophane and triclosan formulations are also occasionally used during outbreaks of staphylococcal infections but these are slower acting and for maximum benefit, several applications may have to be applied (44).

During the surgical scrub, it is necessary to remove all the transient flora and substantially reduce the readily detachable resident flora (Fig. 6.3). To ensure this reduction is achieved and maintained throughout the operation, an antiseptic formulation with a prolonged or sustained effect is required. Tests have shown that the most effective agents are those which contain 60 to 80 per cent alcohol (isopropanol or ethanol) or detergent scrubs containing 4 per cent chlorhexidine, or 7.5 per cent povidone–iodine. Two or more applications of alcohol, with a suitable emollient, is the most effective agent but it cannot be used for hand-cleansing and should therefore be applied after a thorough wash with soap and water (47, 55).

Before the first operation, it is advisable to remove dirt from behind the nails using a sterile nail-brush and scraper. The hands and forearms should then be cleaned and disinfected with a surgical scrub or, if alcohol is to be used, with soap and water. Two minutes is the time usually adopted for a surgical scrub. There is little or no additional benefit in prolonging this activity to 5 or 10 min and persistent scrubbing, or the application of harsh antiseptic detergents, may damage the skin encouraging the proliferation or survival of potentially patho-

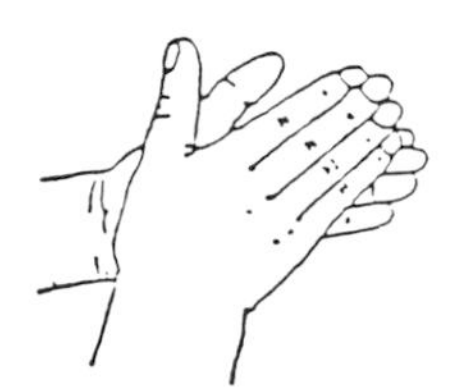
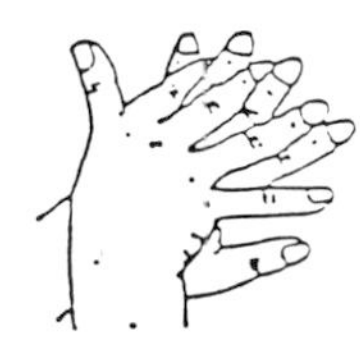
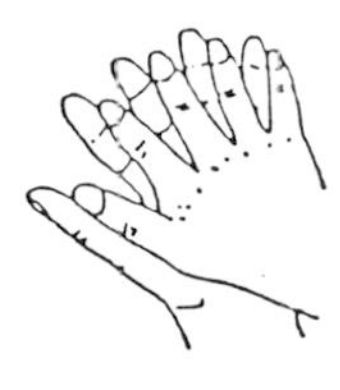

Surgical scrub
For a surgical scrub, the hands are washed with soap or detergent and the nails cleaned with a manicure stick under running water. The nails are then scrubbed using a sterile nail brush and the hands and forearms washed and disinfected using the following hygienic handwash technique. Repeat applications as necessary (four procedures can be completed in two minutes). After aqueous formulations dry the hands thoroughly on sterile towels. Separate towels to be used for hands and forearms.

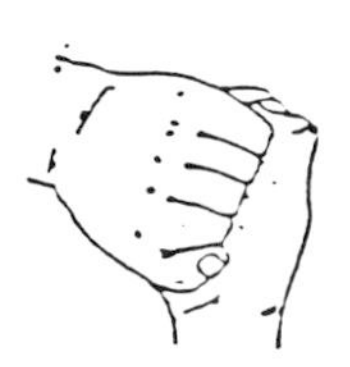
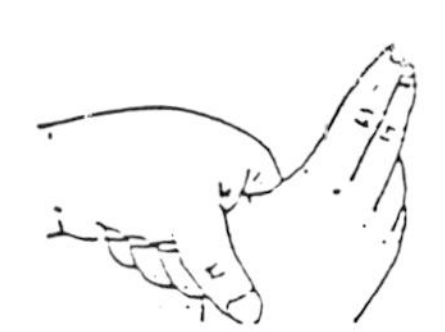
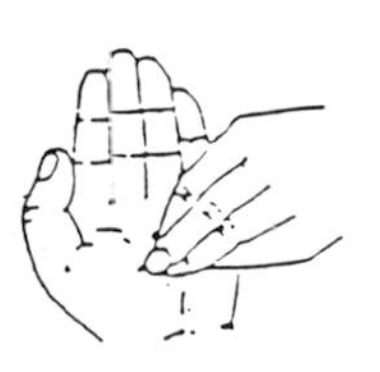

Hygienic hand disinfection

Aqueous formulations—wet hands and wrists apply 3–5 ml of the formulation to the cupped hands and wash hands one or more times using the following procedure, each step consisting of five strokes backwards and forwards. Rinse hands and dry thoroughly.

Alcoholic formulations — apply 3–5 ml of the formulation to the cupped hands and rub in using the following procedure.

Fig. 6.3. Handwashing and disinfection technique.

Table 6.4. Hand hygiene: options.

	Surgical scrub	Hygienic hand disinfection	Social hand wash
WHY	Use antiseptics to remove/destroy transient micro-organisms and substantially reduce detachable resident micro-organisms. A prolonged effect is required	Use antiseptics to remove or destroy all/most transient micro-organisms. A residual effect is preferable.	Use bar or liquid soap to render the hands socially clean and remove transient micro-organisms.
HOW	Scrape/brush nails and apply antiseptic soap or detergent, e.g. chlorhexidine or povidone iodine, to hands and forearms using a defined technique for a minimum of 2 min. Dry hands on sterile towel. Alternatively, clean hands with soap and water and apply two or more applications of an alcohol hand rub.	A thorough or defined wash for 15–30 s with an antiseptic soap or detergent e.g. chlorhexidine, povidone iodine or triclosan. Alternatively, apply an alcohol hand-rub.	A thorough wash with a cosmetically acceptable bar or liquid soap
WHEN	Prior to surgery or invasive procedures, at the discretion of the Infection Control Committee.	During outbreaks of infection, in high risk areas, e.g. isolation units and intensive care or at the discretion of the Infection Control Committee	All other hospital wards and departments

genic micro-organisms (56). As a more effective alternative, cleaning with soap and water followed by two applications of alcohol is highly effective (47). Nail-brushes often become contaminated with Gram-negative bacteria especially when stored moist or in disinfectants. A fresh sterile brush should be used for each surgical scrub. The nozzle of liquid soap/detergent dispensers should be cleaned daily to remove residues and the outside cleaned and dried. Disposable cartridge type dispensers and delivery systems are preferable.

There is a considerable difference of opinion as to which is the best methods of hand and forearm preparation and which formulation to use. The most effective agents for immediate and prolonged effect are those containing chlorhexidine and povidone–iodine (47). These bind well to the skin during the scrub and continue to suppress the growth of bacteria for at least 3 h. Alcohol does not mimic this residual effect but the immediate activity is greater and, as it is more penetrative, it achieves a similar effect.

Should the gloves become damaged and require changing during the course of the operation, blood and other adherent materials must be removed under a running tap, the gloves dried on a sterile towel and disinfected with alcohol. A second pair of gloves may then be donned over the damaged gloves. Some surgeons wear two pairs of gloves if the risk of glove puncture is high but there is little published material to substantiate the value of this procedure. A summary of the hand-washing/disinfection procedure is shown in Table 6.4.

Operation site

A rapid reduction in skin flora is required for the operation site and for the skin prior to an invasive procedure. The most suitable agents are those containing 60 to 80 per cent alcohol (ethanol or isopropanol) (57, 58). Provided the skin is clean, they work rapidly and evaporate leaving the surface dry. The addition of other agents such as dyes, 0.5 per cent chlorhexidine, 1 per cent iodine or 10 per cent povidone iodine (now preferred to iodine as it causes less skin reactions) may help to identify treated areas and may prolong the antimicrobial effect, but they do not appear to enhance significantly the immediate effect.

Antiseptics should be applied to the skin with friction using either a sterile gauze swab or the gloved hand (59). This is most effectively done in the theatre after any shaving or clipping and immediately prior to surgery. The area of application should exceed that of the incision or any possible extensions of it. If diathermy is used, it is important that the alcohol is allowed to dry and is prevented from pooling in the umbilicus, skin folds, or beneath the patient. Pooled alcohol and moist drapes have ignited during diathermy and caused serious flash burns (60).

The application of an effective antiseptic directly before surgery is of paramount importance. However, should the patient be a carrier of a multiresistant, highly virulent or communicable strain, or should they have a pre-existing site of infection elsewhere, a course of pre-operative baths or showers with an effective antiseptic soap or detergent, and the occlusion of the site, is recommended prior to surgery. Chlorhexidine, povidone iodine, hexachlorophane, and triclosan detergents or soaps have all been used for this purpose with some beneficial effect (61). A single pre-operative bath or shower before general surgery would appear to have little or no influence on the incidence of post-operative wound infection (62). However, a course of pre-operative baths or showers with chlorhexidine detergent prior to orthopaedic and vascular surgery (63, 64) has been shown to reduce the incidence of post-operative wound infection and so has bathing with chlorhexidine detergent before and after vasectomy (65).

As is the case with the selection of antiseptics, there is a considerable difference of opinion as to the most effective method of dealing with hair at the site of incision. It would appear that, local clipping or the application of depilatory creams is less damaging to the skin and reduces the risk of post-operative wound infection (66, 51). However, should shaving be necessary, it should be done as late as possible on the day of the operation (67). If hair is to be removed it should be done carefully so as to minimize the risk of skin damage which may induce microbial growth and impair the efficacy of the antiseptics applied immediately before surgery.

Garden soil and faeces may contain clostridial and other spores. These collect behind the nails and on damaged, creased, or folded skin. These spores are particularly tolerant to antiseptics and may prove difficult to remove. The use of nail brushes, detergents, and solvents will help to dislodge this dirt particularly from the nails but heavy faecal contamination of the thighs and buttocks may present a hazard of gas gangrene in patients with poor arterial supply. The use of prophylactic antibiotics substantially reduces this risk. The application of povidone-iodine compresses to the operation site for 30 min may also reduce the risk (68), particularly in patients who are undergoing amputation for diabetic gangrene.

Mucous membranes

There is little evidence in support of the use of antiseptics for the cleaning and disinfection of mucous membranes. Repeated applications of nasal creams containing antibiotics and antiseptics such as Bactroban (Mupirocin) and Naseptin (Neomycin 0.5 per cent and chlorhexidine 0.1 per cent) have been successful in clearing multi resistant and highly communicable strains of *Staph. aureus* from the noses of patients, theatre, and other staff (69) but recolonization often occurs after treatment.

Alcoholic formulations are usually too painful to apply to mucous membranes but have been used in the mouth prior to dental surgery. Antiseptics are soon diluted or inactivated by saliva and consequently have only a marginal effect. Chlorhexidine (0.2 per cent w/v chlorhexidine gluconate) mouth washes are available for oral hygiene and these have been used for the treatment and prevention of gingivitis following periodontal surgery.

The urethra normally has few commensal bacteria but is liable to become contaminated on passage of catheter or other instruments. Disinfection of the urethra before instrumentation is one of the important features of prophylaxis against infections of the urinary tract (70, 71). A 0.02 per cent chlorhexidine solution instilled into the urethra, or applied with lignocaine, will disinfect the meatus prior to cystoscopy or catherization. Cleaning with Savlodil (chlorhexidine 0.015 per cent w/v and cetrimide 0.15 per cent w/v) or a vaginal douche of 0.5 per cent povidone–iodine followed by the use of a 10 per cent povidone iodine gel can be used for the vaginal mucosa. Hibitane obstetric cream containing 1 per cent chlorhexidine gluconate maybe used as an antiseptic lubricant for application to the fingers and vulva prior to vaginal examinations.

References

1. Sterilization and disinfection of heat labile equipment (1986). Central Sterilising Club Working Party Report No. 2. [Available from Hospital Infection Research Laboratory.]
2. Gorman, S. P., Scott, E. M., and Russell, A. D. (1980). A review of antimicrobial activity, uses and mechanism of action of glutaraldehyde. *J. Appl. Bacteriol.*, **48**, 161–90.
3. Babb, J. R., Bradley, C. R., Deverill, C. E. A, Ayliffe, G. A. J., and Melikian, V. (1981). Recent advances in the cleaning and disinfection of fibrescopes. *J. Hosp. Infect.*, **2**, 329–40.
4. Burge, P. S. (1989). Occupational risk of glutaraldehyde. *Br. Med. J.*, **299**, 342.
5. Harrison, D. I. (1991). Control of substances hazardous to health (COSHH) regulations and hospital infection. *J. Hosp. Infect.*, February (suppl. A), **18**, 530–4.
6. Babb, J. R. (1990). Chemical disinfection and COSHH: Safe and effective work practices. *J. Sterile Services Management*, **1**, 10, 9–12.
7. Health and Safety Executive Occupational Exposure Limited Guidance Note EH (40) 91. Environmental Hygiene, London, HMSO, 1991.
8. Tyler, R., Ayliffe, G. A. J., and Bradley, C. R. (1990). Virucidal activity of disinfectants: Studies with the poliovirus. *J. Hosp. Infect.*, **15**, 339–45.
9. Hanson, P. J. V., Gor, D., Jeffries, D. J., and Collins, J. V. (1989). Chemical inactivation of HIV on surfaces. *Br. Med. J.*, **298**, 862–4.
10. Kurth, R., Werner, A., Barrett, N., and Dorner, F. (1986). Stability and inactivation of the human immunodeficiency virus. A review. *Aids Forschung.*, **II**, 601–8.
11. Department of Health and Social Security. Decontamination of equipment, linen or other surfaces contaminated with hepatitis B or human immunodeficiency virus. HN (87)1, London 1987.
12 Hardie, I. D. (1986). Mycobactericidal efficacy of glutaraldehyde based biocides. *J. Hosp. Infect.*, **6**, 436–8.
13. Hanson, P. J. V., Chadwick, M. V., Nicholson, G., Gaya, H., and Collins, J. V. (1988). Mycobactericidal resistance to disinfection in AIDS: whither infection control policies now. *Thorax*, **434**, 850P.
14. Babb, J. R., Bradley, C. R., and Ayliffe, G. A. J. (1980). Sporicidal activity of glutaraldehyde and hypochlorite and other factors influencing their selection for the treatment of medical equipment. *J. Hosp. Infect.*, **1**, 63–75.
15. Ayliffe, G. A. J., Babb, J. R., and Bradley, C. R. (1986). Disinfection of endoscopes. *J. Hosp. Infect.*, **7**, 295–9.
16. Keighley, M. R. B., Makuria, T., Moore, J., and Thompson, H. (1979). Preventing malignant—cell transfer during endoscopic brush cytology. *Lancet*, **i**, 298–9.
17. Duckworth, G. (1988). Non-tuberculous mycobacteria in gastro-intestinal biopsy specimens. *Lancet*, **ii**, 284.
18. Nye, K., Chadha, D. K., Hodgkin, P., Bradley, C. R., Hancox, J., and Wise, R. (1990). *Mycobacterium chelonei* isolation from broncho-alveolar lavage fluid and its practical implications. *J. Hosp. Infect.*, **16**, 257–61.
19. Allen, J. J., Allen, M. O., Olsen, M. M., *et al.* (1987). Pseudomonas infection of the biliary system resulting from the use of a contaminated endoscope. *Gastroenterology*, **92**, 759–63.
20. O'Connor, H. J., Steele, C. S., Price, J., Lincoln, C., and Axon, A. T. R. (1983). Disinfection of gastrointestinal fibrescopes—evaluation of the disinfectants Dettox and Gigasept. *Endoscopy*, **15**, 350–2.
21 Best, M., Sattar, S. A., Springthorpe, V. S., and Kennedy,

M.E. (1990). Efficacies of selected disinfectants against *Mycobacterium tuberculosis. J. Clin. Microbiol.*, **28**, 2234–9.
22. Bond, W.W., Favero, M.S., Petersen, N.J., and Ebert, J.W. (1983). Inactivation of hepatitis B virus by intermediate to high level disinfectant chemicals. *J. Clin. Microbiol.*, **18** 535–8.
23. Kobayoshi, H., Tsuzuki, M., Koshimizu, K., *et al.* (1984). Susceptibility of hepatitis B virus to disinfectants or heat. *J. Clin. Microbiol.*, **20**, 214–6.
24. Tyler, R. and Ayliffe, G.A.J. (1987). A surface test for virucidal activity of disinfectants: a preliminary study with herpes virus. *J. Hosp. Infect.*, **9**, 22–9.
25. Centers for Disease Control. (1985). Recommendations for preventing possible transmission of human T-lymphotrophic virus type III lymphadenopathy associated virus from tears. *MMWR*, **34**, 533–5.
26. Rutala, W.A. (1990). APIC guidelines for selection and use of disinfectants. *Am. J. Infect. Control*, **18**, 99–117.
27. Babb, J.R. and Bradley, C.R. (1991). The mechanics of endoscope disinfection. *J. Hosp. Infect.*, (suppl. A), **18**, 130–5.
28. O'Connor, H.J. and Axon, A.T.R. (1983). Gastrointestinal endoscopy: infection and disinfection. *Gut*, **24**, 1067–77.
29. Working party report—British Society of Gastroenterology. (1988). Cleaning and disinfection of equipment for gastrointestinal flexible endoscopes: interim recommendations of a Working Party. *Gut*, **29**, 1134–51.
30. Working party report—British Thoracic Society. (1989). Bronchoscopy and infection control. *Lancet*, **ii**, 270–1.
31. Babb, J.R., Bradley, C.R. and Ayliffe, G.A.J. (1984). Comparison of automated systems for the cleaning and disinfection of flexible fibreoptic endoscopes. *J. Hosp. Infect.*, **5**, 213–26.
32. Bradley, C.R. and Babb, J.R. (1987). Evaluation of Autodisinfector. *Acta Endoscopica*, **17**, 17–22.
33. Collins, B.J. (1988). The hospital environment: How clean should a hospital be? *J. Hosp. Infect.*, **11** (Suppl. A), 53–6.
34. Bloomfield, S.F. and Miles, G.A. (1979). The antibacterial properties of sodium dichloroisocyanurate and sodium hypochlorite formulations. *J. Appl. Bacteriol.*, **46**, 65–73.
35. Coates, D. (1985). A comparison of sodium hypochlorite and sodium dichloroisocyanurate products. *J. Hosp. Infect.*, **6**, 31–40.
36. Coates, D. and Wilson, M. (1989). Use of sodium dichloroisocyanurate granules for spills of body fluids. *J. Hosp. Infect.*, **13**, 241–51.
37. Coates, D. (1987). A comparison of the tarnishing and corrosive effects of sodium hypochlorite and sodium dichloroisocyanurate disinfectants. *J. Sterile Services Management*, **5**, 19.
38 Shanson, D. (1980). Question and answer: hypochlorite solutions. *J. Hosp. Infect.*, **1**, 88–9.
39. Naggington, J., Sutehall, G.M., and Whipp, P. (1983). Tonometer disinfection and viruses. *Br. J. Ophthalmol.*, **67**, 674–6.
40. Finch, W.E. (1953). A substitute for lysol. *Pharmaceutical J.*, **170**, 59–60.
41. Bloomfield, S.F. and Miller, E.A. (1989). A comparison of hypochlorite and phenolic disinfectants for disinfection of clean and soiled surfaces and blood spillages. *J. Hosp. Infect.*, **13**, 231–9.
42. Fujita, K., Lilly, H.A., Kidson, A., and Ayliffe, G.A.J. (1981). Gentamicin resistant *Pseudomonas aeruginosa* infection from mattresses in a burns unit. *Br. Med. J.*, **283**, 219–21.
43. Price, P.B. (1938). The bacteriology of normal skin: a new quantitative test applied to a study of the bacterial flora and the disinfectant action of mechanical cleansing. *J. Infect. Dis.*, **63**, 301–8.
44. Ayliffe, G.A.J. (1980). Review article. The effect of antibacterial agents on the flora of the skin. *J. Hosp. Infect.*, **1**, 111–24.
45. Lowbury, E.J.L. and Lilly, H.A. (1973). Use of four per cent chlorhexidine detergent solution (Hibiscrub) and other methods of skin disinfection. *Br. Med. J.*, **1**, 510–5.
46. Ayliffe, G.A.J., Babb, J.R., Davies J.G., and Lilly, H.A. (1988) Hand disinfection: a comparison of various agents in laboratory and ward studies. *J. Hosp. Infect.* **11**, 226–43.
47. Babb, J.R., Davies, J.G., and Ayliffe, G.A.J. (1991). Test procedure for evaluating surgical hand disinfection. *J. Hosp. Infect.*, (Suppl. B) **18**, 41–9.
48. Report of a combined working party of the Hospital Infection Society and British Society for Antimicrobial Chemotherapy. (1986). Guidelines for the control of epidemic methicillin resistant *Staphylococcus aureus. J. Hosp. Infect.*, **7**, 193–201.
49. Garner, J.S. and Favero, M.S. (1985). Guidelines for hand washing and environmental control. *Am. J. Infect. Control*, **14**, 110–29.
50. Reybrouck, G. (1986). Review article: Handwashing and hand disinfection *J. Hosp. Infect.*, **8**, 5–23.
51. Cruse, P.J.E. and Foord, R. (1973). A five year prospective study of 23 649 surgical wounds. *Arch. Surg.*, **107**, 206–10.
52. Dodds, R.D.A., Guy, P.J., Peacock, A.M., Duffy, S.R., Barker, S.G.E., and Thomas, M.H. (1988). Surgical glove perforation. *Br. J. Surg.*, **75**, 966–8.
53. Ayliffe, G.A.J., Babb, J.R., and Quoraishi, A.H. (1978). A test for 'hygienic' hand disinfection. *J. Clin. Path.*, **31**, 923–8.
54. Taylor, L.J. (1978). An evaluation of handwashing techniques 2. *Nursing Times*, **74**, 108–10.
55. Lowburry, E.J.L., Lilly, H.A., and Ayliffe, G.A.J. (1974). Preoperative disinfection of surgeons' hands. Use of alcoholic solutions and effects of gloves on skin flora. *Br. Med. J.*, **4**, 369–72.
56. Ojajarvi, J., Makela, P., and Rantasalo, I. (1977). Failure of hand disinfection with frequent handwashing: a need for prolonged field studies. *J. Hygiene*, **79**, 107–19.
57. Lowbury, E.J.L., Lilly, H.A., and Bull, J.P. (1964). Methods for disinfection of hands and operation sites. *Br. Med. J.*, **ii**, 531–6.
58. Davies, J., Babb, J.R., Ayliffe, G.A.J., and Wilkins, M.D. (1978). Disinfection of the skin of the abdomen. *Br. J. Surg.*, **65**, 855–8.
59. Lowbury, E.J.L., and Lilly, H.A. (1975). Gloved hands as applicator of antiseptic to operation sites. *Lancet*, **ii**, 153–6.
60. Department of Health. (1990). Health Circular. Ignition of spirit-based skin cleaning fluid by surgical diathermy setting fire to disposable surgical drapes resulting in patient burns. HC (Hazard) (90)25.
61. Davies, J., Babb, J.R., Ayliffe, G.A.J., Ellis, S.H. (1977). The effect on the skin flora of bathing with antiseptic solutions. *J. Antimicrob Chemother.*, **3**, 473–81.
62. Ayliffe, G.A.J., Noy, M.F., Babb, J.R., Davies, J.G., and Jackson, J. (1983). A comparison of pre-operative bathing with chlorhexidine detergent and non-medicated soap in the prevention of wound infection. *J. Hosp. Infect.*, **4**, 237–44.
63. Brandberg, A., and Andersson, I. (1980). Whole body disinfection by shower-bath with chlorhexidine soap. In *Problems in the control of hospital infection*, pp. 67–70. Royal Society of Medicine International Congress and Symposium Series No. 23. Academic Press and Royal Society of Medicine, London.
64. Brandberg, A., Holm, J., Hammarsten, J., and Schersten, T. (1980). Post-operative wound infections in vascular surgery—effect of pre-operative whole body disinfection by shower-bath with chlorhexidine swab. In *Problems in the control of hospital infection*, pp. 71–75. Royal Society of Medicine International Congress and Symposium Series No. 23. Academic Press and

Royal Society of Medicine, London.
65. Randall, P.E., Ganguli, L.A., Keaney, M.G.L., and Marcuson, R.W. (1985). Prevention of wound infection following vasectomy. *Br. J. Urol.*, **57**, 227–9.
66. Seropian, R. and Reynolds, B.M. (1971). Wound infections after pre-operative depilatory versus razor preparation. *Am. Surg.*, **121**, 251–4.
67. Alexander, J.W., Fischer, J.E., Boyajian, M., Palmquist, J., and Morris, M.J. (1983). The influence of hair removal methods on wound infections. *Arch. Surg.*, **118**, 347–52.
68. Ayliffe, G.A.J. and Lowbury, E.J.L. (1969). Sources of gas gangrene in hospital. *Br. Med. J.*, **ii**, 333–7.
69. Working Party Report. (1990). Revised guidelines for the control of epidemic methicillin-resistant *Staphylococcus aureus*. *J. Hosp. Infect.*, **16**, 351–77.
70. Miller, A., Gillespie, W.A., Linton, K.B., Slade, N., and Mitchell, J.P. (1958). Post-operative infection in urology. *Lancet*, **ii**, 608–12.
71. Falkiner, F.R., Ma, P., Murphy, D.M., Cafferkey, M.T., and Gillespie, W.A. (1983). Antimicrobial agents for the prevention of urinary tract infection in transurethral surgery. *J. Urol.*, **129**, 766–8.

Further reading

Altemeier, W.A., Burke, J.F., Pruitt, B.A., and Sandusky, W.R. (ed.) (1984) *Manual on control of infection in surgical patients.* Edited by American College of Surgeons. Lippincott, Philadelphia.
Ayliffe, G.A.J., Coates, D., and Hoffman, P.N. (ed.) (1984). *Chemical disinfection in hospitals.* Public Health Laboratory Service, 61 Colindale Avenue London. NW9 5EQ.
Lowbury, E.J.L., Ayliffe, G.A.J., Geddes, A.M., and Williams, J.D. (ed.) (1981). *Control of hospital infection: a practical handbook* (2nd edn; 3rd in preparation). Chapman & Hall, London.
Maurer, I.M. (ed.) (1985). *Hospital hygiene* (3rd edn). Edward Arnold, London.

7

Action of antibiotics and the development of antibiotic resistance

SHAHEEN MEHTAR

Introduction

The discovery of antimicrobials in the early 1940s has had a significant impact on infection-related morbidity and mortality. New and more effective antibacterial drugs are continually being discovered for use in clinical practice, and in response, bacteria invent more ingenious ways of surviving in the presence of these potent drugs. And so the battle goes on.

However, to understand the mode of action and development of resistance to antibacterial agents, it is important to become familiar with the relevant components of bacterial structure and metabolism.

Cell structure

The bacterium is surrounded by a protective *capsule* (Fig. 7.1) which is made up of protein or carbohydrate and is under DNA control. The cell envelope has two components: the *cell wall* and the *cytoplasmic membrane*, and lies within the capsule. A prominent *outer membrane* surrounds the cell wall of Gram-negative bacilli but is absent from Gram-positive bacteria; it may be naturally impermeable to certain antibacterials or become so by mutation. The cell wall has a mucopeptide layer (also called murein, or peptidoglycan), which is made up of polysaccharide strands interlinked with short peptide bonds. The *periplasmic space* lies between the mucopeptide strands and contains antibiotic degrading enzymes, such as beta-lactamases, the production of which varies with each species of bacterium.

The *cytoplasmic membrane* lies between the cell wall and the cytoplasm and is held against the cell wall by osmotic pressure. It contains penicillin binding proteins (PBP) which are target sites for the beta-lactam antibiotics (1). The cytoplasmic membrane of Gram-negative bacilli communicates with the periplasmic space and the outer membrane layer via *porins* which allow selective diffusion of nutrients such as carbohydrates and sugars and are also pathways for the entry of certain antibacterials into the cell. Both mutation and plasmids can alter the size of porins and decrease the permeability of antibiotics.

Bacterial protein and DNA synthesis

Deoxyribonucleic acid (DNA) is contained within the nucleus and has genetic control of all specific cellular proteins including enzymes. An intricate enzyme system exists which is crucial to bacterial protein synthesis. Many antibacterials attack different stages of protein synthesis.

An important enzyme, *DNA-dependent RNA polymerase* (transcriptase) co-ordinates the transfer of information from the DNA to the messenger RNA (m-RNA) (Fig. 7.2). On receiving the information m-RNA transcribes a sequence for the amino acid to act as a template for the synthesis of proteins. This length of amino acid sequencing is also known as a

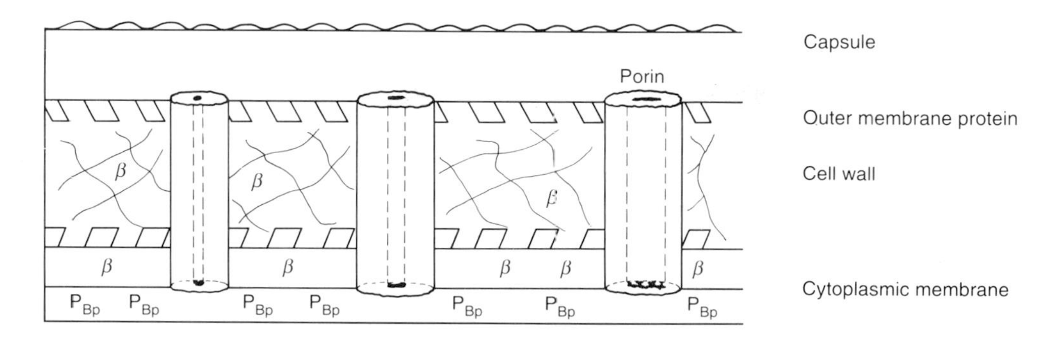

Fig. 7.1. Structure of Gram-negative bacteria cell wall (β = beta-lactamase).

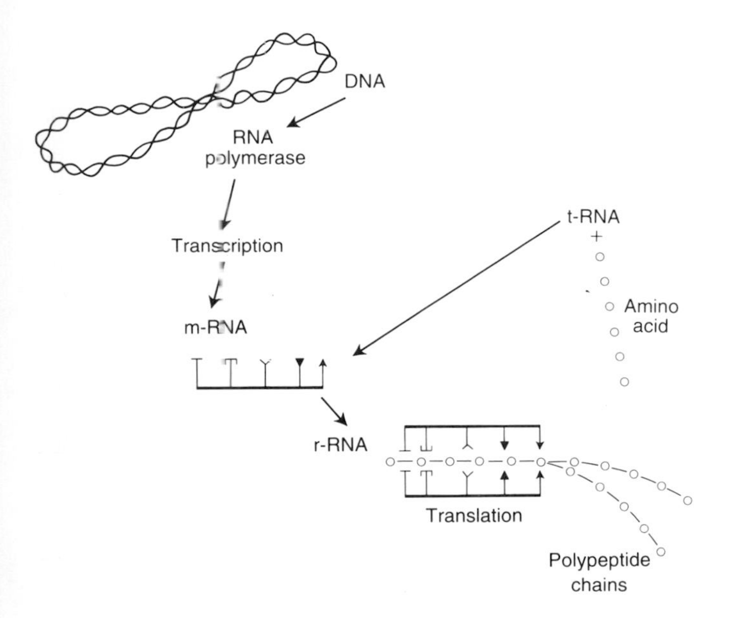

Fig. 7.2. Bacterial protein synthesis.

'codon'. *Transfer RNA* (t-RNA) acts as a carrier of amino acids and transports them to the appropriate sites on the m-RNA; the specific site for amino acid carriage is known as an 'anti-codon'. *Ribosomal RNA* (r-RNA) is crucial to the sequencing and acts as a matrix on which the amino acids join the polypeptide chain in a predetermined arrangement. The m-RNA picks up the amino acid chain and moves it along the t-RNA from a donor site (P site) to a recepient site (A site). This process is known as *translocation*. As the amino acid chain is passed along the template, the 'P site' becomes the 'A site' and so on. This is known as *transpeptidation*, and the whole process is known as *translation*.

Bacterial ribosomes are composed of 70 subunits (S) which differs from mammalian ribosomes which are 80 S. This crucial difference is the reason antibacterials effect only bacterial and not human cellular protein synthesis. Ribosomes may be altered by mutation or by genetic information.

Folic acid metabolism is essential for the synthesis of purine bases, which, in turn, forms an integral part of DNA synthesis. Alteration of the folic acid metabolic pathway can either be effected by natural or acquired mutation, or by genetic control.

Resistance to antimicrobial agents

Bacteria generally become resistant to antibiotics by one or more of the following mechanisms (Fig. 7.3): producing enzymes which degrade or inactivate the drug; alteration of the transport mechanism and cell penetration; alteration of the antibiotic target sites; or by alteration of the metabolic pathways within the cell.

These same mechanisms may be present *naturally*, or may be *acquired* from the same, or another species of bacterium.

Natural resistance

Bacteria may be naturally (or intrinsically) resistant to certain antibiotics because the drug cannot penetrate the organism, or because the necessary transport systems are absent (2). The natural production of beta-lactamase was noted in strains of *Staphylococcus aureus* even before penicillin was 'discovered'. This is understandable because the organisms had been exposed to the natural source of penicillin: a mould *Penicillium notatum*. Antibiotics like sodium fusidate and erythromycin do not penetrate the cell wall of Gram-negative bacilli, whilst other species, such as streptococci and anaerobic bacteria, lack the mechanism necessary to transport aminoglycosides across the cell wall. A small subpopulation of a particular species may mutate naturally (without the presence of antibiotics) but this phenomenon is relatively uncommon and is rarely significant clinically in the absence of antibiotic pressure.

Acquired resistance

Acquired resistance is much more relevant to clinical practice and is greatly influenced by antibiotic prescribing and usage. Acquired resistance to antimicrobials may occur by means of mutation, chromosomally mediated, or most commonly, plasmid mediated by R-plasmids.

Mutation

Mutation is the means by which the bacterium can change a function or amount of a critical target, transport system

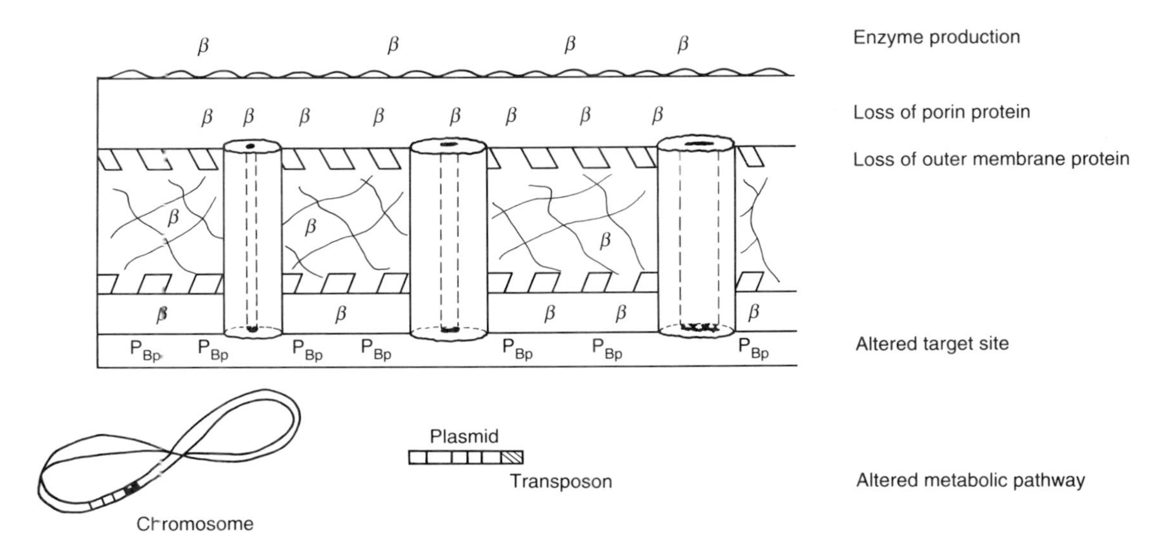

Fig. 7.3. Mechanisms of resistance to antimicrobials (β = beta-lactamase).

or antibiotic-degrading enzymes, e.g. beta-lactamases. The mutational effects on targets such as PBPs, ribosomal protein, DNA or its associated enzymes have serious therapeutic implications.

Genetic resistance

Genetic resistance is usually transmissible, and may be mediated via chromosomes or by plasmids (R-plasmids).

Chromosomal-mediated resistance

Genetic information, which may have originated as a plasmid or transposon, becomes integrated into the cell chromosome, and is passed on to its progeny during cell replication. The commonest example of this is the production of cephalosporinases (beta-lactamase) in *Enterobacter*, *Citrobacter*, and *Morganella* spp. These enzymes may be produced *constitutively* where the bacterium produces low levels of the enzyme continually and sometimes unnoticably, but production increases dramatically when confronted with certain classes of cephalosporins. Alternatively, the enzyme is only produced when the bacterium is faced with a cephalosporin. This *inducible* production is under genetic control and is based on a 'switch on, switch off' mechanism. Occasionally, under continuous cephalosporin pressure, (as seen in prolonged therapy) the gene coding for the enzyme production becomes 'de-repressed', in other words, the 'switch off' mechanism does not work and the organism then constantly produces a large amount of cephalosporinase irrespective of antibiotic stimulus. This is well-recognized in *Enterobacter* spp. but also occurs in other species (3).

Plasmid-mediated resistance

The most common form of antibiotic resistance encountered in hospital practice is plasmid-mediated. Plasmids are extrachromosomal pieces of DNA, capable of self-replication. They can exist independently within a cell or may become integrated into the bacterial chromosome. Plasmid-mediated resistance may be expressed as resistance to one antibiotic (or related group of antibiotics) or to multiple unrelated antibiotics. For example, resistance to ampicillin and to other penicillins may be linked with sulphonamide, trimethoprim, gentamicin, and possibly other aminoglycosides, chloramphenicol, tetracycline, etc. The ease with which these R-plasmids can acquire additional resistance and can be transferred from one bacterium to another, not only within the same species, but to other species as well, is a major cause for concern in hospital epidemiology (4).

Plasmids transfer from cell to cell by transformation, transduction or by conjugation.

Transformation: A piece of DNA is accidently acquired during cell replication and is expressed in the progeny.

Transduction: A plasmid is picked up by a bacteriophage (viruses which infect cellular DNA) and is passed to the next cell. Bacteriophages can also transmit chromosomal resistance.

Conjugation: Plasmids are passed during mating between cells via a sex pilus. (This is the commonest method of transferring plasmids.)

R-plasmids can affect outer membrane protein, porin size, modify target sites, produce modifying or degrading enzymes or can affect metabolic pathways. Further, in association with certain antibiotics, mutation may also be under plasmid control; a mutator plasmid has been reported in association with resistance to the quinolones (5).

Transposons

To complicate matters further, yet smaller pieces of DNA called *transposons* have the capability to link to a plasmid, hop from plasmid to plasmid, and even enter the chromosome without using the cell's recombination system. Transposons code for single or multiple antibiotic resistance and for other aspects of cellular metabolism.

Mode of action of antibiotics and mechanisms of resistance

Antimicrobials affecting the cell wall

The *beta-lactams* are the largest group of antibacterials used in clinical practice. This group includes the penicillins and cephalosporins, and all contain the beta-lactam ring.

Penicillins

Since production of the original penicillin, alteration in the chemical structure has imparted stability to gastric acid (e.g. penicillin V) and permitted expansion of the spectrum of activity by improving the stability to staphylococcal beta-lactamases. The beta-lactamase stable penicillins are known as isoxazolyl penicillins and include cloxacillin, flucloxacillin, and methicillin. In the UK methicillin is used for *in vitro* testing to establish the sensitivity of staphylococci to these antibiotics. There is total cross-resistance with the cephalosporins and therefore methicillin-resistant *Staphylococcus aureus* (MRSA) is by definition, resistant to all penicillins and cephalosporins (6, 7).

Ampicillin and amoxycillin have good activity against Gram-negative bacteria including *Haemophilus* sp. and *Neisseria* sp. but have variable activity against the coliforms. More recently pro-drugs have been introduced which are combined with ampicillin (bacampicillin, talampicillin, etc.) to overcome destruction by gastric acid and thereby increase serum levels.

The 'anti-pseudomonal' penicillins such as carbenicillin and the ureido penicillins (piperacillin, mezlocillin, and azlocillin) are stable to beta-lactamases produced by *Pseudomonas* spp. and other Gram-negative bacilli.

Beta-lactamase inhibitors, such as clavulanic acid, sulbactam, and tazobactam, are penicillins with little or no antibacterial activity of their own, and therefore are marketed in combination with penicillins and cephalosporins. These act by mopping up the beta-lactamases, thus allowing the beta-lactam antibiotics to reach the target sites. They are most active against certain plasmid mediated beta-lactamases, e.g. TEM (the initials of the patient from whose strain this enzyme was first isolated) but less so against the chromosomally mediated beta-lactamases such as the cephalosporinases. There are some differences in tissue stability and spectra of activity between the various inhibitors, but on the whole the clinical outcome is similar.

Cephalosporins

Cephalosporins have developed along similar lines to the penicillins. The terms commonly used are 'first, second, and third generation' cephalosporins. These relate to an increase in spectrum by improved stability to the beta-lactamases produced by Gram-negative bacilli. The earlier cephalosporins were more susceptible to destruction but had better activity against Gram-positive cocci, whilst succeeding generations have been more stable to destruction by beta-lactamases and thus more active against Gram-negative bacteria including *Pseudomonas aeruginosa*. Some have activity against anaerobic bacteria.

More recent developments have included the cephamycins (cefoxitin), latamoxef (moxalactam), carbapenems (imipenem), and the penems; the latter are under clinical trial at present. Of these, imipenem has the broadest spectrum with activity against Gram-negative, Gram-positive, and anaerobic bacteria. Enterococci are uniformly resistant to all the cephalosporins marketed to date, but the most recently developed cephalosporins appear to be more promising.

All beta-lactam antibiotics have a similar mode of action and interfere with cell-wall synthesis. Inhibition of bacterial growth takes place by a direct action on penicillin-binding proteins (PBPs), which leads to growth inhibition, possibly followed by autolysis by endogenous enzymes. The PBPs vary in number and are species specific. They have been most extensively studied in *Escherichia coli* where seven PBPs have been identified. PBP 1a and b are involved in cell elongation; PBP 2 give shape to the bacterium; PBP 3 is associated with cell division. The function of the others is as yet undetermined but they are known to be essential for cell integrity. The beta-lactams selectively act on one or more PBP and therefore alteration of one PBP does not always impart resistance to all beta-lactams, but may effect those acting on the same PBP.

Penicillins essentially act on actively multiplying cells. They do not effect bacteria lacking in cell walls, e.g. spheroplast (cells with deficient cell-walls) or *Mycoplasma* spp. Occasionally, tolerant strains are found during therapy; these strains are inhibited but not killed and may re-emerge after withdrawal of the antibiotic.

Mechanisms of resistance (Table 7.1)

Natural resistance is seen in *Ps. aeruginosa* where certain beta-lactams, such as the penicillins (except the anti-pseudomonal penicillins) and the first and second generation cephalosporins cannot penetrate the cell wall (2).

Acquired resistance is much more relevant to clinical practice and may be due to the following mechanisms.

1. Mutation leading to:
   (a) Alteration of PBPs, thus altering the target sites.

   (b) Decreased permeability due to loss of outer membrane protein and loss of porin proteins. These changes may also effect other beta-lactamases using similar pathways into the cell.
2. Production of beta-lactamases:
   (a) Chromosomally mediated beta-lactamases are usually cephalosporinases, but some penicillinases may also be produced by this mechanism. Some cephalosporins induce more beta-lactamase production than others. Examples of good inducers are cefoxitin, imipenem, and clavulanic acid, while piperacillin and sulbactam are poor inducers of cephalosporinases.

   (b) Plasmid-mediated resistance (R-plasmids) is the commonest form of resistance encountered in clinical practice amongst Gram-negative bacilli. Changes due to R-plasmids are associated with a high level of resistance (64-fold or greater resistant than sensitive strains of the same species). The most common enzyme effected is TEM which effects

Table 7.1. Mechanism of resistance to beta-lactam antibiotics.

Type of resistance	Mechanism	Organism	Antibiotic affected
Natural	Liability to permeate the cell wall	*Ps. aeruginosa*	Most penicillins except anti-pseudomonal pencillins
Acquired	(A) Decreased permeability of the cell wall	Enterobacteriaceae *Ps. aeruginosa*	Imipenem, ceftazidime, other 3rd generation cephalosporins
	(B) Mutation alteration of penicillin binding proteins	*Staph. aureus*	Methicillin (all penicillins and cephalosporins)
		Strep. pneumoniae	Penicillin
		Streptococci (Gp. D and viridans)	Penicillin
		N. gonorrhoeae	Penicillin
		H. influenzae	Broad spectrum beta-lactams
		Ps. aeruginosa	3rd gen. cephalosporins and penicillins
		S. marcescens	3rd gen. cephalosporins and penicillins
	(C) Beta-lactamase production (i) Chromosome mediated (a) Cephalosporinase	*Enterobacter*	Penicillins and cephalosporins except imipenem
		Citrobacter serratia	Not inhibited by clavulanic acid
	(b) Broad spectrum beta-lactamases	*Ps. aeruginosa* *Proteus* (indole +ve) *Enterobacteriaceae*	
	(ii) Plasmid-mediated (TEM commonest)	Enterobacteriaceae *H. influenzae* *N. gonorrhoeae* *Ps. aeruginosa*	Penicillin and cephalosporins inhibited by clavulanic acid

penicillins rather than cephalosporins. This resistance may be linked to other antibiotics or groups of antibiotics such as aminoglycosides, sulphonamides and trimethoprim. R-plasmid mediated beta-lactamases may occur naturally but are usually acquired under antibiotic pressure.

Glycopeptides

Vancomycin, and now teicoplanin, are glycopeptides which have specific activity against Gram-positive organisms, both aerobic and anaerobic, usually independent of resistance to other antibiotics. These antibiotics act by binding irreversibly to the bacterial cell-wall, inhibiting its synthesis and lead to cell death due to autolysis.

Gram-negative bacteria are naturally resistant due to the lack of permeability of the outer membrane and porins. Gram-positive cocci, although rarely resistant to the glycopeptides, may be found to be tolerant, that is they will grow in the presence of the drug. High-level resistance in enterococci has been described recently (8), attributed to plasmid-mediated resistance and associated with high-level gentamicin resistance.

Peptides

Peptides such as bacitracin act by specific inhibition of the second stage of cell-wall synthesis. They may also effect the cytoplasmic membrane causing leakage of the cytoplasm. Bacitracin is too toxic for systemic use and is restricted to topical use only.

Polymyxins

Polymyxins such as colistin, interfere with the outer and cytoplasmic membranes of Gram-negative bacteria leading to leakage of the cytoplasm. Clinically, they were used selectively in severe pseudomonas infection but have been withdrawn in favour of less toxic agents. The main use has been in *Ps. aeruginosa* chest infection in immunocompromised patients where the compound was nebulised into the respiratory tract. None the less, they are effective topical antibacterials because resistance to them is slow to develop.

Gram-positive organisms are naturally resistant to polymyxins, possibly because of the absence of the outer membrane. Resistance in Gram-negative bacilli is by alteration of the outer membrane protein which reduces permeability of the drug but this is rarely encountered.

Antimicrobials affecting protein synthesis

Aminoglycosides and aminocyclitols

(Streptomycin, gentamicin, netilmycin, tobramycin, kanamycin, amikacin, etc.). This is another large group of antibiotics commonly used in clinical practice because of their excellent spectrum of activity against Gram-negative organisms. There is reasonable activity against *Staph. aureus* but a distinct lack of activity against streptococci and anaerobic bacteria. The aminoglycosides are electrostatically bound to the cell membrane at specific sites (9), and are actively transported into the cell by an aerobic, energy-dependent, transfer system. The binding does not occur in streptococci and these antibiotics are not transported into anaerobic organisms. Thus, when aminoglycosides are used in combination with antibacterials which act on the cell wall, e.g. beta-lactams or glycopeptides a synergistic effect is demonstrable because penetration into the cell is facilitated.

Streptomycin has been extensively studied and is a good example of the mode of action of the group. Streptomycin binds to the 30 S ribosome and leads to miscoding of the m-RNA codon so that the wrong amino acids are incorporated; a further effect may be the detachment of the ribosome from m-RNA.

Spectinomycin is an aminocyclitol with a similar mode of action to the aminoglycosides, and marked activity against *Neisseria gonorrhoeae*, which is not effected by resistance of that organism to other antibiotics.

Mechanisms of resistance

Natural resistance is found in streptococci and anaerobic organisms which lack the enzyme system required for transport (10).

Acquired resistance may be due to:

(a) Alteration of the outer membrane, which decreases permeability into the cell, and is usually reflected as resistance to all aminoglycosides.

(b) Mutational alteration of the 30 S ribosome, which may result in resistance to all aminoglycosides. Resistance to streptomycin is a single-step high-level mutation, but resistance to the other members of this group may take longer to develop.

(c) Plasmid-mediated acquisition of enzymes, which modify aminoglycosides so that they are unable to act on the ribosomes. There are ten or more enzymes which modify different aspects of the molecule and effect the various aminoglycosides differently. These are phosphorylating, adenylating, and acetylating enzymes. They are found predominantly in Gram-negative bacilli, but may be also found in Gram-positive cocci. More enzymes affect gentamicin then amikacin. There is total cross-resistance between gentamicin and tobramycin, and between kanamycin and amikacin.

(d) Transposon-mediated acquisition of code for phosphorylating and adenylating enzymes. The transposons can transfer between plasmids or the chromosome. Some transposons code for specific (Tn5), while others code for multiple aminoglycoside resistance (Tn21) (11). Resistance mechanisms are the same for spectinomycin as for the aminoglycosides and may be mutational, plasmid mediated, or chromosomal.

Chloramphenicol

Chloramphenicol is a bacteriostatic drug with a truly wide spectrum of activity covering aerobic Gram-positive, Gram-negative and anerobic bacteria. Its clinical use has been superseded by other, more potent and safer bacteriocidal antibiotics, but it is still useful for specific indications, e.g. enteric fever and bacterial meningitis.

Chloramphenicol inhibits protein synthesis by binding to the 50 S ribosomal subunit, which is essential for transpeptidation at the acceptor site. Actively multiplying cells die rapidly, whilst dormant cells survive for a longer period of time and may regrow after withdrawal of the drug.

(a) *Natural resistance* to chloramphenicol is rarely found apart from *Pseudomonas* sp.

(b) Resistance is acquired by plasmid mediated production of degrading enzymes, acetyl transferases found in a variety of enterobacteriaceae and *H. influenzae*. The enzyme may be constitutive or inducible: both give rise to a high level of resistance. Multiple resistance to chloramphenicol, associated with ampicillin, trimethoprim and sulphonamides, has been reported in approximately 5 per cent of *Haemophilus* spp. isolates (12). Transposons coding for this enzyme have also been identified in *H. influenzae*; decreased permeability by the same mechanism has been reported in *Ps. aeruginosa* and *E. coli* (11).

Macrolides and Lincosamides

Macrolides and Lincosamides are a group of drugs which include erythromycin, and lincomycin (clindamycin) respectively. Recently, there has been renewed interest in the macrolides and clinical trials are in progress with new compounds which are thought to have a superior spectrum of antibacterial activity and a reduced incidence of the common side-effects of abdominal pain and nausea. The spectrum of antibacterial activity extends mainly to the Gram-positive bacteria (except enterococci in the case of lincomycin) and to the anaerobic organisms; they lack activity against Gram-negative bacilli except *H. influenzae*. Macrolides have additional activity against *Mycoplasma* spp. and *Legionella pneumophila*.

Macrolides and lincosamides act by binding to the 50 S subunit of the bacterial ribosome; the difference is that macrolides bind competitively to the donor site thus interfering with translocation, whilst lincomycin and clindamycin affect the peptide initiation stage.

Gram-negative organisms are naturally resistant to erythromycin because the cell wall is impermeable. There may be cross-resistance between erythromycin and lincomycin in *Staph. aureus* and other Gram-positive species. 'Dissociated resistance' is a laboratory phenomenon whereby lincomycin/clindamycin appears resistant when tested in the presence of erythromycin, yet is sensitive when tested alone. Mutational resistance is found (in streptococci) associated with modified target sites (50 S ribosomes). Plasmid-mediated resistance to lincomycin has been reported in *B. fragilis* (13). Plasmid-mediated resistance contributes to macrolide resistance by modifying the target sites.

Fucidic acid

Fucidic acid has marked activity against *Staphylococci* spp. but little activity against other Gram-positive or Gram-negative bacteria. Although it is chemically related to cephalosporin C, there is a marked contrast: it inhibits protein synthesis by interfering with translocation.

The cell walls of Gram-negative bacteria are impermeable to fucidic acid. Resistance in Gram-positive cocci is usually by mutational alteration of the target sites, or is plasmid mediated as reported by Bennett and Shaw (14). Despite usage over many years, the emergence of resistance has been low (4 per cent). This is due partly to the use of this antibiotic in combination with penicillins and partly because of targeted antistaphylococcal therapy.

Tetracyclines

Tetracyclines (chlortetracycline, tetracycline, oxytetracycline, minocycline, etc.) are a group of antibacterial agents with bacteriostatic action which, like chloramphenicol have largely been superceded by more effective antibiotics. Resistance to the tetracyclines has developed amongst both Gram-positive and Gram-negative bacteria and has rendered them less effective in clinical practice. However, they are still effective in chlamydial, mycoplasma, and rickettsial infections. *Ps. aeruginosa* and *Proteus mirabilis* are resistant to tetracycline whilst anaerobic organisms have a variable sensitivity.

Tetracyclines act by binding to the 30 S ribosomal subunit and inhibit enzyme binding of the t-RNA adjacent to the receptor site. They also alter the cytoplasmic membrane, this leads to leakage of the cytoplasm.

Resistance to tetracyclines may be due to a decreased uptake by the bacterium. However, the main mechanism of resistance is plasmid-mediated, usually associated with other antibiotics. Resistance to tetracyclines has been found on transposons (Tn10); chromosomal resistance, linked with erythromycin, chloramphenicol, and spectinomycin, has also been reported in *N. gonorrhoeae* (15).

Mupirocin

Mupirocin is a unique, topical antibiotic recently marketed for the treatment of Gram-positive aerobic infections. It is particularly effective in the eradication of MRSA from carrier sites. No cross-resistance with other major antibiotics has been reported and it is recommended for topical use. It acts by binding reversibly with the enzyme responsible for the incorporation of iso-leucine, thus inhibiting protein synthesis. Chromosomal-mediated resistance in *Staph. aureus* has been reported by Rahman *et al.* (16).

Nitrofurans

Nitrofurans (nitrofurantoin) has been used mainly in the treatment of urinary tract infection. This antibiotic has a reasonable spectrum of activity against Gram-negative and Gram-positive organisms, except *P. mirabilis*. The mode of action is not entirely clear but it is believed to inhibit a number of essential enzymes involved in DNA synthesis, and may even be implicated in DNA damage. Resistance is developed and is due to alteration of the target site, (by mutation or R-plasmids).

Antimicrobials affecting DNA synthesis and associated enzymes

Quinolones

The quinolones are a group of antibiotics which have aroused much interest in recent years. The older members of this group, like nalidixic acid, were used mainly for the treatment of Gram-negative urinary tract infections. However, the newer 4-fluoro quinolones (ciprofloxacin, enoxacin, norfloxacin, pefloxacin, etc.) are very potent Gram-negative antibacterials with some activity against staphylococci, less so against streptococci, and thus far lack activity against anaerobic organisms.

The mode of action of these antibiotics is mainly to inhibit DNA replication by affecting the DNA gyrase (topoisomerases) which are required for supercoiling the strands the DNA. RNA and protein synthesis are secondarily inhibited. There is variable cross-resistance within this class of drugs.

Gram-positive bacteria are not susceptible to nalidixic acid, but the newer quinolones are better able to penetrate the bacterial cells. Mutational resistance by alteration of the target site, the DNA gyrase, is the most frequent mechanism of resistance and is under chromosomal control. Another mechanism whereby bacteria become resistant is alteration of the permeability by loss of the outer membrane proteins (17). The latter has been reported in *Ps. aeruginosa* but to date, no plasmid-mediated resistance to the 4-fluoro-quinolones has been reported.

Rifampicin

Rifampicin is used mainly as anti-tuberculous therapy but is an excellent antistaphylococcal agent in its own right. Apart from activity against Gram-positive organisms, both aerobic and anaerobic, it also has activity against Gram-negative bacteria including *Brucella* spp. It acts by inhibiting RNA polymerase, thus interfering with DNA transcription.

Resistance to rifampicin is by a one-step mutation resulting in alteration of the target site, DNA polymerase. For this reason it is better to use rifampicin in combination with other antibiotics.

Metronidazole

Metronidazole is a widely used drug with activity against anaerobic bacteria, but no activity against aerobic bacteria. It also has activity against *Trichomonas vaginalis* and some activity against *Treponema pallidum*. Despite many years of clinical use, the mode of action is not entirely clear but it is thought that it inhibits DNA synthesis (18). A few metronidazole resistant strains of *B. fragilis* have been reported (19), but its mechanism of resistance was not reported.

Sulphonamides

Sulphonamides were one of the earliest antibacterial agents introduced into clinical practice, but appear to have outlived their usefulness as single agents. Sulphamethoxazole is now used in combination with trimethoprim as co-trimoxazole. They are bacteriostatic drugs with activity against all Gram-positive cocci except enterococci. Most Gram-negative bacilli are sensitive to the sulphonamides, but the susceptibility varies with, and within, each species.

This group of antibiotics act by substrate competition with para-amino-benzoic acid, which is an essential metabolite for folic acid synthesis and thus, indirectly, the purine bases and ultimately DNA synthesis. It is possible that there may be a further site of action on dihydrofolate reductase.

Some streptococci are naturally resistant to sulphonamides because the metabolic pathway is inappropriate for the action of the drug. Gram-negative bacilli become resistant by altering the metabolic pathway, either under control of the chromosome or plasmids, or of a transposon (Tn21).

Trimethoprim

Trimethoprim has long been used in clinical practice, either alone or in combination with sulphamethoxazole. The spectrum of activity of trimethoprim covers Gram-positive cocci (except entercocci, which is variable), Gram-negative bacilli except *Helicobacter pylori* and *Morexella catarrhalis*. It is still widely used in the treatment of urinary tract and chest infections.

Trimethoprim interferes with dihydrofolate reductase, and thus indirectly in the essential enzyme pathway involved in the synthesis of DNA; synergy with sulphonamides is due to blocking of different pathways of folic acid metabolism.

Intrinsic resistance is due either to poor penetration or to a folate reductase with reduced sensitivity to trimethoprim. The latter is seen in *Morexella*, *Neisseria*, and *Brucella* spp.

Chromosomally mediated and plasmid-mediated resistance acts by altering di-hydrofolate reductase with decreased sensitivity to trimethoprim. Resistance carried on transposons is common.

Summary

Emergence of resistance to antimicrobials affects patients in several ways:

(a) The antibiotics required to treat multiply-resistant bacteria are usually more potent, costly and require a parenteral route of administration.

(b) The morbidity, and occasionally mortality, is increased with multiply-resistant bacteria, particularly those involved in nosocomial infections.

(c) The hospital environment becomes colonized with resistant bacteria and the spread of these bacteria is further increased via clinical and non-clinical equipment.

(d) Hospital stay is prolonged, and occasionally further surgical intervention is required.

Rational prescribing of the antibiotic specifically targeted at suspected or proven bacteria, depending on the site of infection, helps to reduce the emergence of resistance. High dosage, short-duration antibiotic prescriptions for prophylaxis and therapy is recommended in both situations. However, it is particularly important that patients are treated on clinical grounds rather than on bacteriology reports (which should be considered as guide-lines should problems arise).

The rotation of antibiotics groups is one of the ways of maintaining antibiotic susceptibility patterns by reducing pressure on the various mechanisms of resistance. A close liaison between the Microbiology Department and the clinicians on antimicrobial susceptibility and advice on alternative antibiotic usage (when necessary) is also useful in retarding the emergence of antibiotic resistance.

References

1. Tomasz, A. (1979). From penicillin-binding proteins to the lysis and death of bacteria. A 1979 view. *Rev. Infect. Dis.*, **1**, 434–67.
2. Bryan, L.E. (1988). General Mechanisms of resistance to antibiotics *J. Antimicrob. Chemother.*, **22**, suppl. A, 1–5.
3. Saunders, C.C. (1983). Novel resistance selected by the new expanded spectrum cephalosporins: A concern. *J. Infect. Dis.*, **145**, 585–9.
4. Casewell, M. (1982). The role of multiple resistant coliforms in hospital acquired infection. In *Recent advances in infection*, Vol. 2 (ed. D.S. Reeves and A.M. Geddes), pp. 231–50. Churchill Livingstone, Edinburgh.
5. Courvalin, P. 1990 Plasmid-mediated 4- quinolone resistance: a real or apparent absence? *Antimicrob. Ag. Chemother.*, **34**, 681–4.
6. Shanson, D.C. (1981). Antibiotic-resistant staphylococcus aureus. *J. Hosp. Infect.*, **2**, 11–36.
7. Thompson, R.L. and Wenzel, R.A. (1982). International recognition of methicillin-resistant strains of *Staphylococcus aureus*. *Ann. Int. Med.*, **97**, 925–6.
8. Uttley, A.H.C., Collins, H., Naidoo, J., and George, R.C. (1988). Vancomycin resistant enterococci, *Lancet*, **i**, 57–8.
9. Bryan, L.E., and Kwan, S. (1983). Roles of ribosomal binding, membrane potential and electron transport in bacterial uptake of streptomycin and gentamicin. *Antimicrob. Ag. Chemother.*, **23**, 835–45.
10. Bryan, L.E. (1984). Mechanism of action of aminoglycoside antibiotics. In *New dimensions in antimicrobial therapy* (ed. In Rook, R.K., and M.E. Sande), pp. 17–36. Churchill Livingstone, New York.
11. Calos, M.P. and Miller, J.H. (1980). Transposable elements. *Cell*, **20**, 579–95.
12. Mehtar, S., and Aminafshar, S. (1983). Antibiotic Resistance amongst various types of haemophilus species. *J. Antimicrob. Chemother.*, **12**, 565–70.
13. Privitera, G., Fayolle, F., and Sebald, M. (1981). Resistance to tetracycline, erythromycin and clindamycin in the *Bacteroides fragilis* group: inducible versus constitutive tetracycline resistance. *Antimicrob. Ag. Chemother.*, **20**, 314–20.
14. Bennett, A.D., and Shaw, W.V. (1983). Resistance to fusidic acid in *E. coli* mediated by the Type 1 variant of chloramphenicol acetyl transferase. A plasmid-encoded mechanism involving antibiotic binding. *Biochem. J.*, **215**, 29–38.
15. Report of a WHO Scientific Group. (1978). *Neisseria gonorrhoae* and gonococcal infections. Ser. No. 616.
16. Rahman, M., Noble, W.C., and Cookson, B. (1989). Transmissible mupirocin resistance in staphylococcus aureus. *Epidemiol Infect.*, **102**, 261–70.
17. Legakis, N.A., Tzouvelekis, L.S., Makris, A., and Kotsifakis, H. (1989). Outer membrane alteration in multi- resistant mutants of Pseudomonas aeroginosa selected by ciprofloxacin. *Antimicrob. Ag. Chemother.*, **33**, 124–7.
18. Edwards, D.I. (1979). Mechanisms of antimicrobial action of metronidazole. *J. Antimicrob. Chemother.*, **5**, 499–502.
19. Ingham, H.R., Eaton, S., Venables, C.W., and Adams, P.C. (1978). Bacteroides fragilis resistance to metronidazole after long term therapy. *Lancet*, **i**, 214.

8

General principles of antibiotic prophylaxis

ERIC W. TAYLOR

Introduction

Surgeons of all specialties will recognize infection as one of the most common complications after an operation, and in many specialties it is one of the most frequent factors in the death of a patient post-operatively. Audit has become an essential requirement in surgical practice in the UK and infection is catalogued in all post-operative audit systems. The value of audit has been demonstrated in Chapter 1 of this book where the results of 100 000 operations over many years have been carefully analysed. Few surgeons can expect to accumulate data of this extent, but each must be aware of the incidence of infection in his own surgical practice, and it is the responsibility of all surgeons to seek to ensure that the incidence of post-operative complications is kept to the minimum. There are many factors which influence the occurrence of post-operative complications, paramount amongst which is surgical technique. Many of the factors which influence endogenous and exogenous contamination have been reviewed in Chapters 2 and 3, and the effect of that contamination is detailed in Chapter 5. All surgeons should strive to reduce their own infection rate but this requires detailed audit as well as attention to surgical technique.

Audit is a complicated and multifaceted exercise embracing analysis of activity, methods, resources, and outcome. Post-operative infection and other complications are part of the outcome criteria of audit, and it is no longer sufficient to review only those complications which occur whilst the patient remains in hospital. In one recent series of 1242 patients 49 (59 per cent) of the 83 post-operative infections only became apparent after the patient had returned home (1). Increasingly there is economic pressure to keep patients in hospital for the shortest period of time, commensurate with safety, and it is not uncommon for clean or clean-contaminated operations to be done as day cases, or with very short periods of in-patient hospitalization. It is frequently on the 7th to 10th day post-operatively that infection presents, utilizing expensive community medical and nursing resources.

Cost of infection

Infection costs lives and it costs money; it causes the patient a great deal of discomfort and inconvenience at the time and may necessitate repeated visits to hospital and additional operations. The patient loses income and there is a considerable cost to the National Health Service or in the society responsible for funding health care. It has been estimated that each infected patient will need to spend an average of four days in hospital (2), and if only one per cent of the 3.3 million operations performed under the National Health Service in the United Kingdom each year became infected, this would mean an additional 132 000 bed days. If the cost of a bed day is now £150 the cost of this aspect of infection is £19.8 million. There are few operations with an infection rate as low as one per cent, and this calculation does not quantify the cost of district nurses time, dressings, etc. once the patient has left hospital. Other, perhaps more realistic, estimates have suggested that the incidence of post-operative nosocomial infection is 5 per cent and that the average increased hospital stay is 7.4 days (3), leading to a cost in excess of £183 million per annum. In 1986 the cost of post-operative infection was estimated at £111 million (4).

Factors influencing post-operative infection

Infection will not occur if bacteria are denied access to a wound. But no matter how strenuously we attempt to exclude bacteria, contamination does occur, either from within the patient (endogenous) or from the environment (exogenous). The degree of contamination of the operation site is the major factor determining the classification of the risk of post-operative infection, and the relationship between bacterial contamination and the incidence of post-operative infection has been dealt with in Chapter 5.

The ability of the body to resist a bacterial challenge is the other major determinant of the incidence of post-operative infection. Despite the pre-operative preparation of the patient, and the precautions taken in the operating theatre, some bacteria gain access to the tissues either from the external environment or from within the patient. A bacterial challenge which would be resisted by most fit, healthy patients may be sufficient to lead to infection, or to sepsis, in a patient with reduced resistance. Factors which reduce the ability of the body to resist bacterial challenge are listed in Table 8.1. Many of the factors relate to the coincident medical condition of the patient and cannot be altered at the time of operation, but there are a number of factors over which the surgeon does have control. Many of these factors have been reviewed in Chapters 4 and 13. However, two are of particular relevance to the use of antibiotic prophylaxis.

Table 8.1. Factors reducing host resistance.

Patient dependent factors	Surgeon dependant factors
Extreme old age	Tissue oxygenation
Obesity	Foreign body implantation
Diabetes	Haemostasis
Cirrhosis	Prolonged pre-operative hospitalization
Malignancy	Prolonged operation time
Malnutrition	Blood transfusion
Leucopaenia	
Steroid therapy	
Antimitotic therapy	

Foreign bodies

As has been demonstrated in Chapter 5 the absolute bacterial count contaminating a wound is an important determinant of whether contamination will lead to infection, yet even more important is the presence of a foreign body. Elek and Conen demonstrated the importance of a foreign body when they showed that 10^6 *Staphylococcus aureus* organisms had to be injected subcutaneously before an abscess would develop in fit healthy individuals, whereas only 10^3 organisms were required when a foreign body was present—in their experiment a silk suture (5). A prosthetic implant is a foreign body and a much lower level of bacterial contamination is necessary to cause infection if a prosthesis is present (6). There has been an increasing awareness of *Staph. epidermidis* or coagulase-negative staphylococci (CNS) as a pathogen causing infection around implanted prostheses. These organisms can hydrolyse the surface of polymers from which prostheses are made, can use the plastic as a food source (7) and have been shown to produce an extracellular slime which may alter bacterial adherence to the prosthesis (8). In addition to CNS a number of other organisms have been shown to be capable of producing a glycocalyx or slime—*Streptococcus viridans*, *Staph. aureus*, *Pseudomonas* spp., and the slime producing strains of these organisms are associated with implant infections to a much greater degree than the non-slime-producing strains (9). Whether this difference is because the slime increases the adherence of the organisms to the prosthesis, or because the biochemistry of the slime is such that it reduces the ability of antibiotics to penetrate the slime and to kill the organisms, remains unclear (10). The slime is known to affect host responses by inhibiting chemotaxis, bacterial engulfment and the oxidation response of the circulating phagocytes (11).

Blood transfusion

Blood transfusion also appears to alter host resistance. The loss of blood during an operation will clearly alter the pharmacokinetics of an antibiotic given for prophylaxis, but blood replacement *per se* may influence the incidence of post-operative infection.

Blood transfusion is expensive and the risks of transfusion reactions, as well as the transfer of hepatitis and the human immunodeficiency virus (HIV) are well known. Intra-operative blood transfusion may reduce the resistance of the body to tumour growth and may increase the incidence of tumour recurrence after operations for malignancy (12–15). Blood transfusion has been used before renal transplantation to reduce the incidence of rejection (16), and evidence is growing that blood transfusion reduces the body's host defence and leads to a higher incidence of post-operative infection (17–21). This change would appear to involve pre-operative as well as perioperative blood transfusion and Spence *et al.* have shown that elective surgery can be done safely in patients with a pre-operative haemoglobin level as low as $6\ g\ dL^{-1}$ if the blood loss is kept below 500 ml (22). This is yet another dimension of surgical technique which is reflected in the morbidity and mortality after an operation. However careful the technique of the surgeon, there will inevitably be operations where blood loss will be such that the patient needs to be transfused, but an awareness of the short-term effect on the body's resistance should impose some caution, and blood should only be transfused when absolutely necessary.

Prophylactic antibiotics

Before the surgeon undertakes any operation it is important to ensure that the patient is adequately prepared, in order to reduce the incidence of endogenous contamination, and that the environment in which he is to undertake the procedure is suitable, to eliminate or to reduce exogenous contamination. However, all surgeons are aware that whatever preparation and precautions are taken bacterial contamination is likely, or may be inevitable, during certain operations, and it is the surgeon's responsibility to try to prevent that contamination progressing to infection, and, of course, subsequently that that infection does not lead to suppuration, sepsis, multiple organ failure, and death.

The role of prophylactic antibiotics is to aid and to support the body's ability to resist the contamination which occurs at the time of operation. Thus if the antibiotic is to work effectively as a prophylactic agent and to prevent infection, it must be administered before or immediately after the bacterial inoculation of the tissues. Where a surgeon thinks it likely that an operation will be contaminated to such an extent that infection may ensue, the antibiotic should be given before the operation commences, and when contamination occurs unexpectedly during the course of the operation the antibiotic should be given immediately. Prophylactic antibiotics are not a substitute for, and will not compensate for, proper patient preparation and selection, nor are they a substitute for good surgical technique. Prophylactic antibiotics will not compensate for technical inadequacy and, if the bacterial challenge is sufficiently high, for whatever reason, or the patient's resistance is sufficiently low, prophylactic antibiotics will not prevent that patient developing infection.

It is important to differentiate 'prophylaxis' and 'therapy'. Prophylactic antibiotics are administered to assist the body's resistance during the period of bacterial contamination. This usually extends for the duration of the operation or posssibly for a few hours thereafter until any bacteria remaining in the wound have been removed by phagocytosis. However, if infection or suppuration has already occurred, as, for example, in the patient with acute appendicitis, it is inappropriate for 'prophylactic' antibiotics to be administered. Host resistance has already been breached, infection has occurred and therapy is indicated.

Indications for prophylactic antibiotics

It has been traditional teaching that antibiotic prophylaxis should be given only if there is likely to be significant contamination of the operative field, or if the patient is at particular risk of infection because of reduced resistance. Where infection and suppuration has already occurred therapy is appropriate over a longer period. Therefore antibiotic prophylaxis should be considered mandatory for all patients undergoing the implant of a prosthesis, for immunocompromised patients undergoing clean operations, for all patients undergoing clean–contaminated operations, and for patients undergoing an operation in which unexpected contamination occurs, where an extended period of administration of the antibiotic, as therapy, may be appropriate.

Clean operations

Despite the traditional teaching outlined above there is now evidence to suggest that prophylactic antibiotics may confer some benefit to patients who are not immunocompromised and who are undergoing clean operations. In a well-constructed trial of 1218 patients undergoing groin hernia repairs and non-implant, clean breast operations, Platt *et al.* have demonstrated a significant reduction in the incidence of nosocomial infection using cefonazid, a second generation cephalosporin (Table 8.2) (23). This paper may prove to have major medico-legal implications and, if the results are confirmed by other equally well-constructed studies of sufficient statistical power, there may need to be a review of surgical practice.

Table 8.2. Prophylactic antibiotics in clean surgery.

		Placebo (n = 614)	Cefonicid (n = 604)
Hernia	Evaluable	311	301
	Wound infection	6	4
	UTI	2	1
	Total	8	5
Breast	Evaluable	303	301
	Wound infection	26	17
	UTI	8	3
	Total	34	20
Total	All infections	50	27 $p < 0.01$

from Platt *et al.* (23).

Prosthetic implant procedures

The number of prostheses implanted into patients has already reached staggering proportions (24) and is rapidly increasing—400 000 joint replacements in 1987 in the USA alone; 120 000 artificial heart valves throughout the world in 1986; 60 000 vascular graft prostheses each year in the USA; 130 000 breast implants, 90 000 in the USA alone. It has been estimated that the cost of infection is increased by 400 to 600 per cent if infection occurs, and this cost has been estimated to be in excess of $100 million for infected joint prostheses alone in the USA each year (25). Cost is important but the pain, repeat operations, and disability are of greater importance to the individual patient.

Implants are usually inserted as clean operations but there may be particular problems when orthopaedic implants are inserted into compound fractures. The risk of infection around the implant should be small (0 to 2 per cent) but when this does occur the results may be disastrous. An infected total hip replacement which ultimately requires a Girdlestone revision is a considerable morbidity, and an infected dacron graft in an aortic aneurysm may lead to the death of the patient (26).

To prove that antibiotic prophylaxis does benefit the patient undergoing an implant procedure is difficult now because a trial of adequate statistical power would require the recruitment of many thousands of patients, and would involve randomization of some patients to a placebo or no treatment group which would no longer be considered ethical. In addition there would be great difficulty in obtaining informed consent from thè patients. Infection in some implants presents late and the follow-up period in such a trial would need to be many years. However, it is now considered normal surgical practice to administer antibiotic prophylaxis whenever a prosthesis is implanted into the body.

Special consideration should also be given to the patient who has already had a prosthesis implanted. These patients should be considered at risk of infection of their prosthesis when they undergo a subsequent operation, just as the patient who has had a heart valve damaged by rheumatic fever is considered at risk of endocarditis. These patients should probably receive antibiotic cover when they undergo an operation or any procedure which may initiate a bacteraemia-dental treatment, urethral catheterization, and sigmoidoscopy with biopsy are probably the most common examples (27).

Choice of antibiotic

The factors which influence the choice of the antibiotic to be used for chemoprophylaxis are listed in Table 8.3. Clearly the antibiotic that is used should have a spectrum of activity sufficiently wide to be effective against the organisms most likely to contaminate the wound. The antibiotic must be capable of being administered in such a way as to ensure that there is a high circulating blood level at the time of the maximal contamination; in practice, this usually means by intramuscular injection at the time of pre-medication or intravenous injection on induction of anaesthesia. Administering the antibiotic after the operation confers no benefit (28), but an antibiotic given during the course of the operation would appear to be as effective as given pre-operatively (29). If there is a need for an antibiotic active against anaerobic bacteria to be given, metronidazole is usually used and this can be given rectally, by suppository, with considerable cost saving, but must be given at least two hours pre-operatively to ensure an adequate blood level.

Table 8.3. Factors influencing the choice of antibiotic for chemoprophylaxis.

Antibacterial spectrum
Route of administration
Frequency of administration
Monitoring of toxicity
Complications
Cost

The pharmacokinetics of the antibiotic used cannot be ignored and if the operation is prolonged for more than two hours, or if there is blood loss in excess of two litres, a second dose of antibiotic should be given. In order to maintain a high circulating blood level, the antibiotic used must have a sufficiently long half-life or, again, an additional dose should be given. The longer half-life of some of the third generation cephalosporins may have the particular benefit of obviating the need for a second dose in this context.

Route of administration

Although intramuscular or intravenous injection is the route most commonly used alternative routes of administration have been advocated. Intra-incisional injection provides a high concentration of the antibiotic at the wound edge as well as an adequate circulating blood level (30–32). A high blood level has also been reported when the antibiotic is used as a lavage of the peritoneal cavity after gastrointestinal surgery. This latter technique, in which tetracycline lavage was used in conjunction with intravenous tetracycline, has been associated with particularly low levels of post-operative infection (33).

Antibiotics have also been given pre-operatively as prophylaxis in an attempt to reduce the gastrointestinal flora and hence the level of contamination that will occur when the bowel is opened. This is the philosophy behind the use of oral antibiotics in elective colorectal surgery which is particularly popular in the USA (34, 35). There is no doubt that this method does reduce the level of contamination at the time of operation, but evidence is increasing that a combination of both pre-operative oral antibiotics and perioperative parenteral antibiotics provides the lowest incidence of post-operative infective complications (36–38).

Duration of administration

In some surgical specialties it has become traditional to administer 'prophylactic' antibiotics for prolonged periods—even up to two weeks, and three- or four-day courses are not uncommon amongst general surgeons (39). Few studies have been conducted to investigate specifically the results of long or short courses of prophylaxis, but Strachan showed no benefit from one pre-operative and a five-day post-operative course of cefazolin when compared with one pre-operative dose alone in biliary tract operations (40). Review of the antibiotic trials published over the recent years shows an increasing trend towards single dose prophylaxis. Even in colòrectal operations, where the risk of infection is highest, no benefit has been demonstrated by continuing the antibiotic cover for more than one dose (41–43) and there is now evidence that prolonging the duration of antibiotic prophylaxis is of no benefit even in those patients who are known to have impaired host defences (44).

Nevertheless, many surgeons have favoured a 'belt and braces' approach and choose to continue to administer antibiotics post-operatively believing that the additional cost, and presumably the additional risks of bacterial resistance, superinfection, pseudomembranous colitis, etc., are outweighed by the benefit to the patient. The cost of prophylactic antibiotics cannot be ignored. There is inevitably a temptation to use the latest, most expensive and most heavily marketed antibiotic when a cheaper agent would be perfectly adequate. But the cost can also be controlled by shortening the duration of the course of prophylaxis and it is of interest to note that in one study where a policy of restricting prophylactic antibiotics to 24 h was enforced, not only was there a considerable cost saving, but the incidence of infection in clean-contaminated operations was lowered from 4.9 to 2.1 per cent (39).

Dangers of antibiotic prophylaxis

The possible dangers or disadvantages of antibiotic prophylaxis are listed in Table 8.4. The administration of any antimicrobial drug will tend to select resistant strains of bacteria. It is inevitable, therefore, that the shorter the course of antibiotic the less likely resistant strains are to be selected and, to date, the author is aware of no study which has demonstrated the emergence of significant resistance following single dose antibiotic prophylaxis.

Table 8.4. Possible dangers of prophylactic antibiotics.

Allergic reactions/anaphylaxis
Drug toxicity
Gastrointestinal upset
Development of resistance
Superinfection

Summary

The risk of infection after a surgical operation is dependent upon the contamination that occurs at the time of operation, and the ability of the body to resist that contamination. Pre-operative patient preparation and careful operative technique will reduce the level of contamination, and appropriate systemic antibiotics given to cover the operative period will assist the body to resist any accidental or inevitable contamination.

Prophylactic antibiotics should be given whenever a prosthesis is to be implanted or has already been implanted into the patient; when the patient is recognized as having reduced resistance to infection; or when a clean-contaminated or contaminated operation if being performed. The role of prophylactic antibiotics in healthy patients undergoing non-implant, clean operations remains open to question.

References

1. Law, D.J.W., Mishriki, S.F., and Jeffrey, P.J. (1990). The importance of surveillance after discharge from hospital in the diagnosis of post-operative wound infection. *Ann. R. Coll. Surg. Engl.*, **72**, 207–9.
2. *Hansard*, 2 July 1986. Written answers. Column 573.
3. Haley, R.W., Schaberg, D.R., Crossley, K.B., Von-Allemen, S.D., and McGowan, J.E. (1981). Extra charges and prolongation of stay attributable to nosocomial infections: A prospective interhospital comparison. *Am. J. Med.*, **70**, 51–8.
4. Department of Health and Social Security. (1988). Hospital infection control: guidance on the control of infections in hospitals. London.
5. Elek, S.D. and Conen, P.E. (1957). The virulence of *Staphylococcus pyogenes* for man. A study of the problems of wound infection. *Br. J. Exp. Pathol.*, **38**, 573–86.
6. Dougherty, S.H. and Simmons, R.L. (1982). Infections in bionic man: The pathobiology of infections in prosthetic devices—Part II. *Curr. Prob. Surg.*, **19**, 265–312.
7. Franson, T.R., Sheth, N.K., Menon, L., *et al.* (1986). Persistent *in vitro* survival of coagulase-negative staphylocci adherent to intravascular catheters in the absence of conventional nutrients. *J. Clin. Microbiol.*, **24**, 559–61.
8. Christensen, G.D., Simpson, W.A., Bisno, A.L. *et al.* (1983). Experimental foreign body infections in mice challenged with slime-producing *Staphylococcus epidermidis*. *Infect. Immun.*, **40**, 407–10.
9. Christensen, G.D., Simpson, W.A., Bisno, A.L. *et al.* (1982). Adherence of slime producing strains of *Staphylococcus epidermidis* to smooth surfaces. *Infect. Immun.*, **37**, 318–26.
10. Hoyle, B.D., Jass, J., and Costeron, J.W. (1990). The biofilm glycocalyx as a resistant factor. *J. Antimicrob. Chemother.*, **26**, 1–6.
11. Johnson, G.M., Lee, D.A., Regelmann, W.E. *et al.* (1986). Interference with granulocyte function by *Staphylococcus epidermidis* slime. *Infect. Immun.*, **54**, 13–20.
12. Burrows, L. and Tartter, P. (1982). Effect of blood transfusion on colonic malignancy recurrence rates. *Lancet*, **ii**, 662.
13. McLinton, S., Moffat, L.E.F., Scott, S., Urbaniak, S.J., and Kerridge, D.F. (1990). Blood transfusion and survival following surgery for prostatic cancer. *Br. J. Surg.*, **77**, 140–2.
14. Blumberg, N., Agarwhal, M.M., and Chuang, C. (1985). Relation between recurrence of cancer of the colon and blood transfusion. *Br. Med. J.*, **290**, 1037–9.
15. Crowson, M.C., Hallissay, M.T., Kiff, R.S., Kingston, R.D., and Fielding, J.W.L. (1989). Blood transfusion in colorectal cancer. *Br. J. Surg.*, **76**, 522–3.
16. Opelz, G., Senger, D.P.S., Mickey, M.R., and Terasaki, P.I. (1981). Effect of blood transfusion on subsequent kidney transplants. *Transplant. Proc.*, **ii**, 253–9.
17. Maitani, S., Nishikawa, T., Hirakawa, A., and Tobe, T. (1986). The role of blood transfusion in organ system failure following major abdominal surgery. *Ann. Surg.*, **203**, 275–81.
18. Jensen, L.S., Anderson, A., Fristrup, S.L. *et al.* (1990). Comparison of one dose *versus* three doses of prophylactic antibiotics, and the influence of blood transfusion, on infectious complications in acute and elective colorectal surgery. *Br. J. Surg.*, **77**, 513–8.
19. Wobbes, T., Bemelmans, B.L.H., Kuypers, J.H.Z., Beerthuizen, G.I.J.M., and Theenwes, A.G.M. (1990). Risk of post-operative septic complications after abdominal surgical treatment in relation to perioperative blood transfusion. *Surg. Gynecol. Obstet.*, **171**, 59–62.
20. Tartter, P.I. (1988). Determinants of post-operative stay in patients with colorectal cancer. Implications for Diagnostic-Related Groups. *Dis. Colon. Rectum.*, **31**, 694–8.
21. Tartter, P.I. (1989). Blood transfusion and post-operative infections. *Transfusion*, **29**, 456–9.
22. Spence, R.K., Carson, J.A., Poses, R. *et al.* (1990). Elective surgery without transfusion: Influence of pre-operative hemoglobin level and blood loss on mortality. *Am. J. Surg.*, **159**, 320–4.
23. Platt, R., Zaleznik, D.F., and Hopkins, C.C. *et al.* (1989). Perioperative antibiotic prophylaxis for herniorrhaphy and breast surgery. *N. Engl. J. Med.*, **322**, 153–60.
24. Sugarman, B. and Young, E.J. (1989). Infections associated with prosthetic devices: Magnitude of the problem. *Infect. Dis. Clin. North Am.*, **3**, 187–98.
25. Salvati, E.A., Small, R.D., Brause, B.D. *et al.* (1984). Infections associated with orthopaedic services. In *Infections associated*

with prosthetic devices (ed. B. Sugarman and E. J. Young) CRC Press, Boca Raton, Fl.
26. Gordon-Smith, I. C., Taylor, E. W., Nicolaides, A. N., Golcman, L., Kenyon, J., and Eastcott, H. H. G. (1978). Management of abdominal aortic aneurysms. *Br. J. Surg.*, **65**, 834–8.
27. Sullivan, P. M., Johnston, R. C., and Kelley, S. S. (1990). Late infection after total hip replacement, caused by an oral organism after dental manipulation. A case report. *J. Bone Joint Surg. (Am.)*, **72**, 121–3.
28. Polk, H. C. and Lopez-Major, J. F. (1969). Post-operative wound infection: A prospective study of determinant factors and prevention. *Surgery*, **66**, 97–103.
29. Bates, T., Siller, G., and Crathern, B. C. *et al.* (1989). Timing of prophylactic antibiotics in abdominal surgery: trial of pre-operative versus an intra-operative first dose. *Br. J. Surg.*, **76**, 52–6.
30. Dixon, J. M., Armstrong, C. P., Duffy, S. W., Chetty, U., and Davies, G. C. (1984). A randomised prospective trial comparing the value of intravenous and pre-incisional cefamandol in reducing post-operative sepsis after operations upon the gastro-intestinal tract. *Surg. Gynecol. Obst.*, **158**, 303–7.
31. Taylor, T. V., Walker, W. S., Mason, R. C., Richmond, J., and Lee, D. (1982). Pre-operative intraparietal (intra-incisional) cefoxatin in abdominal surgery. *Br. J. Surg.*, **69**, 461–2.
32. Taylor, T. V., Dawson, D. L., De Silva, M., Shaw, S. J., Durans, D., and Makin, D. (1985). Pre-operative intra-incisional cefamandole reduces wound infection and post-operative in-patient stay in upper abdominal surgery. *Ann. R. Coll. Surg. Engl.*, **67**, 235–7.
33. Krukowski, Z. H., Stewart, M. P. M., Alsayer, H. M., and Matheson, N. A. (1984). Infection after abdominal surgery: a five year prospective study. *Br. Med. J.*, **288**, 278–80.
34. Nichols, R. L., Condon, R. E., Gorbach, S. L., and Nyhus, L. M. (1972). Efficacy of pre-operative antimicrobial preparation of the bowel. *Ann. Surg.*, **176**, 227–32.
35. Kaiser, A. B. (1986). Antimicrobial prophylaxis in surgery. *N. Engl. J. Med.*, **315**, 1129–38.
36. Lazorthes, F., Legrand, G., Monrozies, X., *et al.* (1982). Comparison between oral and systemic antibiotics and their combined use for the prevention of complications in colorectal surgery. *Dis. Colon Rectum*, **25**, 309–11.
37. Kaiser, A. B., Harrington, J. L., Jacobs, K. J., Mulherin, J. L., Roach, A. C., and Sawyer, J. L. (1983). Cefoxitin *versus* erythromycin, neomycin and cefazolin in colorectal operations. *Ann. Surg.*, **198**, 525–30.
38. Coppa, G. F., Eng, K., Gouge, T. H., Ranson, J. H. C., and Localio, S. A. (1983). Parenteral and oral antibiotics in elective colon and rectal surgery. *Am. J. Surg.*, **145**, 62–5.
39. Scher, K. S., Bernstein, J. M., Arenstein, G. L., and Sorenson, C. (1990). Reducing the cost of surgical prophylaxis. *Am. Surg.*, **56**, 32–5.
40. Strachan, C. J. L., Black, J., Powis, S. J. A. *et al.* (1977). Prophylactic use of cephazolin against wound sepsis after cholecystectomy. *Br. Med. J.*, **i**, 1254–6.
41. Giercksky, K. E., Danielsen, S., Garburg, O. *et al.* (1982). A single dose of tinidazole and doxycycline prophylaxis in elective surgery of the colon and rectum. *Ann. Surg.*, **195**, 227–31.
42. Bergman, L. and Solhaug, J. H. (1987). Single dose chemoprophylaxis in elective colorectal surgery. *Ann. Surg.*, **205**, 77–81.
43. Jagelman, D. G., Fabian, T. C., Nichols, R. L., Stone, H. H., Wilson, S. E., and Zellner, S. R. (1988). Single dose cefotetan *versus* multiple dose cefoxitin as prophylaxis in elective colorectal surgery. *Am. J. Surg.*, **155**, 71–6.
44. Moesgaard, F. and Lukkegaard-Neilsen, M. (1989). Pre-operative cell mediated immunity and duration of antibiotic prophylaxis in relation to post-operative infective complications. A controlled trial in biliary, gastroduodenal and colorectal surgery. *Acta Chir. Scand.*, **155**, 281–6.

9

Definition of infection

ANTHONY L.G. PEEL

Introduction

All surgeons need to maintain an interest in infection despite the significant advances that have been made in antiseptic, prophylactic, and therapeutic antimicrobial chemotherapy, and in operative technique. Patients may present either with established infection which may require operative intervention, or they may undergo surgery and develop infective complications.

The recent importance attached to quality control in surgical practice has emphasized the need for accurate diagnosis and recording of all complications, especially post-operative infection (1). The value of such data will be enhanced if it is based on simple, easily applied, and widely accepted definitions, since fair comparison may then be made between the results after different operative procedures or from different surgical units (2). An attempt has been made to define clinical infection (3) and, although comprehensive, the use of such criteria as 'the attending surgeon's or physician's diagnosis of infection' still has ambiguity and detracts from the value of the report.

In this chapter recommended definitions and criteria for the diagnosis of infection will be advanced based on clinical criteria wherever possible and using laboratory and imaging investigations only to confirm the diagnosis. If the diagnosis is dependent upon laboratory or imaging techniques then the surgeon who does not wish to see infection can avoid doing so by failing to ensure that the appropriate specimens are sent for bacteriological culture, or that the appropriate imaging techniques are requested. Many wound infections present only after the patient has left hospital and it is in this situation that the results of bacteriological studies become unreliable—the general practitioner or district nurse may not take a culture swab, the swab may not be stored at the correct temperature, or may not arrive at the bacteriology department within a reasonable period; and it may not then be plated for a further prolonged period. All these factors conspire to produce false-negative results.

Basis for definitions

Role of clinical evidence, imaging, and laboratory results in the formulation of a definition of infection

Clinical evidence should form the central theme of the definition of infections. Laboratory data can provide confirmation and imaging techniques will give supporting information in appropriate circumstances. A high standard of clinical acumen is desirable in both the prospective and the retrospective assessment of symptoms and signs. The general symptoms and signs of infection include pain, pyrexia in excess of 38 °C, and loss of function. Whenever these are present infection should be suspected. The localized signs of inflammation are well established and have been the hallmark of infection for centuries (since the time of Celsius) — redness, swelling, tenderness, heat, loss of function, and the formation of pus. The results from imaging investigations can provide important supportive evidence particularly when deep infection is suspected. Imaging equipment and techniques have expanded in the past decade and radiology is now supplemented by ultrasonography, isotope scanning, computerized tomography (CT), and nuclear magnetic resonance (NMR) scanning.

Laboratory confirmation of infection depends on the results of microscopy, culture, and antigen/antibody detection tests, but when an organism is identified the differentiation between infection, colonization and contamination may pose problems. Because of this difficulty the culture of an organism is only considered to be essential for the definition of infection in the urinary tract and the central nervous system (CNS).

Hospital- and community-acquired infection

Any infection which was not present or incubating at the time of admission to hospital should be classified as hospital acquired infection (HAI). When doubt exists infection appearing 72 h after admission, or in a patient re-admitted with active infection that results from an earlier hospital admission, should also be classified as HAI. An infection that was already present or incubating at the time of admission to hospital should be classified as community acquired infection (CAI).

Infection in general surgical practice

Most infections in general surgical practice result from contamination by micro-organisms in the intestinal, genito-urinary, or respiratory tracts. Most bacterial infections on surgical wards are post-operative infections, of which the most frequent and important are wound infection, septicaemia, respiratory tract infection, urinary tract infection, and intra-abdominal abscess formation.

Wound infection

A wound is defined as a breach in an epithelial surface which may be surgical or accidental and which includes drain sites but not burns, ulcers, or pressure sores. All wound infections must have either a purulent discharge in, or exuding from, the wound, or there should be a painful spreading erythema indicative of cellulitis around the wound.

The presence of bruising, the formation of a haematoma, and the collection of serum or lymph within a wound may predispose to the development of infection. Certain clinical states can cause the clinician difficulty in deciding whether a wound infection is present. Thus, erythema in the immediate vicinity of the wound may be caused by trauma to the tissues leading to bruising, fat necrosis, or infection, or to a combination of any or all of these. When the erythema is associated with fever, tenderness, oedema, and extension of the margin around the wound, infection is present as cellulitis. The discharge of a few drops of clear fluid from a wound should not be regarded as signifying infection unless it becomes purulent or is accompanied by cellulitis.

The definition of infection in a wound is supported by bacteriological results, both microscopy and culture, but should not be dependent on them. False-negative results of culture may occur and difficulties may be encountered in the interpretation of some cultures leading to a false-positive diagnosis; for example bacteria may be present as a result of contamination or secondary colonization.

Primary and secondary wound infection

In a primary infection the discharge from the wound is purulent. The infection is secondary if that infection follows another complication not directly related to the wound itself; thus the discharge of cerebrospinal fluid, urine, bile, pancreatic juice, gastric, small intestinal, or colonic contents are inevitably contaminated by bacteria either from within the patient or from the environment (4). An anastomosis which dehisces, either because of continued progression of the primary pathology or ischaemia, frequently drains to the laparotomy wound and presents as a secondary wound infection and fistula.

Time-scale

A wound infection should be classified as *early* if it presents within 30 days of operation; *intermediate* if between one and three months of operation; and *late* if presenting more than three months after surgery. Late infection assumes particular importance with regard to implant surgery where it may be difficult to differentiate late primary infection from secondary infection due to haematogenous spread of organisms from another site within the body.

Severity and scoring system

The accurate assessment of the severity of a wound infection is important (5, 6). A wound infection should be classified as *minor* if there is a discharge of pus from the wound without cellulitis, lymphangitis, deep tissue destruction, or systemic disturbance. By contrast a *major* wound infection is defined as the discharge of pus associated with breakdown, partial or complete, and dehiscence of the deep, fascial layers of the wound or when there is evidence of systemic illness accompanying a spreading cellulitis or lymphangitis.

Wilson *et al.* have proposed a scoring system for the assessment of wounds following cardiac surgery based on a point system (6). The points are allocated according to the need for *A*dditional treatment, the presence of *S*erous discharge, *E*rythema, *P*urulent exudate, *S*eparation of the deep tissues, the *I*solation of bacteria and the duration of in-patient *S*tay (ASEPSIS). This has been shown to be reproducible and of value when comparing prophylactic antibiotic regimens in the prevention of wound infection. Application of this system involves daily scoring using features that are easily assessed. Although time and commitment are required, the results when applied to different surgical procedures or to different surgical units, should provide valuable data.

A significant proportion of wound infections will be missed if observation and recording ceases after the patient has left the hospital. In one study, 59 per cent of post-operative wound infections were detected in the community and 43 per cent of all wound infections became apparent more than one week after surgery (7). It should be emphasized that patients undergoing clean, and to a lesser extent clean-contaminated, surgery often leave hospital after a short stay and therefore wound infection is easily overlooked if evaluation ceases at that time. Although the overall incidence of wound infection is higher after contaminated and dirty operations, the majority of these wounds which become infected will be detected due to the patient's longer hospital stay. Assessment at a single out-patient clinic provides limited additional data and, although patient and general practitioner questionnaires improve the quality of the data, there is no doubt that assessment by trained community nursing staff at regular intervals after the patient has left the hospital provides a more accurate picture of the true incidence of wound infection.

Septicaemia

Septicaemia should be diagnosed if rigors occur together with one or more of the following signs: fever higher than 38 °C on more than one occasion in a 24 h period, usually accompanied by hypotension and oliguria. In certain circumstances rigors may not be detected, for example when the patient is under sedation or receiving supported ventilation, or when the rigor occurs at night and is not witnessed by the nursing attendants. Laboratory confirmation of viable micro-organisms (bacteraemia) or their products (exotoxins and endotoxins, antigens or antibodies) in the blood is desirable, but should not be an essential prerequisite to making the diagnosis.

This clinical definition of septicaemia in the absence of the results of blood culture is important since patients with life threatening sepsis require rapid identification and institution of treatment if mortality is to be reduced. However, it is recognized that the presence of fever, shock, respiratory failure, and multiple organ failure may also occur in other conditions such as drug reactions and acute pancreatitis. In addition, even when blood is taken for culture at the appropriate time, the incidence of positive blood culture may be low. In the future it is possible that improvements in the ability to detect endotoxaemia and the role of monoclonal antibodies, particularly against endotoxin and tumour necrosis factor, are likely to be of increasing value in defining the septicaemic state (8).

Lower respiratory tract infection

Infection of the lower respiratory tract includes tracheobronchitis, bronchitis, and broncheolitis, pneumonia, lung abscess, and empyema.

Tracheobronchitis, bronchitis, and broncheolitis

Tracheobronchitis, bronchitis and broncheolitis are defined as the presence of a cough with new or increased production of sputum which may be associated with a fever in excess of 38 °C, bronchospasm, rhonchi, and rales on auscultation. Laboratory evidence to support the diagnosis will include the culture of organisms from sputum, tracheal aspirate on bronchoscopy or a positive antigen test on respiratory secretions. Clinical and radiological evidence of pneumonia is absent.

Pneumonia

Pneumonia should be diagnosed when new or increased production of purulent sputum, usually accompanied by a fever in excess of 38 °C persisting for more than 48 h, occurs together with appropriate clinical signs including tachypnoea, dullness to percussion, increased vocal fremitus, bronchial breathing, and rhonchi. Chest radiography will usually show a new or progressive radiological infiltrate and the diagnosis should be assisted by positive sputum microscopy and bacterial culture whenever possible. For satisfactory laboratory assessment a fresh sample of sputum must be examined microscopically as a routine before initiating antimicrobial therapy. In this way purulence and the significance of organisms cultured can be evaluated. Further laboratory confirmation of infection may be available from positive blood cultures.

Lung abscess or empyema

A lung abscess or empyema is defined as the collection of pus within the lung or pleural cavity respectively. The clinical evidence accompanying an empyema or lung abscess may include impaired respiratory movement and air entry on the affected side with dullness to percussion and reduced breath sounds on auscultation. Radiology may demonstrate lung cavitation in the presence of a lung abscess or accumulation of fluid within the pleural space if an empyema is present.

Urinary tract infection

Urinary tract infection is diagnosed when the presence of micro-organisms in the urinary tract is accompanied by the symptoms and signs of infection. These usually include dysuria, urgency, loin pain, tenderness, pyrexia, pyuria ($>10^5$ WBC/ml urine) and inflammmation of the bladder wall which may be seen at cystoscopy. A bacterial count of in excess of 10^5 organisms/ml is generally considered to be significant in a midstream specimen of urine. Special consideration should be given to a lower bacterial count in specimens obtained by suprapubic puncture or aspirated from a catheter, or when there is a pure growth of a common urinary pathogen such as *Escherichia coli*, *Proteus mirabilis*, coagulase negative staphylococci, *Streptococcus faecalis*, *Klebsiella* spp., *Pseudomonas* spp., and *Acinetobacter*. In these situations a lower number of organisms (10^3/ml) should be considered significant.

In urinary tract infections the laboratory findings are essential to the diagnosis and it is obviously important that the specimens are handled with precision. Difficulties in interpretation may be encountered when multiple organisms are grown or when samples of urine are sent from patients who are already receiving antibiotic therapy. The provision of full clinical details is essential in order to produce accurate reports from the bacteriological results.

Alimentary tract infections

Gastroenteritis

A gastrointestinal infection usually presents with diarrhoea and/or vomiting, sometimes accompanied by colicky pain, pyrexia, and dehydration (3). Other non-infectious causes of gastrointestinal upset, such as therapeutic drug regimens or diagnostic tests must be excluded. When possible, confirmatory laboratory evidence should be obtained which might include microscopic identification of the causative organism or its isolation from culture, detection of antigen or antibody in the faeces, or the detection of an increase in antibody in paired serum samples. In addition to the well-recognized causes, such as infection by *Salmonella* spp., *Shigella* spp., *Staphylococcus aureus*, *Clostridium welchii*, *E. coli*, *Vibrio cholera*, *Giardia lamblia*, and *Entamoeba histolytica*, investigation should be undertaken for four important 'newer' agents: *Campylobacter* spp., *Clostridium difficile*, *Yersinia enterocolitica*, and rota virus (9).

Infections of the alimentary viscera

Infection of the alimentary viscera frequently occurs as a complication of underlying disease and usually presents with clinical symptoms and signs indicative of acute inflammation of the organ concerned, for example acute cholecystitis. In addition to the clinical evidence, support may be obtained from endoscopy, (candida oesophagitis) and imaging techniques, (peridiverticular abscess or empyema of the gallbladder). Confirmation of infection by culture of an organism from aspirate or drainage material, blood or tissue obtained during operation or endoscopy is desirable but, again, should not be considered essential to making the diagnosis.

Viral hepatitis is suspected on clinical grounds with anorexia, nausea, vomiting, a history of blood transfusion in some patients, jaundice, fever greater than 38 °C, tenderness over the liver area, and the diagnosis is supported by abnormal liver function tests with a particularly high elevation of alanine or aspartate transaminases in the early phase. The diagnosis is confirmed by positive virology. Antigen and antibody tests for hepatitis A, B, and C should be performed but other diagnoses: infectious mononucleosis, cytomegalovirus, herpes simplex, adenovirus, and non-viral agents such as leptospirosis, or infection by Gram-negative organisms need to be considered.

Peritonitis

Peritonitis is inflammation of the peritoneum caused by infective agents or toxic substances clinically manifest as abdominal pain, tenderness, and guarding on palpation and subsequent impairment of the alimentary tract functions of motility and absorption. It may be diffuse or localized and this is clinically defined by the severity and extent of the clinical signs. Some of the clinical features may be modified or absent under certain conditions, for example in paraplegic patients, in patients with impaired consciousness, or in those receiving artificial mechanical ventilation. It is desirable that the diagnosis of peritonitis due to bacterial infection is supported by positive cultures of the exudate taken at the time of laparotomy.

Intra-abdominal abscess

An intra-abdominal abscess is the localized collection of infected fluid or pus which may be intraperitoneal (most frequently subphrenic, pelvic, or paracolic), retroperitoneal (perinephric or peripancreatic) or visceral (hepatic or tubo-ovarian) (10). Clinical evidence that an abscess has formed includes pain or discomfort, alimentary dysfunction (anorexia, diarrhoea, jaundice, etc., according to site), weight loss, pyrexia, and a tender mass. Laboratory confirmation by the isolation of bacteria from cultures of the aspirate is desirable. Approriate imaging, especially ultrasonography, will allow confirmation of the diagnosis and the site of the abscess and by accurate localization will permit aspiration and positive identification of the causative agent.

Infection in other surgical specialties

Bone and joint infection

Osteomyelitis should be diagnosed by clinical signs and symptoms: the presence of pain, fever, localized swelling, tenderness, and warmth, and by dysfunction of the appropriate part. There may be overlying skin breakdown and discharge of pus. Laboratory confirmation by identification of the infecting organism(s) from culture of blood, pus, or material obtained by aspiration or at surgery should be obtained if at all possible but should not be considered essential to the diagnosis.

Similarly, infection of a joint should be diagnosed clinically by the presence of pain, fever, swelling, tenderness, warmth, effusion into the joint, and limitation of the range of movement. Laboratory confirmation by microscopy and culture of fluid aspirated from the joint cavity, or biopsy of tissue from the joint capsule should be obtained if possible.

Radiological evidence is of considerable diagnostic value in the later stages of acute infection and in chronic infection. Infection in bones and joints may follow surgery and is classified as *early* and *late*, three months after surgery being the dividing period (11). A diagnosis of early infection should be made in the presence of pain at rest, fever greater than 38 °C persisting for more than 48 h, and should be supported by the isolation of bacteria from cultures when available. Late infection is indicated by pain at rest, an erythrocyte sedimentation rate persistently raised more than 30 mm/h above the preoperative level, radiological changes in bone indicative of infection and the isolation of bacteria from cultures when available.

These definitions may be applied to compound, traumatic injuries and in this context the degree of associated soft tissue injury, peri-osteal stripping, and vascular injury assumes considerable importance in the subsequent management. The culture of Gram-negative organisms is especially significant when there is associated vascular impairment or damage.

Infection following implant surgery

The diagnosis of infection around an implant will to an extent depend on the site and type of prosthesis and thus it is not possible to make an *absolute* generic definition. Infection should be diagnosed in the presence of pain, a fever, local signs of inflammation where the implant is superficial, radiological signs where the implant involves or is adjacent to bone, and an elevated white blood cell count (greater than 11×10^9/L). Important confirmation of the diagnosis may be available by the isolation of organisms from discharging pus, CT guided fine needle aspirate of peri-implant fluid or from blood, but a negative culture does not necessarily negate the diagnosis. Infection is fortunately rare and is frequently diagnosed on presumptive evidence since prophylactic antibiotics in particular make precise bacteriological diagnosis more difficult.

Eye infections

An eye infection should be diagnosed clinically in the presence of pain, visual disturbance, and redness combined with either a purulent discharge or the presence of pus on the surface of, or within, the eye. Confirmatory evidence of bacterial infection should be sought from microscopy and culture of the exudate or discharge.

Ear infections

Ear infections include otitis externa, otitis media, otitis interna, and mastoiditis and should be diagnosed from clinical symptoms and signs: pain, impaired hearing, or balance, pyrexia, localized erythema of the tympanic membrane, or tenderness of the external ear or mastoid process. Confirmation should be sought by the isolation of organisms from purulent discharge or from material obtained by aspiration or at surgery.

Central nervous system infection

Clinical evidence of bacterial infection of the central nervous system (CNS) usually includes general symptoms of infection together with somnolence, pain, and meningism. Laboratory evidence is considered to be critical in making a diagnosis of bacterial infection of the CNS. Micro-organisms should be cultured from the cerebrospinal fluid (CSF), brain tissue or from the contents or wall of a brain abscess. A raised white blood cell count in the CSF in the absence of micro-organisms may also be diagnostic particularly when antibiotics have been administered.

Reproductive system infection

Infection involving the vulva, vagina, uterus, fallopian tubes, and ovaries can occur in the absence of pregnancy, after pregnancy, or following surgery. Clinical symptoms and signs may include pain, dysuria, vaginal discharge, and pyrexia. The diagnosis may be supported by isotopic, ultrasonic, or CT imaging and by endoscopic or laparotomy evidence of acute inflammation or abscess formation. Culture of fluid obtained from the discharge, by aspiration or drainage of pus, or of surgical tissue should be undertaken to isolate the causative organism.

In the male infection may affect the epididymis, prostate, seminal vesicles, or testes. Clinical symptoms and signs include pain, dysuria, pyrexia, and localized tenderness and swelling. Isolation of micro-organisms from blood, urine, or urethral discharge, or from pus or material obtained by aspirate or at surgery should be sought for confirmation.

Role of definition of infection in clinical and research

The importance of quality control in surgery is widely accepted but, in order to assess outcome, the data on which the judgement is made must be sound. The data baselines must be consistent and similar if valid comparisons are to be made and useful deductions drawn. It is against this background that the definition of infection becomes essential. Difficulties in evaluating the effect of sepsis in the Confidential Enquiry into Perioperative Deaths (CEPOD) have already been highlighted, but for the purpose of outcome evaluation such definitions must be clear, concise, easily applied and be widely acceptable to surgeons. Increased awareness of the problem of infection should lead to positive action to reduce it, and thus effect the morbidity for future patients and the financial cost both to the individual patient and to the hospital or health care team (12).

If it is accepted that hospital acquired infection involves an average of four bed days extra hospitalization and that there is a 5 per cent infection rate in acute hospitals at an average cost of £90 per in-patient day (1987) the financial implications can be calculated to give a total approaching £115 000 000 in England (13).

It is important to define the time-scale when assessing the incidence of post-operative infectious complications for audit purposes and the intensity of post-operative monitoring by trained personnel cannot be over emphasized.

A baseline definition alone may be of insufficient detail to allow meaningful comparison for research purposes and it is in this context that scoring systems, by grading the severity of infection, assume considerable importance. Accuracy is fundamental to the critical assessment of infectious complications when comparison is made between different treatment regimens, different surgical procedures, and between surgical units treating patients with defined disease entities. Wound scoring systems are of considerable value in this situation but do not influence the management of an individual patient.

References

1. Devlin, H. B. (1988). Professional audit, quality control, keeping up to date. *Baillière's Clinical Anaesthesiology*, **2**, 299–324.
2. Platt, R., Zaleznik, D. F., Hopkins, C. C. *et al.* (1990). Perioperative antibiotic prophylaxis for herniorrhaphy and breast surgery. *N. Engl. J. Med.*, **322**, 153–60.
3. Garner, J. S., Jarvis, W. I. R., Emon, T. L., Horan, T. C., and Hughes, J. M. (1988). CDC definitions for nosocomial infections 1988. *Am. J. Infect. Control.*, **16**, 128–40.
4. Pollock, A. V., Leaper, D. B., and Evans, M. (1977). Single dose intra-incisional antibiotic prophylaxis of surgical wound sepsis: a controlled trial of cephaloridine and ampicillin. *Br. J. Surg.*, **64**, 322–5.

5. Elebute, G. and Stoner, H.B. (1983). The grading of sepsis. *Br. J. Surg.*, **70**, 29–31.
6. Wilson, A.P.R., Treasure, T., Sturridge, M.F., and Gruneberg, R.N. (1986). A scoring method (ASEPSIS) for post-operative wound infections for use in clinical trials of antibiotic prophylaxis. *Lancet*, **i**, 311–3.
7. Law, D.J.W., Mishriki, S.F., and Jeffrey, P.J. (1990). The importance of surveillance after discharge from hospital in the diagnosis of post-operative wound infection. *Ann. R. Coll. Surg. Engl.*, **72**, 207–9.
8. Bihari, D.J. (1990). Septicaemia—the clinical diagnosis. *J. Antimicrob. Chemother.*, **25**, suppl, 1–7.
9. Shanson, D.C. (1983). Infections and the gut. *Hospital Update*, **9**, 756–63.
10. Nichols, R.L. (1980). Infections following gastro-intestinal surgery: intra-abdominal abscess. *Surg. Clin. North Am.*, **60**, 197–212.
11. Benson, M.K.D. and Hughes, S.P.F. (1975). Infection following total hip replacement in a general hospital without special orthopaedic facilities. *Acta Orthop. Scand.*, **46**, 968–78.
12. Devlin, H.B. (1990). In Surgical Sepsis Problems and Audit: A Report. *Surg. Infect.*, **2**, 13–5.
13. Maynard, A. (1989). Economic aspects of hospital acquired infections. In *Current problems in antibiotic prophylaxis and surgical infection.* Royal Society of Medicine, Round Table Series Vol. 14, pp. 69–77.

10

Diagnosis of 'occult' intra-abdominal infection

STEPHEN J. KARRAN, STUART D. SCOTT, and VALERIE J. LEWINGTON

Introduction

Intra-abdominal infection remains a potentially lethal condition (1–5). In most situations, the diagnosis is relatively easy to establish on clinical grounds, but post-operative intra-abdominal infection can prove a much more difficult problem (6). A carefully taken history will usually give a strong indication of the specific pathology arising within either a particular organ or system. Such knowledge will often prove valuable in predicting the likely microbiological cause of such infection, even before specific localization can be achieved (7).

Careful clinical examination will often increase the diagnostic accuracy by localization of an inflammatory process. In addition, it can be determined whether that process is becoming, or has already become, generalized. Such examination must also attempt to exclude other primary sites of infection, for example within the head and neck or the respiratory or neurological systems, as symptoms and signs may closely mimic those arising from an infective pathology within the abdomen.

Simple blood tests, e.g. for leuocytosis, together with radiological investigations, particularly chest radiographs, must be assessed critically, and, if the clinical diagnosis remains in doubt, cultures of blood and other appropriate specimens are obtained for urgent analysis. It should, therefore, be only a minority of patients who require further and more complex investigations. The use of such investigations is the subject of this review.

Diagnostic pathway

The scheme shown in Fig. 10.1 is a diagnostic policy which will prove satisfactory in the majority of situations. Particular difficulties which may arise post-operatively have already been alluded to. These difficulties may have grave consequences with the remorseless deterioration of the patient, and in this situation the value of a 'high index of suspicion' is particularly important, together with a willingness to proceed to laparotomy without further delay, *despite* the negative findings of the available imaging investigations. On the other hand, the risk of causing potentially lethal small bowel fistulation in patients with dense or ubiquitous adhesions highlights the need to localize any focus of infection as often as possible. This is particularly relevant because of the opportunity to drain such collections by aspiration, guided either by ultrasound (Fig. 10.2) computerized tomography (CT) or, if that should prove impossible, by an extraperitoneal surgical approach which is associated with a lower risk than transperitoneal exploration.

In the post-operative situation there is often a lack of helpful localizing physical signs, and the patient may be deteriorating steadily. Defence mechanisms against infection, however, are often breached through a combination of malnutrition, malignancy or, indeed, therapeutic causes of immunosuppression such as radiotherapy or chemotherapy. The prospect of a 'negative' laparotomy in such a patient is particularly unappealing!

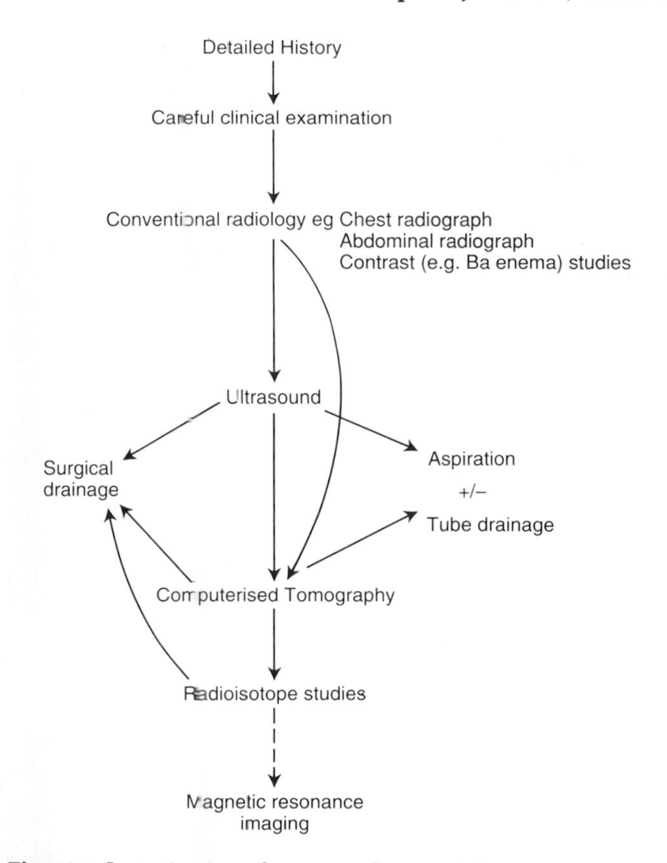

Fig. 10.1 Investigation of suspected intra-abdominal infection.

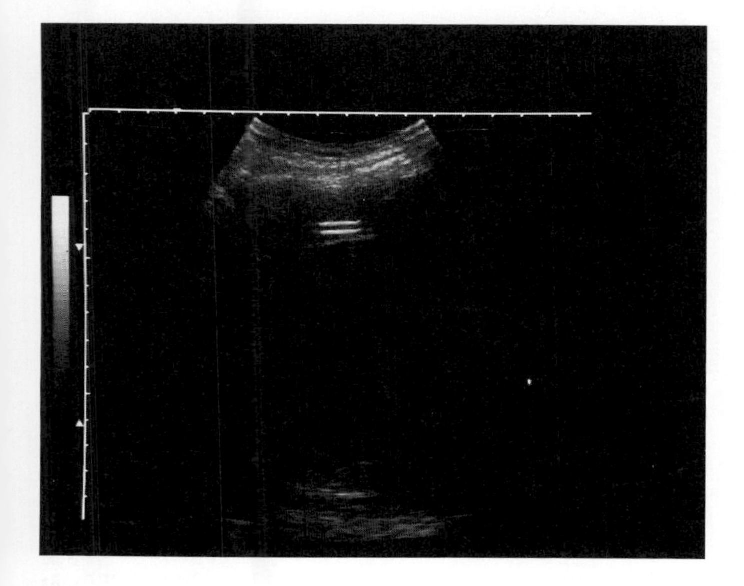

Fig. 10.2 Drain in right subphrenic abscess inserted under ultrasonic guidance.

Features which should raise clinical suspicion of this problem are listed in Table 10.1, but such findings may well, in themselves, fail to point to the abdomen as the source of the infection. In this situation other investigations such as urinary or sputum microscopy, Gram stains and bacterial cultures may prove extremely helpful in identifying the organ or system involved.

Table 10.1. Features suggesting intra-abdominal infection.

History	Pain	
	Nausea	
	Vomiting	
Examination	Tenderness	
	Pyrexia	
	Mass	
	Guarding	
	Rigidity	
	Toxicity	
	Tachycardia	
Investigations	Leucocytosis	
	Raised erythrocyte sedimentation rate	
	Microscopy	of urine and sputum
	Gram staining	
	Cultures (and sensitivites)	

Conventional radiology

Conventional radiological investigations may resolve the diagnostic dilemma in nearly 50 per cent of patients (8). Gas under the diaphragm and supradiaphramatic opacity due to a sympathetic effusion are clear clues to the presence of a subdiaphramatic collection of pus. The diaphragm may also be raised or fixed in this situation. Lack of normal gas shadows in the iliac fossae can indicate a soft tissue mass which, with clinical signs, may suggest abscess formation particularly if displacement of viscera can be seen. Similarly, inflammatory lesions which cause adhesion of small bowel loops may be detected or there may be localized ileus. Diverticulitis is a common cause of this. The normal definition of retroperitoneal structures such as the psoas shadow may also be lost.

Clearly, then, 'plain' radiographs of chest and abdomen usually constitute the first choice of available imaging techni-

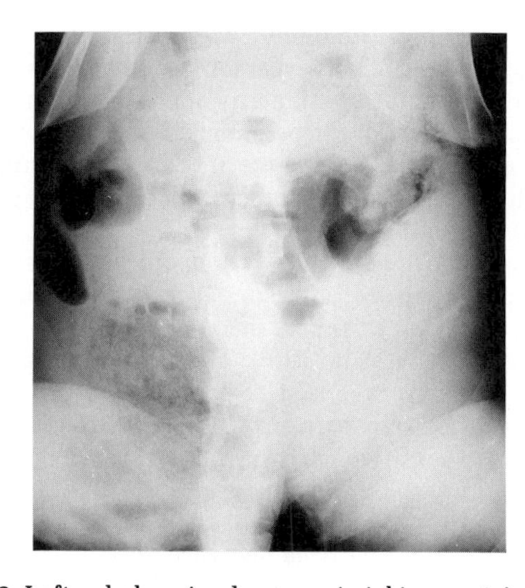

Fig. 10.3 Left subphrenic abscess mimicking gastric shadow.

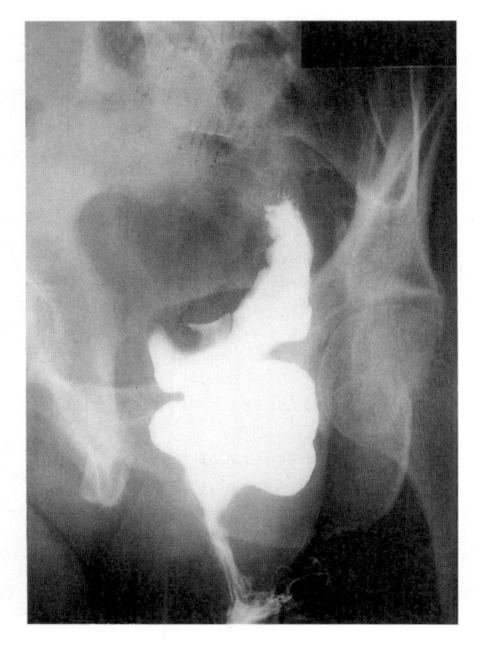

Fig. 10.4 Pelvic abscess displacing rectum.

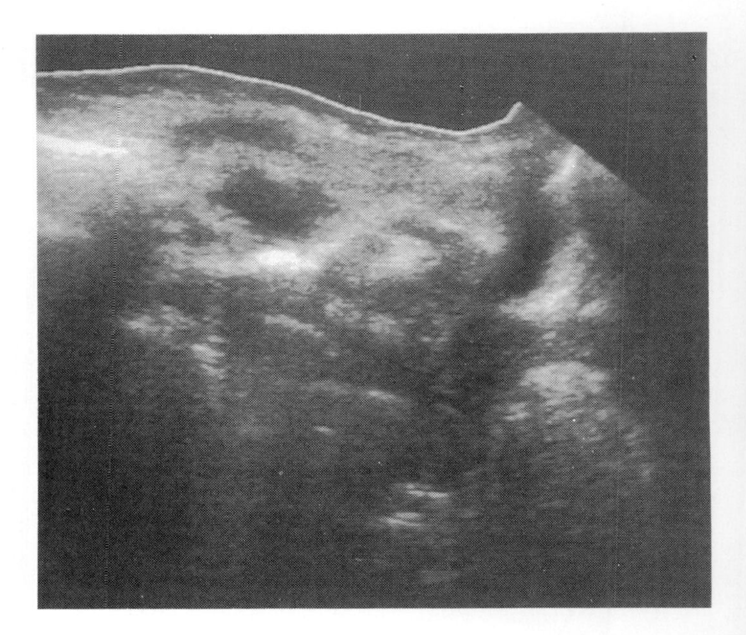

Fig. 10.5 Subcutaneous abscess of anterior abdominal wall demonstrated on ultrasonography.

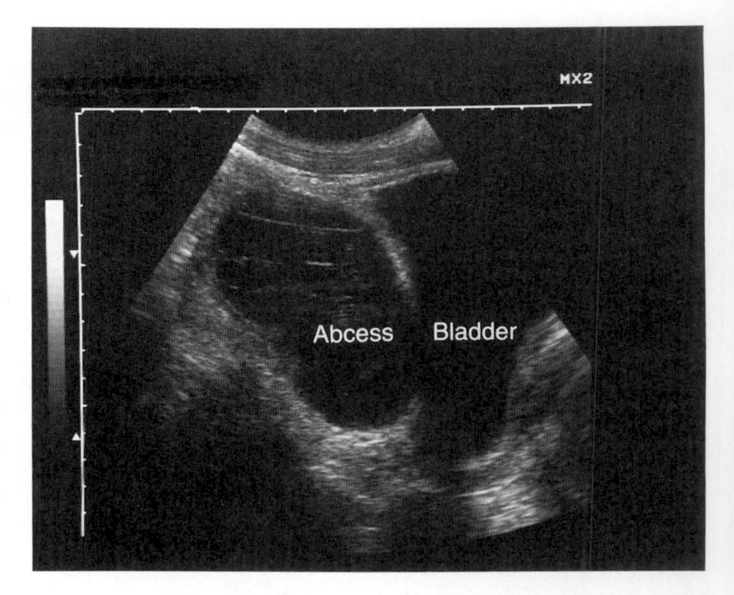

Fig. 10.6 Ultrasound of pelvic abscess.

ques, as such investigations are relatively simple, safe, rapid, and inexpensive. Rectal or oral contrast examinations can on occasion also prove helpful (9) (Figs. 10.3, 10.4).

Ultrasonography

In the last decade ultrasonography has established an enviable role in clinical diagnosis in many areas. It's value in the detection of intra-abdominal infection is one such (10–21). Ultrasonography has the following advantages.

In most hospitals in the UK the facility is now readily available and, because of its portability, the equipment need not necessarily be restricted to the radiological department. Ultrasonography is relatively inexpensive compared with more recently introduced imaging techniques and it is one of the safest of all imaging techniques, with virtually no complications resulting from many years of usage. Because of its non-invasive nature it is particularly appropriate for the investigation of the seriously ill patient. Greater use of portable equipment extends this advantage and, in the investigation of the difficult post-operative problem, these features constitute a particular attraction.

So far as diagnostic accuracy is concerned, as distinct from convenience and safety, ultrasonography is particularly of value in the detection of subcutaneous lesions (Fig. 10.5), and those within the pelvis (Fig. 10.6). The right upper quadrant is another particularly favoured region for diagnostic success (Fig. 10.7). Certain retroperitoneal areas, such as the perirenal region, are also sensitive to ultrasonographic diagnosis.

What, then, are the disadvantages of this major diagnostic technique?

Although these are relatively few, they are still very real. One major disadvantage of this investigation is that is it definitely operator dependent. Even for experienced radiologists a considerable 'learning curve' exists. However, once this is taken into account with suitable training programmes, no major hospital should nowadays be deprived of this important diagnostic facility.

Other difficulties in diagnosis result from the problems caused by overlying gas and clearly this difficulty is particularly relevant in abdominal imaging. Areas which can be notoriously difficult to assess reliably include the mid-abdomen, the left upper quadrant, and those retroperitoneal areas where overlying gas shadows can be expected. However, these problems can often be overcome with the use of multiple scan planes and by the persistence of a skilful operator.

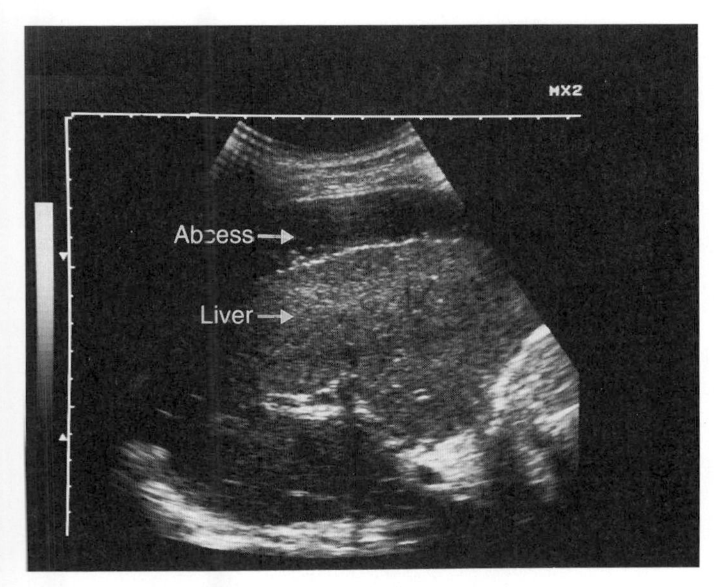

Fig. 10.7 Right subphronic abscess.

Despite these drawbacks, ultrasonography remains the most reliable method for the detection of fluid collections, a property particularly valuable in the diagnosis of abscess cavities.

Therapeutic value of ultrasonographic techniques

One of the additional values of ultrasonography is the opportunity it creates to provide effective therapy at the same time as achieving diagnosis. Abscesses which have been identified can be drained by ultrasonically guided aspiration, though CT can also prove valuable in this way.

Further investigations

When conventional radiology and ultrasonography fail to localize an abscess which has been suspected on clinical grounds, resort must be made to further imaging techniques if the need for a 'blind' laparotomy is to be avoided. These methods include computerized tomography, radioisotope scanning, or even magnetic resonance imaging. Each technique has drawbacks as well as potential advantages and these will now be considered.

Computerized tomography

When ultrasound is inconclusive, CT scanning (21–23) can often localize the site of the abscess. It is usually possible to obtain excellent anatomical detail with this technique and, in particular, inspection of the body wall and retroperitoneal regions can be achieved. Indeed, in many centres this technique has superceded ultrasonography, particularly in difficult clinical situations, e.g. in the presence of overlying gas. The investigation can, however, be impaired by the artefacts produced by surgical clips or other metallic objects. In addition, when contrast opacification of the bowel cannot be achieved, satisfactory image interpretation is made difficult. It is essential to obtain meticulous bowel preparation, as loops of bowel which have not been opacified can either obscure an abscess, or they may themselves be indistinguishable from collections of pus.

There are other disadvantages to this technique, over and above the fact that in many hospitals in the UK it is, as yet, either not available, or access to the facility may be severely restricted. To undertake CT it is always necessary to transport the patient to the radiology department. This may well prove difficult for patients who are severely ill. Compliance by such a sick patient may also be difficult to achieve; lying immobile

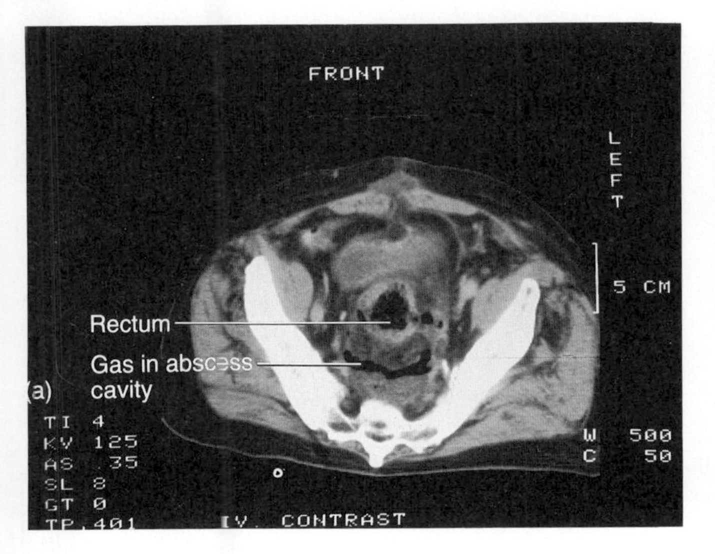

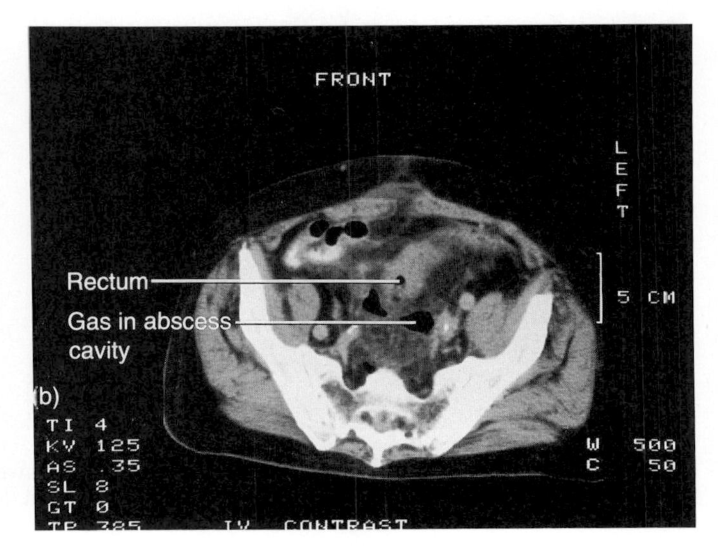

Fig. 10.8 (a) and (b). This patient was pyrexial following an anterior resection for colonic carcinoma. CT shows an abnormal collection of fluid and gas in the presacral space posterior to the rectum (a). Note a number of small collections of gas closely related to the external aspect of the wall of the rectum. On the cut immediately superior (b), collections coalesce into a 'butterfly.' This is the site of the leak from the anastomosis. (Courtesy of Wessex Bodyscanner Unit.)

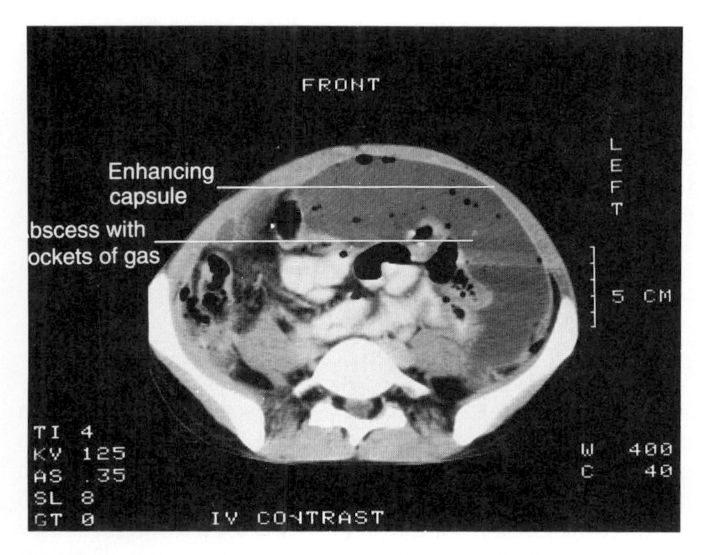

Fig. 10.9. This patient was acutely unwell following right hemicolectomy for Crohn's disease. CT demonstrates a large fluid collection in the left side of the abdomen containing numerous loculated pockets of gas and an enhancing capsule around the collection. This appearance is typical of an abscess. (Courtesy of Wessex Bodyscanner Unit.)

within the scanner is not the most comfortable of procedures! In addition, CT also has the highest radiation exposure of all techniques, and is the most expensive.

Despite these drawbacks, CT has made valuable contributions in this difficult diagnostic area. The results of the investigation are immediately available, and therapeutic needle aspiration of pus with insertion of a tube for subsequent drainage can be effected at the same time. Although both ultrasound and CT can be used when rapid results are required, either in critically ill patients or when there are good localizing signs present, CT is preferable when ileus is present, when drains are *in situ*, or when wounds are left open.

An abscess appears on the CT scan as a low density mass, and in approximately half of the cases abnormal collections of gas can be detected. (Fig. 10.8a, b). Less frequently, rim enhancement may also be seen (Fig. 10.9). As already mentioned, in order to distinguish fluid filled loops of bowel, orally administered contrast medium must be given prior to the investigation. Despite this precaution diagnostic confusion can still be caused by haematomas and seromas. Indeed, even diffuse inflammatory lesions and phlegmons can prove difficult to distinguish from purulent collections. It is always important, therefore, that clinical information be considered carefully in conjunction with the CT findings. As with ultrasonography, CT-directed needle aspiration may be needed to confirm the presence of an abscess (Fig. 10.10a, b). Likewise, such aspiration can precede formal drainage of the lesion once this has been confirmed.

Several studies of the value of computed tomography have indicated diagnostic accuracy of the order of 95 per cent.

Magnetic resonance imaging

As yet there is little experience with this new technique (22). Although it is possible to obtain images which can localize abscesses without the radiation exposure associated with CT scanning, to date it is not a method which is widely available

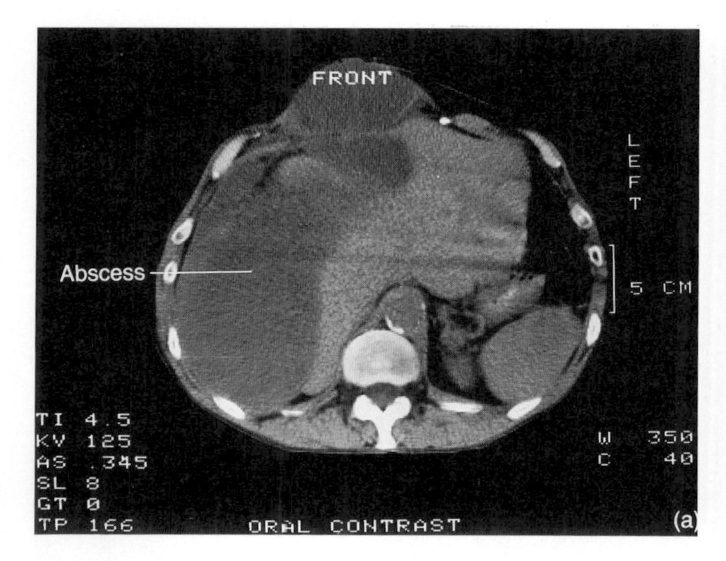

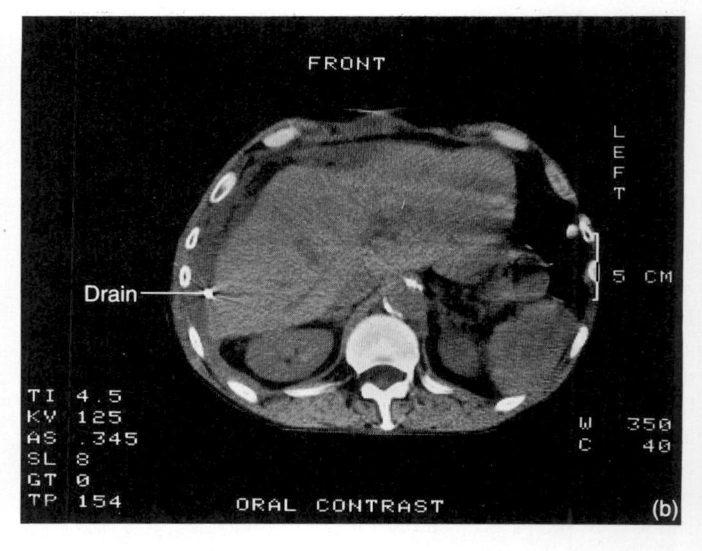

Fig. 10.10 (a) and (b). This patient presented with an increasing swelling on the anterior abdominal wall. He had undergone a prostatectomy 12 months previously, which was followed by a perforated duodenal ulcer which required further surgery. He had been unwell since and had noticed this swelling gradually increasing over the previous few months. His main complaint was of the friction caused by his shirt buttons but he also had felt generally unwell. CT shows a huge collection of fluid in the right subphrenic space extending inferiorly to the right of the liver which was displaced towards the mid line 10.10(a). On some cuts, this collection was shown to be continuous, with the mass in the anterior abdominal wall. Part (b) shows the appearances following percutaneous insertion of a drain using CT guidance. Two litres of pus were drained. (Courtesy of Wessex Bodyscanner Unit.)

in the United Kingdom. In addition, needle aspiration of an abscess is difficult to achieve. It is therefore unlikely to replace the other techniques described in the majority of patients.

Radionuclide imaging

When conventional radiology and ultrasonography have failed to localize a suspected intra-abdominal abscess in a patient who is not critically ill, and CT is either unavailable or unhelpful, radionuclide imaging must be considered (24–49). Various radionuclide procedures are available to detect focal infection. In these techniques, radionuclide labels are attached either to pharmaceuticals or to leucocytes. On injection these complexes become concentrated at the site of infection due to alterations in local blood flow and function.

A range of radiolabelled complexes for the detection of focal infection has been studied. These can be considered in two main categories: labelled white cells (using indium-111 chelates or technetium-99 hexamethylpropyleneamine-oxime ^{99m}Tc HMPAO) and gallium-67 citrate. Neither group is specific for infection, but will target inflammation secondary to infection.

In-111 oxine and tropolone labelled white cells are widely used for infection imaging. Several techniques for cell labelling have been described, important considerations being a high labelling efficiency and care to avoid leucocyte damage during the procedure. The normal distribution of In-111-labelled cells shortly following injection is within the blood pool, spleen and liver. 24-h images show predominant reticuloendothelial activity. Standard imaging protocols include 3-and 24-h spot views, dictated by the clinical history, with 48-h films obtained where necessary.

Abscesses are identified as abnormal focal concentrations of activity, with an intensity greater than that of the liver. Non-specific uptake at sites of inflammation, such as surgical wounds or haematomas is generally less intense than hepatic activity. Early images are useful to identify focal activity as liver activity diminishes with time, whereas abscess uptake increases steadily. Sequential imaging and multiple views are necessary to distinguish an abscess lying in close proximity to the spleen.

The accuracy of In-111-labelled leucocyte imaging is about 85 per cent, and is comparable with that of CT but the technique has several practical disadvantages. The necessity for late films, combined with limited availability of In-111 for emergency use may lead to unacceptable delays in establishing a diagnosis. The technique is, therefore, of limited value for the investigation of critically ill patients. The high energy of In-111 is not suited to modern gamma cameras and image resolution is often poor as a result. Finally, In-111-labelling leads to a relatively high absorbed radiation dose to lymphocytes, leading to possible sublethal chromosome damage.

These disadvantages are overcome by labelling with ^{99m}Tc HMPAO which is now the agent of first choice for localization of occult infection. A highly lipophilic complex, HMPAO diffuses readily across cell membranes, becoming trapped within the cell. Labelling is achieved by incubating ^{99m}Tc HMPAO with a leucocyte suspension, which is then reinjected into the patient. The net result is a pure granulocyte label, since these elements are preferentially labelled and form more stable complexes than other leucocytes.

The normal distribution of ^{99m}Tc HMPAO-labelled leucocytes includes the reticuloendothelial system with renal, urinary, biliary and large bowel activity. Imaging one and four hours post-injection is usually adequate for the diagnosis of focal infection. This has clear advantages in terms of minimizing patient discomfort, reducing camera and radiographer imaging time and allowing management decisions to be reached more rapidly.

The main disadvantage of ^{99m}Tc HMPAO-labelled white cell imaging is significant gut activity resulting from biliary excretion. Early imaging can be used to differentiate between inflammatory bowel disease, physiological bowel activity and focal infection, but it may be difficult to establish whether an abscess communicates with the gut lumen. Under these circumstances, In-111-labelled leucocyte scans are preferable.

Although not of direct relevance to this review, ^{99m}Tc HMPAO is also less satisfactory for thoracic imaging, as, for example, in bronchiectasis, because of the much higher background activity present in the lung.

Gallium-67 citrate is also of value for localizing infection, although its use has declined following the introduction of labelled leucocyte imaging. It has the advantage of simplicity, requiring a single intravenous injection and is thus the agent of choice for centres without facilities for cell labelling. Ga-67 uptake is not mediated solely by leucocyte activity, and it therefore has potential advantages over labelled leucocyte imaging for the detection of chronic infection when leucocyte turnover is slow.

Early images show blood pool and rénal activity with later uptake in the reticuloendothelial system, breast and bone. Like HMPAO labelled white cells, however, ^{67}Ga is excreted in the biliary tree and gut, making image interpretation difficult. Purgatives and delayed images for up to 72 h are advocated but usually impractical in the clinical context of an acutely ill patient. ^{67}Ga is also a tumour imaging agent and is, therefore, even less specific for infection than labelled white cells. Specific antibody labelling *in vivo* will probably prove to be of greater value.

Thus, the principal role of radionuclide scanning is either as a confirmatory investigation, or when ultrasound or CT imaging have failed to identify an abscess cavity strongly suspected on clinical grounds. Increased localized uptake is an indication at least for reassessment of that area by either CT or ultrasound. This is particularly true if infected areas are some distance away from the region which is under clinical suspicion.

Conclusions

Although a detailed history combined with careful clinical examination allows the diagnosis of intra-abdominal infection to be straightforward in most instances, this is not always the case. In the days immediately following major intra-abdominal surgery this problem can be particularly difficult. Even when there is little doubt of the existence of infection with possible abscess formation, it's localization is not always easy.

In these situations, to aid the surgeon, resort must be made to imaging techniques. Although choices between these methods will vary according to local circumstances, dictated largely by the availability of equipment and of expertise, general recommendations can be made. The usual pathway for the clinician has been outlined, with description of some of the more detailed considerations which may be of relevance. In most circumstances this will be the use of conventional radiology, proceeding to ultrasonography; or, increasingly, to CT scanning. When CT is available it should provide answers to most problems so that the necessity for radioisotope investigations should prove infrequent. CT has, therefore, become the technique of choice in many centres for the diagnosis of difficult cases. As yet, magnetic resonance imaging would appear to have little to offer, but developments in this and other imaging techniques should be awaited with interest.

Finally, although the investigation pathway most frequently helpful has been outlined above, it is essential to remember that these investigations are essentially complementary. Decision as to their use must always be guided by the clinical findings. Such decisions can so easily lead to either cure or death of the patient.

References

1. Altemeier, W.A., Culbertson, W.R., Fullen, W.D., Shook, C.D. (1973). Intra-abdominal abscesses. *Am. J. Surg.*, **125**, 71–9.
2. Fry, D.E., Garrison, R.N., Heitsch, R.C., Calhoon, K., Polk, H.C. (1980). Determinants of death in patients with intra-abdominal abscess. *Surgery*, **88**, 517–23.
3. Ochsner, A. and De Bakey, M. (1938). Subphrenic abscess: collective review and analysis of 3,608 collected and personal cases. *Surg. Gynecol. Obstet.*, **66**, 426–33.
4. Ariel I.M. and Kazarian, K.K. (1971). *Diagnosis and treatment of abdominal abscesses*, p. 203. Williams & Wilkins, Baltimore.
5. McDonald, P.J., Taylor, I., Karran, S.J. (1991). Mortality in a University Surgical Unit: What is an avoidable death? *J. R. Soc. Med.*, **84**, 213–16.
6. Rogers, P.N. and Wright, I.H. (1987). Post-operative intra-abdominal sepsis. *Br. J. Surg.*, **74**, 973–5.
7. Geddes, A. Antibiotics for septicaemia. In *Controversies in surgical sepsis* (ed. S.J. Karran), p. 259. Praeger, New York.
8. Meyers, M.A. (1982). Dynamic radiology of the abdomen (2nd edn). Springer-Verlag, New York.
9. Saini, S., Kellum, J.H., O'Leary, H.P. *et al.* (1983). Improved localization and survival in patients with intra-abdominal abscesses. *Am. J. Surg.*, **145**, 136–42.
10. Doust, B.D. and Doust, V.L. (1976). Ultrasonic diagnosis of abdominal abscesses. *Dig. Dis. Sci.*, **21**, 569–76.
11. Taylor, K.J.W., Sullivan, D.C., Wasson, J.F.M., and Rosenfield, A.T. (1978). Ultrasound and gallium for the diagnosis of abdominal and pelvic abscesses. *Gastrointest. Radiol.*, **31**, 281–5.
12. Carroll, B., Silverman, D.M., Goodwin, D.A., and McDougall, I.R. (1981). Ultrasonography and 111-Indium white blood cell scanning for the detection of intra-abdominal abscesses. *Radiology*, **140**, 155–60.
13. Schwerk, W.B. and Durr, H.K. (1981). Ultrasound grey scale pattern and guided aspiration puncture of abdominal abscesses. *J. Clin. Ultrasound*, **9**, 389–96.
14. Joseph, A.E.A. (1985). Imaging of abdominal abscesses. *Br. Med. J.*, **291**, 1446–7.
15. Halasz, N.A. and Van Sonnenberg, E. (1983). Drainage of intra-abdominal abscesses: tactics and choices. *Am. J. Surg.*, **146**, 113–15.
16. Halber, M.D., Daffner, R.H., Morgan, C.L. *et al.* (1979). Intra-abdominal abscess: current concepts in radiologic evaluation. *Am. J. Roentgenol.*, **133**, 9–13.
17. Lundstedt, C., Hederstrom, E., Brisma, J., Holmin, T., and Strand, S.E. (1986). Prospective investigation of radiologic methods in the diagnosis of intra-abdominal abscesses. *Acta Radiol.*, **27**, 49–54.
18. Joseph, A.E.A. and MacVicar, D. (1990). Ultrasound in the diagnosis of abdominal abscesses. *Clin. Radiol.*, **42**, 154–6.
19. Mintz, M.C., Arger, P.H., and Kressel, H.Y. (1983). An algorithmic approach to the radiologic evaluation of a suspected abdominal abscesses. *Seminars in Ultrasound*, **4**, 80–90.
20. Baker, M.E., Blinder, R.A., and Rice, R.P. (1986). Diagnostic imaging of abdominal fluid collections and abscesses. *CRC Crit. Rev. Diagn. Imaging*, **25**, 233–78.
21. Korobkin, M., Callen, P.W., Filly, R.A., *et al.* Comparison of computed tomography, ultrasonography and gallium-67 scanning in the evaluation of suspected abdominal abscess. *Radiology*, **129**, 89–93.
22. Knochel, J.Q., Koehler, P.R., Lee, T.G., and Welch, D.M. Diagnosis of abdominal abscesses with computed tomography, ultrasound and 111-Indium leucocyte scans. *Radiology*, **137**, 425–32.
23. Cohen, J.M., Weinreb, J.C., and Maravilla, K.R. (1985). Fluid collections in the intraperitoneal and extraperitoneal spaces: Comparison of MR & CT. *Radiology*, **155**, 705–8.
24. Zakhireh, B., Thakur, M.L., and Malech, H.L., *et al.* (1979). Indium-111-labelled polymorphonuclear leukocytes: Viability, random migration, chemotaxis, bactericidal capacity, and ultrastructure. *J. Nucl. Med.*, **20**, 741–7.
25. Edwards, C.L. and Hayes, R.L. (1969). Tumour scanning with ^{67}Ga citrate. *J. Nucl. Med.*, **10**, 103–5.
26. Gagliardi, P.D., Hoffer, P.B., and Rosenfield, A.T. (1988). Correlative imaging in abdominal infection: An algorithmic approach using nuclear medicine, ultrasound and computed tomography. *Semin. Nucl. Med.*, **18**, 320–34.
27. Roddie, M.E. (1987). Comparison of white cells labelled with ^{99m}Tc HMPAO and In-111 for imaging inflammation. *Br. J. Radiol.*, **60**, 820.
28. Peters, A.M. Danpure, H.J., Osman, B., *et al.* (1986). Clinical experience with ^{99m}Tc hexamethyl-propyleneamine oxime for labelling leucocytes and imaging infection. *Lancet*, **ii**, 946–9.
29. Thakur, M.L., Segal, A.W., Louis, L., *et al.* Indium-111-labelled cellular blood components: mechanism of labelling and intracellular location in human neutrophils. *J. Nucl. Med.*, **18**, 1020–4.
30. Roddie, M.E., Peters, A.M., Danpure, H.J., *et al.* (1988). Inflammation: Imaging with Tc^{99m} HMPAO-labelled leucocytes. *Radiology*, **166**, 767–72.
31. Mock, B.H., Schauwecker, D.S., English, D., *et al.* *In vivo* kinetics of canine leucocytes labelled with Tc^{99m} HMPAO and In-111 tropolonate. *J. Nucl. Med.*, **29**, 1246–51.
32. Korobkin, M., Callen, P.W., Filly, R.A., *et al.* (1978). Comparison of computed tomography, ultrasonography and gallium-67 scanning in the evaluation of suspected abdominal abscess. *Radiology*, **29**, 89–93.
33. Damron, J.R., Beihn, R.M., and Deland, F.H. (1976). Detection of upper abdominal abscesses by radionuclide imaging. *Radiology*, **120**, 131–4.
34. Doherty, P.W., Bushberg, J.T., Lipton, M.J., *et al.* (1978). The use of Indium-111-labelled leukocytes for abscess detection. *Clin. Nucl. Med.*, **3**, 108–10.
35. Crystal, R.F. and Palace, F. (1984). Indium-111 oxine-labelled

autologous leukocyte scans in the management of colorectal disease. *Dis. Colon Rectum*, **27**, 223–7.
36. Poitras, P., Carrier, L., Chartrand, R., *et al.* (1987). Indium-111 Leukocyte scanning of the abdomen. Analysis of its value for diagnosis and management of inflammatory bowel disease. *J. Clin. Gastroenterol.*, **9**, 418–23.
37. Becker, W., Schaefer, R.M., and Borner, W. (1989). *In vivo* viability of In-111 labelled granulocytes demonstrated in a Sham-dialysis model. *Br. J. Radiol.*, **62**, 463–7.
38. Seabold, J.F., Wilson, D.G., Lieberman, L.M., and Boyd, C.M. (1984). Unsuspected extra-abdominal sites of infection: Scintigraphic detection with Indium-111-labelled leucocytes. *Radiology*, **151**, 213–17.
39. Peters, A.M. (1989). Imaging with white cells. *Clin. Radiol.*, **40**, 453–4.
40. Habibian, M.R., Staab, E.V., Matthews, H.A. (1975). Gallium citrate Ga67 scans in febrile patients. *J. Am. Med. Assoc.*, **233**, 1073–6.
41. Hilson, A.J.W. and Maisey, M.N. (1979). Gallium-67 scanning in pyrexia of unknown origin. *Br. Med. J.*, **ii**, 1330–1.
42. Moir, C. and Robins, R.E. (1982). Role of ultrasonography, gallium scanning, and computed tomography in the diagnosis of intra-abdominal abscess. *Am. J. Surg.*, **143**, 582–5.
43. Saverymuttu, S., Croxton, M.E., Peters, A.M., and Lavender, J.P. (1984).Indium 111 troponolate leucocyte scanning in the detection of intra-abdominal abscesses. *Clin. Radiol.*, **34**, 593–6.
44. Saverymuttu, S.H., Maltby, P., Batman, P., Joseph, A.E.A., and Maxwell, D. (1986). False positive localization of Indium 111 granulocyte in colonic carcinoma. *Br. J. Radiol.*, **59**, 773–7.
45. Ackery, D.M. (1980). Identification and localization of sepsis by radioisotope imaging. In *Controversies in surgical sepsis* (ed. S.J. Karran), Chapter 25, pp. 311–16. Praeger.
46. Taylor, K.J.W., Sullivan, D.C., Wasson, J.F.M., and Rosenfield, A.T. (1978). Ultrasound and gallium for the diagnosis of abdominal and pelvic abscesses. *Gastrointest. Radiol.*, **3**, 281–6.
47. Peters, A.M., Lavender, J.P., Needham, S.G., *et al.* (1986). Imaging thrombus with radiolabelled monoclonal antibody to platelets. *Br. Med. J.* (*Clin. Res.*), **293**, 1525–7.
48. Saverymuttu, S.H., Peters, A.M., Crofton, M.E., *et al.* 111 Indium autologous granulocytes in the detection of inflammatory bowel disease. *Gut*, **26**, 955–60.
49. Saverymuttu, S.H., Peters, A.M., Lavender, J.P. (1985). Clinical importance of enteric communication with abdominal abscesses. *Br. Med. J.* (*Clin. Res.*), **290**, 23–6.

11

The role of the infection control nurse

MARGARET A. WORSLEY

The art of nursing has been reviewed by many authors, and yet there still does not appear to be a clear definition of nursing, either as a skill or as an art. Florence Nightingale said, in 1859, that the very elements of nursing were all but unknown (1). This lady was the first nurse to indicate that nursing should not be limited to a medically derived role. Further, she emphasized 'the proper use of fresh air, light, warmth, cleanliness, quiet, and the proper selection of administration of diet.' This seems to be an excellent framework for the art of surgical nursing more than one hundred years later.

The word 'nursing' itself has different derivations and meanings in different languages, and in some languages there is no word for it at all (2). However, in most countries the function of nurses does have a common core, although in others this may differ widely because of different cultures and economic situations. For example, sick people were cared for in their own homes a long time before nursing became an organized occupation. This has implications for the prevention of surgical infections.

The practice of nursing has been described by Professor Jean McFarlane (3) in the UK acknowledging that all nurses work in collaboration with other health care workers and patients. She stresses three main themes in nursing:

1. Clinical care;
2. Management of care;
3. Teaching.

Such collaboration is an essential element of surgical nursing where the nurse works closely with surgeons and health care workers from many other disciplines to ensure effective patient care.

The original concept of a specialist nurse who would be employed solely for control of infection was described by Brendan Moore in 1959 (4). He and his colleagues introduced and described six main functions of the nurse:

1. Collection and preparation of adequate records.
2. Prompt recognition and disposal of infected patients.
3. Improvement of the liaison between matron and the ward sisters.
4. Checking the performance of ward techniques.
5. Supervision of infection record.
6. Routine checks of staphylococcal carrier-rates in operating theatre staffs, assessment of environmental contamination, efficiency of preventative measures, and research.

Although at that time this appeared to be a clear definition of the specialist role, it could be argued that many of these functions could be carried out by a general nurse. For a variety of reasons the role and specific function of the infection control nurse (ICN) in the UK took many years to develop into a clinical specialty (5).

Many nurses in England were encouraged to sample the environment and to collect records of wound infection without apparently using the information obtained from these practices as the basis for any useful action. Nurses in the USA went through a similar phase but then began to establish hospital infection control programmes. It was noted at that time that the role of the infection control nurse in the USA had much to do with 'effecting behavioural changes and getting people to like and conscientiously implement change' (6).

These nurses were looking at ways of collecting data to provide feedback to the surgeons. Infection control had a relatively high profile in the USA and nurses were appointed in large numbers as epidemiologists.

How then can a trained infection control nurse complement a surgical team in the UK in the prevention and control of surgical infection? It is clear that if the ICN is to achieve any useful purpose in the prevention of surgical infection her activities should be based on practices of proven value. Although experience indicates that, in general, nurses are reluctant to accept research based findings (7), we need to know those factors which increase the risk of surgical infection if we are to enhance the quality of patient care. Most studies (8) reveal an increase in wound infection rate in association with advancing age. Other major risk factors such as diabetes, obesity, and malnutrition are associated with an increase in wound infection rates (9). Pollock (10) states that 'It is equally true that the host's ability to resist infection can be reduced by gross malnutrition, by tissue destruction including clumsy surgery, by prolonged anaesthesia, and by ischaemia, whereas the only proven way of enhancing host resistance is to ensure an adequate supply of oxygenated blood to the tissues'.

Pre-operative nursing care is clearly the responsibility of the primary nurse in charge of the ward, but the ICN can help by acting as a resource to the nursing team to provide information on nursing research which can supplement the planning of nursing care to help to prevent post-operative infection.

Experience indicates that nurses have an important part to play in planning intervention strategies. Such strategies range from skin preparation to care of the patient requiring intravenous nutrition. An example is the surgical patient who needs peripheral venous cannulation. It is said that peripheral venous cannulation is the most commonly performed invasive procedure with the exception of diagnostic venepuncture (11). It is the responsibility of medical and nursing staff to ensure that intravenous therapy is safe and effective for the patient who requires surgery. In 1983 it was reported in a European study that in the UK 15.1 per cent of surgical patients with intravenous devices developed thrombophlebitis. Since 39.9 per cent of all surgical patients had an intravenous device in place, this implies that 6 per cent of all surgical patients have cannula related thrombophlebitis. Fortunately the number of patients with serious infection is much less, 0.8 per cent had bacteraemia (12). Since prevention of infection is an integral part of any invasive, intravenous procedure (13), it is necessary to determine which infection prevention and control measures are considered to be effective on the basis of proven research.

Another example is given by Boore who clearly demonstrated that the patient who is given, in the pre-operative period, a full, comprehensible explanation of what is going to happen as a result of surgery appears to have a less traumatic experience that would otherwise be the case (14). Her study showed a significantly lower incidence of post-operative complications and shorter hospital stay in those patients who were given a carefully planned explanation in the pre-operative period.

Cruse has demonstrated that a full-time surgical research nurse who is in charge of wound surveillance and who observes all wounds during each patient's hospital stay, and after discharge, is effective in the prevention and control of surgical wound infection (15). This data is presented to the individual surgeon at regular intervals (see Chapter 1).

Surveillance

Surveillance is a major component of infection control, although its true value has not yet been completely established. However, as from April 1991 it is likely that many hospitals in the UK will have to provide information at regular intervals on infection rates in surgery. Medical Audit will be a standard requirement for all aspects of patient care (16).

Until now few hospitals in the UK have routinely prepared such information. Its provision will make heavy demands on the time and expertise of the persons responsible: the members of the surgical team, the infection control nurse and the infection control doctor. Before discussing the problems involved it would be useful to consider what surveillance implies. Although the idea of surveillance of hospital acquired infection originated in England, its practice has not been widely accepted here (17).

Bryan and Deever (18) defined two types of surveillance: process surveillance and outcome surveillance. Process surveillance involves the observation, description, and measuring of the process of implementation of infection control policies. Outcome surveillance involves the measurement of the outcome of infection control practices—namely, the infection rate.

Process surveillance is often undertaken by the ICN, although it is clearly within the capability and responsibility of senior nurses in surgical departments. Outcome surveillance is, perhaps, more properly the responsibility of the ICN. However, at the present time in most hospitals in the UK the ICN has little influence on surgical wound infection, most of the action taking place in the operating theatre.

Before examining outcome surveillance as it applies to infection in surgery, it would be worth looking at the aims of surveillance as a whole. In a general review of surveillance of communicable diseases Langmuir (19) stated that there should be regular dissemination of the basic data and its interpretation to all who have contributed to the study and to all others who need to know. He also referred to taking appropriate action when indicated. These comments are pertinent to the particular case of surveillance of surgical wound infection today, to take the most obvious example of surgical infection. Collection of data without taking action on the findings, is not new in infection control as has already been stated, but is likely to confirm the belief that the procedure is a complete waste of time.

Outcome surveillance in the present context implies the establishment of incidence rates: that is the number of new patients infected per 100 discharges or admissions (17). Such incidence rates should not be compared with prevalence rates as given in the results of the National Survey of Infection in Hospitals, 1980 (20). The two rates are obtained by different methods and are not comparable.

Sophisticated methods of hospital-wide surveillance have been described (21); these could be applied to surgical wound infection rates. However, it must be appreciated that such methods will be of no value in a situation where the data collected is often inaccurate and misleading. Several considerations must be borne in mind when calculating incidence rates. Infection rates which relate to all types of operation, pooled together as a single group, are of little value since there will be considerable variation between surgical departments in the types of operations performed. It is usual, in trying to allow for this variation, to consider surgical wound infections in three main groups: clean, clean-contaminated and contaminated (20); in the USA a fourth category—dirty—is added (22). Local considerations may suggest alterations to the precise nature of the categories of operations to be recorded.

When calculating rates of surgical wound infection it would appear relatively easy to establish the denominator: the total number of patients undergoing operations in the various categories. But the numerator—the number of patients infected—is much more difficult to establish, for several reasons.

In the first place it is essential that a clear definition of wound infection is adopted. This is necessary if comparison is to be made with figures from the same unit at different periods, or with figures from different units. A suitable definition is that used in the 1980 National Survey (20), Unfortunately, experience indicates that some workers use their own definition of wound infection, thus making it impossible to compare their data with other data, without drawing misleading conclusions (see Chapter 9).

Different observers may differ in their opinion as to whether a wound is infected or not, although the adoption of standard criteria should decrease the discrepancies. This variation may be eliminated in a particular hospital by having a single observer inspect the wounds. This does not, of course, help when comparing infection rates compiled in different hospitals.

The infection rate may be influenced by the use of different surveillance methods (23).

Many patients do not develop evidence of wound infection until after discharge from hospital (24). If, as usually happens, these patients are not included among those with wound infection the figure for wound infection rate is falsely low. This factor is more likely to be a problem when early discharge is common. Attempts to correct for this factor (17) add considerably to the time and expertise required to compile the statistics.

Furthermore, wound infection on a surgical unit will appear to be low when it is not the practice to take swabs and the identification of infection is laboratory based (23).

Many workers have used the results of surgical wound surveillance in an attempt to reduce the incidence of wound infection by reporting back to surgeons their infection rates along with those of their colleagues, without identifying the latter. This procedure was regarded as one of the essential components of effective infection control in the paper describing the results of the SENIC Project of the Centres for Disease Control of the United States (22). Despite this, Haley, speaking is 1984, reported that the approach was not practised by 'very many hospitals today' (25). More recently, the reporting of surgeon-specific wound infection rates has been criticized by Scheckler as a potentially dangerous and misleading strategy (26).

Systematic surveillance may be used as a valuable research tool. It is clearly of great importance to know what factors increase the risk of infection. Cruse and Foord (27) have described their 10-year prospective study on the epidemiology of wound infection. Also, during the SENIC Project the risk factors for wound infection were studied and four major factors (abdominal operation, operation lasting more than two hours, contaminated or dirty-infected operation, and three or more other concurrent 'diagnoses') were identified (28). Further studies of this type would be valuable in establishing those factors most worthy of further attention. It is clear, from what has been said that a programme of surveillance of surgical wounds requires careful consideration before it is introduced. However, many surgeons who have been involved with research studies will be very familiar with the problems outlined above, since they affect the data for such studies (29).

It would be misleading to suggest that the value of surveillance is universally accepted, even though—as stated above—it will be necessary in many hospitals to provide regular information on infection rates in surgery.

Two extreme views have been expressed. In the SENIC Project (22) surveillance activities, including the reporting of surgical wound infection rates to surgeons, were considered to have played an important part in the reduction of infection rates. 'Control' activities to intervene in the care of patients were also important. 'Intensive surveillance activities' were considered to be an important factor in the prevention of hospital acquired urinary tract infections, including patients with indwelling urinary catheters. High-intensity surveillance was regarded as one of the important factors in the prevention of post-operative pneumonia in surgical patients. On the other hand Casewell (30) was less impressed by the value of energetic surveillance, suggesting that this may well go hand in hand with other factors which favourably influence infection rates.

Rituals in surgery

Many procedures have been introduced into surgical practice over the years. Several of these appear to belong to the category described by Eickhoff as of doubtful or unknown efficiency (31), or can be described more bluntly as rituals. It would require a major study to demonstrate directly any positive value of such practices in reducing infection rates and what work has been done has been based on estimations of the degree of bacteriological contamination, with and without the procedure in question. The following are common examples.

Tacky or antiseptic mats were introduced with the objective of reducing the number of bacteria carried into the operating theatre on trolley wheels or foot covers. It has not been demonstrated that wound infection rates have been reduced by this practice and studies of the extent of bacterial contamination of wheels or foot covers have not shown any convincing evidence that the practice is of any value (32, 33).

Plastic overshoes are still used in many operating theatres. Again there is no evidence that they are of any value (34), on the other hand there is evidence that hands may become contaminated from footwear when donning the overshoes, and hand-washing facilities are not usually provided at the point at which the overshoes are put on.

Changeover trolleys are regarded by many as an essential part of theatre equipment. Again there is no direct evidence that they influence infection rates. Recent work has failed to show any deleterious effect on the environment of the operating theatre if only one trolley is used (35).

Disinfection of the operating theatre floor is still widely practiced, but detergents appear to be equally effective and less likely to damage the floor, especially the seals between sheets of vinyl. Disinfectants should, however, be used if the floor, or any surface, is contaminated with blood or with body fluids (36).

It is now widely accepted that the bacteria that are responsible for infection come from the patient himself or from the operating team, including the non-scrubbed members. It would, therefore, seem sensible to limit the number of staff in the theatre to essential staff, to eliminate any unnecessary movement of staff and opening and closing of doors.

Although it is generally accepted that staff with infected lesions should be excluded from the operating room it is probably not widely appreciated that staff who have had superficial infections such as eczema or otitis externa may apparently be cured but may still carry pathogenic organisms on the skin and be responsible for infection of wounds. This is true even if the person is not a member of the scrubbed team (L. Parker, personal communication). For medico-legal reasons, at the least, there should be close cooperation between the occupational health department and the theatre manager before staff members who have had active infections are allowed to return to work in the operating room.

Conclusions

In the light of changes in the delivery of health care in the UK (16) it will be necessary for all staff involved in the care of the surgical patient to work together to achieve an effective infection prevention strategy for all patients who require surgical intervention. As already indicated the type of surveillance to be adopted warrants careful consideration, interestingly Haley has described a 'sweeping paradigm change in infection control'. He has reported that 'the field is shifting attention to the plight of the patient and away from old hospital-wide surveillance programmes that establish little more than baseline data'. This is indeed a change of direction in the United States and emphasizes that time is well spent examining patient care practices that are based on proven research, and have a measurable outcome.

The ICN can complement the nursing team by providing up to date information on the infection prevention and control literature at regular intervals, arranging seminar presentations in clinical areas; these provide a excellent forum for staff to share recent developments and ideas.

In the field of infection control is it vital that the ICN does not lose sight of the reason for infection prevention and control strategies. She should plan her resources and time to ensure that she provides support for effective patient care.

On the subject of quality and medical and nursing audit as described in the White Paper (16) Pollock (38) states that 'Audit of the quality of life after surgical treatment tends to be neglected by surgeons; it is, however, just as important as audit of morbidity and mortality. Unless our treatments improve the quality of life we are probably doing our patients more good by not operating on them'.

These remarks also apply to all nurses involved in surgical care including the infection control nurse.

References

1. Nightingale, F. (1859). *Notes on nursing*. Harrison & Sons, London.
2. McFarlane, J.K. and Castledine, G. (1982). *A guide to the practice of nursing using the nursing process*. C.V. Mosby, London.
3. McFarlane, J.K. (1975). *Essays on nursing*. King's Fund, London.
4. Gardner, A.M.N., Stamp, M., Bowgen, J.A., and Moore, B. (1962). The infection control sister: a new member of the control of infection team in general hospitals. *Lancet*, **ii**, 710–1.
5. Worsley, M.A. (1988). The role of the infection control nurse. *J. Hosp. Infect.*, **11**(suppl. A), 400–5.
6. Barrett-Connor, E., Brandt, S.L., Simon, H.J., and Dechairo, D.C. (ed.) (1978). *Epidemiology for the infection control nurse*. C.V. Mosby. St. Louis, Missouri.
7. Hunt, M. (1987). The process of translating research findings into nursing practice. *J. Adv. Nurs.*, **12**, 101–10.
8. National Research Council Division of Medical Sciences, Ad Hoc Committee of Trauma. (1964). Post-operative wound infections: The influence of ultraviolet irradiation of the operating room and various other factors. *Ann. Surg.*, **160**(suppl. 2).
9. Cruse, P. (1986). Surgical infection: incisional wounds. In *Hospital infections* (ed. J.V. Bennett and P.S. Brachman). Little Brown, Boston, Mass.
10. Pollock, A.V. (1988). Surgical prophylaxis: The emerging picture. *Lancet*, **1**, 225–9.
11. Peters, J.L., Frame, J.D., and Dawson, S.M. (1984). Peripheral venous cannulation: reducing the risks. *Br. J. Parenteral Therapy*, **5**, 56–68.
12. Nystrom, B., Larsen, S.O., and Dankert, J., *et al.* (1983). Bacteraemia in surgical patients with intravenous devices: A European multicentre incidence study. The European Working Party on Control of Hospital Infections. *J. Hosp. Infect.*, **4**, 338–349.
13. Lonsway, R.A. (1987). *Research, standards and infection control*, Chapter 10, pp. 106–9. National Intravenous Therapy Association.
14. Boore, J.R.P. (1979). *Prescription for recovery*. Royal College of Nursing/Churchill Livingstone, London.
15. Cruse, P. (1988). The psychology of change in health care: preoperative patient assessment and education. In *Proceedings of the Second International Conference on Infection Control*. Infection Control Nurses' Association of Great Britain, London.
16. Department of Health. (1989). *Working for patients*. HMSO, London.
17. Wenzel, R.P. and Streed, S.A. (1989). Surveillance and use of computers in hospital infection control. *J. Hosp. Infect.*, **13**, 217–29.
18. Bryan, C.S. and Deever, E. (1981). Implementing control measures. *Am. J. Infect. Control*, **9**, 101–6.
19. Langmuir, A.D. (1963). The surveillance of communicable diseases of national importance. *N. Engl. J. Med.*, **268**, 182–92.
20. Meers, P.D., Ayliffe, G.A.J., and Emmerson, A.M., *et al.* (1981). Report on the national survey of infection in hospitals. *J. Hosp. Infect.*, **2** (suppl.).
21. Morrison, A.J., Kaiser, D.L., and Wenzel, R.P. (1987). A measurement of the efficacy of nosocomial infection control using the 95 per cent confidence interval for infection rates. *Am. J. Epidemiol.*, **126**, 192–7.
22. Haley, R.W., Culver, D.H., White, J.W., *et al.* (1985). The efficacy of infection surveillance and control programs in preventing nosocomial infections in US hospitals. *Am. J. Epidemiol.*, **121**, 182–205.
23. Surin, V.V. (1988). Effect of different surveillance methods on statistics of post-operative wound infection. *J. Hosp. Infect.*, **11**, 116–20.
24. Reimer, K., Gleed, C., and Nicolle, L.E. (1987). The impact of postdischarge infection on surgical wound infection rates. *Infect. Control*, **8**, 237–40.
25. Haley, R.W. (1985). Surveillance by objective: a new priority-directed approach to the control of nosocomial infections. *Am. J. Infect. Control*, **13**, 78–89.
26. Scheckler, W.E. (1988). Surgeon-specific wound infection rates—a potentially dangerous and misleading strategy. *Infect. Control Hosp. Epidemiology*, **9**, 145–6.
27. Cruse, P.J.E. and Foord, R. (1980). The epidemiology of wound infection—a 10-year prospective study of 62 939 wounds. *Surg. Clin. North Am.*, **60**, 27–40.
28. Haley, R.W., Culver, D.H., Morgan, W.M., *et al.* (1985).

Identifying patients at high risk of surgical wound infection. *Am. J. Epidemiol.*, **121**, 206–15.

29. Walker, A.J., Taylor, E.W., Lindsay, G., *et al.* (1988). A multicentre study to compare piperacillin with the combination of netilmicin and metronidazole for prophylaxis in elective colorectal surgery undertaken in district general hospitals. *J. Hosp. Infect.*, **11**, 340–8.
30. Casewell, M.W. (1980). Surveillance of infection in hospitals. *J. Hosp. Infect.*, **1**, 293–7.
31. Eickhoff, T.C. (1981). Nosocomial infections—A 1980 view: progress, priorities and prognosis. In *Nosocomial infections* (ed. R.E. Dixon), pp. 1–8. Proceedings of the Second International Conference on Nosocomial Infections. Yorke Medical Books.
32. Lowbury, E.J.L., Ayliffe, G.A.J., Geddes, A.M., and Williams, J.D. (1981). *Control of hospital infection: A practical handbook*, p. 165. Chapman & Hall, London.
33. Simmons, B.P. (1982). *Guideline for prevention of surgical wound infections*. Centres for Disease Control, Atlanta, Georgia.
34. Hambraeus, A. and Malmborg, A.-S. (1979). The influence of different footwear on floor contamination. *Scand. J. Infect. Dis.*, **11**, 243–6.
35. Lewis, D.A., Weymont, G., Nokes, C.M., *et al.* (1990). A bacteriological study of the effect on the environment of using a one- or two-trolley system in theatre. *J. Hosp. Infect.*, **15**, 35–53.
36. Ayliffe, G.A.J., Coates, D., and Hoffman, P.N. (1984). Chemical disinfection in hospitals. Public Health Laboratory Service, London.
37. Haley, R.W. (1990). Reported in *Hospital Infection Control* **17**(1): 3–4. American Health Consultants Inc., Atlanta, Georgia.
38. Pollock, A. and Evans, M. (1989). *Surgical audit*. Butterworths, London.

12

Infection scoring systems

BRIAN J. ROWLANDS and PAUL H.B. BLAIR

Introduction

Infection continues to be a major cause of post-operative and post-injury morbidity and mortality in surgical practice. Over the past 20 years many advances have been made in the diagnosis and therapy of surgical infections notably the introduction of new chemotherapeutic agents, radiological innovations such as computerized axial tomography and nuclear scanning, and better patient management in the intensive care setting, utilizing advances in fluid resuscitation, nutritional support, and the treatment of respiratory, hepatic, and renal failure. We now recognize that sequential failure of vital organ systems often precedes death from infection and that successful reversal of this deterioration of metabolic and immune function requires its early recognition and aggressive management. The assessment of innovative methods of diagnosis and treatment has often been difficult due to the heterogeneity of the patient populations being studied, but in recent years a number of scoring systems have been introduced to allow a more meaningful interpretation of data from studies of surgical sepsis. Some of these scoring systems when used sequentially throughout the course of a patient's illness give objective evidence of deterioration or improvement of the clinical condition and allow comparisons of different therapeutic regimen in similar patients. This chapter describes some of the scoring systems currently in use for clinical management and research of surgical sepsis and discusses their application and limitations when applied to individuals and patient populations. It should be noted that all scoring systems are more accurate at predicting death than survival and should mainly be applied to the study of patient populations (1). At the present time, they should not be used to make therapeutic decisions about individual patients although in the future they may be used to determine the most appropriate diagnostic and therapeutic interventions based on an accurate assessment of the degree of disruption of metabolic homeostasis.

What is a scoring system?

Patients with similar illnesses or injuries might be expected to exhibit similar clinical signs and symptoms and to have similar outcomes to a particular therapy. This quite clearly does not happen in clinical practice because each individual patient has a unique metabolic and immunological make-up and responds differently to his pathological derangement and to treatment. A patient with acute appendicitis is usually treated with appendicectomy, but the success of the surgical treatment will depend on the previous health of the patient, the age, time interval between onset of symptoms, and presentation to hospital, whether perforation or diffuse peritonitis are present at the time of the operation and the technical skill of the surgeon and the appropriate use of other supportive therapies such as fluid resuscitation and antibiotic regimen. Thus, even in this simple everyday example of surgical practice there are multiple factors that influence outcome. Study of wound or intra-abdominal infection following treatment of appendicitis is meaningless if these factors are not taken into consideration so that valid comparisons can be made. We can assess the impact of therapeutic regimen on the management of appendicitis prospectively by eliminating as many variable as possible, studying the work of a single surgeon using a standard regimen and stratifying our analysis according to the pathological state of the appendix, e.g. normal, inflamed, suppurative, gangrenous, and perforated. This concept underlies the majority of scoring systems in that they use clinical, pathological, haematological, biochemical, immunological, anatomical, physiological or nutritional parameters, either individually or in combination, to define the patient population under study. Changes in these parameters can be monitored throughout the patient's clinical course to document deterioration or improvement in clinical condition. When a sufficiently large database of individual patients has been accrued and they have been studied over a long enough period, we can then analyse the impact of the original profile on outcome. In addition, we can subdivide patients into similar groups according to predetermined criteria and identify differences in outcome or response to therapy.

There are a number of common clinical conditions in which scoring systems are already used extensively. In surgical oncology we use the tumour–node–metastases (TNM) classification (2) to document the spread of breast cancer into local, regional, and disseminated disease and modifications of Duke's classification (3) similarly define the spread of colorectal tumours. Prognosis is directly related to these pathological scoring systems. The injury severity score (ISS) (4) is used in trauma patients to define the extent of anatomical disruption in six defined areas of the body. Morbidity and mortality are related to ISS. Glasgow Coma Scale (5) assesses the verbal, motor, and sensory response of head injured patients and accurately predicts both survival and long-term disability. The Imrie (6) and Ransome (7) criteria are used as scoring systems to assess the outcome of acute pancreatitis. The Crohn's Disease Activity Index (8) gives some indication of the local and systemic derangements of acute inflammatory bowel disease. Burn injury has traditionally been assessed according to its depth and the body surface area involved, and this information has led to the development of formulae to determine the volume and composition of fluid resuscitation in the immediate post-injury phase (9, 10). A prognostic nutritional index (11) has been used to determine the outcome and need for supplementary nutrition support in patients undergoing gastrointestinal surgery.

The common factor and limitation of all these systems is that they are defined by a particular diagnosis (e.g. trauma, pancreatitis, burn) and do not take into full consideration the extensive disruption to normal physiology and homeostasis that may result from pathological derangement. This is particularly relevant to the study of surgical sepsis and the development of scoring systems that take into account the multifaceted derangements associated with infections due to multiple different micro-organisms, bacteraemia, septicaemia, endotoxaemia, and multiple system organ failure. Any scoring system for use in septic patients with multiple system organ failure has to embrace these derangements of physiology and identify those parameters that most accurately reflect impending organ failure and improved organ function. An example of the application of a simple, physiological scoring system is the Revised Trauma Score that was used in the Major Trauma Outcome Study (12). Three parameters, were assessed as soon after injury as possible and weighted to give an overall score that reflected perfusion, oxygenation, and neurological impairment. This weighted 'physiological' score accurately predicted outcome, and when combined with 'anatomical' score (ISS) was highly discriminatory in predicting survival and death. This information, based on data from 80 544 patients, can now be used as an audit tool in trauma centres and to refine practices to ensure the potential survivors do not die unnecessarily.

If we accept that in septic and infected patients there will be measureable changes in physiological, biochemical, haematological, and other parameters that reflect organ dysfunction and infection severity then we should be able to develop scoring systems that enable us to study similar groups of patients even though their disease process, pathology, infecting organisms and therapy may be different.

Infection scoring systems

These can be classified into three distinct types of assessment:

1. Those that assess the risk factors that predispose to the development of post-operative or postinjury surgical infection, e.g. prognostic nutritional index.
2. Those that assess the amount of anatomical or physiological disruption caused by injury or a pathological process when clinical infection is not present but are capable of predicting the likelihood of clinical infection complicating the subsequent course of the illness, e.g. ISS, APACHE II.
3. Those that assess the physiological effects of established infection and monitor the response of these changes to therapeutic interventions.

Obviously there is some overlap in these categories but it is important to recognize that some scoring systems, particularly those that assess risk factors predisposing to infection, look at objective criteria that describe the patient's condition but are not easily changed (e.g. age, malnutrition), whereas others utilize physiological measurement that may rapidly respond to therapeutic interventions (e.g. oxygenation, haemodynamic parameters). In the patient with established infection the most useful scoring system would therefore be one that embraced parameters that reflect previous state of health, severity of infection, and quality of surgical and medical therapy. The following discussion will amplify some of the limitations and advantages of the various scoring systems in current clinical practice.

Risk factors predisposing to surgical infection

Many of these prognostic scoring systems have developed from initial retrospective studies of patient outcome and then have been used in prospective studies to assess changes in patient outcome following therapeutic intervention (13). Age is a variable that cannot be changed but extremes of age, and in particular old age, is associated with increased post-operative complications. This is probably a reflection of a number of interrelated variables such as impaired immunity, cardiovascular and respiratory disease, and malnutrition. Concurrent diseases such as diabetes, malignancy, cirrhosis, and renal failure also increase complications. Protein-calorie malnutrition often accompanies these conditions and has been shown to be present in up to 50 per cent of general surgical patients

(14). Assessment of anthropometric, biochemical, and immunological measurement may define patients with impaired nutritional status who have a poorer outcome than those who are normally nourished (15). In addition, other factors such as medications which depress immunity (steroids) or lead to other complications (anticoagulants) may have an impact on survival and morbidity. Good aspectic technique, excellent pre- and post-operative care and elective rather than emergency treatment of most conditions have a positive effect on outcome. The classification of surgical procedures into clean, clean-contaminated, contaminated, and dirty accurately predicts the incidence of infective complications ranging from less than 2 per cent in clean cases to 40 per cent in dirty cases (16). Lastly, more complex cases are now being undertaken as surgical techniques and anaesthetic practice have become more sophisticated but these advances often necessitate more invasive monitoring and diagnostic procedures which invariably increase the risks of infection (17).

Several scoring systems have attempted to quantify the risks associated with the above factors. Hill and co-workers (18, 19) have analysed indicators of surgical risk, clinical judgement, and weight loss on surgical outcome and found that weight loss of 10 per cent or more associated with dysfunction of two or more organ systems significantly increased the risk of post-operative septic complications. Mullen and his colleagues describe the prognostic nutritional index (PNI) (11) which related four measurements: serum albumin, serum transferrin, triceps skin-fold thickness, and delayed hypersensitivity response to skin test antigens—to post-operative complications. They classified patients undergoing gastrointestinal surgery into three risk categories: low risk—PNI less than 40; moderate risk—PNI 40–49; and high risk PNI greater than 49; and suggested that perioperative use of nutritional support may improve the outcome of those at highest risk of developing complications (20). The literature contains other examples of assessment of nutritional status and its relationship to outcome but most have been criticized for including measurements such as serum albumin, lymphocyte count, and assessment of immune status that can be affected by other features of disease rather than nutritional status. Patients with malignant disease often have depressed immunity unrelated to cachexia or malnutrition and defects of serum albumin often occur in renal and liver insufficiency. Irrespective of their origin, these biochemical, haematological, and immune measurements do reflect the overall metabolic homeostasis of the patient and the efficiency of organ function so that combinations of measurements are likely to give a more accurate predictor of outcome than single measurements. Addition of other measurements, such as hand grip strength, which is a measurement of muscle function, can increase the predictive power of a prognostic scoring system especially when compared with a group of normal patients in the same hospital community (21).

All these systems of pre-operative assessment need to be used with caution and are not suitable for following patients sequentially through their illness. This is because many of the parameters reflect several factors, e.g. disease process and nutritional status and they rarely change significantly over a short period in response to therapy. Other scoring systems that evaluate the infective process and the response to therapy are more likely to be of use in monitoring progression or resolution of infections and their systemic responses (22).

Anatomical and physiological scoring systems

Many patients who suffer severe injury or develop infective complications quickly manifest signs and symptoms that indicate profound changes in cardiovascular, respiratory, renal, and neurological function. The importance of prompt recognition of these changes and the prompt institution of appropriate therapeutic measures cannot be over emphasized and may have a vital impact on outcome. Thus, a seriously injured patient is more likely to have an optimal outcome to his injuries if resuscitation is commenced soon after injury rather than there being a significant delay. Similarly, patients with perforated peptic ulcer benefit from early resuscitation and surgery, as do patients with intra-abdominal sepsis. Scoring systems that quantify the degree of injury and the derangement of physiology allow us to identify treatment priorities. It is helpful to look at the scoring systems used for trauma and intensive care unit patients to see how they relate to outcome and how their principles may be applied to the surgical patient at risk for developing infection. Trauma patients have a high incidence of infection and much of their post-injury mortality and morbidity can be related to the development of injury related and nosocomial infections.

Glasgow Coma Scale (GCS)

The Glasgow Coma Scale (GCS) was originally described by Teasdale and Jennett in 1974 (5) and is widely used in neurosurgical practice to assess the severity of head injury. It reflects the degree of coma, brain injury, and brain function, by relating three behavioural responses—eye opening, best verbal response and best motor response (Table 12.1). These give a range of scores from 3 to 15 with the highest scores indicating the least impairment of brain function. The GCS is simple to

Table 12.1. Glasgow Coma Scale (GCS).

A. **Eye-opening response**	
Spontaneous	4
To voice	3
To pain	2
None	1
B. **Best verbal response**	
Orientated	5
Confused	4
Inappropriate words	3
Incomprehensible sounds	2
None	1
C. **Best motor response**	
Obeys command	6
Localizes pain	5
Withdraws to pain	4
Flexion to pain	3
Extension to pain	2
None	1

GCS = A + B + C   Range 3–15

Table 12.2. Revised trauma score (RTS).

	Coded value						Product (coded value × weight)
	4	**3**	**2**	**1**	**0**	**Weight**	
Glasgow coma scale	13–15	9–12	6–8	4–5	3	0.9368	A
Systolic blood pressure (mmHg)	>89	76–89	50–75	1–49	0	0.7326	B
Respiratory rate (per min)	10–29	>29	6–9	1–5	0	0.2908	C

RTS = Sum of A + B + C

use and correlates with mortality, morbidity, and Glasgow Outcome Scale (23), the latter reflecting the level of ultimate brain function. The GCS has been incorporated into the Revised Trauma Score which is now widely used for assessing the severity of accidental injury (see below).

The Revised Trauma Score

The Trauma Score (TS) (24) is based on the GCS and assessment of the cardiovascular status (systolic blood pressure and capillary refill) and the respiratory status (respiratory rate and effort). The weighted scores for each variable gives the Trauma Score with a range from 1 (worst prognosis) to 16 (best prognosis) which can be used to evaluate both blunt and penetrating trauma, both in the pre-hospital setting and during triage. It has now been replaced by the Revised Trauma Score (RTS) (25) which uses only three parameters: GCS, systolic blood pressure, and respiratory rate. Coded values for a specific range of each variable are weighted and the sum of the weighted values produces the RTS ranging in value from 0 to 7.8408 (Table 12.2). The RTS is highly correlated with survival and death and has an advantage over TS in that the weighted value assigned to GCS enables it to predict accurately the outcome of head injury in the absence of multiple system injury or severe physiological derangement. When used in conjunction with injury severity score, mechanism of injury (blunt or penetrating), and patient's age it can accurately predict the probability of survival for each patient. It has been used as a valuable research tool in the Major Trauma Outcome Studies (MTOS) in the United States and to audit the efficiency of trauma management in various hospital settings (12). Other scoring systems, e.g. CRAMS scale (26), Hospital Trauma Index (HTI) (27), for trauma triage and management have their advocates and are based on a matrix of anatomical and physiological measurements that reflect severity of injury.

Injury severity score (ISS)

The injury severity score (ISS) (4) is an anatomical scoring system developed for the assessment of multiple traumatic injuries and is based on the Abbreviated Injury Scale (AIS) (28). The ISS is calculated by summing the squares of the AIS scores for the three most significant injuries in different body regions. The six anatomical regions are head and neck; face; thorax; abdomen and pelvis contents; extremities and bony pelvis; soft tissues and burns. The AIS score (1–6) range from minor (1) to maximal or fatal (6) in each region. The maximum ISS is 75 ($5^2 + 5^2 + 5^2$) and an ISS of 16 or more is regarded as major trauma and has a mortality of 10 per cent. The ISS is a reliable predictor of mortality and morbidity, although it has limitations being based entirely on anatomical disruption which may not always be reflected in physiological disturbance of vital organ functions. In addition, it has little practical value at the time of admission, triage, and resuscitation, because the full extent of the anatomical injury is not known at that time. ISS can only be calculated when the full extent of all injuries has been evaluated.

ISS has an excellent correlation with septic complications and mortality in trauma patients. In several studies of antibiotic prophylaxis in patients with penetrating abdominal trauma performed in Houston, ISS was significantly correlated with post-injury wound, intra-abdominal and nosocomial infection and patients with an ISS above 20 were found to be a group that was particularly susceptible to septic complications and death (29, 30). A recent study at the Royal Victoria Hospital Belfast in 108 trauma patients (mean ISS 25) showed that there was an excellent correlation between admission ISS and the development of secondary infection and mortality (Table 12.3). There was also a highly significant correlation between admission ISS and APACHE II scores in these patients. This relationship must be viewed with caution in the young trauma patient whose APACHE II score may not reflect the severity of his injury.

Table 12.3. Comparison of admission injury severity score (ISS), secondary infection, and mortality in 108 trauma patients.

Admission ISS	Secondary infection (%)	Mortality (%)
0–19 (n = 43)	10 (23.3%)	4 (9.3%)
20–39 (n = 56)	18 (32.1%)	12 (21.4%)
greater than 40 (n = 9)	5 (55.6%)	5 (55.6%)

Other scoring systems that rely entirely on anatomical assessment of the full extent of tissue and organ damage have been used in abdominal trauma, and these injury severity indices have a good predictive value. The most useful are the Abdominal Trauma Index (31) and the Penetrating Abdominal Trauma Index (PATI) (32) which are detailed systems for evaluating abdominal trauma but ignore the physiological consequences of these injuries on other regions of the body. The Colon Injury Severity Score (CISS) (33) and Flint Severity Score (34) for colonic injury are similar to the AIS and have been used not only to predict complications but also to determine the appropriate surgical management of the bowel injury.

Acute physiology, age, and chronic health evaluation (APACHE)

APACHE was originally described by Knaus in 1981 to classify patients admitted to intensive care units (35). This scoring system used 34 variables—the acute physiological assessment—obtained during the first 24 h of admission, and an assessment of previous medical history—chronic health evaluation. The physiological assessment included measurements to reflect, cardiovascular, respiratory, renal, gastrointestinal, haematological, metabolic, and neurological function, and whether or not sepsis was present. The APACHE system was tested in a large number of hospitals and was shown to be reliable in describing mortality risk for groups of patients admitted to intensive care units. A subsequent modification by Knaus gave rise to APACHE II scoring system which uses only 12 routine physiological measurements (36). These 12 laboratory values and physical findings (APS-12) are assigned points (0 to 4) dependent on their deviation from the normal range. In addition points are awarded for age above 44 years and for chronic health evaluation. The APS-12 (0 to 60 points), points for age (0 to 6 points) and points for chronic health (0, 2 or 5 points) when added give a range from 0–71 points (Table 12.4). Scores above 40 are uncommon, but those above 30 are associated with a mortality rate of approximately 70 per cent.

In a recent study of 331 patients admitted to the Regional Intensive Care Unit at Royal Victoria Hospital in Belfast, each patient had APACHE II score assessed on admission to the unit. The Range of APACHE II scores was 1–37 and the median was 14. The overall mortality rate was 17 per cent and unit-acquired infection occurred in 19 per cent. For the purposes of a therapeutic trial the patients were randomized according to their admission APACHE II score to four groups (below 10, 10–19, 20–29, 30 and above). There was a progressive increase in mortality and infection rate as the admission APACHE II score rose (Table 12.5). These findings from a mixture of medical, surgical, and trauma patients admitted to a mixed ICU parallel those of Knaus and his colleagues (1985) (36) who showed a close correlation of APACHE II score with subsequent risk of hospital death (many related to septic complications) for 5815 intensive care admission in 13 hospitals. The predictive value of APACHE II may be improved by the use of a weighting factor that reflects the principle diagnosis.

Table 12.4. APACHE II scoring system.

(A) **12 Physiological variables** (0–60 points)

Rectal temperature	Serum sodium
Mean arterial pressure	Serum potassium
Heart rate	Serum creatinine
Respiratory rate	Haematocrit
Oxygenation	White blood count
Arterial pH	Glasgow coma score

(B) **Age points** (0–6 points)

Age (years)	<44	44–54	55–64	65–74	≥75
points	0	2	3	5	6

(C) **Chronic health points** (0, 2, or 5 points)

Severe organ insufficiency—liver, cardiovascular, respiratory, renal

Immunocompromized —therapy or disease that suppresses resistance to infection

(a) for non-operative or emergency post-operative patients—5 points.

(b) for elective post-operative patients—2 points.

APACHE II score is the sum of A + B + C

Table 12.5. Comparison of admission APACHE II score, infective complications and mortality in 331 patients admitted to an intensive care unit.

Admission APACHE II score	Infective complications (%)	Mortality (%)
below 10 (n = 55)	10 (18.2%)	0 (0%)
10–19 (n = 146)	36 (24.6%)	23 (15.8%)
20–29 (n = 47)	13 (27.7%)	10 (21.3%)
30 and above (n = 8)	3 (37.5%)	6 (75%)

Sepsis scoring systems

The systems of scoring discussed above relate to the identification of patients who by virtue of their previous health, severity of illness, or magnitude of trauma have a high likelihood of developing local or systemic septic complications with their attendant problems of multiple system organ failure and subsequent death. In the study of the pathophysiology of sepsis these scoring systems may identify specific groups of patients at risk immediately after the onset of their illness or injury and several days or occasionally weeks may elapse before the development of clinical manifestations of infectious complications. A feature of many studies of antibiotic prophylaxis or therapy in these patients is that they fail to stratify patients prior to randomization into groups with equal risks of developing complications (37). Fortunately, there are now a number of systems, (some of which are already described above) to accomplish the comparison of similar groups and some of these have been developed for use in patients with clinical sepsis.

Sepsis Score

The Sepsis Score was developed by Elebute and Stoner in 1983 (38) to provide a simple method of evaluating the severity of sepsis in patients in a district general hospital. They constructed a list of the clinical features of the septic state and graded four classes of attribute according to severity. The classes chosen were the local effects of sepsis, pyrexia, secondary effects of sepsis, and laboratory data, and a visual linear analogue scale was used to give a spectrum of values from mild to severe. It must be emphasized that assessment of local and secondary effects of sepsis are subjective and their interpretation may vary from unit to unit. The range of scores on this system is 0–45. The grading system was applied to 15 patients, whose clinical course was monitored sequentially. Of the five patients who died, four had a highest sepsis score above 20, while only one of the survivors had a score of 20 or above. Dominioni *et al.* (39) applied this scoring system to a larger number of patients with a variety of infective problems and showed a 20 per cent mortality rate in 64 patients with a score below 20 and an 89 per cent mortality rate in 71 patients above 20. In Belfast, we have used the Sepsis Score for sequential monitoring of ICU patients. In a study of 256 patients, there was a range of admission scores from 0 to 20 (median 4), a strong correlation with admission APACHE II score and an increased mortality with increasing sepsis score (Table 12.6). During their stay in the intensive care unit, clinical deterioration due to septic complications was usually mirrored by changes in both APACHE II and Sepsis Scores.

Table 12.6. Comparison of admission sepsis score and mortality in 256 patients admitted to an intensive care unit.

Admission sepsis score	Mortality (%)
0–4 (n = 121)	12 (9.9%)
5–6 (n = 88)	16 (18.2%)
10–14 (n = 38)	9 (23.7%)
15 and above (n = 9)	2 (22.2%)

Septic severity score

This scoring system was devised by Stevens to represent the magnitude and severity of organ failure (40). He ascribed a score of 1–5 to seven organ systems—lung, kidney, coagulation, cardiovascular, liver, gastrointestinal tract and neurological—to represent degrees of dysfunction in that organ system from mild (1) to severe (5). The septic severity score was derived by squaring the value for each organ and adding the three highest scores. This gave a range of scores from 0 to 75. In his initial study of 35 patients, there was a range of scores from 6 to 67, with an 82 per cent mortality rate above 40 and a 21 per cent mortality rate below 40. Skau *et al.* (41) subsequently showed a strong correlation between increasing mortality rate and increasing score using both the septic severity score and the acute physiological score.

Sepsis score and acute phase proteins

There have been attempts to improve the precision and predictive value of the sepsis scores by the measurement of various acute phase proteins. Dominioni *et al.* (39) found that the initial values of several proteins (alpha-1-glycoprotein, alpha-1-antitrypsin, complement factor B, and complement factor 3) were significantly higher in survivors than non-survivors. From this data they derived a Sepsis Index of Survival (SIS) by stepwise regression analysis using the sepsis score (Elebute and Stoner) and initial plasma value of complement factor B and alpha-1-glycoprotein. An SIS of greater than 150 correctly predicts 88 per cent of survivors and an SIS of less than 50 correctly predicts 86 per cent of non-survivors. Although the addition of acute phase protein measurement may improve predictive value of the sepsis score, the latter still has the greatest impact on survival.

Multiple System Severity of Illness System (MSIS)

This clinical rating system evaluates on-going disease course and severity in septic patients. It uses a combination of scoring systems including APACHE II (See above) and the therapeutic intervention scoring system (TISS) (42) which grades the amount of medical and mechanical support a patient requires, establishing a measure of the therapeutic intensity, and can be used to predict outcome. Jordan *et al.* (43) have shown that MSIS is a more effective indicator of severity of sepsis and more sensitive to the day-to-day changes in clinical status than either the APACHE II or TISS components alone.

Hanover Intensive System (HIS)

The Hanover Intensive System (HIS) (44) evaluates risk factors involving six organ systems—cerebral, cardiovascular, respiratory, gastrointestinal, renal, and immune function—and awards points (up to three) for physiological derangements in each system and additional points for specific therapeutic interventions (use of dopamine or antiarrhythmics) or complications (pneumothorax, anastomotic breakdown). The maximum risk is 32 points. In a study of 215 patients HIS has been shown to be superior to APACHE and TISS scoring systems in predicting lethal outcome at an earlier stage and its advocates suggest that it may have advantages in clinical decision making.

Miscellaneous scoring systems

Two groups from Germany have described scoring systems for severe intra-abdominal infection. The Peritonitis Index Altona (PIA) (45) uses, age, extent of infection, malignancy, cardiovascular risks, and leucopenia to stratify patients. The Mannheim Peritonitis Score (46) includes age, gender, organ failure, cancer, duration of peritonitis, involvement of the colon, extent of spread within the peritoneum, and character of the peritoneal fluid and exudate. Both systems have been shown to be accurate at predicting mortality risk and have been used to identify patients likely to benefit from scheduled reoperation.

Multiple system organ failure (MSOF)

Several studies in the late 1970s (47–49) identified that death following a septic complication often involved the sequential deterioration of organ function most notably, cardiovascular, pulmonary, hepatic, and renal. Fry and associates in 1980 (50) studied 553 patients undergoing emergency surgical procedures and found that failure of two or more organ systems in 30 patients was associated with a mortality rate of 74 per cent. Additional features contributing to morbidity and mortality were stress ulceration, gastrointestinal haemorrhage, disseminated intravascular coagulopathy, coma, malnutrition and abnormalities of substrate metabolism, and homeostasis. The single most important factor related to death was the development of acute renal failure. Clinical variables that are associated with the development of multiple system organ failure are hypovolaemic shock, massive resuscitation, use of blood products, specific organ injury, and clinical sepsis (51). The onset of organ failure is usually sequential commencing with sepsis and pulmonary failure, followed by hepatic, gastrointestinal, and renal failure. The longer organ failure is present the less likely is recovery and the ability of any organ system to withstand failures of perfusion and oxygenation depend on the functional reserve of the organ. Thus patients who already have chronic organ dysfunction, e.g. chronic obstructive airways disease, cirrhosis, are more likely to develop acute deterioration of organ function as a result of their disease, injury or infection. Many of the scoring systems described above are capable of identifying such patients and accurately predicting the outcome of their illness.

Future considerations

Scoring systems should be simple, the data should be easily obtained and analysed, and the numerical score should have a high sensitivity and specificity in different clinical settings. They should embrace anatomical and physiological aberrations and take into account factors such as age, previous health and the effects of therapy. In the future scoring systems should be used in clinical trials of septic patients and in the intensive care unit to select patients for the study, to grade the severity of disease and to statify the risk of mortality. This, together with standardization of the definitions of infection and criteria for its diagnosis, should lead to more meaningful analysis of data, advancement of knowledge and greater understanding of the pathophysiology and management of septic complications (52). Until this information is available, sepsis scoring systems should *not* be used for choosing between therapeutic options in individual patients.

References

1. Dellinger, E.P. (1988). Use of scoring systems to assess patients with surgical sepsis. *Surg. Clin. North Am.*, **68**, 123–45.
2. Bland, K.I. and Copeland, E.M. (1988). Breast: physiologic considerations in normal, benign, and neoplastic states. In *Physiologic basis of modern surgical care* (ed. T.A. Miller and B.J. Rowlands), pp. 1019–56. Mosby, St Louis, Missouri.
3. Dukes, C.E. (1932). The classification of cancer of the rectum. *J. Pathol.*, **35**, 323–32.
4. Baker, S.P., O'Neill, B., Haddon, W. *et al.*, (1974). The Injury Severity Score: A method of describing patients with multiple injuries and evaluating emergency care. *J. Trauma.*, **14**, 187–96.
5. Teasdale, G. and Jennett, B. (1974). Assessment of coma and impaired consciousness: a practical scale. *Lancet*, **ii**, 81–3.
6. Imrie, C.W., Benjamin, I.S., and Ferguson, J.C. (1978). A single centre double blind trial of Trasylol therapy in primary acute pancreatitis. *Br. J. Surg.*, **65**, 337–41.
7. Ranson, J.H.C., Rifkind, K.M., and Turner, J.W. (1975). Prognostic signs and non-operative peritoneal lavage in acute pancreatitis. *Surg. Gynecol. Obstet.*, **143**, 209–19.
8. Best, W.R., Becktel, J.M., and Singleton, J.W. *et al.* (1976). Development of a Crohn's Disease Activity index. National Co-operative Crohn's Disease Study. *Gastroenterology*, **70**, 439–44.
9. Scheulen, J.J. and Munster, A.M. (1982). The Parkland formula in patients with burns and inhalation injury. *J. Trauma*, **22**, 869–71.
10. Demling, R.H. (1987). Fluid replacement in burned patients. *Surg. Clin. North Am.*, **67**, 15–30.
11. Buzby, G.P., Mullen, J.L., and Matthews, D.C. *et al.* (1980). Prognostic nutritional index in gastrointestinal surgery. *Am. J. Surg.*, **139**, 160–67.
12. Champion, H.R., Copes, W.S., Sacco, W.J. *et al.* (1990). The major trauma outcome study: establishing national norms for trauma care. *J. Trauma*, **30**, 1356–65.
13. Dominioni, K., Bianchi, M., and Dionigi, R. (1990). Factors predisposing to surgical infections and identification of patients at risk. *Surg. Res. Comm.*, **9**, 1–7.
14. Hill, G.L., Blackett, R.L., Pickford, I. *et al.* (1977). Malnutrition in surgical patients: an unrecognized problem. *Lancet*, **i**, 689–92.
15. Dionigi, R., Cremaschi, R.E., and Jemos, V. (1986). Nutritional assessment and severity of illness classification systems: a critical review of their clinical relevance. *World J. Surg.*, **10**, 2–11.
16. Cruse, P.J.E. and Foord, R. (1980). The epidemiology of wound infection, a 10 year prospective study of 62 939 wounds. *Surg. Clin. North Am.*, **60**, 27–40.
17. Rowlands, B.J. and Ericsson, C.D. (1986). Surgical Infections. In *Infectious diseases of children and adults, step-by-step approach to diagnosis and treatment* (ed. L.K. Pickering and H. Dupont), pp. 589–613. Addison-Wesley, California.
18. Pettigrew, R.A. and Hill, G.L. (1986). Indicators of surgical risk and clinical judgement. *Br. J. Surg.*, **73**, 47–51.
19. Windsor, J.A. and Hill, G.L. (1988). Weight loss with physiologic impairment. A basic indicator of surgical risk. *Ann. Surg.*, **207**, 290–6.
20. Mullen, J.L., Buzby, G.P., Matthews, D.C., *et al.* (1980). Reduction of operative morbidity and mortality by combined preoperative and post-operative nutritional support. *Ann. Surg.*, **192**, 604–13.
21. Hunt, D.R., Rowlands, B.J., and Johnston, D. (1985). Hand grip strength as an index of nutritional status in surgical patients. *J. Parenteral Enteral Nutrition*, **9**, 701–4.
22. Dominioni, L. and Dionigi, R. (1987). The grading of sepsis and the assessment of its prognosis in the surgical patient—a review. *Surg. Res. Comm.*, **1**, 1–11.
23. Jennett, B., Teasdale, G., Braakman, R., *et al.* (1976). Predicting outcome in individual patients after severe head injury. *Lancet*, **1**, 1031–4.
24. Champion, H.R., Sacco, W.J., Carnazzo, A.J., *et al.* (1981). Trauma score. *Crit. Care Med.*, **9**, 672–6.
25. Champion, H.R., Sacco, W.J., and Copes, W.S. (1989). A revision of the trauma score. *J. Trauma*, **29**, 623–9.
26. Gormican, S.P. (1982). CRAMS Scale: field triage of trauma victims. *Ann. Emerg. Med.*, **11**, 132–5.
27. Champion, H., Sacco, W.J., Hannan, D.S., *et al.* (1980). Assessment of injury severity: the Triage Index. *Crit. Care Med.*, **8**, 201–8.
28. American Association for Automative Medicine: *The Abbreviated Injury Scale (AIS)*—1985 Revision. Des Plaines, Illinois.
29. Rowlands, B.J. and Ericsson, C.D. (1985). Comparative studies of antiobiotic therapy after penetrating abdominal trauma. *Am. J. Surg.*, **148**, 791–5.

30. Rowlands, B. J., Ericsson, C. D., and Fischer, R. P. (1987). Penetrating abdominal trauma: the use of operative findings to determine length of antibiotic therapy. *J. Trauma*, **27**, 250–5.
31. Borlase, B. C., Moore, E. E., and Moore, F. A. (1990). The Abdominal Trauma Index—a critical reassessment and validation. *J. Trauma*, **30**, 1340–4.
32. Moore, E. E., Dunn, E. L., Moore, J. B., *et al.* (1981). Penetrating Abdominal Trauma Index. *J. Trauma*, **21**, 439–45.
33. Nelkin, N. and Lewis, F. (1989). The influence of injury severity on complication rates after primary closure or colostomy for penetrating colon trauma. *Ann. Surg.*, **209**, 439–47.
34. Flint, L. M., Vitale, G. C., Richardson, J. D. *et al.* (1981). The injured colon. *Ann. Surg.*, **193**, 619–23.
35. Knaus, W. A., Zimmerman, J. E., Wagner, D. P., *et al.* (1981). APACHE acute physiology and chronic health evaluation: a physiologically based classification system. *Crit. Care Med.*, **9**, 591–7.
36. Knaus, W. A., Draper, E. A., Wagner, D. P., Zimmerman, J. E. (1985). APACHE II: a severity of disease classification system. *Crit. Care Med.*, **13**, 818–29.
37. Solomkin, J. S., Dellinger, E. P., and Christou, N. V. (1987). Design and conduct of antibiotic trials. *Arch. Surg.*, **122**, 158–64.
38. Elebute, E. A. and Stoner, H. B. (1983). The grading of sepsis. *Br. J. Surg.*, **70**, 29–31.
39. Dominioni, L., Dionigi, R., Zanello, M., *et al.* (1987). Sepsis score and acute phase protein response as predictors of outcome in septic surgical patients. *Arch. Surg.*, **122**, 141–6.
40. Stevens, L. E. (1983). Gauging the severity of surgical sepsis. *Arch. Surg.*, **118**, 1190–2.
41. Skau, T., Nystrom, P. O., and Carlsson, C. (1985). Severity of illness in intra-abdominal infection. *Arch. Surg.*, **120**, 152–8.
42. Keane, A. R. and Cullen, D. J. (1983). Therapeutic intervention scoring system—update. *Crit. Care Med.*, **11**, 1–9.
43. Jordan, D. A., Miller, C. F., Kubos, K. L., and Rogers, M. C. (1987). Evaluation of sepsis in a critically ill surgical population. *Crit. Care Med.*, **15**, 897–904.
44. Lehmkuhl, P., Jeck-Thole, S., and Pichlmayr, I. (1989). A new scoring system for disease intensity in a surgical intensive care unit. *World J. Surg.*, **13**, 252–8.
45. Teichmann, W., Wittmann, D. H., and Andreone, P. A. (1986). Scheduled reoperations (etappenlavage) for diffuse periotonitis. *Arch. Surg.*, **121**, 147–52.
46. Wacha, H., Linder, M. M., Feldmann, U., *et al.* (1987). Mannheim peritonitis index. Prediction of risk of death from peritonitis. Construction of a statistical and validation of an empirically based index. *Theoret. Surg.* **1**, 169–77.
47. Baue, A. E. (1975). Multiple progressive or sequential systems failure, a syndrome of the 1970's. *Arch. Surg.*, **110**, 779–81.
48. Eiseman, B., Beart, R., and Norton, L. (1977). Multiple organ failure. *Surg. Gynecol. Obstet.*, **144**, 323–6.
49. Polk, H. C. and Shields, C. L. (1977). Remote organ failure a valid sign of occult intra-abdominal infection. *Surgery*, **81**, 310–3.
50. Fry, D. E., Pearlstein, L., Fulton, R. L., *et al.* Multiple system organ failure. *Arch. Surg.*, **115**, 136–40.
51. Fry, D. E. (1988). Multiple system organ failure. *Surg. Clin. North Am.*, **68**, 107–22.
52. Nystrom, P. O., Bax, R., Dellinger, E. P., *et al.* Proposed definitions for diagnosis, severity scoring, stratification and outcome for trials on intra-abdominal infection. *World J. Surg.*, **14**, 148–58.

13

Infection and sepsis: a review of multiple organ failure and abacterial sepsis

PER OLOF NYSTRÖM

Introduction

Recent research has increased our understanding of sepsis immensely. Interest used to be centred on the specific micro-organisms of a septic focus that could be treated by surgery and antibiotics. However, a major area of interest now is the commensal microflora that is seen to invade the body from the gut. In a sense, the entire perspective has been changed from study of the infecting micro-organisms and the appropriate antibiotic treatment, to study of cell and tissue responses during surgery and acute illness. Multiple organ failure, the septic state, transient immunodeficiency, and gut-origin nosocomial infection are all end-stage attributes of advanced sepsis. An intriguing feature is that many of these patients do not display abscess pathology when investigated by computed tomography scan, ultrasound, or exploratory laparotomy. Indeed, we now realize that the patient's septic state may preclude him from producing an abscess (1).

It is widely believed that patients with severe sepsis follow a common pathway, centred around the 'activated macrophage'. Although a unifying theory may eventually be developed, the multitude of events makes it impossible to describe the severely septic patient in one dimension. Rather there are series of events which seem to be linked, and several such chains can be identified. What follows is an attempt to outline multiple organ failure (MOF), transient immunodeficiency, and gut-origin infection as the extended development of body responses that are already operative in less advanced disease states. These are parallel developments which are not always the result of bacterial infection but infection will be a complication of such severe illness. It will be stressed that ischaemic tissue injury is an important common finding, and that recent advances in scoring methods provide a measure of case severity.

It is traditional to equate sepsis with infection which is unfortunate. The term infection should be used aetiologically for disease that is caused by both proliferation of microbes and their invasion of body spaces. Sepsis designates the physiologic response to illness, which may be infection, but essentially is the host response to any severe illness. It is characterized by fever, hypotension, diminished oxygenation and leucocytosis among other signs of disturbed physiology. When sepsis continues over days and weeks it is appropriately called the septic state.

The concept of severe sepsis

Severe sepsis is a rather vague term that lends itself to several interpretations. Obviously there are two immediate components: extensive local pathology and extensive physiologic disturbance. Pathological anatomy and pathophysiology usually correlates in a patient. But physiology is much easier to measure, and grading physiological variables is more precise than grading pathological anatomy (2).

Study of the patient's physiology will reveal information about the homeostasis, which must be kept within certain limits to be compatible with survival from disease. This implies that both a measure of deranged homeostasis, and the time it takes to normalize the homeostasis, relates to the prognosis. The less deranged the patient is and the sooner the physiology can be normalized the better will be the prognosis. The relationship of homeostasis to prognosis is particularly relevant when grading severity of illness. This approach was assumed in the APACHE II (acute physiology, age, and chronic health evaluation) severity of disease index (3). The major component of this index is the acute physiology score, APS, which in its present form is composed of twelve physiology variables (3). The physiology variables have been carefully weighted such that each additional point increases the patient's risk of death in a near linear fashion. We may, somewhat arbitrarily, define severe illness as any acute disease state which is associated with at least 10 per cent mortality risk, despite adequate treatment.

Identification of severely septic patients

In infected surgical patients the APACHE II and APS values that carry at least a 10 per cent mortality risk are about 8 and 5 points respectively, on admission to the intensive therapy unit (ITU). The APS is favoured for following the patient's course as this score closely reflects the pathophysiology that is treated. The prognosis is dependent on how quickly the total treatment can change the APS towards zero. We found an average mortality of 57 per cent in a group of 63 patients with severe intra-abdominal infection, defined as an APS of at least 8 points on the admission to the ITU. Scores were obtained daily for up to 14 days, or until the patient died, if within this period. Those who improved their score by at least 20 per cent during the observation period had a mortality of 19 per cent whereas those who had the same or an increased APS had a mortality of 76 per cent. This statistically significant difference in outcome resulted despite an equal mortality risk on admission to ITU with APACHE II scores of 18 in both groups. The majority developed a septic state with MOF. Almost invariably, their temperature rose to above 38.5 °C within a week, regardless of whether another septic focus developed or not. There was no relationship between outcome and the number of relaparotomies, courses of antibiotic therapy, or frequency of positive blood cultures. These factors increased in frequency the longer the patient remained alive. Similar results have been reported by others (4, 5).

The patient's course is also related to whether the operation successfully dealt with the septic focus. In a group of 271 patients with intra-abdominal infection, the mortality was 17 per cent in those reported to have a successful first operation (89 per cent of all operations) but 60 per cent in patients with an unsuccessful operation. However, there was a difference in the extent of the pathology which was accompanied by a significantly higher APACHE II score and which accounted for some of the difference in outcome (Wittmann, personal communication).

Mechanisms of multiple organ failure

The clinical syndrome

Baue was the first to bring failed organ function of the lung, liver, intestine, and kidney together into a single entity which, as he stated it, was to become 'a syndrome of the 1970s' (6). Its immediate recognition among surgeons was the result of modern intensive care, which allowed patients to survive long enough for this syndrome to become the experience of every surgeon involved with treating severely ill patients. It was easy to observe failure of individual organs such as lung, kidney, and liver but more subtle functions such as coagulation, metabolism, or neuro-endocrine regulation can also fail (7). Thus it became evident that MOF represented a more basic underlying disease state, which involved homeostatic mechanisms. The number of recognized failures and their definitions varied according to the preferences of each research group (6–12). Definitions included a mixture of physiologic, diagnostic, and therapeutic information which makes the subject hard to penetrate. Some definitions recognized that MOF nearly always involves a disrupted regulation of the homeostasis. It is, therefore, better measured as a graded response examples of which are the MOF score (13), the sepsis severity score of Stevens (14), and of Border *et al.* (4).

The ideal method to score MOF is probably an improved version of the acute physiology score of the APACHE system. It would consist only of basic physiology that can be measured objectively. The variables would be weighted such as to create a cardinal scale where each additional point increases the case severity at equal increments of risk. In our experience the APS, with 12 variables, recorded daily, accurately describes the course of patients with MOF. Any patient with an APS of five or higher during three consecutive days has at least one failed organ by traditional definitions. The new APS of the forthcoming APACHE III (15) will probably provide an even better measurement of the disease states presently understood by the rather dubious terms of multiple organ failure and septic state. Such a score would considerably advance research within this field as patient studies then can be better compared (16).

Patient outcome in MOF relates to the number of failed organs. Mortality is 10 to 30 per cent in single failure but increases steeply to 90 per cent with failure of three organs. Mortality increases further as the failure persists. It is our experience that these results can translate into APS values, measured daily.

Infection was immediately assumed to be a predominant cause of MOF and the search for 'uncontrolled infection' became the major factor in the management of these patients (9, 17). Only slowly did new insight begin to change this perspective as it became evident that, with more stringent definitions of infection, many patients developed MOF without infection. Treating the infection did not prevent or reverse the MOF. The situation became even more confounding when it was discovered that non-bacterial challenge could cause a similar syndrome in experimental animals (see Section 13.7). The term 'generalized autodestructive inflammation' was given as a descriptive term for MOF by Goris *et al.* (11) who suggested that it is inflammation, not infection, that causes MOF. Bacteria and endotoxin have again become important considerations as our understanding of the phenomenon of bacterial translocation has developed (see later).

Tissue hypoperfusion, hypoxia, and acidosis

The relationship between oxygen delivery to tissues and oxygen consumption is the basic concept of shock pathophysiology. Under normal circumstances the oxygen demand of cells is well below the delivery of oxygen. As delivery decreases during shock, cells may compensate by increasing the extraction of oxygen until cells at the venous end of a capillary circuit reach their critical demand and switch to anaerobic metabolism, which generates lactate production and acidosis. The critical levels of oxygen delivery and oxygen consumption vary with the patient's condition and the type of tissue. In septic patients the oxygen delivery can be inadequate in spite of the increased cardiac output usually seen in such patients (18). An oxygen supply demand is found in septic patients at higher levels of oxygen delivery than in healthy subjects. The reason for this increased demand is that the inflamed tissue generates oxygen needs that cannot be met under the circumstances. The septic patient who suffers a circulatory collapse, as is often the case with the neglected post-operative patient, is challenged by an abruptly decreased delivery in a situation where supply may already be insufficient. This is the septic shock.

Lately, the effects of hypoperfusion and hypoxia on splanchnic circulation and the epithelium of the intestines, liver, gall-bladder, and pancreas have been studied extensively. The splanchnic circulation receives 15 to 20 per cent of the cardiac output. There exists an autoregulation of intestinal blood flow which keeps the flow fairly constant, with changes of perfusion pressure between 80 and 160 mmHg (19). About 75 per cent of the blood flow through the small intestine is directed to the mucosa–submucosa. The arterial supply to each villus consists of one or two single vessels running in the core without branching. Close to the tip of the villus the artery branches into a dense, subepithelial network of capillaries and venules. This anatomy results in a countercurrent exchange mechanism which produces increasing osmolarity towards the tip, reaching as high as 800 mOsm (19). As blood flow decreases through the villi in shock, and oxygen delivery is diminished, there will be more time for counter current exchange of oxygen which presumably results in insufficient oxygen supply to the epithelium towards the tip of the villus. These changes of the microcirculation are influenced by various mediators that can decrease or increase splanchnic blood flow. Angiotensin II and vasopressin are extremely potent vasoconstrictors of the splanchnic bed (20) as are platelet activating factor (21), thromboxane and some prostaglandins (22). Tumour necrosis factor (TNF) produces haemodynamic changes that are characteristic of clinical sepsis (23). These include acutely diminished hepatic blood flow (24). Patients with established sepsis, and hyperdynamic circulation, have increased hepatic blood flow, but also a commensurately increased oxygen consumption which means that the liver cells can still have a flow dependent oxygen consumption (25, 26).

Patchy cell injury

In virtually every animal shock model lesions of the intestinal epithelium will be observed. The lesions start by the epithelium lifting from the basement membrane. A subepithelial space is created which gradually expands from the tip down the sides of the villus. With still more severe hypoxia sloughing of the epithelium produces micro-ulcerations of the villus tip, or blunting of the entire mucosal structure (27, 28). These lesions, which begin to appear after 20 min of total ischaemia or less than 2 h of partial ischaemia, are augmented by the generation of oxygen-free radicals upon reperfusion. The reperfusion injury can be blocked by inactivation of the mucosal xanthine oxidase activity (29) and is also related to the attraction of polymorphonuclear leukocytes to the injured mucosa (30). The same types of cellular injury can be seen in gastric mucosa and colon mucosa.

In patients these lesions have also been found in liver (31), gall-bladder (32), and pancreas (33) following a period of ischaemia. The cell injury can be subclinical but identified on biopsy or autopsy. Nuytinck *et al.* (34) studied the particular tissue injury of patients that died after trauma, with or without MOF. They found that haemorrhage and pathological accumulation of PMN's (polymorphonuclear neutrophil) were common findings in lung and liver in both those who died within 24 h of trauma and those who died later. The kidneys showed various degrees of vacuolar nephrotubulopathy. These changes could be seen even in patients who had not presented with shock or had not developed MOF.

Failed organ function

From the above evidence it seems likely that the acutely ill patient can develop ischaemic cell injury of lung, kidney, and all viscera due to low flow hypoxia, or by cellular oxygen consumption that is locally flow dependent even with the increased cardiac output of sepsis. Resident macrophages and endothelial cells would be activated and release inflammatory mediators. The resulting ischaemic inflammation attracts PMNs that increase the oxygen consumption at the inflammation site and add to the cellular injury by their release of oxygen radicals and proteolytic enzymes. The tissue injury is microscopical and patchy with all stages of cellular injury seen, from cell death to loss of proper function only. It is probable that the cell injuries can develop over hours to days, but more commonly they are the result of the initiating trauma with shock, or the hypoperfusion of acute illness. Depending on the extent and magnitude of these patchy cell injuries to organs it would be possible to explain both the immediate and delayed expression of individual organ failure, as well as the sequence of failure of the MOF syndrome. An explanation is still needed, why, in patients with minor degrees of cell injury, the injury does not heal but develops into organ failure. This problem will be considered later.

Mechanisms of transient immunodeficiency

Action of mediators

The cytokines are a group of protein cell regulators, variously called lymphokines and monokines. They are involved in immunity and inflammation where they regulate the amplitude and duration of responses. They are produced after activation by many cell types and exert their action transiently and locally by binding to cell surface receptors that are specific for each type of cytokine. They are predominantly a signal system of macrophages, and of T and B lymphocytes, for cell to cell interaction, each cell type having diverse secretion profiles and expression of the receptors relating to the activation state of the cell (35, 36). More than one hundred clones of leucocytes, T and B lymphocytes and macrophages have been identified (37). The cells are transformed, replicated, matured and mobilized by the cytokine stimuli to play their role in inflammation, immunity, and tissue healing.

All the cytokines have growth factor activity but some also have the ability to inhibit cell growth (35). The major known cytokines are tumour necrosis factor (TNF), platelet activating factor (PAF), interferons (IFN), interleukins (IL), lymphotoxin (LT), and macrophage colony stimulating factor (M-CSF). Various other growth factors are of the same type and can have very diverse effects on inflammation and its resolution. One notable example is the transforming growth factor (TGF) (38). The interplay within this complexity will generate the physical signs of disease in the patient. As an example, TNF, IFN and IL-1 and IL-2 are all capable of inducing fever (23, 35, 39, 40).

The eicosanoids are lipid mediators produced from arachidonic acid released from cellular membranes by phospolipase. The phospolipases are themselves bound, in inactive form, in the cell membranes but are released upon tissue injury. The arachidonic acid is metabolized by the cyclooxygenase pathway (prostaglandins, thromboxanes) or the lipoxygenase pathway (leucotrienes) by virtually every tissue except T-lymphocytes which lack these enzymes (41). The eicosanoids serve primarily as intercellular signals and are associated with the activation and regulation of a variety of biological systems. They are abundantly produced by macrophages and monocytes and are hence involved with inflammation and immunity. Prostaglandins are immunoregulatory because of their ability to alter the intracellular ratio of cAMP/cGMP. Activation of cAMP synthesis relative to cGMP causes activation and function of both T-helper and T-suppressor cells. T-helper cells seem more responsive to lower concentrations of prostaglandin E (PGE) while higher concentrations, and prolonged influence of PGE, activates the T-suppressor subset (42). Whereas the cytokines are regarded as specific mediators of cellular activity, the prostaglandins may be regarded as regulators of these mediators.

The interaction of cytokines with eicosanoids is, indeed, a complex relationship. Levels of both are usually elevated in trauma and other severely ill patients (43–45). PGE is a potent inhibitor of blastogenic response in lymphocyte cultures. There is some data to demonstrate that an increased PGE_2 production will block the production or expression of interleukins (IL-1, IL-2), interferon, and TNF (41). This has been assumed to be a major mechanism to quench the immunological and inflammatory reactions (46). A correlation has been observed between the levels of TNF of monocytes and both the severity of illness and the number of septic episodes (47, 48), but the same authors found that PGE_2 levels were also increased. They were, therefore, unable to confirm assumptions of TNF down-regulation by PGE_2. Using a long-acting derivate of PGE Waymack and Yurt (49) were unable to demonstrate decreased survival in a rat model with 30 per cent burn or *Escherichia coli* peritonitis. Nor was inflammation diminished. Both unstimulated and stimulated blastogenesis were increased. These studies seem to refute the hypothesis that PGE_2 is largely the mediator responsible for impaired immune response in severe illness.

Activation of the macrophage and down-regulation of inflammation and immunity

Macrophages are abundant throughout the body with three large collections in the intestine, the liver (Kupfer cells), and the lung (alveolar macrophage). The macrophage is a primary target cell and effector cell for immunology and inflammation (50). Its diverse repertoire includes immediate responses such as engulfment and killing of bacteria, making it a first-line defence to intraperitoneal bacteria, and more slow responses such as presenting antigen to T-cells for the production of immunglobulin by B-cells. It is also a major elicitor of inflammatory responses (an immediate reaction) and controls wound healing. Macrophages are important for chemotaxis, and localization of inflammation, at times leading to continuing destructive processes. The macrophage exerts its action by production and secretion of signal molecules which provoke numerous responses among other cells and this makes the macrophage important for both host defence and homeostasis.

It is not entirely clear what is meant by activation of the macrophage. The classical meaning is 'destruction' but a more diverse interpretation is appropriate as many of the macrophages' actions depend on their precise state of activation (50). Nor is it entirely clear what is meant by down-regulation of immunity and inflammation. It has been interpreted as failed mobilization of various cell populations of lymphocytes, impaired spontaneous or stimulated mitogenic activity, impaired or excessive production of cytokines, or impaired production of antibodies. It is generally understood that the deficiencies are detrimental and methods to correct them are assumed to be the way we should be treating severely septic patients in the future. One might speculate, as the body expresses these deficiencies so quickly, that they would be better regarded as adaptive mechanisms which increase the chance of survival in the reasonably ill or traumatized patient.

Mechanisms of disturbed wound healing

The incisional wound of the severely ill patient notoriously fails to heal properly, causing it to dehisce, especially after a second exploration of the abdomen (51). It is often attributed to infection but a closer examination of such wounds reveals a lack of responsiveness of the tissues. The wound margin is without reddening and there is little oedema. The subcutaneous fat may look as if the wound had been created the same day. Typically, the muscular layer is necrotic, through which the sutures have cut. There is no pus in such wounds but usually some opalescent fluid. Over the following days, or even weeks, as long as the patient remains in a septic state, it can be seen that individual lobes of subcutaneous fat turn necrotic while adjacent lobes are alive. There will be no granulation tissue but the fat continues to have a dull appearance. Over time, the skin epithelium will begin to cover the uppermost half centimeter of the wound with a thin epithelial surface. Obviously, epithelial cells can proliferate to some extent while the mesenchymal cells are more sensitive and fail to proliferate. A striking feature is that necrotic and live tissue exist side by side without provoking classical signs of inflammation. There will be no granulation tissue until the patient begins to recover. The turning point may be quite sudden. The same reaction can occasionally be observed within the abdomen.

Recently, Mastboom *et al.* (52) described their experience of 53 small bowel perforations which they considered non-iatrogenic. On six occasions they observed two lesions in the same patient and twice there were three lesions. The patients had been treated with planned relaparotomy for severe intra-abdominal infection. They had been subjected to from four to twenty operations. The perforations appeared at a time, relative to the relaparotomy, that they could not reasonable be attributed to missed perforations during the procedure. The authors concluded that the reason was unknown.

In a young, previously healthy trauma victim (APACHE II score of 17) with several laparotomies the author has experienced a perforation of the small intestine one week after the last operation. At laparotomy a punched out perforation was seen but there was no surrounding inflammation. The hole was sutured but leaked again after a further week, at which time it was brought out as a stoma. This patient then developed an abdominal wound dehiscence with exactly the appearance as described above.

It is important to speculate about the significance of these observations, and its cause. It is evident that the observations represent failed wound healing but the important feature seems to be that slight mechanical trauma of live tissue can create a discrete cellular injury, which probably happens at every operation, but these patients cannot repair their injury. Instead, the cells die and the tissue breaks down after about a week. It is an intriguing thought that the same mechanism is operative in MOF where substantial evidence points at cellular injury caused by the hypoperfusion and hypoxia of trauma and severe illness. The transient immunodeficiency would impair healing of injured tissue whatever its cause.

Immunodeficiency and wound healing

We must next consider the evidence for immunoregulation of wound healing. The macrophage is assumed to be a key cell in control of wound healing (53, 54). It secretes a number of regulatory signal substances. Prostaglandin E, which, it would appear, down regulates immunocompetence, was detected in high concentration of burn wounds (43). More recent studies have revealed that the eicosanoid profile in normal healing of rat colon anastomosis displayed a shift towards lipoxygenase products over cyclooxygenase products within one day, with a peak on day 8 (55). The macrophage was assumed to be the source of the lipoxygenase products. Prostaglandin E was not increased in the anastomosis. In another study of the healing colonic anastomosis, injections of PGE_1 impaired mobilisation of inflammatory cells to the anastomosis which resulted in a preserved collagen content of the anastomosis (56). The explanation might be that ischaemic inflammation of a suture line normally attracts neutrophils which release proteolytic enzymes that cause disintegration of the injured tissue as part of the remodelling of the normal healing process (57).

Wound healing is enhanced in nude mice that lack a normal T-cell system (58). Antibody depletion of T-helper and T-suppressor subsets in immunocompetent mice showed that loss of the T-helper cells was of no consequence for wound healing, whereas depletion of T-suppressor cells augmented the healing as measured by wound strength and hydroxyproline deposition (59). The results can be interpreted to mean that the macrophage initiates healing but the suppressor cell subsequently attenuates the stimuli to create the perfect scar.

Various cytokines, and growth factors, are present in wound fluid. The notable exception seems to be IL-2 (60). Fluid from healing wounds, ten days old, contained substances that increased the mortality of mice subjected to peritonitis by caecal ligation and puncture (61). This fluid from the normal healing process was a strong inhibitor of lymphocyte mitogenesis but it was devoid of TNF, INF, and TGF activity, indicating that the wound macrophage had been deactivated. The deposition of TNF, TGF, and platelet-derived growth factor (PDGF) in experimental wounds in rats revealed that TNF had no enhancing effect on wound healing and antagonized the stimulating effect of TGF, whereas it had no such diminishing effect on PDGF stimulation (62). Both TGF and PDGF accelerated healing of experimental wounds (63).

Wound healing must be seen as the integrated action of a number of growth factors and inflammatory mediators secreted by various cell populations within the wound. It appears that growth factors have narrow window concentrations within which they promote the healing process but their appearance in different concentrations, or at other time intervals, may delay or impair healing by antagonizing other factors. It is a reasonable assumption that mediators which trigger the inflammatory response, such as PAF and TNF, would delay the healing process for as long as the inflammation is active. Spill over of immunosuppressive wound fluid into the systemic circulation might, under certain circumstances, be a mechanism for systemic immunosuppression (61, 64). It is easily seen that a patient with extensive cellular injury throughout the splanchnic bed, as a result of the precipitating shock, is at risk of failure of healing of the epithelial layers, and therefore may have lost barrier function and other specialized function of the organs for extended periods of time. While we understand some of the normal wound healing processes the mechanisms that bring about a failed healing are far from clear. Studies of wound healing in the immunocompromised host, especially in models of sustained inflammation, would contribute to the understanding.

Mechanisms of nosocomial infection

Gastrointestinal hypomotility

The normal intestine has several motor patterns (65). Every surgeon knows that even minor intra-abdominal disease or a simple ceoliotomy may cause an ileus for several days. The precise mechanisms involved with this 'atonia' are not well understood. It can be mitigated by epidural anaesthesia and hence control by the central nervous system is involved. A number of drugs, notably opiates, will disturb the motility of the intestines (66). It is also strange that acute illness outside the abdomen can cause paralysis of the intestines. We may therefore infer that acute illness *per se* can adversely affect the intestines, possibly through mediators that are released by the disease. Finally, the grossly distended and swollen intestines resulting from generalized peritonitis are an obviously failed organ.

Loss of mucosal barrier function

The digestion of food necessitates a selective barrier that allows absorption of nutrients but excludes larger molecules that could be toxic or allergenic. The barrier normally allows the passage of molecules in descending frequency up to at least 1338 daltons (67). It appears to be a normal phenomenon that small amounts of large molecules pass the intestinal mucosa and are handled by the clearing mechanisms of the body (68). Such molecules pass through tight junctions between cells rather than through the enterocyte absorptive mechanisms. The barrier is very sensitive and easily disrupted in disease (69–74), by starvation (75) and by parenteral nutrition (76). An increased uptake of lactulose, a probe substance, was detected in burn patients without circulatory defects as early as 16 to 30 h post-burn (77). A single dose of parenteral endotoxin given to humans disrupted the barrier (78). When the barrier is broken there exists the potential for transgression of live intestinal flora and infection (79).

Bacterial overgrowth

The normal gut is capable of preventing overgrowth of microflora through its motility. In germ-free mice the motor pattern is slower but is restored when the intestine is colonized (80). A possible explanation is that the motility responds to microbial metabolites such as short chain fatty acids (81, 82). The acidity of the stomach is the important determinant of gastric colonization (83, 84). Systematic studies of the flora associated with severely ill patients, with MOF, displayed an almost exclusive aerobic flora dominated by *E. coli*, *Klebsiella* spp., enterococcus, *Staph. epidermidis*, *Pseudomonas*, and *Candida* (85). This flora was detectable in large numbers in the proximal intestinal tract in patients (13) and in experimental animals (86).

The flora is qualitatively different from the flora of secondary peritonitis where anaerobic organisms are common. The reasons for this change of flora, which occurs with both duration and severity of disease, is speculative. Review of the animal experiments on bacterial translocation shows that it is the aerobic flora which increases and this explains part of the problem. The change towards a multiresistant flora of staphylococci, *Klebsiella*, *Pseudomonas*, and fungi is partly a result of the practice of treating all severely ill patients with broad-spectrum antibiotics for extended periods of time.

Bacterial translocation

Bacterial translocation is the process by which live bacteria transgress the intestinal mucosa to reach mesenteric lymph nodes or the portal and systemic circulation. Studies of these processes, in both animals and humans, show that it is indeed a common phenomenon (69, 70). It is a graded result of loss of barrier function, decreased motility, and the resulting bacterial overgrowth. The slightest injury will allow endotoxin to be detected in portal blood and live bacteria in mesenteric lymph nodes. With still more severe injury the bacteria will appear in portal blood and systemic circulation in significant numbers (87, 88). The bacteria are trapped in lungs, liver, kidney, and spleen where they can be detected (89).

It is almost certain that the bacteria transgress the intestinal wall at the level of the small intestine. In most models the initiating trauma has produced mucosal injury of the villi of the ileum, usually of grade 2–3 of Park's classification, i.e. subepithelial space or mucosal lifting along the sides of villi. There is also evidence of some mucosal loss in the caecum. Most studies show an overgrowth of about 2 logarithms of predominantly *E. coli* in the caecum but there are studies to demonstrate bacterial overgrowth of the small intestine at an early stage of the disease (86). It is a reasonable hypothesis that, since aerobic Gram-negative flora dominates the small intestine, an overgrowth of this flora is more likely here and is then propelled to the caecum where it has been detected. It is otherwise rather difficult to explain the selective overgrowth of aerobic flora in the first part of colon where normally anaerobic flora dominates. The anaerobic flora does not translocate except in very severe mucosal injury (69, 70, 90). The precise mechanism by which the bacteria cross the wall is not entirely clear. Evidence has been presented that the bacteria are engulfed by macrophages and carried to the lymph nodes (69) but the initial process can also be passage through the enterocyte itself (91). These two mechanisms both seem to be operative in minor disease.

Bacteriology of severe illness

The severely septic patient has a predominance of aerobic flora (12, 85). Apart from being the result of bacterial translocation another pathomechanism should be considered. The typical anaerobic infection is an abscess. Anaerobic bacteria do not invade tissue or enter cells but provoke a local tissue response that creates the abscess within which a suitable milieu for proliferation of anaerobic bacteria is established. The aerobic bacteria, on the other hand, have the capacity to invade tissue, adhere to cells, and to penetrate cells. These species subsequently proliferate in interstitial spaces, on cell surfaces, or within cells. The difference in pathogenic mechanisms was clearly demonstrated in animal experiments which showed that the mortality from peritonitis was caused by the invasiveness of the aerobic flora (92). In the immunosuppressed patient, with diminished wound healing capacity, an abscess may not form, but proliferation of aerobic bacteria can be enhanced within non-responsive tissues. The inherent pathogenic mechanisms of aerobic and anaerobic bacteria, and the paralysis of the immune system may be important explanations for the almost total preponderance of aerobic infection.

Probably of less importance is the modulating effect of antibiotic treatment. The imidazoles, commonly used in the treatment of surgical infection, are extremely potent against anaerobic flora, which is almost uniformly sensitive to this group of antibiotics. But there will always be a shift, and replacement by resistant flora, with every antibiotic directed against the aerobic flora. Taken together, the above mechanisms would explain the emergence of nosocomial infections with multiresistent aerobic flora.

Gut-origin nosocomial infection

Suspicion has arisen that the typical flora identified with various infective episodes are, in fact, derived from the gastrointestinal tract. Observations by Du Molin (93) implicated microaspiration along the nasogastric tube as a major cause of hospital aquired pneumonia. It was demonstrated that secondary infections can be prevented with oral, non-absorbable antibiotics in neutropenic patients (94). A concept of 'colonization resistance' was developed in which the aerobic intestinal flora is suppressed by antibiotics but the anaerobic flora is retained to prevent colonization with new, potentially pathogenic flora. This treatment has been called selective decontamination of the digestive tract, SDD. (See Chapter 36.) The treatment has three components. A triple combination of non-absorbable antibiotics via the nasogastric tube, the same antibiotics applied as an ointment to the oropharynx, and intravenous antibiotic prophylaxis with a cephalosporin is given. Stoutenbeek *et al.* (95, 96) demonstrated that the rate of superinfection was much lower in polytrauma patients on SDD in intensive care. The results have been confirmed by Ledingham *et al.* (97). Respiratory tract infection seems to be particularly lowered but septicaemia, urinary tract infection and wound infection rates were also greatly diminished. It is only the secondary infections that can be prevented. The odd result is that patient outcome was not altered.

The effects of SDD can be interpreted against the overgrowth by aerobic flora in the stomach and small intestine, together with the transgression of this flora through the walls of the intestine. This is the sequel of severe illness, not its cause. Many of these patients have nasogastric tubes, enteric fistulas, or enterostomas. The patient is besieged by highly contaminated enteral secretions, rich in aerobic flora. The flora will appear at every location and particularly will invade intravenous lines, endotracheal tubes, and urinary tract catheters to colonize and eventually cause infection at these sites (98). SDD, which lowers the concentration of microflora within the intestines, may delay or prevent the process but the damage to the epithelium of various organs in severe illness has already occurred. Therefore SDD cannot be expected to alter patient outcome significantly.

The abacterial sepsis syndrome

The role of uncontrolled infection as the primary cause of MOF began to be questioned in the 1980s. It was soon realized that MOF developed in patients with primary infection as well as in patients with no obvious infection, such as acute pancreatitis or trauma. Indeed, most patients with a high severity score from acute disease develop persisting failure of at least one organ.

In patients with MOF after intra-abdominal infection it was difficult to see a cause beyond the infection although it became evident that infection was not always present at the time of MOF, and that MOF was not reversed by drainage of an abscess (99, 100). Goris *et al.* (11) compared patients who had MOF after intra-abdominal infection with those who had MOF after trauma. The sequence in which organs failed was similar and independent of infection. Septicaemia is seen in less than one-third of trauma patients with MOF, and usually only after about two weeks (4, 10, 11). The conclusion, therefore, is that MOF is not primarily caused by infection but that MOF invites infection. MOF is almost invariable associated with a septic response which also is independent of infection (5).

It became necessary to develop models of abacterial sepsis to study the nature of 'multiple organ failure—septic state' without infection. Zymosan is a glycoprotein from the cell wall of baker's yeast. It is a potent activator of complement by the alternate pathway and generates an inflammatory response *in vivo* that can be beneficial in low doses (101), but in high dose causes a deleterious systemic response. In two similar studies (102, 103) zymosan was injected intraperitoneally into rats. The rats displayed typical signs of sepsis, and multiple organ malfunction developed over the first week. These responses were qualitatively identical in germ-free rats but less pronounced. The normal rats showed bacterial translocation with positive cultures of peritoneal fluid, retroperitoneal lymph nodes, and portal blood. In surviving animals the percentage of positive cultures decreased as time elapsed. Both investigators found identical microscopic changes in the failed organs. These consisted of congestion, vacuolization of epithelium, and accumulation of inflammatory cells. In addition, the lungs showed areas of haemorrhage, and the mucosa of the small intestine showed blunting of villi. Zymosan given in much lower dose to mice also resulted in bacterial translocation and typical changes of villi on histologic examination (75).

These studies seem to show that systemic inflammation is the bridge linking the typical changes of the epithelium of lung, kidney, liver, and intestine. The epithelium is rendered incapable of its specialized function, and hence these organs fail. The destruction of the epithelium of lung and intestine are obviously more deleterious in the early phase. Pulmonary failure is the earliest and most common failure seen in the ITU. Loss of the gastrointestinal barrier and translocation of bacteria have consistently been shown to occur within hours of onset of acute illness, but have not been clinically recognized as a form of organ failure in patients.

Conclusions

There is now convincing evidence that ischaemic cellular injury of abdominal viscera, kidney and lung is the main problem leading to MOF. The injury is sustained early in the disease process but continues to develop over hours or days as ischaemic inflammation ensues. Altered secretion and responses to cytokines, eicosanoids and growth factors bring about an adaptive down regulation of immunity and inflammation. Its major sequel is the failure to heal cell damage or to reconstruct the texture and function of highly specialized organs. To prevent this high-risk condition it is mandatory to prevent hypovolaemic shock and tissue oxygen deficiency. Once this condition has developed, treatment must be aimed at excising or draining any focus of localized diseased tissue, abscess or necrosis, and possibly to supress the intestinal flora thus preventing further seeding of microbes from the intestinal tract. The aim is to obtain a 'clean', haemodynamically stable patient, and a period of alert observation while the immune 'paralysis' fades away and healing capacity is restored.

References

1. Rotstein, O.D. and Meakins, J.L. (1990). Diagnostic and therapeutic challenges of intra-abdominal infections. *World J. Surg.*, **14**, 159–65.
2. Pointing, G.A., Sim, A.J.W., and Dudley, H.A.F. (1987). Comparison of the local and systemic effects of sepsis in predicting survival. *Br. J. Surg.*, **74**, 750–2.
3. Knaus, W.A., Draper, E.A., Wagner, D.P., and Zimmerman, J.E. (1985). APACHE II: A severity of disease classification system. *Crit. Care Med.*, **13**, 818–29.
4. Border, J.R., Hasset, J., LaDuca, J., *et al.* (1987). The gut origin septic states in blunt multiple trauma (ISS = 40) in the ICU. *Ann. Surg.*, **206**, 427–48.
5. Marshall, J. and Sweeney, D. (1990). Microbial infection and the septic response in critical surgical illness. Sepsis, not infection, determines outcome. *Arch. Surg.*, **125**, 17–23.
6. Baue, A.E. (1975). Multiple, progressive, or sequential systems failure: a syndrome of the 1970s. *Arch. Surg.*, **110**, 779–81.
7. Baue, A.E. (1990). Historical perspective. In *Multiple organ failure: pathophysiology and basic concepts of therapy* (ed. E. Deitch), pp. 1–12. Thieme Medical Publishers, New York.
8. Eiseman, B., Beart, R., and Norton, L. (1977). Multiple organ failure. *Surg. Gynecol. Obstet.*, **144**, 323–6.
9. Fry, D.E., Pearlstein, L., Fulton, R.L., and Polk, H.C. Jr. (1980). Multiple system organ failure: the role of uncontrolled infection. *Arch. Surg.*, **115**, 136–40.
10. Faist, E., Baue, A.E., Dittmer, H., and Heberer, G. (1983). Multiple organ failure in polytrauma patients. *J. Trauma*, **23**, 775–87.
11. Goris, R.J.A., te Boekhorst, T.P.A., Nuytinck, K.S., and Gimbrère, J.S.F. (1985). Multiple organ failure—generalized autodestructive inflammation. *Arch. Surg.*, **120**, 1109–15.
12. Knaus, W.A., Draper, G.A., Wagner, D.P., and Zimmerman, J.G. (1985). Prognosis in acute organ system failure. *Ann. Surg.*, **202**, 685–93.
13. Marshall, J.C., Christou, N.V., Horn, R., and Meakins, J.L. (1988). The microbiology of multiple organ failure. The proximal gastrointestinal tract as an occult reservoir of pathogens. *Arch. Surg.*, **123**, 309–15.
14. Stevens, L.E. (1983). Gauging the severity of surgical sepsis. *Arch. Surg.*, **118**, 1190–2.
15. Wagner, D., Draper, E., and Knaus, W. (1989). Development of APACHE III. *Crit. Care Med.*, **17**, (suppl.), S 199–S 203.
16. Nyström, P.O., Bax, R., Dellinger, E.P., *et al.* (1990). Proposed definitions for diagnosis, severity scoring, stratification, and outcome for trials on intra-abdominal infection. *World J. Surg.*, **14**, 148–58.
17. Polk, H.C. Jr., and Shields, C.L. (1977). Remote organ failure: a valid sign of occult intra-abdominal infection. *Surgery*, **81**, 310–3.
18. Vincent, J.-L. and van der Linden, P. (1990). Septic shock: particular type of acute circulatory failure. *Crit. Care Med.*, **18** (suppl. 2), S 70–S 74.
19. Lundgren, O. (1989). Physiology of the intestinal circulation. In *Splanchnic ischemia and multiple organ failure* (ed. A. Marston, G.B. Bulkley, R.G. Fiddian-Green, and U.H. Haglund), pp. 29–40, Edward Arnold, London.
20. Porter, J.M., Sussman, M.S., and Bulkley, G.B. (1989). Splanchnic vasospasm in circulatory shock. In *Splanchnic ischemia and multiple organ failure* (ed. A. Marston, G.B. Bulkley, R.G. Fiddian-Green, and U.H. Haglund), pp. 73–88. Edward Arnold, London.
21. Binnaka, T., Yamaguchi, T., Kubota, Y., Hirohara, J., Mizuno, T., Sameshima, Y. (1990). Gastric hemodynamic disturbance induced by hemorrhagic shock in rats: role of platelet activating factor. *Scand. J. Gastroenterol.*, **25**, 555–62.
22. Lefer, A.M. and Bitterman, H. (1989). Eicosanoids: their role in splanchnic ischemia and shock. In *Splanchnic ischemia and multiple organ failure* (ed. A. Marston, G.B. Bulkley, R.G. Fiddian-Green, and U.H. Haglund), pp. 214–27. London, Edward Arnold.
23. Michie, H.R., Guillou, P.J., and Wilmore, D.W. (1989). Tumour necrosis factor and bacterial sepsis. *Br. J. Surg.*, **76**, 670–1.
24. Schirmer, W.J., Schirmer, J.M., and Fry, D.E. (1989). Recombinant human tumor necrosis factor produces hemodynamic changes characteristic of sepsis and endotoxemia. *Arch. Surg.*, **124**, 445–8.
25. Dahn, M.S., Wilson, R.F., Lange, P., Stoen, A., and Jacobs, L.A. (1990). Hepatic parenchymal oxygen tension following injury and sepsis. *Arch. Surg.*, **125**, 441–3.
26. Dahn, M.S., Lange, P., Wilson, R.F., Jacobs, L.A., Mitchell, R.A. (1990). Hepatic blood flow and splanchnic oxygen consumption measurements in clinical sepsis. *Surgery*, **107**, 295–301.
27. Chiu, C.J., McArdle, A.H., Brown, R., *et al.* (1970). Intestinal mucosal lesions in low-flow states. I. A morphologic, hemodynamic and metabolic reappraisal. *Arch. Surg.*, **101**, 478–83.
28. Park, P.O., Haglund, U., Bulkley, G.B., and Fält, K. (1990).

The sequence of development of intestinal tissue injury after strangulation ischemia and reperfusion. *Surgery*, **107**, 574–80.
29. Deitch, E.A., Bridges, W., Baker, J., *et al.* (1988). Hemorrhagic shock-induced bacterial translocation is reduced by xanthine oxidase inhibition or inactivation. *Surgery*, **104**, 191–8.
30. Vedder, N.B., Fouty, B.W., Winn, R.K., Harlan, J.M., and Rice, C.L. (1989). Role of neutrophils in generalized reperfusion injury with resuscitation from shock. *Surgery*, **106**, 509–16.
31. Vickers, S.M., Bailey, R.W., and Bulkley, G.B. (1989). Ischemic hepatitis. In *Splanchnic ischemia and multiple organ failure*. (ed. A. Marston, G.B. Bulkley, R.G. Fiddian-Green, and U.H. Haglund), pp. 261–7. Edward Arnold, London.
32. Haglund, U. and Arvidson, D, (1989). Acute acalculus cholecystitis. In *Splanchnic ischemia and multiple organ failure* (ed. A. Marston, G.B. Bulkley, R.G. Fiddian-Green, and U.H. Haglund), pp. 269–72. Edward Arnold, London.
33. Clemens, J.A., Bulkley, G.B., and Cameron, J.L. (1989). Ischemic pancreatitis. In *Splanchnic ischemia and multiple organ failure* (ed. A. Marston, G.B. Bulkley, R.G. Fiddian-Green, and U.H. Haglund), pp. 273–7. Edward Arnold, London.
34. Nuytinck, H.K.S., Offermans, X.J.M.V., Kubat, K., and Goris, R.J.A (1988). Whole-body inflammation in trauma patients. An autopsy study. *Arch. Surg.*, **123**, 1519–24.
35. Balkwill, F.R. and Burke, F. (1989). The cytokine network. *Immunology Today*, **10**, 299–303.
36. Mitchison, N.A. (1989). Supression. *Immunology Today*, **10**, 392–3.
37. Knapp, W., Rieber, P., Dörken, B., Schmidt, R.E., Stein, H., Borne, A.E.G. (1989). Towards a better definition of human leucocyte surface molecules. *Immunology Today*, **10**, 253–9.
38. Wahl, S.M., McCartney-Francis, N., and Mergenhagen, S.E. (1989). Inflammatory and immunomodulatory roles of TGF-β. *Immunology Today*, **10**, 258–61.
39. Michie, H.R., Spriggs, D.R., Manogue, K.R. *et al.* (1988). Tumor necrosis factor and endotoxin induce similar metabolic responses in human beings. *Surgery*, **104**, 280–6.
40. Fong, Y., Moldawer, L.L., Shires, G.T., and Lowry, S.F. (1990). The biological characteristics of cytokines and their implication in surgical injury. *Surg. Gynecol. Obstet*, **170**, 363–78.
41. Goldyne, M.E. (1988). Lymphocytes and arachidonic acid metabolism. *Prog. Allergy*, **44**, 140–52.
42. Plescia, O.J. and Racis, S. (1988) Prostaglandins as physiological immunoregulators. *Prog. Allergy*, **44**, 153–71.
43. Arturson, G. (1977). Prostaglandins in human burn-wound secretion. *Burns*, **3**, 112–8.
44. Faist, E., Mewes, A., Baker C.C., *et al.* (1987). Prostaglandin E_2 (PGE_2) dependent supression of interleukin-alpha (IL-2) production in patients with major trauma. *J. Trauma*, **27**, 837–48.
45. Miller-Graziano, C.L., Fink, M., Jia Yan Wu, Szabo, G., and Kodys, K. (1988). Mechanisms of altered monocyte prostaglandin E_2 production in severely injured patients. *Arch. Surg.*, **123**, 293–9.
46. Green, D.R. and Faist, E. (1988). Trauma and the immune response. *Immunology Today*, **9**, 253–5.
47. Takayama, T.K., Miller, C., and Szabo, G. (1990). Elevated tumor necrosis factor-alfa production concomitant to elevated prostaglandin E_2 production by trauma patients' monocytes. *Arch. Surg.*, **125**, 29–35.
48. Puyana, J.C., Rode, H., Gordon, J., Meakins, J.L., Chartrand, L., and Christou, N.V. (1988). Lack of cytokine-induced skin reaction correlates with acute physiology score and mortality in patients receiving intensive care. *Arch. Surg.*, **123**, 1474–6.
49. Waymack, J.P. and Yurt, R.W. (1988). Effect of prostaglandin E on immune function in multiple animal models. *Arch. Surg.*, **123**, 1429–32.
50. Adams, D.O. (1989). Molecular interactions in macrophage activation. *Immunology Today*, **10**, 33–5.
51. Lévy, E., Palmer, D.L., Frileux, P., *et al.* (1988). Septic necrosis of the midline wound in post-operative peritonitis. *Ann. Surg.*, **207**, 470–9.
52. Mastboom, W.J.B., Kuypers, H.H.C., Schoots, F.J., and Wobbes, T. (1989). Small-bowel perforation complicating the open treatment of generalized peritonitis. *Arch. Surg.*, **124**, 689–92.
53. Leibovich, S.J. and Ross, R. (1975). The role of the macrophage in wound repair: a study with hydrocortisone and antimacrophage serum. *Am. J. Pathol.*, **78**, 71–91.
54. Browder, W., Williams, D., Lucore, P., Pretus, H., Jones, E., and McNamee, R. (1988). Effect of enhanced macrophage function on early wound healing. *Surgery*, **104**, 224–30.
55. van der Ham, A.C., Kort, W.J., Bijma, A.M., Zijlstra, F.J., Vermeer, M.A., and Jeekel, J. (1990). Eicosanoid profile of healing colon anastomosis and peritoneal macrophages in the rat. *Gut*, **31**, 807–11.
56. Terzoglu, T., Sonmez, Y.E., and Eldegez, U. (1990). The effect of prostaglandin E1 on colonic anastomotic healing: a comparison study. *Dis. Col. Rect.*, **33**, 44–8.
57. Högström, H., Haglund, U., and Zederfeldt, B. (1990). Tension leads to increased neutrophil accumulation and decreased laparotomy wound strength. *Surgery*, **107**, 215–9.
58. Barbul, A., Shawe, T., Roter, S.M., Efron, J.E., Wasserkrug, H.L., and Badawy, S.B. (1989). Wound healing in nude mice: a study on the regulatory role of lymphocytes in fibroplasia. *Surgery*, **105**, 764–9.
59. Barbul, A., Breslin, R.J., Woodyard, J.P., Wasserkrug, H.L., and Efron, G. (1989). The effect of *in vivo* T-helper and T-supressor lymphocyte depletion on wound healing. *Ann. Surg.*, **209**, 479–83.
60. Ford, H.R., Hoffman, R.A., Wing, E.J., Magee, D.M., McIntyre, L., and Simmons, R.L. (1989). Characterization of wound cytokines in the sponge matrix model. *Arch. Surg.*, **124**, 1422–8.
61. Lazarou, S.A., Barbul, A., Wasserkrug, H.L., and Efron, G. (1989). The wound is a possible source of posttraumatic immunosuppression. *Arch. Surg.*, **124**, 1429–31.
62. Steenfos, H.H., Hunt, T.K., Scheuenstuhl, H., and Goodson, W.H. (1989). Selective effects of tumor necrosis factor-alfa on wound healing in rats. *Surgery*, **106**, 171–6.
63. Mustoe, T.A., Landes, A., Cromack, D.T., *et al.* (1990). Differential acceleration of healing of surgical incisions in the rabbit gastrointestinal tract by platelet-derived growth factor and transforming growth factor type beta. *Surgery*, **108**, 324–30.
64. Barbul, A., Fishel, R.S., Shimazu, S., Damewood, R.B., Efron, G. (1984). Inhibition of host immunity by fluid and mononulear cells from healing wounds. *Surgery*, **96**, 315–9.
65. Ehrlein, H.J., Schemann, M., and Siegle, M.L. (1987). Motor patterns of small intestine determined by closely spaced extraluminal transducers and videofluoroscopy. *Am. J. Physiol.*, **253**, G 259–G 267.
66. Fox, J.E.T. and Daniel, E.E. (1987). Exogenous opiates: their local mechanisms of action in the canine small intestine and stomach. *Am. J. Physiol.*, **253**, G 179–G 188.
67. Tagesson, C., Andersson, P.Å., Andersson, T., Bolin, T., Källberg, M., and Sjödahl, R. (1983). Passage of molecules through the wall of the gastrointestinal tract. Measurement of

intestinal permeability to polyethylene glycols in the 634–1338 dalton range. *Scand. J. Gastroenterol*, **18**, 481–6.

68. Bjarnason, I. and Peters, T. J. (1987). Helping the mucosa make sense of macromolecules. *Gut*, **28**, 1057–61.
69. Wells, C. L., Maddaus, M. A., and Simmons, R. L. (1988). Proposed mechanisms for the translocation of intestinal bacteria. *Rev. Infect. Dis.*, **10**, 958–79.
70. Deitch, E. A. (1990). The role of intestinal barrier failure and bacterial translocation in the development of systemic infection and multiple organ failure. *Arch. Surg.*, 125: 403–4.
71. Wilmore, D. W., Smith, R. J., O'Dwyer, S. T., Jacobs, D. O., Ziegler, T. R., and Wang, X. D. (1988). The gut: a central organ after surgical stress. *Surgery*, **104**, 917–23.
72. Deitch, E. A., Sittig, K., Li, M., Berg, R., and Specian, R. D. (1990). Obstructive jaundice promotes bacterial translocation from the gut. *Am. J. Surg.*, **159**, 79–84.
73. Deitch, E. A. (1989). Simple intestinal obstruction causes bacterial translocation in man. *Arch. Surg.*, **124**, 699–701.
74. Jones, W. G., Minei, J. P., Barber, A. E., *et al.* (1990). Bacterial translocation and intestinal atrophy after termal burn wound sepsis. *Ann. Surg.*, **211**, 399–405.
75. Deitch, E. A., Ma, W. J., Ma, L., Berg, R. D., and Specian, R. D. (1990). Protein malnutrition predisposes to inflammatory-induced gut-origin septic states. *Ann. Surg.*, **211**, 560–8.
76. Alverdy, J. C., Aoys, E., and Moss, G. S. (1988). Total parenteral nutrition promotes bacterial translocation from the gut. *Surgery*, **104**, 185–90.
77. Deitch, E. A. (1990). Intestinal permeability is increased in burn patients shortly after injury. *Surgery*, **107**, 411–6.
78. O'Dwyer, S. T., Michie, H. R., Ziegler, T. R., Revhaug, A., Smith, R. J., and Wilmore, D. W. (1988). A single dose of endotoxin increases intestinal permeability in healthy humans. *Arch. Surg.*, **123**, 1459–64.
79. Ziegler, T. R., Smith, R. J., O'Dwyer, S. T., Demling, R. H., and Wilmore, D. W. (1988). Increased intestinal permeability is associated with infection in burn patients. *Arch. Surg.*, **123**, 1313–9.
80. Caenepell, P. H., Janssens, J., Vantrappen, G., Eyssen, H., and Coremans, G. (1989). Interdigestive myoelectric complex in germ-free rats. *Dig. Dis. Sci.*, **34**, 1180–4.
81. Kamath, P. S., Phillips, S. F., and Zinsmeister, A. R. (1988). Short-chain fatty acids stimulate ileal motility in humans. *Gastroenterology*, **95**, 1496–502.
82. Finch, A., Phillips, S. F., Hakim, N. S., Brown, M. L., and Zinsmeister, A. R. (1989). Stimulation of ileal emptying by short-chain fatty acids. *Dig. Dis. Sci.*, **34**, 1516–20.
83. Muscroft, T. J., Deane, S. A., Youngs, D., Burdon, D. W., and Keighley, M. R. B. (1981). The microflora of the post-operative stomach. *Br. J. Surg.*, **68**, 560–4.
84. Driks, M. R., Craven, D. E., Celli, B. R., *et al.* (1987). Nosocomial pneumonia in intubated patients given sucralfate as compared with antacids or histamine type 2 blockers. The role of gastric colonization. *N. Engl. J. Med.*, **317**, 1376–82.
85. Rotstein, O. D., Pruett, T. L., and Simmons, R. L. (1986). Microbiologic features and treatment of persistent peritonitis in patients in the intensive care unit. *Can. J. Surg.*, **29**, 247–50.
86. Marshall, J. C., Christou, N. V., and Meakins, J. L. (1988). Small-bowel overgrowth and systemic immunosupression in experimental peritonitis. *Surgery*, **104**, 404–10.
87. Rush, B. F., Redan, J. A., Flanagan, J. J., *et al.* (1989). Does bacteremia observed in hemorrhagic shock have clinical significance. *Ann. Surg.*, **210**, 342–7.
88. Redan, J. A., Rush, B. F., Lysz, T. W., Smith, S., and Machiedo, G. W. (1990). Organ distribution of gut-derived bacteria caused by bowel manipulation and ischemia. *Am. J. Surg.*, **159**, 85–90.
89. Redan, J. A., Rush, B. F., McCullough, J. N., *et al.* (1990). Organ distribution of radiolabeled enteric *Escherichia coli* during and after hemorrhagic shock. *Ann. Surg.*, **211**, 663–8.
90. Steffen, E. K., Berg, R. D., and Deitch, E. A. (1988). Comparison of translocation rates of various indigenous bacteria from the gastrointestinal tract to the mesenteric lymph node. *J. Infect. Dis.*, **175**, 1032–8.
91. Alexander, J. W., Boyce, S. T., Babcock, G. F., *et al.* (1990). The process of microbial translocation. *Ann. Surg.*, **212**, 496–510.
92. Bartlett, J. G., Onderdonk, A. B., Louie, T., Kasper, D. L., and Gorbach, S. L. (1978). Lessons from an animal model of intra-abdominal sepsis. *Arch. Surg.*, **113**, 853–7.
93. Du Moulin, C. G., Paterson, D. G., Hedley-Whyte., J., Paterson, D. G., and Lisbon, A. (1982). Aspiration of gastric bacteria in antacid-treated patients: a frequent cause of post-operative colonisation of the airway. *Lancet*, **ii**, 242–5.
94. Guiot, H. F. L., van den Broek, P. J., van de Neer, J. W., and van Furth, R. (1983). Selective antimicrobial modulation of the intestinal flora of patients with acute nonlymphocytic leukemia: a double blind placebo controlled study. *J. Infect. Dis.*, **147**, 615–23.
95. Stoutenbeek, C. P., van Saene, H. K. F., Miranda, D. R., Zandstra, D. F., and Langreher, D. (1987). The effect of oropharyngeal decontamination using nonabsorbable antibiotics on the incidence of nosocomial respiratory tract infection in multiple trauma patients. *J. Trauma*, **27**, 357–64.
96. Stoutenbeek, C. P., van Saene, H. K. F., Miranda, D. R., Zandstra, D. F., and Binnendijk, B. (1984). The prevention of superinfection in multiple trauma patients. *J. Antimicrob. Chemother.*, **14** (suppl.) B, 203–11.
97. Ledingham, I. McA., Eastaway, A. T., McKay, I. C., Alcock, S. R., McDonald, J. C., and Ramsay, G. (1988). Triple regimen of selective decontamination of the digestive tract, systemic cefotaxime, and microbial surveillance for prevention of acquired infection in intensive care. *Lancet*, **i**: 785–90.
98. Meakins, J. L., Wicklund, B., and Forse, R. A. (1980). The surgical intensive care unit: current concepts in infection. *Surg. Clin. North Am.*, **60**, 117–32.
99. Norton, L. W. (1985). Does drainage of intra-abdominal pus reverse multiple organ failure? *Am. J. Surg.*, **149**, 347–50.
100. Sutherland, F. R., Temple, W. J., Snodgrass, T., and Huchcroft, S. A. (1989). Predicting the outcome of exploratory laparotomy in ICU patients with sepsis or organ failure. *J. Trauma*, **29**, 152–6.
101. Browder, W., Williams, D., Pretus, H., *et al.* (1990). Beneficial effect of enhanced macrophage function in the trauma patient. *Ann. Surg.*, **211**, 605–12.
102. Goris, R. J. A., Boekholtz, W. K. F., van Bebber, I. P. T., Nuytinck, J. K. S., and Schillings, P. H. M. (1986). Multiple organ failure and sepsis without bacteria. *Arch. Surg.*, **121**, 897–901.
103. Steinberg, S., Flynn, W., Kelly, K., *et al.* (1989). Development of a bacteria-independent model of the multiple organ failure syndrome. *Arch. Surg.*, **124**, 1390–5.

14

Is it worthwhile reducing hospital infection rates?

ALAN MAYNARD

Introduction

Hospital-acquired infections (HAI) reduce the quality of life of patients and may threaten their lives. Furthermore such infections consume scarce resources which could be used to treat other patients in need of beneficial procedures. Despite these obvious effects of HAI data about their incidence and prevalence are incomplete and the cost-effectiveness of the many competing procedures to reduce these infections is largely unknown.

The purpose of this chapter is to discuss whether it is worthwhile to reduce hospital-acquired infection rates and, if so, by how much. After a review of the evidence about the incidence, prevalence and cost of HAI some competing interventions to reduce the level of HAI are identified. Simple techniques of economic evaluation can be deployed to determine whether a programme to prevent HAI is worthwhile and, if it is, how much resource should be deployed. The cost of infection control may increase as its volume rises and thus it may be too expensive to eradicate all HAI: there is an efficient level of control, beyond which scarce economic resources will be wasted on infection control which could yield greater health benefits if used elsewhere in the National Health Service (NHS).

Information about the costs and benefits of infection control are of great importance to health care purchasers. Whether the purchaser of health care is private (e.g. BUPA or the Blue Cross/Blue Shield insurers in the USA) or public (e.g. NHS budget holders or US Federal budget holders for Medicaid, for the poor, or Medicare, for the elderly) their interests are the same: is it worthwhile to reduce hospital infection rates, and if so, by how much should these rates be reduced?

Incidence, prevalence, and cost of hospital-acquired infections

There have been numerous studies of HAI and these show a remarkable similarity in terms of incidence and prevalence. The economic effects of HAI have recently been reviewed (1). An average incidence of 5 per cent and a prevalence of 10 per cent disguises a range of between 5.9 and 13.5 per cent for prevalence (2).

The most comprehensive study was SENIC (the Study of the Efficacy of Nosocomial Infection Centre) carried out by the USA Center for Disease Control (CDC) in 1975–76. This found 5.7 infections per 100 admissions in a sample of 338 hospitals (13). They estimated that HAI in 1975–76 may have numbered 3.6 to 4 million and there was a slow upward trend in the incidence of the problem. This trend was, the authors argued, associated with invasive and more complex operations, new strains of antibiotic resistant organisms, and hospital 'economics' which had depleted infection control programmes. Meers *et al.* surveyed 18 186 patients in 43 hospitals and found a prevalence of HAI of 9.2 per cent, with infections of the urinary tract, surgical wound and respiratory tract being the most common (2).

The resource consequences of HAI are significant. Using CDC data it has been estimated that the costs of increased hospitalization due to the infection of 1.7 million patients was over $1 billion (in 1973–74 prices) (4). Using SENIC data, Larson and Oram estimated that 60 000 deaths were caused, or contributed to, by hospital acquired infections and that these infections cost $4 billion annually in the USA (5). The average additional length of stay appears to be 4 to 10 days in the USA (6).

In the UK, the government's view is that HAI usually generates 4 days of additional hospitalization. Thus with a 5 per cent infection rate, 950 000 lost bed days per year (in 1986) cost the NHS £111 million (7). Small scale specific studies have found high infection rates for particular groups of patients (8).

It is possible to reduce infection rates and the costs they impose in a variety of ways which appear to be 'proven', e.g. sterilization, hand-washing/disinfection, isolation procedures, non-touch dressing techniques, closed urinary drainage system, perioperative antibiotic prophylaxis for certain procedures, and disinfection of respiratory therapy equipment. Some other interventions are of unproven benefit, e.g. disinfection mats, plastic shoe covers, ultraviolet lights, disinfection of floors, walls and sinks, laminar air-flow systems, and antibiotic prophylaxis for certain procedures.

However, whatever combinations of proven and unproven control techniques produce the greatest benefit, at least cost is now known. Many of the studies of competing techniques or combinations of techniques in infection control produce incomplete measures of both their benefits to society and their costs. To remedy these deficiencies more prospective studies, using a randomized control design, are needed.

One reason why such studies are necessary is that, although most NHS hospitals monitor infection rates, there is little scrutiny of their resource consequences. Thus data about quarterly variations in infections, their types and the speciality in which they were detected can be acquired from NHS monitoring systems. However, these data are linked neither to the resource consequences in hospitals (e.g. additional bed days) or in the community (e.g. increased use of GP services and drugs after discharge), nor to the impact of such infections on the quality of life of patients.

From the evidence available it is apparent that the incidence of HAI is about 5 per cent and that these events consume considerable amounts of resources which could be used to care for and to cure other, untreated patients. Previous studies have often examined the costs and benefits of control policies in a superficial manner. The two crucial questions need to be answered: is it worthwhile to control hospital infections *and* how much scarce resource should be allocated to controlling these infections?

The role of economic evaluation

Types of economic evaluation

Economic evaluation is a tool-kit of techniques which can be used to identify, measure and value, to differing extents, the costs (what society gives up) and the benefits (what society gains in terms of health) of competing health care interventions, one of which is the control of HAI.

In Fig. 14.1 inputs, processes and outcomes are identified separately. Inputs are made up of two types of cost: direct costs (DC) that arise from the provision of care by all public (e.g. hospital and general practioners) and private (carers and families) agencies; indirect costs (IC) are the consequences of the patient withdrawing from the labour force for treatment (production foregone and the costs of pain and suffering).

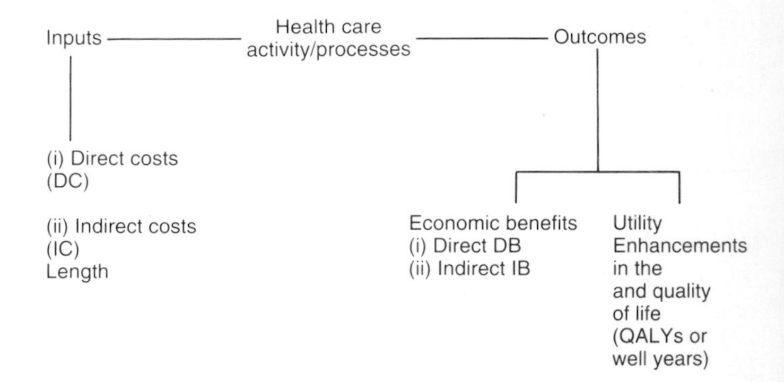

Fig. 14.1. Economic evaluation.

Inputs are combined to produce health care processes (e.g. bed days or consultations) which produce beneficial outcomes. These outcomes can be measured either in terms of economic benefits (the reverse of DC and IC, e.g. the hospital costs saved and the production gain acquired due to cure) or in terms of utility, enhancements in the length and quality of life (e.g. quality adjusted life years or QALYs).

The differing types of economic evaluation incorporate these elements to varying degrees: the characteristics of the alternative techniques are set out in Table 14.1. The simplest form of economic evaluation is cost minimization analysis. The purpose of this approach is to identify alternative means of achieving a given therapeutic end and costing the alternatives (i.e. identify, measure, and value both DC and IC in Fig. 14.1). In this type of analysis there is no attempt to measure outcomes which are *assumed* to be identical. Many of the economic evaluations carried out in the area of HAIs seek to identify the costs of control policies.

Table 14.1. Types of economic evaluation.

Type of economic evaluation	How are costs measured?	How are outcomes measured?
Cost minimization	£ (pounds)	Assumed equal
Cost-effectiveness	£ (pounds)	In different units e.g. life-years saved, infected days avoided
Cost-benefit	£ (pounds)	In money terms (£)
Cost-utility	£ (pounds)	In a single measure of the attributes of health (e.g. a QALY or well year)

A major defect of the cost minimization approach is that the benefits of the alternative control policies are not identical. Cost effectiveness analysis is used to identify the costs of the alternatives but couples this analysis with some measure of outcome. The objective of this approach is to identify the costs of alternative interventions in achieving some given outcome, e.g. the cost per infected day avoided, of alternative intervention such as using a prophylactic antibiotic and 'doing nothing' (i.e. usual practices).

This type of analysis is very useful in identifying which infection control intervention produces an infected day avoided at least cost. However, NHS and purchasers in other health care systems need to decide also whether to invest in infection control, or in hip replacements or any one of many thousand other interventions. The results of cost–effectiveness analysis do not give us data on these choices because the outcome measures are not comparable: what is the relative value of an infected day avoided as compared with an additional week of life following renal dialysis?

There are two ways of producing information which facilitates choices across specialties. Cost–benefit analysis is rarely carried out in health care because of the difficulties involved in identifying, measuring and valuing many of the indirect costs and benefits (IC and IB), e.g. pain and suffering arising from infections. However, this approach can be used partially. For instance, Shapiro and his colleagues built their analysis of the use of an antimicrobial prophylactic (cefazolin) for patients undergoing abdominal hysterectomy on the evaluation of direct and indirect costs and benefits (DC and DB) showing that the drug arm of the trial cost, on average over $100 less than the control arm which used a placebo, i.e. the increased drug costs (DC) reduced hospitalization costs (DB) (9).

An alternative to cost–benefit analysis is cost–utility analysis where a generic measure of health status, such as a QALY, is used to measure outcome. This approach involves costing the alternative treatments (e.g. drug and placebo) and identification of the cost of producing one year of good quality life (a QALY) by each route.

Which form of economic analysis should be used? It depends on the question being addressed by the evaluator. Increasingly the demands of purchasers and the contracting process in the NHS will require evaluators to determine which alternatives give the best return (i.e. the lowest cost of producing a QALY)? To answer this question cost utility analysis is needed. However, if the arguments for infection control policies are to be based on cost savings the simpler approaches (i.e. cost minimization and cost-effectiveness) may suffice.

Questions to be asked of economic evaluations

Whatever technique of economic evaluation is used there are a set of questions which must be asked of the design.

1. What is the question? Are the costs (and benefits) to be measured from the perspective of the hospital, the health care system, the patient, the carer, or society? Daschner pointed out that, in Germany, hospital managers were not interested in reducing the costs of HAIs because the insurers paid for additional bed days without questioning whether they were the minimum possible (10).

Economists prefer to evaluate the costs to society, but most studies in the field of HAIs examine only the hospital costs. This may be adequate if the study demonstrates that the intervention yields cost savings, inclusion of non-hospital, patient, and carer costs will usually enhance these savings. However, if the intervention generates increased costs it may still be beneficial if it also generates benefits to other, non-hospital agencies such as the patient and carers. Such an intervention can only be evaluated adequately in a cost–utility or more complete cost–benefit study.

2. What are the alternatives? An obvious option with which to compare an intervention to reduce infection is the 'do nothing' alternative. Weinstein *et al.* (11) and Shapiro *et al.* (9) compared alternative drug treatments. Platt *et al.* (12) and Persson *et al.* (13) compared drugs with changes in surgical technique or hygiene controls. Given that there are many ways in which infection control can be changed each component of the overall control 'package' needs to be evaluated separately. This is a costly approach and *ad hoc* rules to determine the allocation of scarce evaluative resources might include, as Daschner suggests (10), prioritization in relation to high cost infections, high cost patients, and high cost patient care.

3. What costs and benefits are included? A major issue in costing is that, typically, studies are restricted only to hospital costs. Infections may also create considerable post-hospital costs in primary care and in the family. Better control may reduce these costs and also improve the quality of life for patients. These latter costs also tend to be ignored. As a consequence 'best practice' in evaluation should include the identification of all relevant costs and benefits even if not all these costs and benefits are also measured and valued. This approach facilitates the identification of the interstices in a study and the evaluation of its strengths and weaknesses.

4. What study design should be used? Augmenting clinical trials with economic components has many advantages. However, there are large variations in hospital length of stay and other economic and quality of life measures and, as a consequence, the identification of statistical differences in the two arms of a trial may require large sample sizes. Furthermore some intervention, for instance changes in operating theatre ventilation, can only be evaluated using before and after studies.

5. Marginal analysis. Scarce health care resources should be allocated amongst competing treatments according to two rules:

Rule 1.
Should an investment be made? Investment should be made in an activity if the total benefits (TB) exceed its total costs (TC) i.e. if $TB > TC$ invest; if $TC > TB$ do not invest.

Rule 2.
How much should be invested in any activity? If Rule 1 leads to investment (i.e. $TB > TC$) it should continue until the cost of an additional unit of investment (the marginal cost, MC) is equal to the benefit obtained from that investment (the marginal benefit, MB). Thus if $MB > MC$, invest more until $MB = MC$; if $MC > MB$, invest less until $MC = MB$.
This rule means that the volume of investment in any activity is determined by identifying how much extra is gained by a small increase in the activity (MB) and how much extra is given up by that small increase in activity (MC).

This focus is particularly important in infection control. Relatively simple and cheap measures may reduce the infection rate, but beyond this further 'units' of control may be bought at an increasing cost. How far should this investment in infection control go? There is an efficient level of infection control (where MC = MB) and this will not be zero, i.e. it will be too expensive to get rid of all infections.

In identifying the margins (MB and MC) in any study it is important to distinguish between fixed and variable costs. If infection controls reduce the length of patient stay what is saved? If the bed and staff are merely unused the savings to the hospital to be derived from reducing the length of stay may be slight.

6. Sensitivity analysis. Any analysis is usually built on a series of assumptions. Small changes in these assumptions may or may not have significant effects on the results if any evaluative study. This must be tested for by sensitivity analysis.

Overview

There are different types of economic evaluation and a number of very useful studies have already been undertaken to determine the costs, and benefits, of competing infection control policies. As more clinical studies are undertaken the inclusion of economic components is increasing and this type of analysis is illuminating what types of controls are worthwhile and how much resource should be allocated to these beneficial but costly procedures.

Who cares whether infection control is efficient?

As a consequence of the reforms of the NHS in 1991 purchasers will seek the most cost-effective care with greater diligence and if they can identify providers with low infection rates and lower costs then contracts may be let to them. These 'market pressures' will make it increasingly prudent for clinicians to establish infection control guidelines based on the findings of evaluation. Such guide-lines will assist managers, whether they are in the public or private sectors, as they strive to fund appropriate infection control programmes and rationalize hospital bed provision in a world of scarce resources.

References

1. Currie, E. and Maynard, A. (1989). *The economics of hospital acquired infections*. Discussion Paper 56. Centre for Health Economics, University of York.
2. Meers, P.D., Ayliffe, G.A.J., Emmerson, A.M. *et al.* (1981). Report on the survey of infection in hospitals. 1980. *J. Hosp. Infect.*, **2**, Suppl, 1–51.
3. Haley, R.W., Culver, D.H., White J.W. *et al.* (1985). The nationwide nosocomial infection rate: a new need for vital statistics. *Am. J. Epidemiol.*, **121**, 159–67.
4. Haley, R.W. (1978). Preliminary cost benefit analysis of hospital infection control programmes (the SENIC project). In *Proven and unproven methods in hospital infection control* (ed. F. Daschner). Germany.
5. Larson, E., and Oram, L.F. (1988). Nosocomial infection rates as an indicator of quality, *Med. Care*, **26**, 676–84.
6. Haley, R.W. (1986). *Managing hospital infection control for cost effectiveness: a strategy for reducing infectious complications*, American Hospital Association, Chicago.
7. Department of Health and Social Security. (1988). *Hospital infection control: guidance on the control of infections in hospital.* DHSS, London.
8. Davis, T.W. and Cottingham, J. (1979). The cost of hospital infection in orthopaedic patients, *J. Infect.*, **1**, 329–38.
9. Shapiro, M., Schoenbaum, C., Therib, I.B. *et al.* (1988). Cost benefit analysis of antimicrobial prophylaxis in abdominal and vaginal hysterectomy. *J. Am. Med. Assoc.*, **249**, 1290–2.
11. Daschner, F. (1989). Cost effectiveness in hospital infection control: lessons for the 1990s, *J. Hosp. Infect.*, **13**, 325–6.
12. Weinstein, M.C., Read, J.L., and Mackay, D.N. (1986). Cost effective choice of antimicrobial therapy for serious infections. *J. Gen. Int. Med.*, **1**, 352–63.
13. Platt, R., Polk, B.E., Murdock, B., and Rosner, B. (1989). Prevention of catheter-associated urinary tract infection: a cost benefit analysis. *Infect. Control. Hosp. Epidemiol.*, **10**, 60–4.
14. Persson, U., Montgomery, F., Carlsson, A., Linderen, B., and Ahnfelt, L. (1988). How far does prophylaxis against infection in total joint replacement offset its cost, *Br. Med. J.*, **296**, 99–102.

15

Infection in the accident and emergency department

GRAHAM PAGE and THOMAS BEATTIE

Definition of superficial infection

This can be defined as infection involving the skin and subcutaneous tissues. It can occur at four levels: *Subcuticular* between the epidermis and dermis; *Intracutaneous* at the level of the dermis; *subcutaneous*; *collar stud*, subcuticular communicating with subcutaneous.

Aetiology

Bacteriology

The predominant organism encountered in superficial infection seen in the Accident and Emergency Department is *Staphylococcus aureus*. This is now almost invariably penicillin resistant. *Streptococcus pyogenes* is seen less commonly, but is still very sensitive to penicillin. Ano-rectal, pilonidal, and finger nail infections usually yield a mixed flora of *Escherichia coli, Proteus* spp., *Pseudomonas aeruginosa, Strep. faecalis*, and anaerobic organisms.

Defence impairment

Many factors influence the ability of the body to resist infection (see Chapter 4). Most are not relevant to the Accident and Emergency Department, but diabetes mellitus commonly predisposes to superficial infection and should always be excluded. Immune system dysfunction caused by the human immunodeficiency virus (HIV) should increasingly be considered.

Pathology and clinical signs

Diffuse inflammation presents as cellulitis without suppuration and is the earliest sign of superficial infection. If an appropriate antibiotic is administered at this stage complete resolution may be achieved. Pus formation is usually heralded by a persistant point of tenderness despite 24 to 48 h antibiotic therapy. The pyogenic membrane round an abscess cavity limits the spread of infection, but it also prevents antibiotic from reaching the area. The classical teaching of waiting for fluctuation before drainage is performed is unnecessary, since fluctuation does not occur until extensive soft tissue necrosis has occurred.

Complications

Spread to deeper structures

Infection may spread to deep structures by *lymphatic* spread giving rise to lymphangitis and lymphadenitis or by *blood-borne* spread giving bacteraemia or septicaemia. This may lead to metastatic infection in deeper organs, of which the most serious example is infection of the nose and face which can lead to cavernous sinus thrombosis (see Chapter 26). Alternately there may be *direct* spread after trauma to the infected lesion.

General principles of treatment

Antibiotics

There is still a widespread belief that antibiotics will resolve pus formation and to blame them as ineffective if this does not occur. If administered at the cellulitic stage, complete resolution is possible, but not once pus has formed. At this stage incision, drainage, and removal of the pyogenic membrane are also necessary. Once an abscess is present, an antibiotic will limit the spread of surrounding cellulitis and help localization. Once the pyogenic membrane has been removed the antibiotic can enter the abscess cavity and help to clear residual infection. Topical antibiotics have no useful role in superficial infections.

The antibiotics usually administered for infection caused by *Staph. aureus* are flucloxacillin 500 mg four times a day or erythromycin 500 mg twice daily. If *Strep. pyogenes* is suspected phenoxymethyl penicillin 500 mg four times a day is administered. Perineal infections, or situations where mixed organisms are likely to be present are usually treated with co-amoxyclav 500 mg three times a day. Metronidazole 400 mg three times a day is added if anaerobic organisms are thought to be present. If the patient cannot be relied upon to take oral medication, or if the infection is widespread, admission to hospital and intravenous antibiotic therapy are indicated.

It is not always possible to predict the antibiotic sensitivity of the infecting organism, and virtually never appropriate to wait for the results of bacteriological culture. Careful assessment should be made after 24 h of antibiotic administration. Significant regression of the cellulitis means that the antibiotic is working satisfactorily, even if there is a persistant point of tenderness.

Incision and drainage

It is important to be sure of the exact site of pus formation before draining an abscess. This is manifest by a point of persistant tenderness following administration of an appropriate antibiotic. If the pus has not localized, antibiotic administration and immobilization of the affected part should continue until a point of persistent tenderness is well defined. The purpose of incising an abscess is to remove pus and necrotic material, to decompress the area and to establish drainage. Incisions are made at the point of maximum tenderness along Langer's skin crease lines. Once pus is encountered, a swab is taken for bacteriological culture and antibiotic sensitivity. The incision is then enlarged to expose the whole abscess cavity and the pus removed with gauze on sinus forceps. The pyogenic membrane surrounding the abscess cavity is removed with gauze or, if necessary, sharp dissection. Antibiotics should be continued for 72 h after drainage to sterilize the cavity.

Primary closure

Primary suture of an abscess cavity has been advocated once the pyogenic membrane has been removed and where there is sufficient laxity of the surrounding tissues. The dead space is obliterated by using sutures of monofilament nylon or polypropylene. There is no doubt that in expert hands this can give very good results and greatly hasten healing, but it's unsupervised use by inexperienced surgeons is questionable.

Drains

Drainage is usually achieved by converting a linear incision into an ellipse. Tulle gras may be laid between the wound edges to prevent apposition. Drains are seldom required and frequently do not work.

Anaesthesia

Insufficient thought is frequently given to anaesthesia. Removal of the pyogenic membrane is necessary to ensure rapid healing. The use of ethyl chloride spray to permit quick incision and decompression of an abscess is mentioned only to be condemned. Most abscess cavities require drainage under general anaesthesia in order to break down the pyogenic membrane adequately. The use of local anaesthetic infiltration in cellulitic tissue is dangerous because the hyperaemia leads to fast entry into the circulation. In addition satellite abscess formation frequently results. However, digital anaesthesia block can, be used provided there is no cellulitis proximal to the proximal interphalangeal joint. Plain lignocaine without adrenalin is used, since adrenalin can give severe vasospasm and lead to gangrene of the digit. Subcuticular abscess drainage requires no anaethesia and can be dealt with using a sharp pair of scissors.

Use of tourniquets

A tourniquet can make the task of incision and drainage of abscess cavities in superficial tissues easier and safer especially where important anatomical structures must be avoided, e.g. in the hand. A pneumatic tourniquet is used with the usual strict precautions. Fingers and toes can be dealt with using fine rubber tubing applied tightly round the base of the digit and fastened with artery forceps. It is, of course, essential to ensure that the touriquet is removed on completion of the operation.

Resting the inflamed area

Immobilization is frequently forgotten, but has several advantages. It assists localization of pus, may prevent haematogenous spread, and helps to reduce discomfort. Limbs should be elevated to reduce swelling. A sling is the usual method of immobilizing the upper limb. Hands are best splinted in the position of function using a volar splint of Plaster of Paris.

Dressings

The saucerized abscess cavity can be packed lightly with gauze containing sodium hypochlorite solution for the first 24 h only. Thereafter dry gauze is placed directly over an abscess cavity. A generous layer of cotton wool followed by a crepe bandage is applied. Initially the dressing is changed daily. Depending on the size of the cavity and the amount of soakage, the interval can be gradually increased as healing occurs.

Specific superficial infections

Boil (furuncle) and carbunculosis

A boil is caused by staphylococcal infection of a hair follicle or sebaceous gland in any hirsute part of the body. Cellulitis of the hair follicle produces a localized area of inflammation. Resolution may occur at this stage ('blind boil'), or progress to suppuration and tissue necrosis forming the core of the boil, which eventually becomes conical in shape. After a few days, the skin commonly gives way and the boil discharges. If extensive abscess formation takes place the condition is known as carbunculosis. There is usually subcuticular pus formation with honeycombing of the subcutaneous tissue. This can be complicated by sloughing of large areas of skin and subcutaneous tissue. Flucloxacillin or erythromycin if prescribed early enough may prevent boil formation and in the established situation diminish the surrounding cellulitis and prevent infection of the neighbouring hair follicles ('cropping'). Boils seldom require incision, and carbuncles usually require only sharp scissor removal of the subcuticular abscess component, without anaesthesia.

Infected sebaceous cyst or inclusion dermoid (Fig. 15.1)

There is usually a history of a pre-existing swelling in the area which becomes increasingly painful and inflamed. Treatment follows the general principles already outlined and particular efforts are required to remove the wall of the cyst to prevent recurrence. This frequently requires sharp dissection.

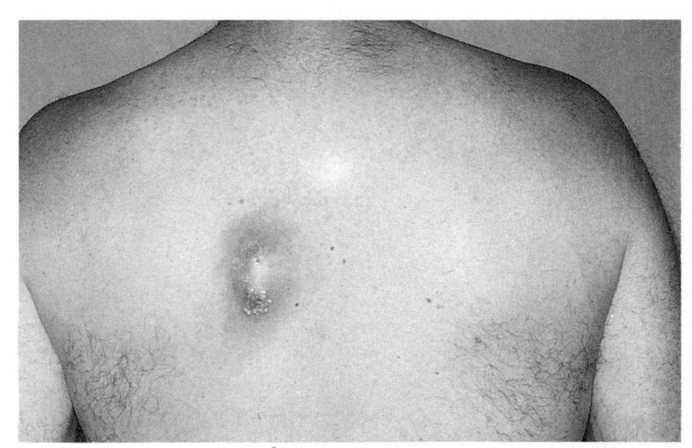

Fig. 15.1. An infected sebaceous cyst of back. (See plate section.)

Bursitis (olecranon, pre- and infra-patellar) (Fig. 15.2)

Adventitial bursae overlie the elbow, and the pre- and infrapatellar areas of the knee. These can become chronically irritated giving a serous effusion or traumatized giving a haemorrhagic effusion. Infection can supervene giving a purulent effusion. Treatment follows the general principles and frequently excision of the bursal sac is necessary to prevent the wound discharging chronically.

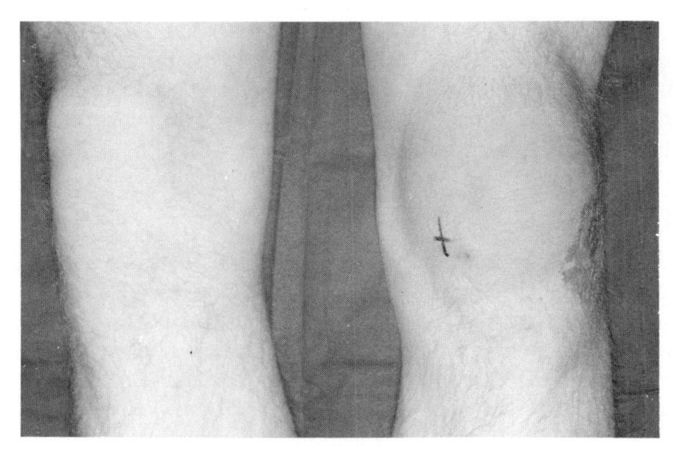

Fig. 15.2. An infected pre-patellar bursa. (See plate section.)

Axillary abscess (Fig. 15.3)

Axillary abscess is usually due to infection of the hair follicles or the apocrine glands. People who regularly shave the axilla or who have excessive sweating from the axillary glands (hydradenitis) are particularly liable. Recurrent infection is not uncommon. Ocassionally, large areas of 'acne conglobulata' form giving a honeycomb abscess formation. Rarely the abscess is caused by lymphadenitis secondary to infection in the upper limb. Cutaneous or pulmonary tuberculosis should not be forgotten and, if necessary, a chest radiograph taken. Treatment follows general principles, usually requiring incision under general anaesthesia with the patient's hand placed under his head. Care is taken to avoid the neurovascular structures in the area. If tuberculosis or lymphadenitis is present, tissue should be sent for histological examination, as well as pus for microbiological culture.

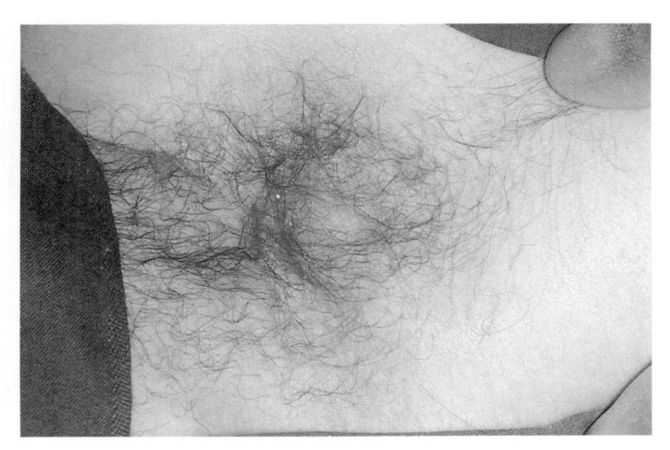

Fig. 15.3. Axillary abscess. (See plate section.)

Pilonidal abscess (Fig. 15.4)

A pilonidal sinus may occur on almost any part of the body, but it is most common in the midline of the natal cleft at about the level of the coccyx. Pilonidal sinus usually affects obese hairy males who drive lorries or jeeps hence the term 'jeep bottom'. It is caused by loose hairs in the natal cleft penetrating the skin in the midline and forming a cavity lined by stratified squamous epithelium. Infection is usually with mixed organisms and treatment with co-amoxyclav in the early cellulitic stage may be effective, but to eradicate the problem, the sinus should be laid open and the hair removed.

Ano-rectal abscess

There are four main types of ano-rectal abscess: perianal; ischiorectal; submucous/intermuscular; pelvirectal.

Only the first two are commonly seen in the Accident and Emergency department. Inflammatory bowel disease (IBD) in the form of ulcerative colitis and Crohn's disease predisposes to these abscesses and a history of IBD should be actively sought in all presentations of ano-rectal infection. If there is such a history, the patient should be referred to a general or colorectal surgeon. The causative organisms are usually mixed enterobacteria. Ano-rectal abscess formation should be dealt with energetically since, if neglected, sinus formation or fistulation into the anal canal can occur. A fistula-in-ano is a cause of recurrent perianal infection.

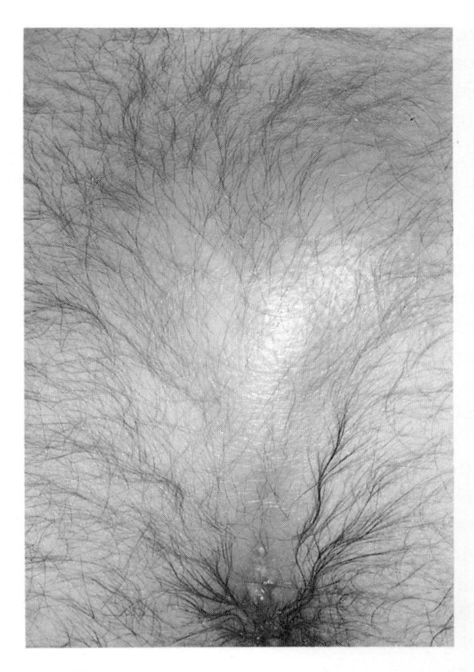

Fig. 15.4. Pilonidal abscess of natal cleft. (See plate section.)

Perianal abscess is usually the result of infection in a hair follicle or it may arise in a thrombosed perianal haematoma. It is superficial to the external sphincter. It usually presents as an established abscess with a cherry-sized, round, cystic lump at the anal verge inferior to the pectinate line. Rectal examination is normal and, if gently performed painless.

Ischiorectal abscess lies in the ischiorectal fossa and usually arises from an infected deep anal gland which spreads laterally. The fat which fills the space has a poor blood supply and readily becomes infected. Rarely the infection is blood- or lymph-borne. It usually presents as a brawny, indurated, tender area in the ischiorectal fossa. Systemic upset with pyrexia is common. Rectal examination shows a swelling on one side and is very painful.

These abscesses should be treated under general anaesthesia with the patient in the lithotomy position, and the bowel emptied pre-operatively, if necessary with an enema. Rectal examination may reveal a nodule which represents the possible internal opening of a fistula. The lower bowel is inspected with a sigmoidoscope looking for evidence of inflammatory bowel disease. The abscess is drained in the normal manner and an overlying ellipse of skin removed. A biopsy of the wall is sent for histological examination. The dressing is held in place using a T bandage. Post-operatively particular attention is paid to prevent constipation. The patient has a bath after each bowel movement.

Ingrowing toenail (Fig. 15.5)

The nail of the great toe is most commonly affected, and the problem is most frequently seen in teenagers. Infection is caused by lack of hygiene, wearing unsuitable, tight footwear and by incorrect nail cutting. To prevent ingrowing, the nail should be cut straight across so that the edges project beyond the skin fold. Typically the affected side is tender on palpation and chronic pyogenic granulation tissue is present. A variety of treatments have been proposed, but it is worth trying simple removal of the nail initially since the condition is frequently self-limiting. The nail is removed under local or general anaesthesia by inserting a sturdy pair of artery forceps under one side of the nail and removing it with a twisting action. The granulation tissue at the site of ingrowth is removed using a curette. The raw area is dressed with tulle gras. Chiropody is useful as the nail regrows in an attempt to prevent further ingrowing. However, if the nail again ingrows lateral wedge excision of the nail and nail bed, or full ablation of the nail bed can be achieved using phenol, or by surgical excision (Zadik's operation). Antibiotic therapy is rarely necessary.

Hand infections

Hand infections are common presentations because the hands are very exposed to trauma. The thick skin of the palm and the ventral aspect of the fingers masks the presence of infection and pus formation, and also prevents pus from escaping. Immobilisation of infected hands in the position of function using a volar slab of Plaster of Paris and elevation of the limb are important in the successful treatment of all hand infections. Physiotherapy helps to regain function and to ensure an early return to employment.

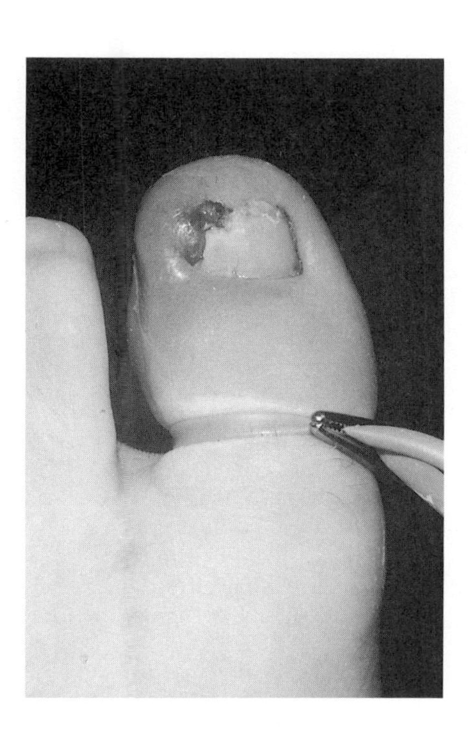

Fig. 15.5. Infected ingrowing toenail. (See plate section.)

Paronychia (Fig. 15.6)

A paronychia is a subcuticular or intracutaneous infection of the nail fold by mixed organisms. It may be in either the superficial or deep aspect (or both) of the nail-fold and may spread under the nail. It seldom spreads into the subcutaneous tissue. Although it is a subcuticular infection, anaesthesia is usually required to drain the infection. A digital anaesthetic block and a fine rubber tourniquet round the base of the digit is usually used. The nail fold is separated from the nail and the abscess drained in the usual way. If there is pus under the nail, the nail should be removed as well.

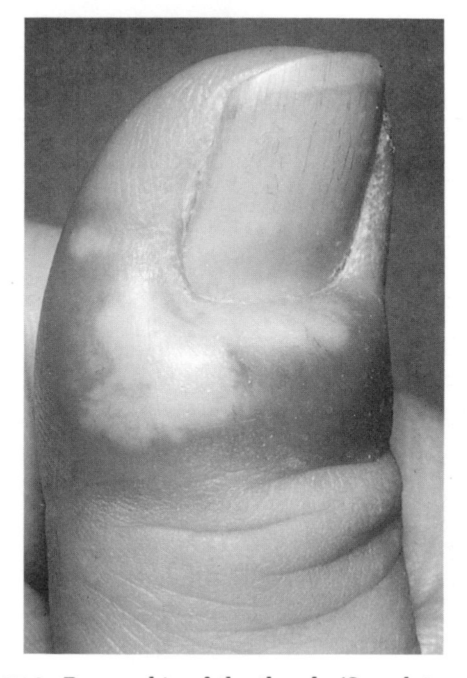

Fig. 15.6. Paronychia of the thumb. (See plate section.)

Pyogenic granuloma (Fig. 15.7)

A pyogenic granuloma is a chronic staphylococcal infection of the nail-fold. It has the appearance of a chronic, granulomatous, red, soft, warty lesion which bleeds easily. It is removed using a digital anaesthetic block and a fine rubber tourniquet and the lesion should be sent for histological examination. The base of the lesion should be thoroughly curetted.

Pulp abscess (Fig. 15.8)

There are dense fibrous bands attaching the skin of the pulp of the finger to the periosteum. These, in combination with the presence of thick skin, allow no space for the presence of pus—hence pyogenic infections of this area are exceedingly painful. The proximity of the terminal phalanx make osteomyelitis a possible complication. Initial cellulitis presents as a bright red colour which changes to a dusky shade as localization takes place. Usually, pus formation cannot be seen, but is manifest by a point of persistent tenderness. Incision at this point is indicated, and is usually carried out under a digital anaesthetic block with a fine rubber tourniquet clipped round the base of the finger. A transverse or slightly oblique incision

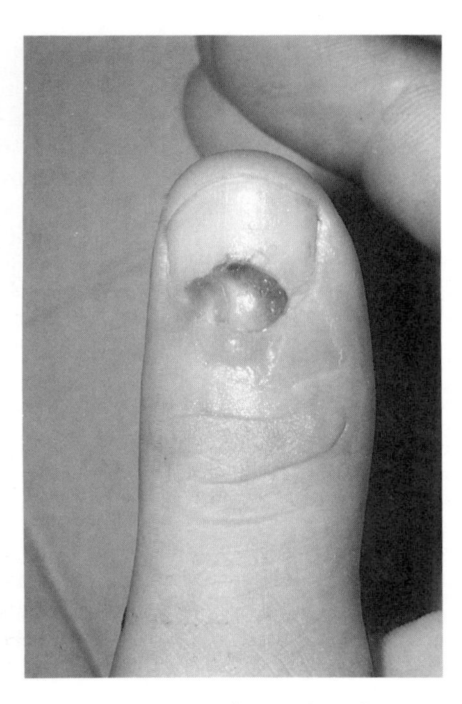

Fig. 15.7. Pyogenic granuloma. (See plate section.)

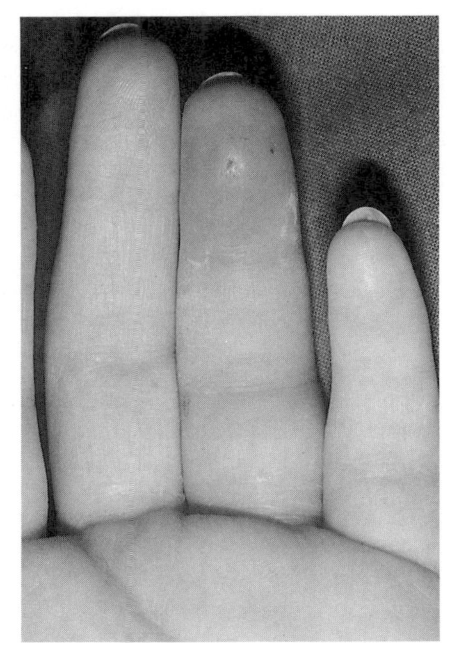

Fig. 15.8. Pulp abscess of ring finger. (See plate section.)

is used. The cavity is drained and the wall saucerized in the normal way. A pair of dissecting forceps is used to feel the underlying bone of the terminal phalanx. Any roughness indicates early osteomyelitis and, if present, a three week course of antibiotic therapy is given.

Herpetic pulp infection

Pulp infection may be caused by the herpes simplex virus and it is important to differentiate this infection from a pyogenic pulp abscess. The condition never requires incision and should be treated with antiviral agents; acyclovir tablets 200 mg five times daily, combined with topical application of acyclovir cream. Diagnosis can be confirmed by aspiration of a vesicle and electron microscopy of the aspirate which will confirm the presence of the virus.

Apical abscess

Apical abscess occurs at the tip of the finger, under the free edge of the nail. It shares the propensity of a pulp abscess to spread to the terminal phalanx.

Web space abscess

Web space abscess occurs on both the ventral and dorsal aspect of a web between the fingers. It commonly arises from a infected cut or callosity at the base of a finger. Pus may track around the sides of the fingers and force them apart with much swelling. More than one web space may be involved. Treatment under general anaesthesia and a pneumatic tourniquet, is by a transverse incision. Care should be taken to safeguard the digital nerves on the ventral aspect.

Erisipeloid of Rosenbach (Fig. 15.9)

Erysipelothrix rhusiopathiae is prevalent wherever fish, poultry, pigs, or game are processed. Erysipeloid is commonly known as 'fish poisoning' or 'fish hand'. The hands of these workers are constantly receiving minor trauma from fish fins, teeth, knives, machines, and fish boxes. This breaches the skin and allows the organism to enter.

Usually the patient cannot recall a specific injury to the hand. The skin lesion starts with a sensation of heat and subsequently becomes itchy, tight, and painful. The pain is described as being prickly. The lesion is initially pink, changing

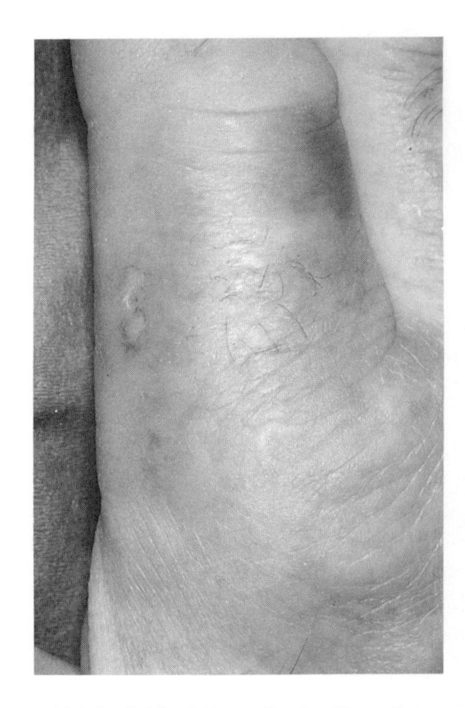

Fig. 15.9. Erisipeloid of Rosenbach. (See plate section.)

to red and later assumes a violaceous colour. Slight pain and stiffness in adjacent joints is common. There is a notable absence of pus formation although, occasionally, erysipeloid becomes secondarily infected. Erysipeloid is usually self-limiting. It spreads for a few days, the advancing edge being slightly raised, whilst the centre fades and slight desquamation occurs. Incision and drainage is virtually never required. A useful local dressing is ten per cent ichthammol in glycerine. Pyogenic infection is treated with erythromycin.

Orf (Fig. 15.10)

Orf is a viral infection transmitted from sheep and found in shepherds and those who handle these animals. The lesion consists of a purplish, red raised area containing flecks of yellow and is often given the popular name of 'Strawberry'. It usually resolves by spontaneous regression after about a week. Antibiotics are not necessary. The lesion should be washed with a weak antiseptic twice a day to prevent secondary infection. Surgical interference is contraindicated.

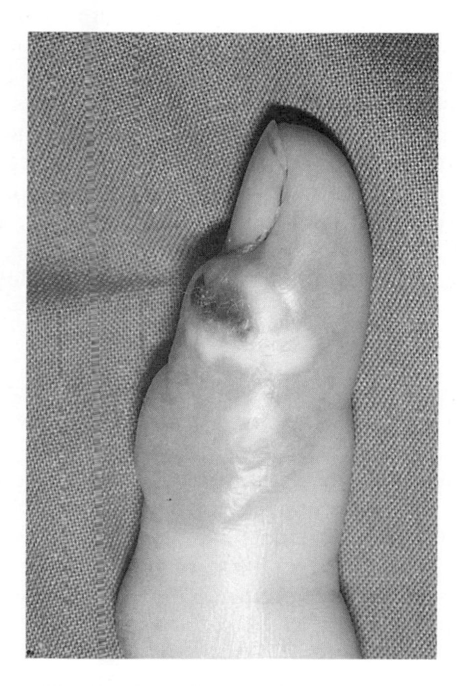

Fig. 15.10. Orf. (See plate section.)

Suppurative tenosynovitis

Suppurative tenosynovitis is now much less common than it used to be. It is important to remember the anatomy of the long flexor tendon sheaths to the fingers. The flexor tendons are enclosed in synovial sheaths where they pass deep to the flexor retinaculum, and also in the fibrous flexor sheaths. In the carpal tunnel, the tendons of flexor digitorum superficialis and profundus are enclosed in a common sheath beside the sheath containing the tendon of flexor pollicus longus. These two sheaths may communicate and both extend 2–3 cm proximally into the forearm, posterior to the tendons. Distally they extend to the terminal phalanx only in the thumb and little finger. The remainder of the common sheath is interrupted in the palm. Separate synovial sheaths reappear in the fibrous flexor sheaths of the middle three fingers. The continuity of the common synovial sheath with that in the little finger and the thumb allows infection to spread rapidly from these digits to the carpal tunnel.

Suppurative tenosynovitis is caused by a penetrating wound breaching the sheath. It does not result from overlying soft tissue infection unless there is inoculation of the sheath at the same time as the soft tissue. Injudicious drainage of a subcutaneous abscess may also lead to penetration of the sheath. There are two main forms: generalized—caused by *Strep. pyogenes* and localized (segmental) caused by *Staph. aureus.*

If a tendon sheath becomes inflamed, it distends with fluid. In the thumb and little finger, distension can extend to 2–3 cm proximal to the flexor retinaculum. With the other fingers the distension can only extend as far as the metacarpal heads. If the tendon sheath infection is not vigorously treated, ischaemia may cause necrosis and, eventually, the tendon snaps.

Symptoms are severe pain over the segment of tendon sheath involved. There may be systemic upset in the generalized form. Frequently there is little or no swelling, or erythema of the overlying skin. The affected finger is held flexed and there is tenderness over the part of the sheath involved. Active movement is grossly diminished and painful, and passive extension is resisted.

Treatment is with flucloxacillin and penicillin combined with rigid immobilization—usually bed rest with the arm elevated and the hand splinted in the position of function by a volar Plaster of Paris slab. If there is not rapid resolution of the symptoms and signs, the sheath is surgically explored under general anaesthesia using a pneumatic tourniquet. The sheath is exposed, taking care to avoid damage to the neurovascular bundles, opened longitudinally and any fluid expressed. A swab is taken for bacteriological culture and sensitivity. The sheath is irrigated using a mixture of saline with penicillin and flucloxacillin. In the generalized form, both the proximal and distal ends may require to be opened in order to irrigate the whole sheath effectively. Subsequently the skin is loosely closed, leaving the sheath opened. Antibiotics, rest, and elevation are continued until the infection subsides. Active exercises, supervised by a physiotherapist, are thereafter started as soon as possible.

Septic arthritis of finger joints

Septic arthritis is associated with extreme pain in the joint, particularly if it is moved passively. Crepitus may be felt and there may be a discharging sinus. Radiological examination shows rarefaction of the bone around the joint only in advanced cases.

Distal interphalangeal (DIP) joint

Septic arthritis of the DIP joint is usually due to penetrating injury. Osteoarthritis in the elderly appears to predispose to infection when not caused by injury. The organism can be determined by aspiration of the joint. Treatment is usually with three weeks antibiotic therapy. If arthrodesis appears to be inevitable, the joint is splinted in 10 degrees of flexion. Amputation of the terminal phalanx may be the best treatment in the elderly.

Proximal interphalangeal (PIP) joint

Infection of the PIP joint is frequently associated with cat bites. The cat's mouth harbours the organism *Pasturella multocida*. They have long, thin teeth which readily penetrate tendon sheaths and joint capsules, particularly the PIP joint. The antibiotic of choice is tetracycline or Septrin. Surgical drainage is frequently necessary.

Metacarpal phalangeal (MCP) joint

There are a large number of organisms in the healthy human mouth including anaerobic bacteria. Although normally commensals within the mouth, many of these organisms are virulent pathogens if inoculated into skin, subcutaneous tissue, tendon sheaths, or joints. A common injury seen in the Accident and Emergency Department is a septic arthritis of the MCP joint. This occurs as a result of a fist fight, in which the knuckle makes contact with the upper incisor teeth causing a penetrating injury of the joint. (Fig. 15.11). Frequently the diagnosis is missed because the patient does not admit to being in a fight. Radiological examination may show fragments of tooth within the joint.

The usual antibiotics are penicillin and co-amoxyclav, to which metronidazole may be added if required. Surgical exploration and irrigation of the joint is frequently necessary. Post-operative elevation in the position of function and mobilization carefully supervised by a physiotherapist is important.

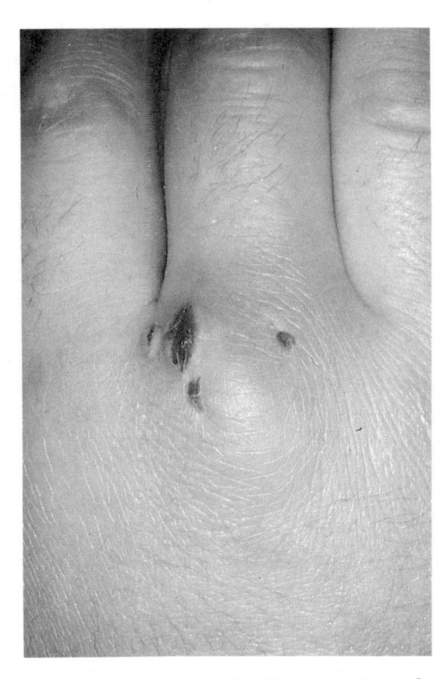

Fig. 15.11. Teeth marks over MCP joint. (See plate section.)

Palmar and complex palmar abscess

A palmar abscess lies subcutaneously, superficial to the palmar aponeurosis, whereas a complex palmar abscess extends deep to it. The flexor tendon sheaths are seldom involved unless inoculated at the same time. Treatment follows general principles. A tourniquet is necessary if drainage is indicated in order to avoid damage to the tendon sheaths, nerves and vessels in the area.

Mid palmar and thenar space abscess

The palmar aponeurosis sends a septum posteriorly which becomes continuous with the fascia covering the palmar surface of the adductor pollicus and the two medial interosseus spaces. Posterior to the flexor tendons and their enclosing sheath is the mid palmar space. The thenar space is the compartment containing adductor pollicus and is lateral to the mid-palmar space. Infection of these spaces is very rarely seen since the advent of antibiotics. It is usually due to puncture wounds affecting the tendon sheaths which become infected and, if neglected, this spreads to the spaces.

Dog bites

Dog bites produce puncture wounds or stretch lacerations. Treatment is by normal principles of wound care with tetanus prophylaxis. The possibility of rabies should also be considered. Although the disease does not yet exist in animals in the UK, it is prevalent abroad. It affects other carnivorous animals as well as dogs. The mode of infection is usually a bite, but a lick on an area of broken skin can transmit the virus. Any contact with a suspected rabid animal in an area where the disease is prevalent should be taken very seriously. This is particularly important in people who travel by air. Treatment, if suspected, is urgent and consists of a course of human diploid cell vaccine and human rabies immunoglobulin.

Snake bites

The only common snake-bite in the UK is from the adder (*Vipera berus*). In most cases venom is not injected. If venom has been injected, local swelling begins within 30 min and spreads proximally over the next 24 h. Systemic poisoning, manifested by persistent hypotension, abnormal bleeding, and electrocardiographic abnormalities, is exceedingly rare. Antivenom is used only if there is systemic poisoning. Local limb swelling is treated symptomatically by elevation. Infection virtually never occurs.

Seal bites

Seal bites may be contaminated a variety of organisms including anaerobic bacteria. Treatment consists of thorough cleaning and antibiotic therapy with a combination of erythromycin and metronidazole.

Tetanus

Aetiology

Tetanus is caused by a Gram-positive bacillus—*Clostridium tetani*. It is found mainly in soil and decaying material, and is also present in the gut of man and animals in an inactive spore-bearing form. The spores can survive for long periods in dust. It is most prevalent in soil that has been manured with farm animal, particularly horse, dung. Approximately 50 per cent of the soil in the UK is contaminated with the organism and the disease is due to exotoxin production from the active form. Anaerobic conditions are necessary for the production of the active form. Deep puncture wounds with necrotic muscle produce the ideal culture medium for the active form.

Epidemiology

Farmers, gardeners, sewage workers, slaughterhouse workers, and butchers are particularly liable to have wounds contaminated with tetanus spores. Operations on the lower colon, and road traffic accidents similarly, have a risk of introducing the spores into wounds.

Pathology

Truly anaerobic conditions are necessary to convert the tetanus spore-bearing form into the active exotoxin-producing form. Many wounds are contaminated with spores, but few develop the disease. Anaerobic conditions are produced by necrotic muscle, coincidental infection with pyogenic organisms, clothing, and the presence of soil containing calcium salts and silicate in the wound. The exotoxin itself produces anaerobic conditions, perpetuating continued production. The active tetanus bacilli do not disseminate into the body, but the exotoxin is believed to travel to the motor end-plate of muscle, and thereafter it passes between nerve fibres to the anterior horn cells of the spinal cord. These cells are irritated, leading to tonic muscle spasms.

Prevention of tetanus

There are four lines of attack: wound debridement; active immunization; passive immunization; antibiotic therapy.

Wound debridement

This is probably the most important defence against tetanus. The wound is thoroughly and energetically debrided paying strict attention to surgical principles. Any muscle which does not readily contract when pinched with dissecting forceps, or bleed when cut, should be excised.

Active immunity

Active immunity must be developed before a wound is sustained if it is to be effective. Active immunization is achieved using tetanus toxoid (tetanus toxin plus formalin which is adsorbed on to aluminium hydroxide) 0.5 ml given by intramuscular or deep subcutaneous injection.

Infants in the UK are offered a primary course of three injections (usually combined with diphtheria and pertussis vaccine) starting at the age of two months with an interval of one month between each dose. Reinforcing doses are given prior to school entry at about 5 years and again when leaving school at 15 years. Thereafter reinforcing doses at 10-yearly intervals are sufficient to maintain protection.

Children over ten years and adults who have not been previously immunized should receive a primary course of three injections of tetanus toxoid, given with intervals of one month between each dose. Reinforcing doses at 10-yearly intervals are sufficient to give lifelong protection.

It is believed that a booster or reinforcing dose of tetanus toxoid given at any time after a properly administered primary course will rapidly produce a high level of immunity. Occasionally, local reactions occur consisting of swelling at the site of injection. However, systemic reactions, are rare but may result from excessive and irrational administration of toxoid. Routine tetanus immunization has been offered since 1961, and patients should be given a record of their tetanus immunizations.

After a full primary course, those who sustain wounds require tetanus toxoid only if the last injection was more than ten years previously. Patients with tetanus prone wounds are given human tetanus immunoglobulin in addition.

Passive immunity

If active immunity is not developed at the time of sustaining a wound, the use of tetanus toxoid does not protect the patient from tetanus. In these patients passive immunity should be conferred, using 250 units of human tetanus immunoglobulin (Humotet). This is prepared by refining the plasma of actively immunized humans. Passive immunity lasts about six weeks. A course of active immunization should be started at the time of administration of the immunoglobulin. It cannot be mixed in the same syringe and should be injected at a different site. Patients with an impaired immune response (HIV positive or those on immunosuppressive therapy) may not respond to toxoid and the criteria for administration of human tetanus immunoglobulin should be modified bearing this in mind.

Antibiotics

Antibiotics destroy the active form of *Cl tetani*. The main drugs used are penicillin, erythromycin, and tetracycline; a five day course should be given. If the patient is deemed unreliable about taking oral antibiotics, intramuscular administration should be considered.

Prognosis

The severity of tetanus is related to the incubation period. Mortality is 80 per cent if the incubation period is less than 10 days, falling to 10 per cent if the incubation period is more than 21 days.

Treatment of tetanus

The tonic muscle spasms are controlled by paralysing the patient and instituting mechanical assisted ventilation. It may be several weeks before the exotoxin is eliminated. Prolonged mechanical ventilation is necessary and the patient requires to be in an intensive therapy unit. Human tetanus immunoglobulin and large doses of penicillin are administered.

Further reading

1. *British National Formulary*. British Medical Association.
2. Duerden, B.I., Reid, T.M.S., Jewsbury, J.M., and Turk D.C.

(1988). *A new short textbook of microbial and parasitic infection*. Edward Arnold, London.

3. Forrest, A. P. M., Carter, D. C., and Macleod, I. B. (1990). *Principles and practice of surgery* (2nd edn). Churchill Livingstone, Edinburgh.
4. Laurence, D. R. and Bennett, P. N. (1987). *Clinical pharmacology* (6th edn). Churchill Livingstone, Edinburgh.
5. Mills, K., Morton R., and Page G. (1984). *A colour atlas of accidents and emergencies*, pp. 48–68.

16

Trauma

SEAN P.F. HUGHES

Introduction

Injuries to bone and soft tissues are an increasing problem, due mainly to the rise in road traffic accidents, affecting particularly those between the ages of 18 and 40 years. Also there appears to be an increase in the incidence of fractures of the neck of the femur in the elderly population. Fractures in general can be considered in these categories: those involving long bones, those involving joints, and those involving flat bones.

Fractures involving long bones

The principles of treatment of fractures that involve a long bone, for example either the femoral shaft or a metacarpal bone, are to enable union to occur, to prevent non-union and to discourage malunion.

Fractures involving joints

When fractures involve joints, particularly a weight-bearing joint such as the upper tibial surface of the knee joint, the cartilaginous surface may be disrupted. It is apparent that hyaline cartilage cannot repair itself when damaged, but reforms as fibrocartilage. If this occurs in a weight bearing joint the fibroartilage undergoes degeneration under load and results in osteoarthritis (1). Hence the aim of treatment is to reduce to the minimum the area of fibrocartilaginous formation.

Fractures involving flat bones

When the skull or the pelvis is involved in a fracture, the prime concern may be the loss of blood, which occurs in association with these fractures, along with the management of the injuries to related structures, such as the brain in skull fractures, or the bladder in pelvic fractures.

Principles of treatment

The principles of treatment of a fracture are: reduction, immobilization, and rehabilitation.

A fracture needs to be reduced accurately so that the bone can reform. The haematoma which forms at the fracture site is followed by an inflammatory response, which in turn is associated with cartilage formation, bone formation, and remodelling (2). Further work has shown that there is also an early vascular response to the fracture whereby capillary recruitment and increased bone blood flow occurs (3, 4). This vascular response brings the solutes and factors that are necesary for the fracture healing process. These include oxygen and the solutes calcium and phosphate together with growth factor, bone morphogenic protein (5), and others yet to be identified. In addition it is also now apparent that an osteoprogenitor cell,

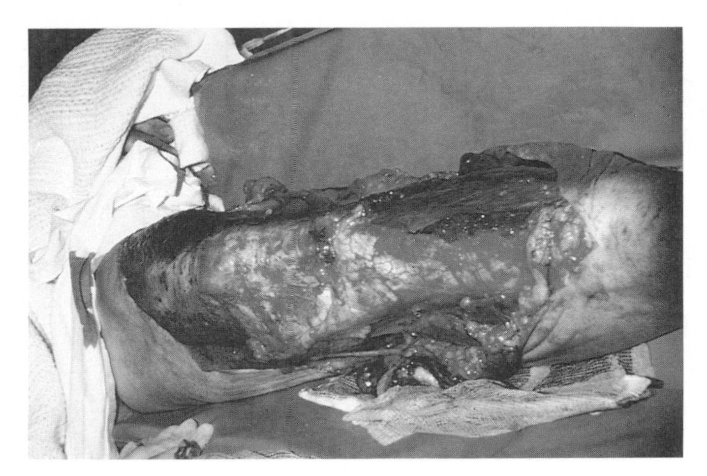

Fig. 16.1. An open fracture of the leg as a result of a road traffic accident. (See plate section.)

present within the tissues, responds to these factors resulting in the production of osteoblasts and osteocytes.

Recent work has shown that this vascular response has an important role in the fracture healing process. The nutrient artery and the periosteal vessels are involved, and this peristeal response is vital for the fracture healing process (6). This work has confirmed previous findings and interpretation (7–9).

The mechanical environment plays an important role in the fracture healing process, particularly the act of loading the fracture which stimulates the fracture healing response (10). Pead and Lanyon have demonstrated that bone cells have a memory which is stimulated by load and hence the mechanical environment is a vital part of fracture healing (11).

Fractures of bone must not be considered in isolation. The fracture involves a biological tissue and produces a biological response. Many bones are involved in weight bearing and the mechanical environment must also be considered when treating a fracture.

Classification

Until recently, fractures were classified according to their appearance, and were classified as either compound or closed. This method did not recognize the importance of damage to other tissues and hence Gustillo and Anderson's classification of open fractures is an important milestone in fracture management (12):

Type 1 — puncture wounds, less than 1 cm of skin is destroyed;

Type 2 — laceration, more than 1 cm is involved;

Type 3 — extensive damage to soft tissues including muscle, skin, and neurovascular structures.

Type 3 is further subdivided into:

3a in which there is associated soft tissue damage;

3b in which there is extensive bone and soft tissue damage;

3c in which there is vascular damage;

On the basis of this classification it is now possible to record and compare different treatment programmes, bearing in mind that the fracture is not the only event and that the soft tissue may be severely damaged, thereby impairing the vascular response to the fracture and delaying fracture healing.

In closed fractures Oestern and Tscherne have produced an equally important classification which is used for identifying the extent of the bone damage and the soft tissue involvement (13).

Management of a patient with an open fracture

When a patient presents with an open fracture it is important to exclude any other life-threatening injuries (Fig. 16.1). Steps need to be taken to ensure that the patient has an airway and has an adequate circulation. The state of a head injury needs to be assessed, as does the extent of a coincidental abdominal or chest injury.

It is important for fracture healing that there is an adequate circulatory volume. If the vascular response is shut down because of impaired or inadequate peripheral circulation, the fracture response will be retarded and may progress to non-union. After the patient has been resuscitated, the wound can be examined and the extent of the injury noted, along with the involvement of associated tissues.

The wound should be covered with a sterile dressing at this stage and, after radiological investigation, arrangements made to take the patient to an operating theatre as soon as possible.

Antibiotic therapy

Patients with open fractures should receive antibiotic therapy. The evidence for this has been clearly established by the experience of surgeons dealing with these fractures. Prior to adequate surgery and antibiotic therapy, amputation was a common outcome of an open fracture. These wounds are contaminated at the time they arrive in hospital and they should be considered contaminated even if they are brought to the operating theatre within 6 h of injury (14).

The main type of organisms isolated from open fractures include: *Staphylococcus aureus*, coagulase negative staphylococcus, *Streptococcus* spp., *Escherichia coli*, *Pseudomonas*

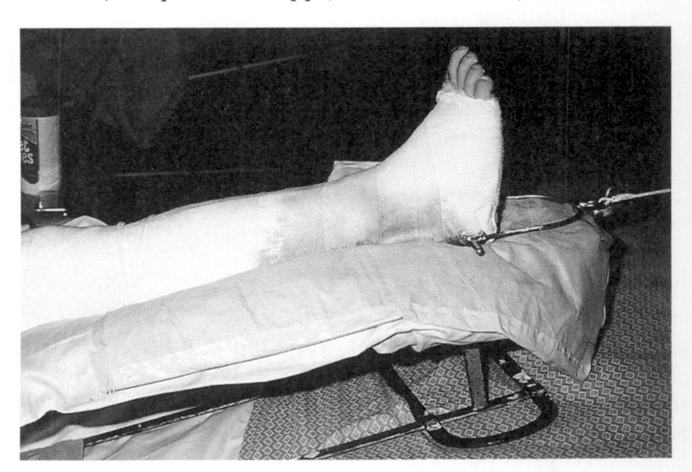

Fig. 16.2. Traction and plaster for a distal open tibial fracture. (See plate section.)

spp., *Proteus* spp., *Klebsiella* spp., together with anaerobic bacteria, in particular *Clostridia* spp. *Pseudomonas* spp. are particularly prevalent in Type 3c open fractures.

There is no doubt that high-dose intravenous antibiotic therapy should be administrated as soon as the patient arrives in the accident room. This applies to all open fractures, irrespective of type, as *all open fractures are contaminated* (15). Failure to administer antibiotics will jeopardize the patient's fracture, and indeed in certain circumstances their life, from either gas gangrene or overwhelming infection.

Administering high-dose antibiotics provides good tissue concentrations within a very short time (16). However, delay or low dosage does not provide high concentration in the tissues (17) and therefore there is every reason to give high doses on admission, particularly after the circulation has been restored and the blood flow has returned to the limb.

The choice of antibiotic depends upon the environment in which the accident occurred (18). For example, farm injuries carry a high risk of contamination by anaerobic organisms which may not be apparent in an urban environment. However, the regimen that has been adopted by the author is a combination of cefuroxime—a second generation cephalosporin effective against staphylococci; benzyl penicillin—for its activity against clostridia; and ceftazidime—a third generation cephalosporin effective against Gram-negative organisms.

These antibiotics are administered to patients with open fractures according to the following regimen:

Type 1	Cefuroxime 1.5 g IV on admission only. Benzyl penicillin 1 mega-unit IV.
Type 2	Cefuroxime 1.5 g IV on admission and continued 6 hourly for 48 h. Benzyl penicillin 1 mega-unit IV, and continued 6 hourly for 48 h.
Type 3a and 3b	Cefuroxime 1.5 g IV on admission and continued for up to 5 days. Benzyl penicillin 1 mega-unit IV and continued for 5 days.
Type 3c	Cefuroxime and benzyl penicillin as for Types 3a and 3b, ceftazidime 1 g IV on admission and continued for 5 days.

Wound debridement

Wound debridement is an important part of the management of all open fractures, even Type 1. The patient is taken to the operating theatre where the wound is cleansed with an appropriate antiseptic, the skin edges are excised and any dead tissue including muscle is removed. All dead or devitalized bone must be removed. It is unwise to be tempted to leave a piece of bone behind if it has been devitalized, no matter how large, as it will be a source of infection and produce horrendous results. It is far better to remove the dead bone and then bone graft the area either immediately or later. It is also important to irrigate the whole wound and it is normal practice to use copious quantities (up to 4 litres) of 0.9 per cent saline or Ringer's lactate.

Stabilization of the fracture

Once the wound is clean the fracture must be stabilized. There is a variety of methods available but essentially these include external fixation with Plaster of Paris, traction, or external fixation systems; or internal fixation with solitary screws, plate and screws, or intramedullary systems. Each system has its advocates and enthusiasts (19–22). In the author's view there are certain overall problems and clear advantages.

Plaster of Paris is a simple system for treating a fracture provided the joint above and the joint below are immobilized. However, in an open fracture the fracture site cannot be visualized and hence the wound cannot be inspected, unless a window is made in the plaster. Also as the swelling resolves, the fracture tends to displace within the plaster. Immobilizing the joint above and below causes quite significant joint stiffness, seriously affecting rehabilitation. Traction allows better visualization of the fracture site, but, because the method of fixation is not strong, there is a tendency for the fracture to displace, and this will affect union (Fig. 16.2).

Extensive soft tissue stripping is required to place and screw a plate across a fracture and this is not desirable, particularly in view of our understanding of the fracture healing process. Although the method of fixation is excellent in most fractures, the degree of trauma that can be caused to the soft tissues alone throws into question its role in open fractures.

However, external fixation of fractures using one of the many frames of single bars available has revolutionized the management of open fractures and indeed is now the gold standard of many treatment programmes (Figs. 16.3, 16.4).

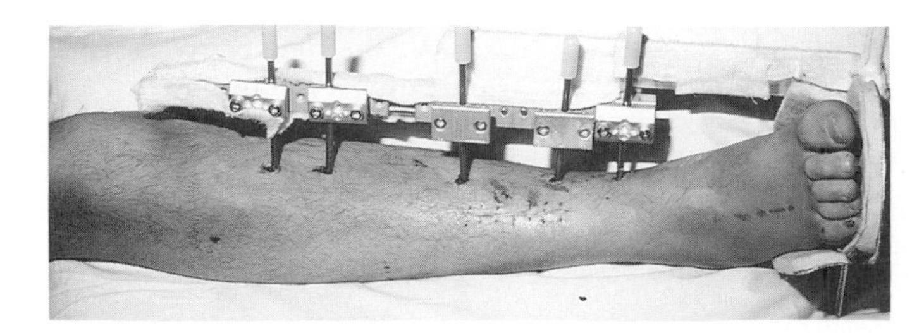

Fig. 16.3. Sukhtian–Hughes external fixation, single bar system, for an open tibial fracture. (See plate section.)

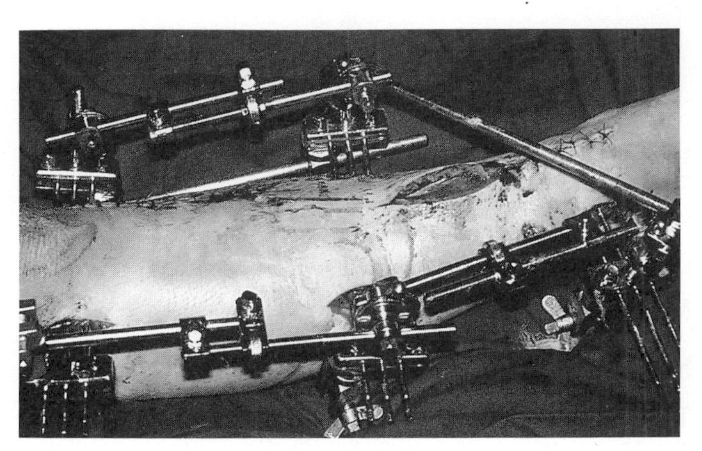

Fig. 16.4. Hoffman external frame for an open tibial fracture. (See plate section.)

The fracture can be adequately stabilized by using external fixation, and the joints above and below the fracture kept mobile from the first post-operative day. Skin cover is relatively easy to achieve by this means. The only problem is to decide when the external fixation system should be removed. This can be a real problem, particularly with the more rigid systems that are available, and there may be little in the way of callus 12 weeks after a fracture in which external fixation has been applied. Maurer *et al.* found that external fixation of open tibial fractures followed by intramedullary nailing 8 weeks later was contraindicated if pin tract infection was present (23).

Court-Brown *et al.* have advocated the use of intramedullary locking nails in the treatment of open fractures (22). This type of surgery carries a high risk of infection but, when practised by those skilled in the technique, produces excellent results.

However, if great care is not taken with this form of treatment amputation may be inevitable. Hence interlocking nail treatment of open fractures, whilst innovative and producing really impressive results, clearly should not be used unless the surgeon has had training in their application.

Wound cover

Following the fixation of the fracture it is of equal importance to obtain adequate skin cover (Fig. 16.5). Methods currently available include split skin grafts, myocutaneous flaps, or artificial skin cover such as Xenoderm®. If the wound is small, skin cover can be completed 48 h later by *delayed primary skin closure*, or by a *delayed split skin graft*.

The involvement of the plastic surgeons at the early stages of fracture management, that is at the time of the original injury, is vital, so that planned treatment can be initiated and the appropriate skin cover obtained. Under no circumstances should the wound be closed under tension.

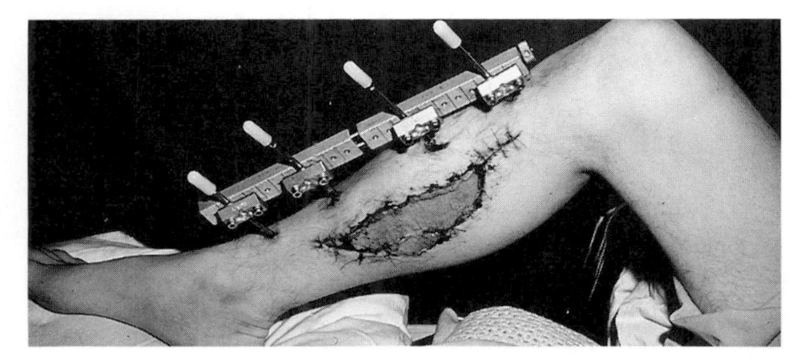

Fig. 16.5. Split skin graft for an open fracture. There is a Sukhtian–Hughes external fixation system in place. (See plate section.)

Management of complications

Non-union

The end result of treatment of a long bone fracture will be evidence of union, as defined by the ability of the patient to bear weight in a lower limb fracture, without pain or disability, along with radiological evidence of union of the fracture. This normally takes three to six months after a fracture of the lower limb. In those patients who have sustained open fractures there is a prolonged period of healing.

Infected non-union

The risk of non-union varies according to the type of the open fracture. The risk of infected non-union is particularly high in those patients who have sustained type 3b and 3c injuries (Fig. 16.6).

Incidence of infection

Gustilo has reported the incidence of infection to be 0 per cent in Type 1 open fractures, 1.8 per cent in Type 2 and 10.2–18.4 per cent in Type 3 (24). In these patients there is not only an unstable fracture but there is also evidence of osteomyelitis, which accentuates the non-union. Hence treatment of the infection in these patients is important if the fracture is to progress to union.

The organisms commonly isolated are those previously mentioned as contaminants of the original fracture. Gram-positive and Gram-negative organisms, particularly *Psuedomonas* spp. and *Proteus* spp. predominate.

Treatment follows the lines already laid down for the early management of the open fracture:

1. Ensure adequate vascularity and viability of all the tissues. This is achieved by surgical removal of all dead and non-viable tissue, especially scar tissue.
2. Ensure adequate antibiotic therapy is administered, based upon the pathogenic organisms identified within the deep tissues.
3. Stabilize the fracture. This may be achieved either by external fixation or by means of an interlocking nail.
4. Encourage bony union, using a bone graft if necessary.
5. Provide adequate and viable skin cover, usually by means of a myocutaneous flap (Fig. 16.7). This type of flap brings with it not only the skin for cover, but also the muscle which provides an increase in the blood supply to the fracture site and hence brings about union of the fracture.

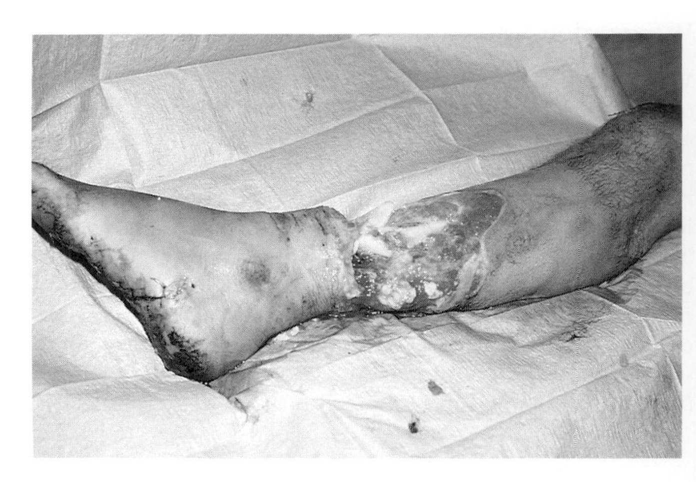

Fig. 16.6. Infected non-union of the tibia. (See plate section.)

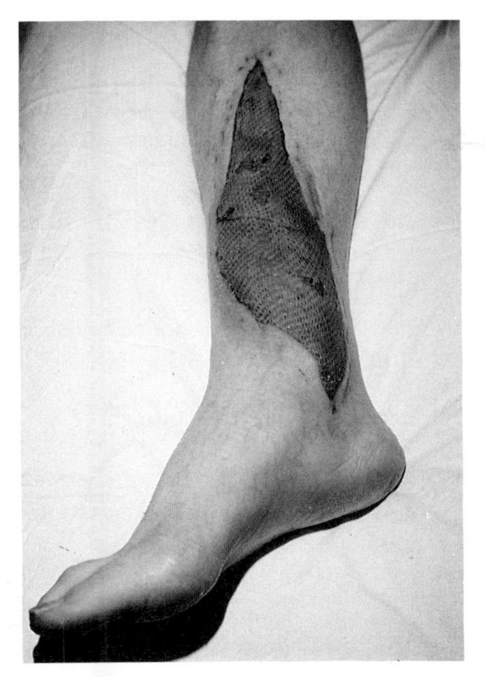

Fig. 16.7. A myocutaneous flap for a distal tibial fracture. (See plate section.)

Amputation

In some patients, even these measures are unsuccessful, and amputation may be necessary. The difficult decision is whether to ampute early or late. Early amputation seems logical in a severely damaged lower limb, where the vascular supply is grossly impaired and the risk of infection is high. Even after many months of conservative treatment in hospital amputation may be necessary when all surgical means have failed to salvage the limb.

Caudle and Stern (25) reviewed 62 type III open fractures and found that in eleven patients with type III A, none required amputation; of 42 with type III B, seven required amputation, whilst in nine patients with type III C, seven had secondary amputation and the two who avoided amputation had poor results.

Clearly, therefore, early amputation is worth considering in type III C open fractures.

Management of closed fractures

Oestern and Tscherne have produced a classification of soft tissue injuries associated with fractures (13).

C0 – Simple fracture configuration with little or no soft tissue injury.
C1 – Superficial abrasion; mild to moderate soft tissue damage; severe fracture configuration.
C2 – Deep contaminated abrasion with local damage to skin or muscle, moderately severe fracture configuration.
C3 – Extensive contusion or crushing of skin or destruction of muscle. Severe fracture.

Internal fixation of C1, C2, and C3 fractures can still present a major problem, particularly if there is not firm adherence to the principles of clean surgery. Low velocity C0 fractures, such as occur after a simple fall, probably do not warrant prophylactic antibiotic cover provided that there is adequate respect for the soft tissues at the time of operation. In a study of 54 patients sustaining low velocity fractures and treated by internal fixation, 25 received cefuroxime 1.5 g IV and 29 no antibiotic. There was no infection in the antibiotic group but three patients in the control group developed infection ($p = 0.24$) (26).

However, the use of interlocking nails in those high velocity injuries, particularly C2 and C3, probably does warrant antibiotic prophylaxis, although this topic has, as yet, not been adequately addressed and awaits a controlled prospective trial.

In fractures of the femoral neck, particularly in the elderly, there is a known risk of deep infection after surgery for fixation of the fracture. Table 16.1 indicates the results of antibiotic trials in fixation of fractured neck of femur.

Infection after this injury causes prolonged hospitalization and there is an 18 per cent mortality at 3 months for femoral neck fractures, which is associated with the general condition of the patient prior to the fracture (30). However, a recent prospective trial has demonstrated that single dose prophylactic

Table 16.1. Incidence of infection in fractured neck of femur.

Author	Antibiotic	Infection comment
Boyd *et al.* (27) 417 patients	Nacfillin 48 h	Wound infection 0.8% (treated) 4.8% (control)
Tengve and Kjellander (28) 140 patients	Cephalothin and Cephalexin 48 h	Wound infection 1.8% (treated) 16.9% (control)
Burnett *et al.* (29) 307 patients	Cephalothin 72 h	Major wound infection 0.7% (treated) 4.7% (control)
McQueen *et al.* (30) 502 patients	Cefuroxime Single dose	Deep wound infection 1.6% (treated) 2.7% (control)

Table 16.2. Antibiotic prophylaxis in proximal femoral fractures.

	Placebo	Cefuroxime	
Patients entered	256	246	
Age (years)	78.7	79.7	
Intracapsular fracture	127	127	
Extracapsular fracture	129	119	
Infection			
Superficial	33	25	
Deep	7	4	
Total infection	40 (15.6%)	29 (12.0%)	n.s.

Adapted from McQueen *et al.* (30)

antibiotics do not appear to have an effect on the overall incidence of wound infection, (30) and further trials are still necessary in this area (Table 16.2).

Conclusions

Without doubt infection following a fracture is a major problem. Open fractures are best treated by long established principles. Bone should not be considered an isolated structure, care must be given to the associated tissues. The blood supply to bone is vitally important and needs to be maintained as it is the source of the factors that promote the fracture healing process (32). Equally important is fracture stabilization which enables the mechanical environment to play its role. Failure to abide by these principles can result in disaster for even the mildest of open fractures.

Similar principles hold for closed fractures, particularly when an open reduction is contemplated. Once the fracture is exposed to the outside environment there is a risk of contamination by pathogenic organisms and this can result in osteomyelitis.

Orthopaedic practice has progressed a great deal since the days when amputation was advocated at the first sign of limb infection, but only because certain principles are now accepted. If we lose sight of these basic principles, careful handling of the tissues and an understanding of the biology of bone, all the advanced technology available will be useless, and the patient's condition will be far worse in the long term.

References

1. Mankin, H.J. (1984). The articular cartilages, cartilage healing and osteoarthritis. *Adult orthopaedics* (ed. R.L. Cruess and W.R.J. Rennie). Churchill Livingstone, New York.
2. Ham, A.W. and Cormack, D.H. (1979). *Histology*, Lippincott, Philadelphia.
3. Paradis, G.R. and Kelly, P.J. (1975). Blood flow and mineral deposition in canine tibial fractures. *J. Bone Joint. Surg. (Am.)*, **57**, 220–6.
4. Hughes, S.P.F., Lemon, G.J., Davies, D.R., Bassingthwaighte, J.B., and Kelly, P.J. (1979). Extraction of minerals after experimental fractures of the tibia in dogs. *J. Bone Joint. Surg. (Am.)*, **61**, 857–66.
5. Urist, M.R. (1972). Osteoinduction in undermineralized bone implants modified by chemical inhibition of matrix enzymes. *Clin. Orth.*, **87**, 132–7.
6. Strachan, R.K., McCarthy, I., Fleming, R., and Hughes, S.P.F. (1990). The role of the tibial nutrient artery. Microsphere estimation of blood flow in the osteotomised canine tibia. *J. Bone Joint. Surg. (Br.)*, **72**, 391–4.
7. Trueta, J. (1957). The normal vascular anatomy of the humeral head during growth. *J. Bone Joint. Surg. (Br.)*, **39**, 358–94.
8. Brookes, M., Elkin, A.C., Harrison, R.G., and Heald, C.B. (1961). A new concept of capillary circulation in bone cortex. *Lancet*, **i**, 1078–81.
9. Rhinelander, F.W. (1968). The normal microcirculation of diaphyseal cortex and its response to fracture. *J. Bone Joint. Surg. (Am.)*, **50**, 784–800.
10. Goodship, A. and Kenwright, J. (1985). The influence of induced micromovement upon healing of experimental fractures. *J. Bone Joint. Surg. (Br.)*, **67**, 650–5.
11. Pead, M.J. and Lanyon, L.E. (1989). Indomethacin modulation of load-related stimulation of new bone formation *in vivo*. *Calcif. Tiss. Int.*, **45**, 34–40.
12. Gustilo, R.B. and Anderson, J.T. (1976). Prevention of infection in the treatment of one thousand and twenty five open fractures of long bones. *J. Bone Joint. Surg. (Am.)*, **58**, 453–8.
13. Oestern, H.J. and Tscherne, H. (1984). Pathophysiology and classification of soft tissue injuries associated with fractures. In *Fractures and soft tissue injuries* (ed. H. Tscherne and L. Gotzen). Springer–Verlag, Berlin.
14. Robinson, D., On, E., Hadas, N., Halperin, N., Hofman, S., and Bolder, I. (1989). Microbiologic flora contaminating open fractures: its significance in the choice of primary agents and the likelihood of deep wound infection. *J. Orthop. Trauma*, **3**, 283–6.
15. Pastakis, M.J. and Wilkins, J. (1989). Factors influencing infection rate in open fracture wounds. *Clin. Orthop.*, **243**, 36–40.
16. Hughes, S.P.F., Dash, C.H., Benson, M.K.D., and Field, C. (1978). Infection following total hip replacement and the possible prophylactic role of Cephaloridine. *J.R. Coll. Surg. Edinb.*, **23**, 9–12.
17. Pollard, J.P., Hughes, S.P.F., Evans, M.J., Scott, J.E., and Benson, M.K.D. (1979). Concentration of flucloaxacillin in femoral head and joint capsule in total hip replacement. *J. Antimicrob. Chemother.*, **5**, 721–6.
18. Merritt, K. (1988). Factors increasing the risk of infection in patients with open fractures. *J. Trauma*, **28**, 823–7.
19. Ellis, H. (1958). The speed of healing after fractures of the tibial shaft. *J. Bone Joint. Surg. (Br.)*, **40**, 42–6.
20. Haines, J.F., Williams, E.A., Hargadon, E.S., and Davies, D.R.A. (1984). Is conservative treatment of displaced tibial shaft fractures justified? *J. Bone Joint. Surg. (Br.)*, **66**, 84–8.
21. Court-Brown, C.M., and Hughes, S.P.F. (1985). Hughes external fixator in treatment of tibial fractures. *J.R. Soc. Med.*, **78**, 830–7.
22. Court-Brown, C.M., Christie, J., and McQueen, M.M. (1990). Close intramedullary tibial nailing: its use in closed and Type I open fractures. *J. Bone Joint. Surg. (Br.)*, **72**, 605–11.
23. Maurer, D.J., Merkow, R.L., and Gustilo, R.B. (1989). Infection after intramedullary nailing of severe open tibial fractures initially treated with external fixation. *J. Bone Joint. Surg. (Br.)*, **71**, 835–38.
24. Gustilo, R.B. (1982). In *Management of open fractures and their complications*, Vol. IV (ed. C.B. Sledge). Saunders, Philadelphia, Penn.
25. Caudle, R.J. and Stern, P.J. (1987). Severe open fractures of the tibia. *J. Bone Joint. Surg. (Am.)*, **69**, 801–7.
26. Hughes, S.P.F., Miles, R.S., Littlejohn, M.A., and Brown, E. (1991). Is antibiotic prophylaxis necessary for internal fixation of

low energy fractures? *Injury*, **22**, 111–13.
27. Boyd, R.J., Burke, J.F., and Colton, T. (1973). A double-blind clinical trial of prophylactic antibiotics in hip fractures. *J. Bone Joint. Surg. (Am.)*, **55**, 1251–8.
28. Tengve, B. and Kjellander, J. (1978). Antibiotic prophylaxis in operations on trochanteric femoral fractures. *J. Bone Joint. Surg. (Am.)*, **60**, 97–9.
29. Burnett, J.W. Gustilo, R.B., Williams, D.N. *et al.* (1980). Prophylactic antibiotics in hip fractures. *J. Bone Joint. Surg. (Am.)*, **62**, 457–64.
30. McQueen, M.M., Littlejohn, M.A., Miles, R.S., and Hughes, S.P.F. (1990). Antibiotic prophylaxis in proximal femoral fracture. *Injury*, **21**, 104–6.
31. Foubister, G. and Hughes, S.P.F. (1989). Fractures of the femoral neck: a retrospective and prospective study. *J.R. Coll. Surg. Edinb.*, **34**, 249–52.
32. Hughes, S.P.F., McCarthy, I.D., and Hooper, G. (1986). The vascular system in bone. Its importance and relevance to clinical practice. *Clin. Orthop.*, **210**, 31–6.

Further reading

1. Gustilo, R.B. (1982). In *Management of open fractures and their complications* (ed. C.B. Sledge). Saunders, Philadelphia, Penn.
2. Coombs, R. and Fitzgerald, R.H., Jr. (ed.) (1989). *Infection in the orthopaedic patient.* Butterworths, London.
3. Hughes, S.P.F. and Fitzgerald, Jr, R.H. (1986). *Musculoskeletal infections.* Year Book Medical Publishers, Chicago.
4. Gustilo, R.B., Gruninger, R.P., and Tsukayama, D.T. (1989). *Orthopaedic infection: diagnosis and treatment.* Saunders, Philadelphia, Penn.

17

Gunshot wounds and war surgery

MICHAEL S. OWEN-SMITH

Introduction

Gunshot wounds are one of the greatest causes of morbidity and mortality throughout the world. War wounds occur not only in times of war, but whenever and wherever weapons of war are used. Peace time assaults usually involve hand held and sharp instruments and low-velocity hand-guns. Military weapons, whether they be rifles, machine guns, or explosive devices cause a different type of injury especially when the missile travels at high velocity. Wounds inflicted by low-velocity hand-guns, knives, or other penetrating weapons can usually be managed by standard surgical procedures. If, however, these same procedures are applied to high-velocity bullet wounds or explosive blast injuries the results can be disastrous.

A glance at the newspapers or television will confirm that limited wars and terrorist activity has become an inevitable accompaniment of life today. All surgeons must now be prepared to receive and treat patients wounded by the weapons of war. In order to do this they must understand how the different types of missiles and explosives cause wounds, how to assess this damage and how to treat them in the most effective way. It is only by understanding the physical phenomena of missile wounding that the surgeon appreciates what makes these wounds so different from other forms of trauma and why they have to be treated by special methods. These methods have stood the tests of time, are based upon millions of battle casualities and are ignored to the peril of the patient and the humiliation of the surgeon.

Bullet wounds

When a bullet strikes the body the damage depends on the size, shape, stability, and velocity of the missile, and on the structures of which it comes into contact. Bullets can be divided into rifle or high-velocity, and pistol or low-velocity. What do we mean by high-velocity? In the UK the accepted definition depends on the velocity of sound in air which is 340 m/s (1100 ft/s). This simple definition was chosen because something peculiar happens to the mechanism of injury to the body caused by a bullet at about the speed of sound. New physical phenomena come into play with high-velocity bullets that cause wounding effects of a different order of magnitude.

Hand-guns may be revolvers or automatics, but they all fire a fairly heavy bullet at relatively low velocities of about 150–300 m/s (500–1000 ft/s). A typical military rifle fires a bullet of about 10 g at a velocity of over 800 m/s (2600 ft/s). This velocity is very much greater than that of bullets from hand-guns. Rifles of this type are not new, they have been in existence for well over 100 years. Recent developments in military rifles have led to smaller bullets fired at even higher velocity. For example the 5.56 mm Colt Armalite Rifle fires a very light weight bullet of 3.4 g at a velocity of about 1000 m/s

(3250 ft/s). The armies of the world are in the process of replacing their existing rifles with these light assault rifles as typified by the Colt Armalite, the Warsaw Pact AK-74 rifle, and the new rifles adopted by the United Kingdom, Germany, and France.

The motion of the bullet in flight, and within the tissues after impact, depends on its size, shape, composition and above all, its stability and velocity. In the tissues density and elasticity are the most important factors which influence the retardation of the missile. Spinning the bullet by means of rifling the barrel of the gun gives it stability and this increases the range and accuracy. Rifle bullets are used for accurate target shooting at ranges of over 1000 m and have been known to kill at 2000 m.

The soft tissues of the body are very similar to water, in that they are approximately 800–900 times as dense as air and whenever a bullet hits tissues it becomes more unstable. Tissues of increasing density cause greater retardation of the missile and therefore greater energy is released to cause damage. Retardation is not only directly proportional to the presenting area of the bullet but is also proportional to the cube of its velocity, thus if a bullet fragments on striking the body, as happens with many of the newer small-calibre bullets, the presenting area will be increased, retardation will be more rapid and a greater proportion of the bullets energy will be transferred to the tissues to create a larger wound. The longer the wound track the greater the chance for a bullet to become unstable in its path thereby creating greater damage. A wound in the body occurs from the transfer of energy from the bullet to the tissues penetrated. When a bullet is stopped completely by the tissues it penetrates, the energy liberated must be equal to the total kinetic energy of the bullet. A stable, perforating bullet with a short wound track may use up only 10–20 per cent of its actual strike energy in creating a wound. An unstable bullet of the same mass and velocity will always give up a much greater proportion of its energy thereby creating a more severe wound in the same tissues and over the same length wound track. Fragmentation of the bullet has a similar effect in creating larger wounds when compared with a non-fragmenting bullet.

Mechanism of injury

A bullet can cause injury in the following three ways: laceration and crushing of tissues; shock waves; temporary cavitation and stretching of tissues.

Laceration, crushing, and stretching of tissues

When the missile penetrates the tissues they are crushed and forced apart, this is the principal effect of low-velocity missiles travelling at up to 340 m/s (1000 ft/s). The crushing and laceration caused solely by the passage of the missile are not serious unless vital organs or major blood vessels are directly injured. Only those tissues that have come into immediate contact with the missile are damaged and the wound is comparable to those caused by hand held weapons such as knives. No significant energy is transmitted to tissues surrounding the wound track and the damage seen at operation is all the damage that has occurred, with nothing being hidden.

Shock waves

Whilst the missile forces a track through solid tissues it compresses the medium in front of it and this region of compression moves away as a shock wave with spherical form. The velocity of this shock wave is approximately that of sound in water, 1500 m/s (4800 ft/s). These shock waves can cause damage at a considerable distance away from the wound track when they traverse fluid–gas interfaces where there is a considerable change in the specific gravity of the medium. They can also be transmitted along fluid filled tubes such as arteries and veins to cause damage at a distance. However, rather like the pressure wave from a lithotripter, provided that no gas filled cavities are traversed, damage from shock waves is of little significance.

Temporary cavitation—violent stretching of tissues

This phenomenon usually only occurs with high-velocity bullets or fragments and is the main reason for their immensely destructive effects. When the penetrating missile releases its energy rapidly, it is absorbed by the local tissues, which are accelerated violently forwards and outwards thereby stretching them. Due to their inertia, the tissues take a perceptible time to get moving and then the momentum created causes them to continue to move after the passage of the missile. Thus, a large cavity is created which is approximately 10–15 times the diameter of the missile. This cavity has a subatmospheric pressure and is connected to the outside by entry and exit holes. Bacteria from the outside together with clothing and debris are actively sucked into the depths of the wound. The cavity rapidly collapses over a few milliseconds in pulsatile fashion leaving a narrow permanent cavity which is the cavity that may be seen at operation.

It is the cavitation–stretch phenomenon that accounts for the 'explosive' nature of high-velocity missile wounds. The greater the energy that is imparted to the tissues the greater will be the size of the temporary cavity and the more extensive the damage. Soft tissue will be pulped, small blood vessels will be disrupted and bone may be shattered without being hit directly. Since the larger blood vessels are more elastic they may be pushed aside, nevertheless, the blood vessels may well suffer damage to the intima at a distance from the wound even though there is no external sign of injury. Thrombosis and stasis in vessels in the hours following the injury further increase the volume of dead tissue and plasma leaks from the damaged vessels causing a tense oedema and further compressive ischaemia. This large amount of dead tissue inextricably mixed with bacteria and debris actively sucked in from the environment is the specific pathological entity known as the high-velocity missile (HVM) wound.

The cavitation phenomenon takes place in all tissues whether they be the limb, abdomen, chest, or head. Some tissues are much more sensitive to the cavitational changes than others. In general, the damage is directly proportional to the density of the tissue and therefore homogeneous tissues like muscle, liver, spleen and brain are very sensitive whereas the light tissue such as the lung, which is mainly filled with air, are resistant.

The damage is also inversely in proportion to the amount of elastic fibres present; for example, skin and lung are remarkably resistant to such damage, whereas bone is very sensitive. Evidence that there has been a temporary cavity is demonstrated by the zone of bruising which occurs around the permanent track of the experimental wound. This zone of damaged muscle has an abnormal colour, does not contract when pinched and does not bleed when cut. These appearances are characteristic, can be readily demonstrated to the uninitiated and are an accurate estimate of the death of muscle. This volume of dead tissue is surrounded by a zone of stretched, damaged, but recoverable tissues.

Pistol bullets have a relatively low amount of energy available to cause damage. In general this occurs only at fairly close ranges and the damaging effects are very limited at ranges at 50–100 m. All rifle bullets have an incredible amount of available energy, although this energy decreases with increasing range, nevertheless they have great wounding power even at distances of many hundreds of metres. If the bullet fragments on impact, all the energy will be used up in creating horrendous wounds.

The external appearances of a bullet wound can be deceptive. If the bullet enters or leaves skin end-on, then it will commonly leave a small hole, irrespective of the severe damage it may cause during its passage of the tissues. If the bullet enters or, more commonly, leaves the skin sideways then the hole in the skin will be large and ragged.

In an experimental rifle bullet wound, a volume of tissue approximately 500 ml, or the size of a fist, is damaged. This large amount of dead tissue, uniformly and grossly contaminated with bacteria and debris from the surface, is characteristic of the high velocity missile wound.

All accidental wounds are contaminated but this is particularly true of HVM wounds as they contain a mass of pulped tissue with a gross amount of debris and bacteria. Clostridia spores are normally carried on the skin and clothing and most infections resulting from these organisms are endogenous. In wounds containing dead tissue, particularly muscle, the conditions are ideal for the development of clostridial myonecrosis or gas gangrene. This is a clinical diagnosis, not a bacteriological one, and is the one condition which, above all other infections, must be prevented. This infection was the main reason why the principles of thorough wound excision and delayed primary closure were made mandatory in war surgery. This mandatory treatment must now be extended to include all HVM wounds.

Explosive blast injuries

Explosives are substances which, when detonated, are changed almost instantaneously from solid or liquid form into a vast volume of gas. The body can be damaged by three separate physical phenonema associated with the explosive blast: fragments from the bomb; blast pressure waves; blast wind.

The fragments which come from an explosive device travel at high velocity. They are not streamlined like bullets and therefore, at a distance from the explosion they become low-velocity missiles. In war-time, more than three-quarters of all injuries are caused by fragments from explosive devices and, similarly, home made bombs which are packed with nails, screws, ball bearings and other debris can create a large number of injuries.

The blast pressure wave is created by explosive gases compressing the surrounding air. The zone of compression moves away from the site of the explosion at high speed as a sphere of rapidly increasing radius. Although the pressure wave does not last for long it can reach very high pressures of thousands of pounds per square inch. Like sound waves, pressure waves will flow over and around an obstruction so that someone hiding behind a wall may be affected by a pure pressure wave. These waves are similar to radio waves in that they will pass right through the body and it is only those parts which contain air or gas which are damaged. The ears, the lungs, and the gas-containing viscera are damaged in that order of vulnerability.

The blast wave or mass movement of air, is caused by the displacement of air by the vast volume of explosive gases. This rushes away from the explosion at high speed, in excess of the speed of Concorde in flight. According to the velocity of the wind, the body may simply be blown over, thrown many metres or thrown against the surrounding environment, causing acceleration and deceleration injuries. Closer to the explosion, the blast wind may simply blow pieces off the body. All variations occur in proportion to the violence of the explosion and velocity of the blast wind. In a massive explosion, the body may be totally disintegrated and atomized. Lower levels may cause total disruption of the body or it may be blown into a few or more pieces. Lesser levels will cause traumatic amputation, varying from the whole of the limb to parts of the limb or a digit. These traumatic amputations are quite common after explosions. When they occur in confined spaces, up to a quarter of all the dead and seriously injured victims may have traumatic amputations.

Principles of surgery of war wounds

All bullet wounds involve soft tissues and most of them will involve damage to other structures in the limbs or to the deeper structures and organs of the head and trunk. Treatment of the dirty soft tissue wound is a two-stage procedure: the first operation is excision of the wound, and the second operation is delayed primary closure.

Wound excision

Wound excision is the process whereby the dead, damaged, and grossly contaminated tissue, is thoroughly excised. This leaves an area of healthy tissue with a good blood supply capable of combating residual surface infection – provided the wound is not closed. The technique of wound excision is as follows: clothing, dressing, and splints are carefully removed and a sterile gauze pad is held over the wound. The skin over a large surrounding area and the whole circumference of the limb or the body is cleansed with detergent, shaved, dried, and then painted with antiseptic such as chlorhexidine or povidone-iodine. In the case of multiple wounds, those on the posterior aspects of the body and limbs should be dealt with before those on the anterior aspect in order to minimize turning the patient. Skin is remarkably viable and very resistant to damage by crush or stretch, it should be treated as conservatively as possible, only the minimal amount of skin should be excised from the edges of the wound; rarely will more than 1 mm be required to be removed, except when the skin is grossly pulped.

The skin and subcutaneous tissues should be incised generously in order to get to the depth of the wound. In the limb the incision should be along the long axis, but not over subcutaneous bone or across flexion creases. The subcutaneous fat and the shredded superficial fascia are always contaminated and must be excised in a generous fashion. The deep fascia must be incised along the length of the incision. This fasciotomy is an essential step that allows wide and deep retraction without tension and enables the depth of the wound to be exposed. It may be necessary to add transverse cuts to the deep fascia in order to improve access. Undamaged fascial compartments may well need decompression to avoid post-operative ischaemic changes where the muscles swell in response to trauma. Dead muscle must be thoroughly excised because this is the ideal medium for clostridial infection leading to gas gangrene. The track of the missile is seen at operation, but this track is surrounded by dead muscle and it is this volume of tissue which must always be excised completely. The finger placed in the wound and swept around the cavity will give a good idea of the size of the cavity and the amount of dead tissue that is likely to need excision.

All muscle that is not healthy and red, and that does not contract and bleed when it is cut must be excised with scissors until healthy, contractile bleeding muscle is reached. Each wound must be evaluated individually and great care must be taken not to excise viable tissues by over-enthusiastic, incompetent surgery. Recent publications have alleged that lesser procedures such as fasciotomy and minimal excision are better than thorough excision of clinically dead muscle in wounds of the limbs. This repeats earlier published animal work using minimal surgical methods in high-energy missile wounds. In practice, in human missile wounds with high-energy transfers (usually HVM wounds) this has not been successful. In the experience of almost every war surgeon there have been more problems from not excising sufficient dead muscle tissue rather than taking too much. Each wound must be examined and dealt with on its merits in relation to tissue that has been destroyed or damaged. There must be no pre-judgement before operation reveals the extent of the wound.

The edges of the wound should be retracted and dirt, debris, fragments of missiles, and blood clot are removed from the sides and depths of the wound. Gentle and copious irrigation with saline will wash out most of the residual debris. The wound should be explored with the finger to identify any foreign body and unexpected deep recesses in the wound. All organic matter must be removed, but it is not essential to spend too much time spent searching for metallic foreign bodies. Haemostasis must be by firm pressure with warm packs and ligatures using fine thread, silk, or polyglycolic acid sutures at the bleeding point. These must be picked up accurately in order to leave as little dead tissue as possible in the wound, and diathermy coagulation should not be used for the same reason.

The widely opened deep fascia, which has been freely incised, should be left open to allow post-operative oedematous and congested tissue to swell without tension and so avoid interference with the blood supply. All wounds should be left open, without suture of the skin or deep structures, with the following exceptions.

1. *The face and neck and genitalia.* These wounds *may* be closed primarily after primary wound excision but there is no absolute need to do so.
2. *Soft tissues of the chest wall.* These wounds must be excised and healthy muscle should be used to close sucking chest wounds in order to establish an air tight closure. The skin should be left open.
3. *Head injuries.* The dura is closed directly by temporalis fascia graft and the galea and skin closed by rotating flaps to provide cover.
4. *Hand injuries.* Some injuries may be closed primarily but usually these should be left open for delayed primary closure. All viable tissues must be preserved for this simplifies the reconstruction procedures. Tendons and nerves should be covered by healthy tissue.
5. *Joints.* The synovial membrane should be closed, but if this is not possible the capsule alone should be closed. However, little harm seems to be done in practice if the joint cannot be closed securely.
6. *Blood vessels.* Those blood vessels that have been repaired primarily or by vein graft should be covered by viable muscle.

The widely opened wound is simply covered by a layer of dry gauze and this in turn is covered by a bulky absorbent dressing. The aim of the dressing is to draw inflammatory fluid out of the wound and into the dressing. Tulle gras or other paraffin dressing should not be used and the wound should not be packed in any way with a dressing since this will form a plug and prevent the easy outflow of inflammatory fluid. The whole dressing should be kept in place by sticky tape and it is important that this dressing must not go completely round a limb. In all cases where there has been an extensive soft tissue wound of the limb there should be effective immobilization, this is best done with splints, well-padded plasters that must be split down to the skin at the time the plaster is applied, by plaster slabs or, of course, by external fixation.

Delayed primary closure

If the wound resulting from an HVM injury has been thoroughly excised there should be no necessity for further inspection until the time comes for closure. If there is a specific indication – such as excessive pain, oedema, or signs of infection – then it may be necessary to inspect the wound in the operation room under a general anaesthetic. It is usually an indication that wound excision is incomplete and further excision of dead tissue will be necessary. When initial wound excision has been adequate the open wound should be closed on the fourth or the fifth day. Practical experience and experimentation has demonstrated that this is the optimum time and that primary healing should be obtained in more than 90 per cent of all cases. The sutures should be fine so that tension is avoided, dead space must be obliterated and drains avoided whenever possible, or used for twenty four hours only. Split skin grafting may well be required in combination with suturing.

Regional wounds

Wounds of limbs

About 60 to 75 per cent of all missile wounds and blast injuries involve the upper and lower extremeties and, therefore, such a wound is usually the first type of missile wound the surgeon is called upon to treat. Management of a compound fracture is similar to that of the soft tissue wound already described, but with the special addition of injury to bone and associated injuries to blood vessels and nerves. Bone is commonly shattered into a number of pieces. Tiny fragments without any attachment should be discarded but all other fragments with periosteum or muscle attachment should be cleaned thoroughly, using a sharp curette and copious irrigation, and replaced. Any large attached fragments should be cleaned and replaced, and the major bone ends brought roughly into line. The soft tissues are excised as has already been described. Repair of any major blood vessel to the limb must be performed at that earliest stage of the operation, as failure to do this jeopardizes the survival of the limb. Venous repair should precede arterial repair. Severed nerves are marked and their positions noted and the same is done with damaged tendons, but no attempt should be made at primary repair in either case. Internal fixation of bone should not be done in these injuries even when required to protect an accompanying arterial anastomosis because of the gross contamination and unacceptable risk of infection. External fixation using pins placed through normal tissue above and below the fracture is often the treatment of choice. After delayed primary closure, and when primary wound healing has taken place, further procedures on the bone, nerves or tendons can be done at leisure.

Vascular injuries

Injuries to major blood vessels require immediate surgical treatment if the tissues supplied by there vessels are to be salvaged. Most acute vascular injuries which come to surgical repair involve peripheral vessels, because very few patients with major vessel injury in the abdomen or chest cavity survive to reach hospital. Time is at a premium with vascular injuries, the vessels should be repaired and the blood supply to the peripheral tissues restored as soon as possible and in any case within six hours. At operation, wound excision has to follow control of haemorrhage. The damaged ends of the vessel are trimmed until macroscopically normal vessel is reached and 20–40 ml of heparinized saline is injected distally. If free back bleeding is not obtained, a size 3 or 4 Fogarty balloon catheter should be passed and withdrawn before injecting heparinized saline. The deep veins are as important to repair as arteries and similar methods should be used. A simple laceration of a vein caused by a low-velocity missile can be repaired by lateral suture. A vessel that has been severed, or has had a segment destroyed by HVM must be repaired, using autogenous vein graft. Synthetic prostheses should not be used because of the grave and unacceptable risk of infection. Usually, a reversed saphenous vein graft is used and anastomoses are made obliquely in order to gain maximum diameter, using 5/0 or 6/0 atraumatic sutures. After repair the vessels are covered by healthy muscle, a fasciotomy is usually performed, and the wound left open for delayed primary closure.

Chest wounds

Direct damage to the chest from penetrating wounds may involve the chest wall, lungs, mediastinal contents, heart, and diaphragm. The lung itself is remarkably resistant whereas the heart and mediastinal contents are extremely susceptible to missile damage. It is essential that the pleural and pericardial spaces be kept empty, and that normal pressures be maintained. This requires release of tension pneumothorax, aspiration of the pericardium for cardiac tamponade, closure of an open pneumothorax, stabilization of the flail chest, and drainage of a large pneumothorax or haemothorax. Bleeding from penetrating chest wounds is usually from intercostal or internal mammary vessels. The lung itself does not usually bleed to any great extent and massive haemorrhage from major pulmonary vessels is rapidly fatal. The basis of treatment is withdrawal of the bloodstained effusion from the pleural space and replacement of the measured blood loss.

If clinical examination reveals signs of blood or air in the pleural space a wide-bore intercostal drainage tube should be inserted through the lateral chest wall, in the mid-axillary line, for removal of blood or fluid. This should be attached to a Heimlich one-way valve and thence to a drainage bag. Underwater seal suction drainage should be applied as soon as is practicable. A chest radiograph should be taken afterwards to confirm the location of the tube and the evacuation of the pleural space, and also to locate any foreign bodies. The tube may be removed when there is no longer any evidence of air leak, the lung is fully expanded, and when air and fluid are no longer present in the pleural cavity. An accurate record should be made of the amount of blood lost though the chest drain. War experience has shown that over 85 per cent of all penetrating and perforating wounds of the chest may be managed by closed-tube thoracostomy.

Thoracotomy is required for specific indications: continued intrathoracic bleeding; massive and continuing air leakage; abdomino-thoracic injury; injury to the mediastinal contents; cardiac wounds; sucking wound of the chest; large wounds of the chest wall with a defect.

Most chest wounds can be dealt with through the standard postero-lateral thoracotomy. Bleeding from the lung usually ends once the lung has been inflated and comes into contact with the chest wall, but in some lung wounds ligation of bleeding vessels and oversewing of a small segment of the lung may be necessary. Pulmonary resection is seldom required. Major chest wall defects should be closed by swinging a flap of a local muscle such as latissimus dorsi or pectoralis major.

Abdominal wounds

Penetrating missile wounds of the abdomen require urgent treatment. A patient who has been wounded in the abdomen is almost certain to die unless he is operated upon. Small calibre bullets and HVM fragments from explosive devices may produce minute superficial wounds which can be associated with amazingly severe internal damage. Early operation is mandatory as part of the resuscitation process; the commonest cause of death is haemorrhage, and this requires treatment at the earliest possible moment, whereas the closure of intestinal leaks is less urgent. After passing a catheter into the bladder a full laparotomy incision should be made; for severe injuries a generous full mid-line incision is quickest and best. Haemorrhage is dealt with first, followed by repair of all perforations of the alimentary tract.

Perforations of the small bowel and stomach may be closed by suture in the usual fashion. Resection of small bowel should be performed when the group of perforations is so close that their repair would overlap or when the injury is on the mesenteric border; end to end anastomosis should be done by the surgeon's usual technique and the result should be good.

Wounds of the colon occur almost as frequently as those of the small bowel; they are usually more serious because the blood supply is not so good and the contents of the large bowel escape more readily and are highly infective. Perforations of the colon should be looked for most carefully because those in the fixed portions and those in the mesenteric aspects of the transverse colon are difficult to demonstrate and can easily be missed. The colon must be mobilized in order to get a good view of it; any part of the wall of the colon which is contused or discoloured should be considered for repair, resection, or exteriorization. There are three basic methods of treating colon injuries caused by missiles: exteriorization of the damaged or repaired colon; repair by suture, with or without proximal colostomy; resection, with or without primary anastomosis.

Due to difficulties with its liquid contents the right colon should not be exteriorized, but the transverse and descending colon are readily exteriorized and this method is still very useful on occasions, particularly under field conditions when post-operative care is minimal. The method of treatment used will depend on the severity of damage to the colon that is discovered at laparotomy. Major disrupted segmental damage caused by a HVM wound should be treated by resection and the formation of a colostomy, or ileostomy, and a distal mucous fistula. Moderate wounds should be treated by resection, anastomosis, and proximal defunctioning colostomy. A damaged section of transverse or left colon may be mobilized and exteriorized as a large loop colostomy. Finally simple repair of perforation should be reserved for the uncomplicated, low-velocity wound with minimal damage to the colon and no complicating factor.

Thorough peritoneal toilet and lavage with warm saline or antibiotic solution such as tetracycline 1 g per litre should be followed by thorough dependent drainage and closure of the laparotomy wound, using looped nylon or other form of retention suture. Good pelvic drainage can be achieved by excision of the tip of the coccyx, placing drains well up in the space between the sacrum and rectum. Wounds of the rectum should be treated by repair or resection and anastomosis, thorough drainage, and the formation of an efficient defunctioning colostomy. This means either dividing the sigmoid and bringing the two ends out as separate colostomy and mucous fistula or by closing the distal end and bringing the proximal end out as a colostomy in the fashion of Hartmann's operation. The distal rectal segment should be irrigated and thoroughly cleansed at the time of initial surgery and adequate drainage of the retro-rectal space provided.

Liver injuries should be treated by excision of the damaged tissue, haemostasis and very thorough drainage. Wounds of the spleen are treated by splenectomy. Pancreatic injuries require repair and thorough drainage if it is minor or involving the head of the pancreas, whereas severe injuries of the body or the tail require resection and drainage.

Infection in war wounds

All war wounds are grossly contaminated and will inevitably become infected unless treated quickly and correctly. Ideally these wounds should be treated surgically by excision of the damaged tissue within 6 h. Up to this time the wound is simply contaminated but delay allows invasive infection to become established and successful treatment becomes less likely.

The major threat to a patient with a war wound is the development of gas gangrene. Clostridia are sensitive to penicillins, erythromycin and tetracyclines and penicillin is the antibiotic of choice. Despite the great therapeutic use of antibiotics in infected wounds, they are no substitute for adequate excision of dead tissues and general surgical principles such as faecal diversion. All soft-tissue wounds should therefore receive benzylpenicillin 1–5 million units IV as soon as possible after wounding and 6 hourly thereafter for 24 h. Abdominal wounds should be treated by penicillin as above together with an appropriate antibiotic for colonic organisms such as metronidazole plus a cephalosporin or ureidopenicillin.

Mortality

The mortality from missile wounds and explosive blast injury is high. Even when the best facilities are available, together with a short evacuation time, the mortality is of the order of 18 per cent. If relatively minor injuries are excluded, the mortality rises to between 20 and 25 per cent, and if high-velocity penetrating or perforating missile injuries alone are included, the mortality rate exceeds 30 per cent. Mortality is four to five times higher for high-velocity wounds than for low-velocity and stab wounds. The important factors that influence mortality and morbidity rates are:

- the type of missile, whether high- or low-velocity
- the part of the body that is hit
- the organs that are damaged
- the delay before surgery

All these variables must be clearly separated and defined

before any comparison of various series of gunshot wounds is made. The principles of management of high-velocity missile wounds is based upon the treatment of millions of patients and the experience of many thousands of surgeons. These principles and simple methods work. They have stood the test of time, and many patients have had to suffer in the past when surgeons have had to relearn these principles the hard way in every war, or every situation that involves high-velocity missile wounds.

Further reading

1. Dufour, D., Owen-Smith, M.S., and Stening, G.F. (ed.). (1988). *Surgery for victims of war*. International committee of the Red Cross, Geneva.
2. *Field Surgery Pocket Book*. (1981). HMSO, London.
3. Janzon, B. (1983). *High energy missile trauma*. University of Göteborg, Sweden.
4. *N.A.T.O. Emergency War Surgery*. (1975). First revision. US Government Printing Office, Washington, DC.
5. Ordog, G.J. (ed.). (1988). *Management of gunshot wounds*. Elsevier, New York.
6. Owen-Smith, M.S. (1981). *High velocity missile wounds*. Edward Arnold, London.
7. Rich, N.M. and Spencer, F.C. (1978). *Vascular trauma*. Saunders, Philadelphia, Penn.
8. Swan, K.G. and Swan, R.C. (1980). *Gunshot wounds: pathophysiology and management*. PSB Publishing, Littleton, Mass.

18

Gas gangrene

E. PAXTON DEWAR

Introduction

Gas gangrene is an acute, spreading infection of muscle caused by bacteria of the *Clostridium* species, the main pathogenic organisms being *Clostridium perfringens*, *Clostridium septicum*, and *Clostridium novyi*. The rapid spread and severity of the infection is due to the powerful toxins produced by these organisms.

Gas gangrene should be considered neither a disease of the past nor peculiar to war wounds or other forms of trauma. Some 50 per cent of patients presenting with gas gangrene have no history of trauma and, despite advances in treatment by surgery, antibiotics and hyperbaric oxygen, the morbidity and mortality remain high, possibly because of lack of awareness. The condition is invariably fatal if untreated and successful management is dependent upon anticipation of the problem and early therapeutic intervention.

Terminology

The term gas gangrene is synonymous with *necrotizing myositis* and *clostridial myonecrosis* and all fulfil the definition of gas gangrene. However, because organisms other than *Clostridium* spp. produce gas in the tissues, a confusing nomenclature has evolved regarding necrotizing soft tissue infections which may confound the unwary if only because of the interchange of terminology. In particular, the terms 'necrotizing fasciitis', 'clostridial gangrene', 'synergistic', and 'streptococcal gangrene' need clarification.

Necrotizing fasciitis is a rapidly progressive necrosis of fascia (1) caused by multiple, mainly enteric, organisms. Crepitus may be present due to gas in the tissues in 50 per cent of patients in the absence of *Clostridium* spp. (2).

Clostridial gangrene is a necrotizing cellulitis which involves clostridial organisms but is associated with other Gram-positive and Gram-negative organisms in up to 75 per cent of cases (2, 3). Crepitance is present in about 50 per cent of patients only and in a similar percentage the source of the infection is the gastrointestinal (GI) tract rather than trauma.

Synergistic gangrene is an erythematous cellulitis that progresses through vesicle formation to necrotic ulceration. Clostridial organisms are not involved and the name arises from the synergistic action of streptococci and staphylococci described by Meleney (4). It is associated with either trauma or post-operative wounds.

Streptococcal gangrene, as the name implies, is caused by various strains of haemolytic streptococcus. It presents as a diffuse spreading cellulitis associated with thrombosis of the cutaneous vessels, usually as a result of trauma.

Aetiology

Gas gangrene is caused by organisms of the *Clostridium* species. These Gram-positive, anaerobic, spore forming bacilli produce a variety of exotoxins which, in the right environment, are severely damaging to human tissues.

The commonest causative organism is *C. perfringens* but *C. novyi* and *C. septicum*, although less common, are also important aetiological agents. Often more than one species is isolated and in addition to the three commonest species others such as *C. histolyticum*, *C. bifermentans*, and *C. sporogenes* are occasionally found.

Soil and the GI tract of humans and animals are the natural environment of these saprophytes whose growth is dependent in the main upon strict anaerobic conditions. The presence of oxygen not only inhibits the growth of the bacteria but also affects production of exotoxins by the bacteria. Factors that operate to reduce available oxygen in wounds such as dead tissue, tissue ischaemia, and foreign bodies all potentiate the proliferation of the *Clostridium* spp. and the production of the toxins.

Historically, gas gangrene has presented in large numbers in wartime and therefore is classically associated with battlefield injuries. However, nowadays some 50 per cent of patients who develop gas gangrene have not sustained trauma but the infection either occurs spontaneously or after elective surgery (5). After trauma the source of infection is usually exogenous contamination whereas after elective surgery endogenous clostridia from the GI tract are the most likely source. In spontaneous cases, where there has been no trauma or surgery, the underlying primary diagnoses have included large bowel pathology, particularly carcinoma, peripheral vascular disease, diabetes, and cholecystitis.

Elective surgery

Recognition of those patients most at risk after elective surgery should lead to appropriate prophylactic measures being taken to reduce the chances of endogenous contamination.

Surgeons should be aware of the presence of *Clostridium* spp. in human faeces and the spores on the skin, particularly from the waist down. Care should be taken prior to major surgery especially of the lower limbs where there may be reduced oxygen tension and ischaemia of the tissues, particularly in the elderly and those with peripheral vascular disease. Skin preparation, as normally practised, is insufficient to kill the clostridial spores but numbers may be reduced by more prolonged preparation with antiseptics such as povidone -iodine. In addition there should be high tissue levels of antibiotic before and during surgery. Intravenous penicillin is the drug of choice for this purpose.

Trauma

The wound is already present in traumatized patients and in addition to possible contamination from endogenous sources, exogenous contamination from soil or clothing must be considered. If a wound is contaminated by foreign bodies or if the trauma has resulted in devitalized tissue then the likelihood of proliferation of gas gangrene bacilli is greatly increased. In crush injuries and low- velocity missile wounds the area of devitalized tissue will be apparent but it must be remembered that the temporary cavitation caused by a high-velocity missile results in ischaemia to the tissues far beyond the defined track of the missile with a consequent increase in the risk of gas gangrene.

In such patients the aim of prevention is to produce an environment which is not conducive to the multiplication of the bacteria. Prophylactic penicillin in high dose should be commenced immediately and the casualty transferred to a surgical facility where excisional surgery can be performed as soon as possible. These two measures are complementary but the surgery is of the greater importance.

The use of antitoxins in prophylaxis has not been widely accepted as allergic reactions may be severe and the risk-to-benefit ratio is poor (6).

Microbiology

Louis Pasteur first described *Clostridium butyricum* in 1861 and since then more than 150 species of clostridia have been recognized. Some 40 to 50 of these have been identified in human faecal flora. (6). The *Clostridium* spp. are Gram-positive, anaerobic, spore-forming, putrefactive bacilli which may be motile or non-motile depending on the species. Whilst most are soil contaminants they can also be isolated from the GI tract and skin. The putrefaction and decomposition of the body after death are in part due to such clostridia as *C. perfringens* and *C. sporogenes* entering the blood and tissues at the time of death.

C. perfringens is the main causative agent of gas gangrene in man and was originally identified by Welch and Nuttall (6, 7) hence its original nomenclature *C. welchii*. *C. septicum* and *C. novyi* also cause classical gas gangrene being both toxigenic and proteolytic like *C. perfringens*.

C. histolyticum, *C. bifermentans*, and *C. sporogenes* are less pathogenic and have mainly proteolytic rather than toxigenic properties by which they augment infection. Other species such as *C. sordelii*, *C. tertium*, and *C. butyricum* are usually only wound contaminants.

Clostridium perfringens, *C. septicum*, and *C. novyi* are the major opportunistic pathogens causing gas gangrene and have a wide range of toxic activities. Each produces between 4 and 12 toxins (labelled alpha, beta, gamma, etc.). Many of the toxins are characterised by specific enzymatic activities, thus *C. perfringens* produces phospholipase C, collagenase, hyaluronidase, and deoxyribonuclease and its lethal potential is due to the alpha toxin, phospholipase C.

The clostridia bacilli, straight or slightly curved rods, are large with rounded ends. Different forms occur in culture such as filaments, club forms and spindle shapes, the latter giving the genus its name, a clostridium being a little spindle. Though some are microaerophilic the majority are true obligate anaerobes and all are capable of producing spores which can survive the most adverse conditions. The spores are the most important factor in the transmission of the bacteria from contaminated soil to wounds, but vegetative forms can be recovered from soil and may also be involved in wound contamination.

Pathogenesis

In a wound contaminated by clostridia the development of gas gangrene (clostridial myonecrosis) depends upon the organisms having an environment conducive to their growth. In damaged tissue, be it post-traumatic or post-surgical, the vascular supply is inevitably compromized and tissue oxygen tension (pO_2) is lowered. If, for whatever reason, the pO_2 is lowered significantly then the anaerobic clostridia will thrive.

In traumatic wounds the infection usually results from contamination by soil or clothing, though trauma involving the GI tract is another source. In post-operative wounds the source may be the skin or the GI tract and in criminal abortion the damaged uterine muscle is contaminated by clostridia from the perineal skin causing uterine muscle necrosis. In spontaneous cases metastatic myonecrosis may be caused by a breach in the large bowel mucosa usually associated with a neoplasm. Other spontaneous cases have occurred in patients where diabetes, peripheral vascular disease, or large bowel abscesses have been the underlying pathology.

In healthy tissue, with a normal pO_2, the anaerobic bacilli and spores cannot resist phagocytosis, are unable to grow, and cannot produce toxins. Therefore the risk factors which predispose to the development of gas gangrene are those that cause a low pO_2 in the tissues such as impaired blood supply, residual devitalized tissue, and the presence of foreign bodies or old blood clot subsequent to the original trauma.

The toxins are produced once the infection is established in the devitalized muscle. A rapidly progressive process ensues with the toxins spreading to surrounding muscle which, though previously healthy, will have become oedematous in response to the initial devitalized focus. The oedema results in a further reduction in blood supply to the area and a consequent lowering of tissue pO_2. The toxins compound the insult by killing muscle and extending the area of necrotic tissue in which the clostridia can flourish, produce yet more toxins and continue the spreading process along tissue planes.

Increasing oedema and the consequent tissue ischaemia not only result in further lowering of pO_2 but also prevent the inflammatory response by limiting the ingress of polymorphs. The fulminant phase of the process is now under way and, untreated, the infection will come to involve whole muscle groups. As a result of the rapidity of spread the patient may develop fulminant toxaemia in as little as 12 hours in the most severe cases.

Clostridial contamination of the traumatised uterine muscle in criminal abortion causes the specific entity of uterine myonecrosis. However, the mechanisms by which the organisms gain access to the blood stream, settle upon apparently healthy muscle distant from the source, and initiate spontaneous necrosis of this muscle—metastatic myonecrosis—are not readily apparent.

Incidence

The true incidence of gas gangrene is difficult to estimate. Historically it was associated with war wounds, grossly contaminated with clothing, faecal material and soil, that were not properly treated. It was very common on the battlefields of Europe during the First World War, 1914–18, but less so in the Second World War, 1939–45, as medical teams were better organized. The incidence partly reflects the time taken for the injured person to reach a surgical facility following trauma. There were very few cases amongst American servicemen in Vietnam where evacuation helicopters were used, and in the Falkland Islands campaign it was virtually non-existent because of the short evacuation time and the highly organized and aware medical teams (8). The advent of appropriate antibiotics since the Second World War has contributed greatly to prophylaxis and treatment. However, the incidence has increased in civilian practice in recent years because of the increase in urban terrorism and the development of high velocity weapons.

Overall gas gangrene is a relatively rare condition and its occurrence depends upon a number of factors—not least the presence of viable organisms and tissues conducive to bacterial multiplication. The potential for infection is substantially increased by a number of risk factors (Table 18.1). The proximity of the wound to a source of faecal bacteria, such as occurs after hip surgery, lower limb amputation in the presence of ischaemia and peripheral vascular disease, the degree of contamination with foreign objects and dirt and the presence of wounds involving large muscle masses as in the buttocks, thighs, and shoulders all predispose to gas gangrene. Certain types of injury also present high risk, including crush injuries, burns, and compound fractures, particularly if there is associated vascular damage.

Table 18.1. High-risk factors in gas gangrene.

Wounds of large muscle
Crush injury
Compound fracture
Burns
Severe wound contamination
Hip surgery
Ischaemia
Lower limb amputation
Peripheral vascular disease

Estimates of the incidence of gas gangrene have varied from up to 1000 patients per year in the United States (9) to 56 patients over a two-year period in 55 British hospitals after clean elective operations (10). If this latter figure is extrapolated to include post-traumatic and 'spontaneous' presentation there would be over 3000 cases a year in the United States of which 35 per cent would be following elective clean surgery (5).

Prevention

The mortality in established gas gangrene is between 10 and 30 per cent (5) and therefore prevention is an important consideration in an attempt to reduce the incidence, morbidity, and mortality. The approach to prevention depends upon whether the patient is at risk from a traumatic or non-traumatic situation. In the former both exogenous and endogenous sources of contamination may be implicated but in the latter only the endogenous source is likely.

Clinical features

The incubation period of gas gangrene is not usually greater than four days, maybe less than 24 h and, not uncommonly, is as short as 6–12 h. The clinical features are both local and systemic and the chronological development of the signs and symptoms from the outset is very rapid.

Local signs

The first local symptom is the sudden onset of severe unremitting pain that increases in severity disproportionately to the extent of the wound or incision. This is rapidly followed by changes in the appearance of the wound. The overlying skin becomes blanched, stretched, and oedematous prior to discolouration which may be purple, blue, bronze or grey. Subsequently, haemorrhagic bullae, frank necrosis, and an extending margin of erythema develop (Fig. 18.1). Although gas may be present in the tissues, crepitation is often not a prominent sign until late in the process when it is associated with exquisite tenderness over the area. The wound classically emits a sweet odour, and produces a brown watery discharge.

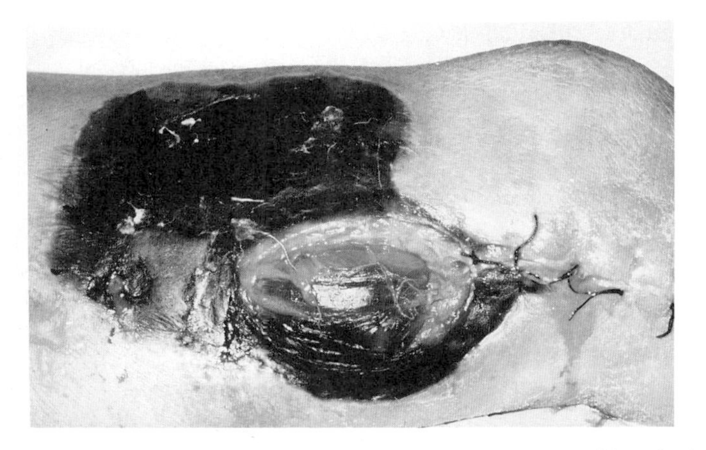

Fig. 18.1. Gas gangrene of the leg demonstrating blanched oedematous skin, purple discoloration, haemorrhagic bullae, frank necrosis, and an extending margin of erythema. Tight skin sutures and brown watery discharge are also shown. (See plate section.)

Systemic changes

The patient develops a low or moderate pyrexia initially but becomes sweaty and has a tachycardia in excess of that expected with the degree of pyrexia. Although apparently alert and orientated but restless, paradoxically the patient exhibits signs of indifference to his situation despite often having a sense of impending doom. Toxic delirium develops late. Hypotension, jaundice, and renal failure occur in the later stages of the disease and death may ensue in less than 48 hours.

Diagnosis

The diagnosis of gas gangrene is based upon three major factors: an awareness of gas gangrene as an entity, a high index of suspicion, and accurate clinical assessment. The diagnosis must be made on clinical grounds as quickly as possible because rapid progression of the myonecrotic process can result in death within hours if inappropriately treated. Haematological, radiological, and microbiological investigations play only a minor part in the initial diagnosis but can provide important confirmation.

A history of trauma with wound contamination, particularly in missile injuries and especially high-velocity missile injuries, or a history of recent surgery followed by an unexpected and very sudden deterioration in the condition of the patient should alert the clinician to the possibility. Additional risk factors such as peripheral vascular disease or hypotension, resulting in reduced tissue perfusion generally and locally, should increase the level of suspicion. Mechanical causes of reduced blood flow such as tight skin sutures, marked abdominal distension, and constricting plaster casts or bandages should heighten suspicion. The diabetic, immunodeficient, or already infected patient is also at greater risk.

Thus alerted, a thorough and accurate clinical examination to elicit any of the clinical features previously described must be performed immediately. All positive findings must be assiduously recorded to establish a baseline of information. Treatment must not be delayed whilst waiting for the results of investigations, and serial examinations and monitoring, all fully recorded, form part of the continuing assessment.

The differential diagnoses—necrotizing fasciitis, necrotizing cellulitis, synergistic gangrene, and streptococcal gangrene—must be considered as in any clinical assessment. In the majority of patients these alternatives do not produce such rapid deterioration or such severe toxicity as gas gangrene.

Even the presence of gas in the tissues with myonecrosis does not necessarily mean a diagnosis of gas gangrene. Other organisms such as *Proteus* spp., *Escherichia coli*, *Klebsiella* spp., *Pseudomonas* spp., and *Bacteroides* spp. can present a similar picture (11).

Gram staining of the wound discharge or exudate, if possible obtained from deeper parts of the wound, may demonstrate many large Gram-positive bacilli with or without spores. A paucity of polymorphs exists in contrast to the findings in the other possible diagnoses where, in addition, the predominant bacteria may be Gram-positive cocci.

Other, non-bacterial, causes of gas in the tissues—recent previous surgery, the direct effects of trauma, high pressure air hose injury, and barotrauma—should be considered, but these are not normally associated with the profound constitutional disturbances seen in gas gangrene.

Culture of necrotic tissue, wound slough, or discharge is too slow for diagnostic purposes (48–72 h often being required for growth in culture) and does not necessarily confirm a diagnosis of gas gangrene because non-pathogenic colonization of wounds by clostridia is not uncommon.

Characteristically *C. perfringens* appear as thick rectangular bacilli on Gram staining and only rarely are spores present. Scanty Gram-positive bacilli with oval subterminal spores sug-

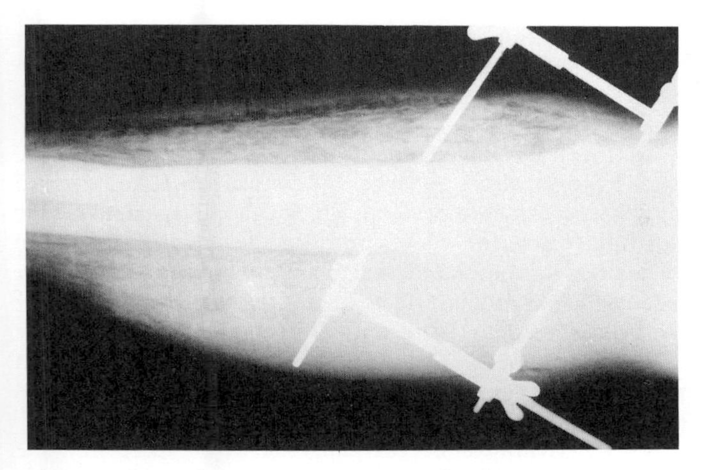

Fig. 18.2. Gas in the tissues presenting a feathery appearance on radiography.

gest *C. novyi* as the causative organism, whilst the irregularly staining pleomorphic leaf-shaped so-called 'citron bodies' suggest *C. septicum*. The organisms can be more accurately differentiated by testing with specific antisera, but accurate laboratory identification does not alter the requirement for urgent treatment.

Radiological examination may show small amounts of gas in early lesions but, whilst the absence of gas does not preclude the diagnosis of gas gangrene, its presence is not pathognomonic. Gas may not be present at any stage or may only appear late in the disease process. If present, a feathery appearance rather than discrete bubbles suggests spread between muscle fibres and is a more positive indication of gas gangrene (Fig. 18.2).

Management

The management of gas gangrene is based upon antibiotics, excisional surgery, and hyperbaric oxygen. The effectiveness of serum therapy has not been proven and the risks of allergic reactions are as yet unacceptable. Clinical experience has shown that wound excision alone does not significantly lower the morbidity or mortality, and that antibiotics alone do not prevent gas gangrene if the wound is not correctly excised.

Various vogues in treatment have been proposed over the years suggesting that antibiotics, surgery, or hyperbaric oxygen, alone or in any combination, give equally successful results, but the larger clinical series point to the fact that it is a combination of all three which gives the most effective results (5, 9, 12).

Survival rates of 95 per cent have been demonstrated with the combined therapy in animal models compared with 70 per cent survival after surgery and antibiotics without hyperbaric oxygen (13). Survival using antibiotics alone was 50 per cent, and if surgery or hyperbaric oxygen were used singularly then the survival rate was zero. The survival rate using the combined therapy in humans is normally between 70 to 80 per cent (5).

In addition to these specific aspects of treatment these severely ill patients require intensive supportive care to counteract the effects of the complications such as shock, blood loss, dehydration, acid–base imbalance, haemolytic anaemic, and secondary infection.

Antibiotic therapy

Antibiotics form a major part of the specific treatment of gas gangrene and complement surgery and hyperbaric oxygen. They are not a substitute for adequate surgery.

Penicillin remains the drug of choice for both treatment and prophylaxis though in severely ill patients many would use combination antibiotic therapy, with penicillin, aminoglycosides, and clindamycin as the most likely choices (12). Penicillin therapy should be of high dosage in an attempt to obtain therapeutic levels in the relatively avascular tissues. Doses of 20–40 million units intravenously per day are required.

Penicillin should still be considered even in those patients reported to be sensitive to penicillin. If there is a convincing history of penicillin allergy an alternative antibiotic should be administered until sensitivity testing has been performed but only approximately 10 per cent of those reputed to be allergic will actually be so. The alternatives to penicillin therapy are tetracycline in a dose of 2–4 g intravenously per day, although clostridia have developed some resistance to this antibiotic (14). Clindamycin, erythromycin, and chloramphenicol have all been used successfully in the past. With the advent of metronidazole in the treatment of anaerobic bacterial infections, many would advocate the inclusion of this drug as concomitant treatment to cover other anaerobic organisms such as *Bacteroides fragilis*, which may also be present (6, 15).

Antibiotic therapy must be instituted early in the disease process and a sufficiently high dosage must be administered to penetrate ischaemic tissues.

Surgery

The surgical treatment of gas gangrene is of paramount importance but, alone, is less beneficial than when combined with antibiotic and hyperbaric oxygen therapy. The terminology of the actual surgical process varies but the two terms most commonly used are wound excision and wound debridement. Excision of the wound is more apt but undoubtedly the most descriptive term is wound *parage* (to pare—to cut away the edges). Whatever term is used wound excision must be radical and uncompromising. There is no evidence, other than in an animal model using an uncomplicated, uncontaminated wound of the leg in which treatment was started 30 min from the time of wounding, to suggest that anything less is adequate (16).

The wound is laid open so that all dirt and foreign bodies can be seen and removed. This process is then followed by lavage of the wound with copious quantities of normal saline and hydrogen peroxide. All haematomata must be completely evacuated and all non-viable tissue must be excised.

It can be difficult to decide exactly how much muscle is, in fact, viable. Careful assessment of the muscle, in particular its consistency, colour, contractility, and capillary bleeding when cut, is most important. If there is any doubt then the tissue should be excised. Absolute haemostasis should be achieved and the wound should be dressed with loose gauze dressings so that drainage is not compromised. Primary closure should not be contemplated.

The wound should be redressed as often as is necessary to prevent it bathing in its own exudate, and at each dressing change the wound should be thoroughly inspected and any further necrotic tissue fully excised. This process continues until all evidence of gas gangrene has been eliminated and the wound commences to heal.

It is unlikely that any form of delayed primary suture will be appropriate in such wounds, which should be allowed to heal by granulation, with the option to apply skin grafts at a later date. In the seriously ill patient with gas gangrene affecting one or more limbs, the decision may have to be made between continued muscle excision and amputation of the affected extremities.

Hyperbaric oxygen

Hyperbaric oxygen is the third element of the specific treatment regimen for gas gangrene, and complements surgery and antibiotic therapy. Hyperbaric oxygen was first used successfully in the early 1960s (17) and has become more widely used in the treatment of gas gangrene as it has become more commonly available. There is little convincing evidence that hyperbaric oxygen reduces mortality rates significantly, but its use may result in a more clear demarcation of devitalised tissue and thus assist decision-making during wound excision. It also produces a more rapid relief of the systemic toxicity associated with the disease (15, 18). However, it is important to state that surgery should not be delayed whilst awaiting transfer of the patient to a hyperbaric unit.

Hyperbaric oxygen therapy requires special equipment, close monitoring, and experienced supervision. It should be remembered that oxygen is toxic and that there are risks involved. The patient is placed in a special pressurized chamber which is equipped so that close monitoring of the patient can be maintained. One hundred per cent oxygen is breathed at varying pressures, the most common being 2.5 atmospheres (36.7 p.s.i.) for 1–2 h, 3 times a day. Using this regimen a tissue PO_2 of 250 mmHg can be achieved, the normal being between 30–40 mmHg (19).

Oxygen toxicity has not proven to be a problem with these regimens. The risks associated with hyperbaric oxygen, apart from oxygen toxicity, include barotrauma (particularly otic barotrauma), decompression sickness, lung damage, and, of course, fire hazard. Bilateral myringotomy has been advocated as prophylaxis against otic barotrauma (15).

Depending upon the progress made by the patient it is likely that hyperbaric oxygen therapy will be required for at least four days although the frequency of administration may be reduced from three times to twice a day as the condition improves. Isolation in the chamber can prove a problem to the patients, particularly when their systemic toxicity clears and their neurosensorium returns to normal. Diazepam sedation may be required.

Hyperbaric oxygen has been reported to be bactericidal *in vitro* and bacteriostatic *in vivo* (20, 21). However, its major benefit is almost certainly the reduction of spore germination and the inhibition of toxin production, or the inactivation of toxins already produced in the tissues (22). The alpha toxin of *C. perfringens* is stable even in an hyperoxygenated environment.

Another important action of this form of therapy is that the tissue hypoxia, which enhances the disease process, is reversed allowing peroxides to develop, which can kill or inactivate the clostridia. Catalase, which is produced by necrosing tissue and by blood in haematomata, inactivates peroxides and therefore reduces their beneficial effects against the bacteria. Surgery, by removing necrotic tissue and all haematomata, therefore reduces the amount of catalase available and, in conjunction with hyperoxygenation of the tissues, allows for increased production of peroxides with consequent benefit.

For the treatment of gas gangrene to be successful, the combined modalities of antibiotics, surgery, and hyperbaric oxygen, with their individual and synergistic contributions, offer the best chance to the patient. The clinician must be aware of the possibility of gas gangrene if he is to make an early diagnosis and initiate immediate, aggressive intervention. Nevertheless, gas gangrene still has a mortality rate of between 20 and 30 per cent and the morbidity associated with life-saving wide excisional surgery is not inconsiderable. However, rehabilitation can produce remarkable functional results in muscle groups which have been severely affected. Undoubtedly the worst prognosis is associated with delay in diagnosis or commencement of treatment, the presence of shock or secondary infection, and factors which compromise the resistance of the patient such as concomitant illness, immune deficiency, and old age. In these patients, the clinician must be particularly aware that gas gangrene can occur, prophylaxis should be considered, and therapy should be early and adequate.

References

1. Bacter, C. R. (1972). Surgical management of soft tissue infections. *Surg. Clin. North Am.*, **52**, 1483–98.
2. Freischlag, J. A., Ajalat, G., and Busuttil, R. W. (1985). Treatment of necrotizing soft tissue infection. *Am. J. Surg.*, **149**, 751–5.
3. Caplan, S. and Kluge, R. M. (1976). Gas gangrene. *Arch. Intern. Med.*, **136**, 788–91.
4. Meleney, F. L. (1924). Haemolytic streptococcus gangrene. *Arch. Surg.*, **9**, 17–35.
5. Hart, G. B., Lamb, R. C., and Strauss, M. B. (1983). Gas gangrene. *J. Trauma*, **23**, 991–1000.
6. George, W. L. and Finegold, S. M. (1989). Clostridial infections. In *Textbook of internal medicine* (ed. W. N. Kelley), pp. 1557–62. Lippincott, Philadelphia, Penn.
7. Welch, W. H. and Nuttall, G. H. (1892). A gas-producing bacillus capable of rapid development in blood vessels after death. *Bull. Johns Hopkins Hosp.*, **3**, 81–91.
8. Jackson, D. S., Batty, C. G., Ryan, J. M., and McGregor, W. S. P. (1983). The Falklands War: Army field surgical experience. *Ann. R. Coll. Surg. Engl.*, **65**, 281–5.
9. Hitchcock, C. R., Demello, F. J., and Haglin, J. J. (1975). Gangrene infection: New approaches to an old disease. *Surg. Clin. North Am.*, **55**, 1403–10.
10. Parker, M. T. (1969). Post-operative clostridial infection in Britain. *Br. Med. J.*, **3**, 671–6.

11. Bessman, A.N., and Wagner, W. (1975). Non-clostridial 'gas gangrene'. Report of 48 cases and review of the literature. *J. Am. Med. Assoc.*, **233**, 958–63.
12. Hirn, M. and Niinikoski, J. (1988). Hyperbaric oxygen in the treatment of clostridial gangrene. *Ann. Chir. Gynecol.*, **77**, 37–40.
13. Demello, F.J., Haglin, J.J., and Hitchcock, C.R. (1973). Comparative study of experimental Clostridium perfringens infection in dogs treated with antibiotics, surgery and hyperbaric oxygen. *Surgery*, **73**, 936–41.
14. Johnstone, F.R.C. and Cockcroft, W.H. (1968). Clostridium welchii resistance to tetracycline. *Lancet*, **i**, 660–1.
15. Gibson, A. and Davis, F.M. (1986). Hyperbaric oxygen therapy in the management of clostridium perfringens infections. *NZ Med. J.*, **99**, 617–20.
16. Fackler, M.L., Breteau, J.P.L., Courbil, L.J. *et al.* (1989). Open wound drainage versus wound excision in treating the modern assault rifle wound. *Surgery*, **105**, 576–84.
17. Brummelkamp, W.H., Hogendijk, J., and Boerema, I. (1961). Treatment of anaerobic infections (clostridial myositis) by drenching the tissues with oxygen under high atmospheric pressure. *Surgery*, **49**, 299–302.
18. Larson, H.E. (1987). Botulism, gas gangrene and clostridial gastrointestinal infections. In *Oxford textbook of medicine* (ed. D.J. Weatherall, J.G.G. Leadingham, and D.A. Wassell), pp. 273–4. Oxford University Press, Oxford.
19. Wells, C.H., Goodpasture, J.E., Horrigan, D.J. *et al.* (1977). Tissue gas measurements during hyperbaric oxygen exposure. In *Proceedings of the Sixth International Congress on Hyperbaric Medicine* (ed. G. Smith), pp. 118–24. Aberdeen University Press.
20. Hill, G.B. and Osterhout, S. (1972). Experimental effects of hyperbaric oxygen on selected clostridial species: I. *In-vitro* studies. *J. Infect. Dis.*, **125**, 17–25.
21. Hill, G.B. and Osterhout, S. (1972). Experimental effects of hyperbaric oxygen on selected clostridial species: II. *In-vivo* studies in mice. *J. Infect. Dis.*, **125**, 26–35.
22. Demello, F.J., Hashimoto, T., Hitchcock, C.R., and Haglin, J.J. (1970). The effect of hyperbaric oxygen on the germination and toxin production of Clostridium perfringens spores. In *Proceedings of the Fourth International Congress of Hyperbaric Medicine*, Tokyo (ed. J. Wada and T. Iwa), pp. 276–81. Igaku Shoin, Tokyo.

19

Antibiotic prophylaxis in the gastrointestinal tract

T. VINCENT TAYLOR

Introduction

Despite the plethora of antibiotics available to us, the number of which is increasing almost by the week, septic complications remain today the most common cause of death following gastrointestinal (GI) surgery. Prophylactic antibiotics are of proven value in GI surgery; their use has been shown to reduce infections of the wound and peritoneum and also associated respiratory tract and urinary tract infections, though possibly not to reduce post-operative mortality (1–3). In the USA approximately one-third of hospitalized patients receive antibiotics and, of these, up to one-half receive prophylactic antibiotics, primarily for surgical procedures (4). In GI surgery many surgeons now use prophylactic antibiotics for all operative procedures, even clean procedures such as highly selective vagotomy. For clean–contaminated procedures such as cholecystectomy the role of prophylactic antibiotics is now well-proven and for contaminated colorectal operations the use of appropriate antibiotic prophylaxis is mandatory. Along with the use of prophylactic antibiotics in GI surgery there are, in appropriate situations, indications for other methods of reducing bacterial counts in relation to surgery and these may involve mechanical preparation and the use of antiseptics. A further important factor in reducing infection is meticulous surgical technique.

It was pointed out by Pollock as recently as 1988, that 'no amount of antibiotic, however potent, can compensate for clumsy operating and hypoxic conditions' (5).

The only proven way of enhancing host resistance is to ensure an adequate supply of oxygenated blood to the tissues that are contaminated by bacteria (6). Factors which increase the risk of wound infection are malnutrition, prolonged operations, dehydration and poor tissue perfusion, old age, immunosuppression, cancer chemotherapy, and blood transfusion (7). We have learned over the years that when the appropriate antibiotic is administered, with optimal timing and duration of therapy by a suitable route, antibiotic prophylaxis is not only valuable but failure to use it in an increasing number of clinical situations in the GI tract surgery is now regarded as negligent (8).

The principles of prophylaxis are: to avoid or minimize bacterial contamination, to use antibiotics intelligently, and to do nothing to compromise the host's ability to defeat invaders (9). Pertinent questions relating to the use of prophylactic antibiotics, many of which remain to be solved in certain situations, are the length and duration of prophylaxis; the route of administration; the choice of agent, given the type or even location of surgery; and the prevention of complications solely attributable to inappropriate antibiotic usage. One of the problems when selecting an appropriate antibiotic for prophylaxis is the interpretation of clinical trials reported in the literature. In a review of 131 clinical trials of systemic antibiotic prophylaxis only 18 per cent were found to be appropriately designed and to give meaningful data (10).

As in other branches of surgery, the effect of prophylaxis is most easily, accurately, and appropriately studied in GI surgery by assessing wound infection. The establishment of intra-peritoneal infection requires a much larger inoculum of bacteria, it is uncommon and is usually due to a major intra-abdominal surgical problem such as dehiscence of the suture line. In general, an inoculum of 1×10^5 bacteria when introduced into the wound may induce infection whereas in the peritoneum it is many times more, and the risk is increased many fold by the presence of a foreign body, or by ischaemic or devitalized tissue. It has been estimated that septic complications of GI surgery double the average hospital stay with a comparable increase in costs. A number of factors unrelated to the use of antibiotics influence the development of post-operative wound infection. These have been outlined elsewhere in this book but are: the length of hospitalization, in particular pre-operative stay (11); shaving the abdomen (12); pre-operative bathing with hexochlorophane; the use of drains and pre-operative preparation by the surgical team.

The use of drains in GI surgery remains a controversial issue. Skin bacteria are frequently found on the interior of abdominal drains thus introducing the 'two-way street' concept of drainage and access. Magee (13) demonstrated that the presence of either silastic or latex Penrose drains in experimental wounds dramatically enhanced the wound infection rate even in the presence of sub-infective doses of bacteria. It has long been known that, in general terms, the presence of a foreign body within the tissue acts as a nidus for infection and renders eradication of that infection almost impossible until the foreign body has been removed. It has been concluded that the use of abdominal drains is unwarranted and indeed may be dangerous practice. The matter remains controversial, but when they are used, drains should be placed through sites other than the primary surgical incision to decrease the incidence of subsequent wound infection. Closed suction drainage is the method of choice when abdominal wound drainage is indicated (14).

Goals in effective prophylaxis

In GI surgery large numbers of organisms can be rapidly released into the tissues. The ability of these organisms to cause infections depends upon the type, the pathogenicity, and on the multiplicity of organisms that are present. The interaction between the different organisms and the time that these are present before the antimicrobials reach the tissues is important.

Infection is common after GI surgery, with *Escherichia coli* and a variety of streptococci from the endogenous flora, chiefly *Streptococcus faecalis* being the predominant pathogens. *Staphylococcus aureus* remains a problem. Anaerobic bacteria alone are relatively uncommon as a single source of infection, as are *Proteus* and *Pseudomonas* spp.. Mixed infections, however, are much more common than those due to a single organism and here anaerobic organisms often predominate. When a large number of organisms are present it is probable that there will be a great diversity of organism species and that the infection rate will be higher. Here, anaerobic organisms are the predominant normal flora of which *Bacteroides fragilis* comprises only 13 per cent, but in cultures from post-operative infections this species is present in 83 per cent. This organism has a greater, if only opportunistic, potential to cause infection.

The most damaging combination of organisms following GI surgery is that of Gram-negative rods and anaerobes. When *E. coli* is combined with *B. fragilis* the life phase and growth of the *B. fragilis* is dramatically reduced allowing the two organisms to grow together, thus reducing the local oxygen supply and hence promoting growth of *B. fragilis* synergistically. Under these circumstances coliforms are usually isolated from blood in the event of septicaemia and bacteroides from any abscesses which occur later.

Choice of antibiotics

Controversy still exists over the choice of individual agents, the dose, the duration of administration, the route of administration, the toxicity, and the cost of prophylaxis. The ability of the organisms released into the tissues when the GI tract is opened to produce infection, depends upon type, pathogenicity and the multiplicity of the organisms present (15). The interaction between the different organisms and the time that these are present before the antimicrobials reach the tissue are also important. Ideally, antimicrobial prophylaxis has to be given before the organisms gain access to the tissues, and delay of more than four hours eliminates all benefits (16). It is possible that the production of a biofilm or 'slime' by an organism protects that organism from the antibiotic. This is an area which is currently undergoing investigation.

As infections in GI surgery are usually produced by multiple organisms, often acting synergistically (17), it is important that a broad spectrum antibiotic or combination of antibiotics should be used prophylactically. When there is heavy gut colonization by anaerobic bacteria, as in the colon, it is essential that the prophylactic antibiotic used is active against these organisms. Despite bacterial synergy, prophylaxis must be aimed at preventing infection by both anaerobic and aerobic bacteria. In addition to endogenous organisms it must be remembered that *Staph. aureus* and other exogenous organisms may act alone or in concert with the endogenous organisms to produce infection (18). Many of these patients have had various types of catheters introduced and, therefore, run the risk of *Staph. epidermidis* infection.

Spread of infection in GI surgery is most commonly produced by *E. coli* which may give rise to a Gram-negative septicaemia. Other organisms with a tendency to spread through the blood stream are *Bacteroides*, *Pseudomonas* spp., streptococcus and clostridia. Hence the strategy used to prevent or treat early septicaemia must be to use a broad spectrum antibiotic (19).

In choosing the antibiotic a relatively long serum half-life is an obvious advantage for prophylactic use. However, in biliary prophylaxis where anaerobic bacteria are less likely to be present and operations are often of short duration, such longer term cover is less important (20). Antibiotic resistance has increased considerably in recent years. This is particularly true in the case of methicillin resistant *Staph. epidermidis* and resistance can be transferred from these organisms to *Staph. aureus*. In long-standing, overwhelming surgical infections resistance to the newer antimicrobials; cephalosporins, beta-lactams, and quinolones occurs, particularly with organisms such as pseudomonas, enterobacter, and staphylococci. Thus caution is required in the employment of new antibiotics and the overuse of single agents (21). Attempts to reduce the development of resistance have been made by using differing agents for prophylaxis and for treatment, or by using different agents in rotation. These attempts are, however, unlikely to be effective as resistance frequently arises to multiple agents, and cross-cover occurs. Such considerations do much to promote the shortest effective duration of prophylactic antibiotics (22).

In determining the efficacy of our prophylactic agents we are subject to the inherent delay in culturing the organisms. Attempts have been made to predict the infective organisms by simple direct microscopy of operative samples, or by gas liquid chromatography. These have proved disappointing and further attempts are being made which employ sophisticated techniques of computerized imaging, or DNA probes, to identify early the offending organism.

Kinetics of the prophylactic agent

In choosing an appropriate antibiotic for the particular type of gastrointestinal surgery being undertaken kinetic considerations are important. The half-life (t½) of the drug should be considered in the light of the expected duration of the operation. Some agents demonstrate the 'post-antibiotic effect' whereby there is persistent suppression of bacterial growth after only limited exposure to an antibiotic. This bacteriostatic phase may persist for several hours after the plasma concentration of the drug has fallen to values below the minimum inhibitory concentration (MIC) (23).

Route of administration

Patients undergoing elective GI surgery will have fasted for at least six hours prior to their operation. They may absorb oral antibiotics poorly, or may be vomiting, and almost invariably will have a paralytic ileus post-operatively for at least 24–48 h. The route of administration of the antibiotic is of fundamental importance. The clinician is attempting to achieve a high, safe level of antibiotic in the serum and soft tissues, in the peritoneal cavity and particularly in the wound. As the major aim of antibiotic prophylaxis is to reduce wound infection it is tissue levels in the wound which are perhaps of greatest importance. These high levels of the chosen antimicrobial should ideally be present from the outset of the operation and adequate concentration should be maintained until well after the wound has been closed.

Some of the early trials of antibiotic prophylaxis employed the installation of antibiotic into the abdominal wound by either injection or spray at the time of surgical closure and agents have been introduced into the peritoneal cavity on completion of the procedure. Topical antibiotics may be applied to surgical wounds in sprays, dry powders, or by irrigation through drains. Although very high levels of antibiotic can be achieved along the wound, organisms introduced into that wound during the time of operation will have had the opportunity to multiply and become established, thus placing greater demands on the prophylaxis. Intramuscular injection of the agent in appropriate dosage gives adequate serum, and ultimately tissue, levels with sustained levels in the serum due to continuing absorption from the injection site. Optimal timing of the intramuscular injection is important and serum levels become adequate usually between 15 and 30 min after the injection. These levels should have been achieved by the time the intestine is opened.

From the time of Halsted, surgeons have irrigated wounds with saline during operations (24). This has recently been extended to incorporate antiseptics in the saline which may be introduced into the peritoneal cavity (25–27). These agents are almost certainly less effective than an appropriate parenteral antibiotic.

Matheson and co-workers in Aberdeen combined an intravenous injection of tetracycline 500 mg pre-operatively with irrigation of the peritoneal cavity and parietes with one litre of a 0.1 per cent tetracycline solution and produced remarkably low rates of infection (28). However, Pollock and co-workers found that a single pre-operative intravenous dose of latamoxef produced better prophylaxis than intra-peritoneal 0.1 per cent tetracycline alone (29).

The oral route is less commonly used for antibiotic prophylaxis presently. The administration of antibiotic prophylaxis orally may predispose to super-infection and pseudo-membranous colitis and may also increase the risk of emergence of bacterial resistance to the drugs used. Use of suppositories can be valuable. For example, metronidazole suppositories have been shown to provide useful prophylaxis for appendicectomy.

The intravenous route delivers all of the antibiotic into the peripheral compartment and, following bolus injection, serum levels become optimal in minutes, thereafter falling off more rapidly than with the intramuscular route. Intravenous administration is essential for emergency cases where peritoneal contamination exists prior to surgery but this is therapy not prophylaxis. Where major surgery is prolonged for more than three hours a second bolus of intravenous injection may be indicated.

Recently prophylactic antibiotics have been administered in intra-abdominal or thoracic intestinal surgery by the preincisional technique (30, 31). Here the chosen antibiotic, diluted in about 20 ml of water, is infiltrated uniformly along the length of the intended incision. The injection is given immediately after intubation in the anaesthetic room, a fine disposable spinal needle being employed. The antibiotic is thus deposited into the fat and musculature along the whole length of the wound some 10 to 15 min before the incision is made. This method delivers extremely large concentrations of antibiotic into the wound at the start of the operation which are maintained throughout the procedure. From the large bolus injection infiltrated over a large area, serum levels rapidly rise and are again well-maintained as the process of absorption continues. The peripheral tissues receive the antibiotic from the serum at a rate of somewhere between that achieved with an intramuscular and an intravenous injection.

Clearly the chosen route of administration must be taken into consideration along with the pharmacodynamics of the drug and its antimicrobial action. Strategies vary in their mechanism of action and efficacy, for example, quinolones and aminoglycosides have marked concentration-dependent bactericidal activities with the rate of bacterial killing increasing with higher peak drug concentrations (32). By contrast, most beta-lactams show little concentration dependence and, for the most part, the killing of bacteria is related to the duration of effective drug levels.

Antibiotics used in gastrointestinal prophylaxis

Cephalosporins

The cephalosporins are the most commonly prescribed antibiotics in GI surgical prophylaxis. They are popular because of their broad antimicrobial coverage and relative lack of toxicity. They are effective against penicillinase producing *Staph. aureus*. The disadvantages of the first generation cephalosporins were: limited or no activity against enterococci and pseudomonas; poor cerobrospinal fluid penetration; and excessive nephrotoxicity when combined with aminoglycosides. The cephalosporin nucleus has a beta-lactam ring like the penicillins and is, therefore, susceptible to degradation by beta-lactamases. The latest generation are resistant to all or most Gram-negative beta-lactamases. Three generations of the drug now exist with cefuroxime being the most widely used. Most are ineffective against the anaerobic bacteria, in particular, *B. fragilis*, though cefoxitin, which has been popular in the USA, has some activity against these organisms. Newer agents with extended spectra are ceftazidime and cefotaxime, the former is effective against pseudomonas. All of these agents have been shown to be effective in both biliary and colorectal prophylaxis.

Penicillins

The older antibiotics in this range have never been widely used for prophylaxis in GI surgery, though of these amoxycillin is effective against *Strep. faecalis*. Many strains of *E. coli* and some strains of *Proteus mirabilis* produce beta-lactamases which destroy ampicillin and amoxycillin. The recently available broad spectrum acylureido penicillins have been shown to be useful as prophylactic agents as an alternative to the cephalosporins. In general terms the penicillins have a shorter half-life, narrower spectrum, and a higher risk of allergy and resistance than cephalosporins. Fourth generation broad spectrum penicillins: mezlocillin, piperacillin, and azlocillin, which are all derivatives of ampicillin, have been used successfully in prophylaxis. They have, however, little advantage over third-generation penicillins; they are only bactericidal in high doses and resistance may emerge during relatively short-term drug therapy. Co-amoxyclav, the combination of amoxycillin with clavulanic acid, has been widely and successfully used in GI surgery prophylaxis. The clavulanic acid is a weak antibacterial but a potent inhibitor of many beta-lactamases, although not those produced by enterobacter or *Pseudomonas* species.

Erythromycin

This drug used to be commonly used in combination with neomycin as oral bowel preparation. Its range is somewhat narrow though in addition to major activity against Gram-positive organisms it is also active against the bacteroides and *E. coli*. Erythromycin base is not absorbed from the GI tract and is still used extensively with neomycin as pre-operative bowel preparation and prophylaxis before colorectal surgery in the USA.

Aminoglycosides

This group of drugs have been widely used in prophylaxis before GI surgery, particularly before major, high-risk surgery. These agents are very effective against aerobic Gram-negative bacteria including those that are nosocomially acquired. The main three in current use are gentamicin tobramycin and netilmicin, all of which have a similar basic chemical structure. Tobramycin has been claimed to be less ototoxic then gentamicin. It is more active against *Ps. aeruginosa* and less active against other Gram-negative bacilli. They are highly bactericidal, penetrating the cell wall and membrane and binding to 30S bacterial ribosomes. They have been widely used for short-term prophylaxis in GI surgery, particularly colorectal surgery. When used in combination with a penicillin and metronidazole this form of triple therapy provides excellent broad-spectrum prophylaxis. The long-term use of these drugs requires careful monitoring of the blood levels to avoid ototoxicity and nephrotoxicity.

Metronidazole

This drug has been very widely used in gastrointestinal surgery because of its strong cidal activity against anaerobic bacteria including *B. fragilis* and other bacteroides species. As it is not active against the common aerobic bacteria it should be used in combination with another antibiotic. The drug is very safe to use and has little apparent risk of resistance. In recent years its intravenous use has formed the mainstay of prophylaxis against anaerobic organisms in colorectal surgery in Britain. In the USA, clindamycin and lincomycin have found greater favour.

Other beta-lactam antibiotics

Aztreonam is a monocyclic beta-lactam antibiotic with an antibacterial spectrum limited to Gram-negative aerobic bacteria including *Ps. aeruginosa*. It has been used as an alternative to the aminoglycosides in biliary, small and large intestinal surgery. Imipenem, a carbapenem, is the first thienamycin beta-lactam antibiotic. In view of its very broad spectrum of activity which includes aerobic and anaerobic Gram-positive and Gram-negative bacteria, it has excellent potential for use as a prophylactic antibiotic. The drug is partially inactivated in the kidney by enzymatic activity and is, therefore, administered in combination with cilastatin, a specific enzyme inhibitor which blocks its renal metabolism. There have been few side effects following its use, the most significant of which are hypersensitivity and GI upset. The drug has been shown to have a major therapeutic value in established infection relating to visceral perforations. It is expensive, and because of this it is not commonly the first choice of agents although it retains its efficacy when used as a single agent for major GI surgery such as total colectomy, mucosal proctectomy, ileal reservoir formation, and ileo-anal anastomosis.

Strategies employed

When considering prophylaxis for a surgical procedure on a particular area in the GI tract, the surgeon must assess whether there are any unrelated conditions which make the patient particularly susceptible to infective complications such as valvular heart disease or the presence of prosthetic heart valves; these patients should always be given antibiotic prophylaxis to prevent bacterial endocarditis. Immunosuppressed patients, those with malignancy and probably all patients with respiratory problems should be given prophylactic antibiotics even if clean surgery is to be performed. The evidence that prophylactic antibiotics prevent or reduce post-operative respiratory infections is not strong. Many surgeons including the author would extend this philosophy further and use single shot prophylaxis of a suitable antibiotic for all gastrointestinal procedures including those classified as clean such as highly selective vagotomy. In forming a strategy for prophylaxis the clinician must ask:

1. Can the most likely infective organism be named?
2. Can the sensitivity be predicted?
3. Can the period of susceptibility to the organism be defined? (33–35)

Which operations need antibiotic prophylaxis?

Before considering the appropriate antibiotic regimen for a specific operation, the viscus must be clean and empty in order to reduce the risks of parietal contamination during the procedure. Operations on the mouth and pharynx are preceded by removal of dental plaque and repair or extraction of carious teeth. These precautions are also important for those with valvular heart disease. Operations on the oesophagus require pre-operative oesophagoscopy with aspiration of the contents if there is mechanical obstruction to the oesophageal lumen. For all major GI procedures the stomach should be emptied by nasogastric aspiration and, if stenosis is present, by gastric lavage. Recovery from upper GI operations may be aided by mechanical clearance of the colon. The small intestine is prepared by fasting prior to surgery. There are numerous ways of mechanically cleansing the colon provided that it is not obstructed. The author's preference is to use 'Go-Lightly', which when taken orally over a 24-hour period prior to surgery produces excellent mechanical cleansing, and in a physiological way. Two sachets of Picolax and a phosphate enema probably work as well.

Oesophago-gastric surgery

The normal oesophagus contains a few oropharyngeal and upper respiratory tract organisms, thoracotomy predisposes to chest infection and most patients who undergo oesophageal resection are treated in an intensive care unit. The number of organisms present is many times greater if there is an oesophageal stricture (36). The bacteria responsible are a mixture of aerobic and anerobic organisms, with a tendency to an overgrowth of enterobacteriaceae, enterococci and *Strep. viridans*. One to three dose intravenous prophylaxis with a cephalosporin, such as cefazolin or cefuroxime, with metronidazole is adequate prophylaxis and has been shown to reduce infective complications. Similar prophylaxis should be used for gastric surgery for whilst the stomach and duodenum normally contain few organisms, if the pH of the gastric juice rises above 4 and if there is pyloric obstruction, gastric bleeding or gastric carcinoma, enterobacteriaceae, enterococci, and anaerobic organisms can multiply and lead to endogenous contamination (37, 38). Some 80 per cent of wound infections after resection for gastric carcinoma are caused by an organism present at the time of operation. Wound infection occurs in over 90 per cent of patients with more than 10^6 organisms in the stomach at the time of operation if no prophylaxis is given. Patients with bile reflux gastritis invariably have large numbers of organisms in the stomach, but gastric contents in patients with recurrent ulcer are usually sterile.

Many gastric surgical procedures have been associated with a high risk of post-operative infective complications (39, 40). Selective antibiotic prophylaxis has been recommended in gastric surgery in patients with hypochlorhydria, and those taking H_2-receptor antagonists and similar drugs (41, 42). Details of post-operative infective complications and the micro-organisms found in primary infections were reported recently in 750 gastric operations performed between 1972 and 1986 at the Karolinska Institute (43). The overall rate of primary infections was 23 per cent. The infection rates were related to the diagnosis and to factors that could influence the colonization of the stomach. In a recent study, patients with high or normal acid output were compared with those with decreased acid output or impaired gastric motility, and with those with low acid output and either bleeding or a tumour. The majority of micro-organisms from the primary infections in all three of these groups of patients belonged to the normal oropharyngeal microflora. Micro-organisms were isolated from the stomach much more commonly in the hypochlorhydric, bleeding, and tumour groups. Anergy has been studied in gastric cancer patients using the multitest technique and was found to be more common (76 per cent) in gastric cancer patients than controls (43 per cent) (44). This method of instant multipuncture involves injection of seven antigens and a glycerine control. Patients were assessed at 48 h after injection into the forearm.

Biliary tract surgery

In health the gall-bladder and pancreas are sterile but if these organs are inflamed they can release pathogenic bacteria, enterobacteriaceae, enterococci, anaerobic bacteria. *Strep. faecalis*, *Klebsiella*, and occasionally *Clostridium welchii*. When stones are present in the gall-bladder alone the incidence of infected bile is 30 per cent, the presence of common bile-duct stones increases the prevalence of these biliary organisms to 70 per cent. There is a threefold increase in the rate of wound infection if the common bile duct is opened, and infections are particularly liable to occur when T-tubes are used. Obstructive jaundice, repeat surgical procedures and increasing age increase the incidence of infection. Thus bile is infected in at least 30 per cent of elective operations and 90 per cent of emergency procedures (45). All biliary operations should be covered by at least a single intravenous dose of a beta-lactam antibiotic (46). During endoscopic retrograde cholangio-pancreatography (ERCP) there is a risk of septicaemia and pancreatitis and, therefore, a single dose of antibiotic prophylaxis is recommended. Little remains known about the microflora in pancreatic disease.

Anergy has also been studied in patients with biliary lithiasis. A prospective study of the cell mediated immune response was performed in 212 controls and 216 patients undergoing surgery for biliary lithiasis. Delayed hypersensitivity response was again assessed using the multitest method. No difference was seen in the delayed hypersensitivity response between controls and patients with uncomplicated cholilithiasis. Relative anergy has been reported in those with acute cholecystitis and there was also a difference between patients with icteric and non-icteric choledocholithiasis. The presence of jaundice was associated with anergy and a good correlation existed between the anergic state and the development of post-operative infective complications (47).

In a recently reported study, 644 patients undergoing biliary surgery received ampicillin 2 g and sulbactam 1 g iv (48). The accuracy of the presence of 'high risk factors' was compared with the occurrence of infection. Organisms were cultured from the bile of 121 (19 per cent) patients in whom the incidence of infective complications was 22 per cent compared with 2 per cent in those with sterile bile ($p < 0.001$). Fifty-four per cent of those with positive bile cultures were assessed as being of 'low risk'; the incidence of colonization of bile was 32 per cent in the high risk and 14 per cent in the low risk groups. Pre-operative assessment of high-risk factors does not predict bile colonization, the latter being the factor most strongly associated with infective complications after biliary surgery. It was recommended, therefore, that antibiotic prophylaxis is essential in all biliary surgery.

Two-hundred patients undergoing biliary surgery were recently randomized to receive either cefazolin or sulbactam ampicillin, both given intravenously (49). No difference emerged in terms of efficacy of prophylaxis overall but in jaundiced patients infection was less common with sulbactam/ampicillin. The overall infection rate was 24 per cent in jaundiced patients and 7 per cent in non-jaundiced ($p = 0.004$). In another study of 200 patients ceftriaxone 2 g IV was compared with amoxycillin/clavulanate 1200 mg IV pre-operatively (50). Post-operative wound infections following biliary surgery occurred in 4 per cent of each group with a similar distribution of organisms: *E. coli*, *Klebsiella*, and *Proteus*. Both post-operative pyrexia and chest infections were less common and there was a shorter hospital stay in the ceftriaxone group. The improved results with ceftriaxone were attributed to the sustained action of this antibiotic which prevents proliferation of bacteria in atelectatic foci.

Cefmetazole, a new broad-spectrum parenteral cephamycin antibiotic has been compared with cefoxitin in 78 high-risk patients undergoing elective cholecystectomy (51). The risk factors used here were: acute cholecystitis, choledocholithiasis, hyperbilirubinaemia, hyperamylasaemia, age over 60 years, and diabetes mellitus. The two antibiotics had similar efficacy in preventing post-operative infection which only occurred in two patients.

In a large study of 1451 patients undergoing gastric or biliary surgery cefotaxime ($n = 722$) was compared with cefoxitin ($n = 729$). Wound infection occurred in 3.3 per cent of the cefotaxime group and 7.6 per cent of those given cefoxitin ($p < 0.002$). The major factor influencing infection rates in this study was the length of the operation. Infection prolonged hospital stay by three days, showing an advantage on cost-benefit analysis for the use of cefotaxime (52).

Predictive factors for bactibilia in acute cholecystitis have been addressed in 49 patients (53). Pyrexia (> 37.3 °C), raised bilirubin (8.6 μmol/L) and white cell count (> 14×10^9/L) were the best predictors of bactibilia. These authors advocated single-dose antibiotics for all except those with two or three predictive factors of bactibilia, who should receive more prolonged prophylaxis.

In a study of 86 patients who had emergency exploration of the biliary tree, 55 had septic shock pre-operatively (54). Predictive factors for cholangitis were identified (relative risk) as concomitant medical problems (4.5); pH less than 7.4 (3.5); bilirubin more than 90 μmol/L (3.1); platelet count less than 150×10^9/L (2.9) and serum albumin less than 30 g/L (2.9). Clearly under these circumstances prolonged antibiotic therapy is necessary.

A recent study has addressed the question of drainage after cholecystectomy (54). Drains were omitted in 248 patients, 122 had closed suction drains and 124 had Penrose drains. The incidence of subhepatic or subphrenic bile collections and of chest infections was not significantly raised in the group without drains. There was no difference in hospital stay between the two groups. Therefore it was considered that simple elective cholecystectomy is safe without peritoneal drainage.

Despite this evidence for the routine use of prophylactic antibiotics in all biliary operations a questionnaire sent to 25 per cent of consultant surgeons in the U.K (90 per cent reply rate) showed that only 56 per cent used prophylactic antibiotics for elective cholecystectomy (56). Eighty-four per cent used them for emergency cholecystectomy, peritoneal drains were used by 75 per cent.

Small bowel and colorectal surgery

Heavy bacterial contamination is much more likely to follow an incision into the terminal ileum, colon, or rectum where there are high concentrations of aerobic and anaerobic bacteria. Here parietal contamination from spillage from the open viscus can be minimized by inserting large swabs soaked, for example, in aqueous betadine to isolate the abdominal wound. Some surgeons prefer a plastic ring drape for this purpose but the evidence that either prevention influences the incidence of post-operative infection is not strong.

A large number of studies atest to the efficacy of prophylactic antibiotics at appendicectomy, without prophylaxis wound infection occurs in 10 to 30 per cent and intra-abdominal abscess in 2 to 3 per cent (57). Infections may only become manifest after the patient has been discharged from hospital. A large Danish multicentre study reported that the incidence of wound infections, but not of intra-abdominal abscess, was reduced by single-dose pre-operative antibiotic prophylaxis in 1735 patients (58). A recent study failed to show any additional advantage for the use of ampicillin and gentamicin together with metronidazole (59). In patients with gangrenous or perforated appendicitis, a reduced surgical infection has been recorded in patients who receive topical ampicillin in addition to intravenous clindamycin (60). Single-dose metronidazole suppositories have been shown to be effective. A single, intravenous dose of metronidazole is probably the treatment of choice for uncomplicated appendicitis with the addition of a cephalosporin and the use of multiple doses for those with gangrenous appendicitis or frank peritonitis where a therapeutic course of antibiotics is indicated.

Small bowel resection should receive similar, single dose antibiotic prophylaxis with a cephalosporin and metronidazole. Some surgeons prefer to use either a broad-spectrum acylureido penicillin or an aminoglycoside in preference to a cephalosporin.

Despite good mechanical preparation of the bowel, it must be regarded as negligent not to use antibiotic prophylaxis in colorectal surgery. Attitudes towards the use of antibiotics have changed greatly in recent years from a three or even five day course of pre-operative oral antibiotics to a single, intravenous dose of antibiotic given at the time of induction of anaesthesia. The prolonged use of oral antibiotics should be abandoned in view of the risks of complication (61). Poorly absorbed oral antibiotics have little or no role, for it is felt that there is at least a theoretical risk of overgrowth of *Clostridium difficile* or *Strep. milleri* (62, 63). Both of these organisms can have dangerous consequences, particularly the latter, in the form of multiple metastatic abscess formation.

Optimal mechanical preparation of the bowel is achieved by confining the patient to oral fluids only for the pre-operative 24 h and administration of two sachets of Picolax or oral polyethylene glycol during that time followed by a phosphate enema on the morning of surgery (64). A sachet of Picolax contains sodium picosulphate 10 mg, magnesium oxide 3.5 g and citric acid 12 g. In the emergency situation when operating upon unprepared bowel intra-operative antegrade colonic irrigation may permit immediate resection and primary anastomosis of obstructed lesions of the left colon and may also be considered for left colonic perforation or haemorrhage (65). Intra-operative colonic irrigation with povidone iodine has been reported to be effective in 367 patients (66).

Although few surgeons outside the USA now use oral antibiotic prophylaxis alone in colorectal surgery, it is possible to achieve low rates of infection with their use (67). Intravenous cefoxitin is as effective as a combination of oral erythromycin, neomycin, and cefazolin together with intravenous cefazolin in colorectal surgery (68). In a study of 250 patients reported in 1988, however, the addition of pre-operative oral neomycin and erythromycin to perioperative parenteral cefoxitin significantly reduced the incidence of intra-abdominal abscess and anastomotic dehiscence (69). Probably the most popular antibiotic regimen used in colorectal surgery is an aminoglycoside (gentamicin) and metronidazole given intravenously at induction of anaesthesia and at 8 and 16 h post-operatively. Keighley and his colleagues, in a prospective randomized trial of 93 patients undergoing elective colorectal surgery, reported that systemic metronidazole and kanamycin were more effective than these drugs given orally (63). Lau and his colleagues reported 194 patients, divided into three groups, receiving either oral neomycin and erythromycin systemic metronidazole and gentamicin or both oral and systemic regimens (70). The incidence of post-operative complications was 27.4 per cent, 11.9 per cent, and 12.3 per cent respectively. Those patients receiving oral antibiotics alone were shown to have a significantly higher risk of post-operative infection compared with the other two groups. It was concluded that systemic antimicrobial prophylaxis was safer and more effective than oral prophylaxis.

There has been an increasing tendency to replace the aminoglycosides by one of the newer cephalosporins. Aminoglycoside resistant flora occur in 65 per cent of patients undergoing colorectal surgery but these resistant organisms were considered to be of little importance as potential pathogens (71).

Recent studies of intravenous antibiotics in colorectal surgical prophylaxis have claimed that the use of aztreonam resulted in less infection than gentamicin but no difference was seen between co-amoxyclav and either mezlocillin or metronidazole plus gentamicin (72–74). A number of studies have also shown that cefoxitin alone reduces wound infection (75, 76). In a study to assess the value of topical ampicillin prophylaxis in elective colorectal surgery 193 patients received cefotaxime 2 g IV at the start of operation and two further doses in the next 12 h (77). At the time of wound closure they were randomized to receive a local instillation of ampicillin or not. The wound infection rate was not affected by ampicillin. A large study of 907 patients showed that single-dose cefotaxime plus metronidazole was of equal efficacy to a standard, three-dose regimen of cefuroxime plus metronidazole in preventing wound infection after colorectal surgery. In this study there was no difference in mortality or in the incidence of other post-operative complications.

Risk factors for infectious complications in patients undergoing colorectal surgery include age greater than 40 years, the presence of cancer, the administration of antibiotics more than 60 min before surgery, the duration of operation and patients undergoing rectal procedures (78). Ileal pouch procedures for ulcerative colitis are often long operations in the presence of a badly diseased and inflamed bowel. The author employs a three dose regimen of intravenous imipenem beginning immediately pre-operatively and pelvic irrigation with a 0.1 per cent tetracycline solution.

Duration of prophylaxis

The minimum duration of perioperative antimicrobial prophylaxis has not been completely clarified. In a prospective randomized trial to compare triple dose mezlocillin with triple dose cefuroxime plus metronidazole there was no significant difference in either the total number of operation related infections or in the incidence of severe wound infection (79). It has been shown, however, that single dose pre-operative cefotaxime was as effective as multiple-dose cefoxitin (80). In two controlled trials of single-dose prophylaxis with cefotetan, the wound infection rate was similar irrespective of whether the patient received single-dose cefotetan, two doses of cefotetan or cefazolin and metronidazole for 24 h (81, 82). On economic grounds, the single dose of cefotetan alone is recommended.

Strachan has recently addressed the question of 'when is one dose of antibiotic not enough?' in an excellent review article (83). The efficacy of short-duration cephalosporin cover was demonstrated by Polk some 20 years ago (84). The use of single-dose intravenous prophylaxis has been slow to gain widespread acceptance and most current texts recommend continuing therapy for 24–72 h whilst emphasizing the risks of more prolonged therapy. Gastrointestinal operations have a decisive risk period for bacterial innoculation of around two to three hours at the most and should be adequately covered by a single dose of a suitable antibiotic.

Multiple dosage is indicated for operations which last more than three hours and those where the blood loss exceeds two litres. In addition, Strachan has identified specific areas where he considers three doses may still be required: in cholangitis; following biliary bypass for major bilio-pancreatic resection; and in major colonic surgery. If a single antibiotic is used in colorectal prophylaxis then either augmentin or imipenem could be used. Virtually all other drugs require to be given in combination, and metronidazole should be one of these agents. In those patients with either intestinal obstruction or peritoneal contamination, three doses should be adequate provided that surgery has been efficient and is combined with peritoneal lavage. Pollock has recently shown that single-dose pre-incisional intraparietal infiltration with augmentin halved the incidence of wound infection compared with single dose intravenous administration of augmentin in 624 patients undergoing GI operations.

Wider adoption of prophylaxis

Surveys of antibiotic prophylaxis in GI surgery in Scotland have been carried out in 1980 and 1985 (85). In 1980 21 per cent of surgeons used antibiotics routinely at cholecystectomy compared with 53 per cent in 1985. The number of surgeons using antibiotics at appendicectomy increased from 49 per cent to 79 per cent over this five-year period; whereas in colorectal surgery, the corresponding figures were 95 per cent and 98 per cent. This study also showed a major swing in the last five years towards the use of a single-dose prophylaxis.

Conclusions

Prophylactic antibiotics have a proven role in GI surgery and should always be used where any part of the digestive tract is to be opened. Adequate pre-operative preparation is essential. The importance of meticulous care in handling the tissues and performing adequate surgery cannot be overemphasized. The intravenous or the pre-incisional, intraparietal routes are superior to other methods of administration. Single-dose prophylaxis with one or two antibiotics should be standard except where surgery is prolonged over three hours, is major, or requires transfusion of more than two litres of blood, or is incomplete, i.e. the pathology is not completely excised at a single session. In more complicated situations, prophylaxis will need to be continued for 24 h or rarely 72 h. More prolonged prophylaxis may be required for those with valvular heart disease and for selected patients who are being nursed in an intensive care unit.

References

1. Pollock, A. V. (1988). Surgical prophylaxis—the emerging picture. *Lancet*, **i**, 225–8.
2. Hirschman, J. V. and Inui, T. S. (1980). Antimicrobial prophylaxis: a critique of recent trials. *Rev. Infect. Dis.*, **2**, 1–20.
3. Hunt, T. K. (1981). Surgical wound infection—an overview. *Am. J. Med.*, **70**, 712–8.
4. Veterans Administration Ad Hoc. Interdisciplinary Advisory Committee on Anti-Microbial Drug Usage. (1977) Prophylaxis in surgery. *J. Am. Med. Assoc.*, **237**, 1241–55.
5. Pollock, A. V. (1987). *Surgical infections*, pp. 180–5. Edward Arnold, London.
6. Chodak, G. W. and Plaut, M. E. (1977). Use of systemic antibiotics for prophylaxis in surgery: a critical review. *Arch. Surg.*, **112**, 326–34.
7. Russell, R. C. G. (1987). Surgical technique. *Br. J. Surg.*, **74**, 763–4.
8. Kaiser, A. B. (1986). Antimicrobial prophylaxis in surgery 1979. *N. Engl. J. Med.*, **315**, 1129–38.
9. Wangensteen, O. H. and Wangensteen, S. D. (1978). *The rise of surgery from empiric craft to scientific discipline*. Dawson, Folkestone, Kent.
10. Keighley, M. R. B. and Burdon, D. W. (1979). *Antimicrobial prophylaxis in surgery*. Pitman Medical, London.
11. Cruse, P. J. E. and Foord, R. (1980). The epidemiology of wound infection—A ten-year prospective study of 62, 939 wounds. *Surg. Clin. North Am.*, **60**, 27–40.
12. Leader. (1968). Aseptic methods in the operating suite. *Lancet*, **i**, 705–9.
13. Hunt, T. K. (1981). Surgical infections—an overview. *Am. J. Med.*, **70**, 712–8.
14. Shapiro, M., Munoz, A., Tager, I. G., Schoenbaum, S. C., and

Polk, B.F. (1982). Risk factors for infection at the operative site after abdominal or vaginal hysterectomy. *N. Engl. J. Med.*, **307**, 1661–6.

15. Stone, J.J., Hooper, C.A., and Kolls, L.D. (1976). Antibiotic prophylaxis in gastric, biliary and colonic surgery. *Ann. Surg.*, **184**, 443–52.
16. Bates, T., Siller, G., and Crattern, B.C. (1989). Timing of prophylactic antibiotics in abdominal surgery. *Br. J. Surg.*, **76**, 52–6.
17. Stone, H.H., Hainey, B.B., Kolb, L.D., Geheber, C.E., and Hooper, C.A. (1979). Prophylactic and preventive antibiotic therapy. *Ann. Surg.*, **189**, 691–9.
18. Bethune, D.W., Blower, R., and Parker, M. (1965). Dispersal of Staphylococcus aureus by patients and surgical staff. *Lancet*, **i**, 480–3.
19. Eykyn, S.J. (1988). The prophylactic use of antibiotics in surgery. *Surgery*, **55**, 1304–7.
20. Crossley, K. and Gardner, L.C. (1981). Antimicrobial prophylaxis in surgical patients. *J. Am. Med. Assoc.*, **245**, 722–6.
21. Shapiro, M., Townsend, T.R., Rosner, B., and Kass, E.H. (1979). Use of antimicrobial drugs in general hospitals. *N. Engl. J. Med.*, **301**, 351–5.
22. Lant, A.F. (1982). Factors affecting the action of drugs. In *Scientific foundations of anaesthesia*. (3rd edn) (ed. C.F. Schurr and S. Feldman), pp. 425–50.
23. Vogelman, B.S. and Craig, W.A. (1985). Post-antibiotic effect. *J. Antimicrob. Chemother.*, **152**, 373–8.
24. Dunphy, J.E. (1975). Wound irrigation versus debridement. *Ann. Surg.*, **181**, 12A.
25. Gilmore, O.H.A. and Sanderson, P.J. (1975). Prophylactic interparietal povidone iodine in abdominal surgery. *Br. J. Surg.*, **62**, 792–9.
26. Galland, R.B., Mosley, J.G., Saunders, J.H., and Darrell, J.H. (1977). Prevention of wound infection in abdominal operations by pre-operative antibiotics or povidone infection. *Lancet*, **ii**, 1043–5.
27. Bird, G.G., Bunch, G.A., and Croft, C.B. (1971). Topical noxytiolin antisepsis. Report of a controlled trial. *Br. J. Surg.*, **58**, 447–8.
28. Krukowski, Z.H., Stewart, M.P., Alsayer, H.M., and Matheson, N.A. (1984). Infection after abdominal surgery: five year prospective study. *Br. Med. J.*, **288**, 278–80.
29. Sauven, P., Playforth, M.J., Smith, G.M.R., Evans, M., and Pollock, A.V. (1985). Single dose antibiotic prophylaxis of abdominal surgical wound infection: a trial of pre-operative latamoxef against pre-operative tetracycline lavage. *J.R. Soc. Med.*, **9**, 137–41.
30. Armstrong, C.P., Taylor, T.V., and Reeves, D. (1982). Pre-incisional intraparietal injection of cephamandole: a new approach to wound infection prophylaxis. *Br. J. Surg.*, **69**, 459–60.
31. Taylor, T.V., Walker, W.S., Mason, R.C., Richmond, J., and Lee, D. (1982). Pre-operative intraparietal intraincisional cefoxitin in abdominal surgery. *Br. J. Surg.*, **69**, 461–2.
32. Roosendaal, R., Bakker-Woudenberg, I.A.J.M., and Van den Berg, J.C. (1985). Therapeutic efficacy of continuous versus intermittent administration of ceftazidine in experimental Klebiselle pneumonia in rats. *J. Infect. Dis.*, **152**, 373–8.
33. Pollock, A.V., Froome, K., and Evans, M. (1978). The bacteriology of primary wound sepsis in potentially contaminated abdominal operations. *Br. J. Surg.*, **65**, 76–80.
34. Kelly, M.J. and Warren, R.E. (1978). The value of an operative wound swab sent in transport medium in the prediction of lateral clinical wound infection. *Br. J. Surg.*, **65**, 81–88.
35. Armstrong, D., and Smith, R. (1974). Prophylactic antibiotics in surgery. *Clin. Bull.*, **4**, 97–101.
36. Kippax, P.W. and Thomas, E.T. (1966). Surgical wound sepsis in a general hospital. *Lancet*, **ii**, 1297–300.
37. Brooks, J.R., Smith, H.F., and Peese, F.B. (1974). Bacteriology of the stomach following vagotomy. *Ann. Surg.*, **179**, 859–62.
38. MacGregor, A.B. and Ross, P.W. (1972). Bacterial content of gastric juice. *Br. J. Surg.*, **59**, 443–5.
39. Lewis, R.T. (1977). Wound infection after gastroduodenal operations: a 10-year review. *Can. J. Surg.*, **29**, 435–40.
40. Gatehouse, D., Dymock, F., Burdon, D.W., Alexander-Williams, J., and Keighley, M.R.B. (1978). Prediction of wound sepsis following gastric operations. *Br. J. Surg.*, **65**, 551–4.
41. Hares, M.M., Hegarty, M.A., Warlow, J., *et al.* (1981). A controlled trial to compare systemic and intraincisional cefuroxime prophylaxis in high risk gastric surgery. *Br. J. Surg.*, **68**, 276–80.
42. Nichols, R.L., Webb, W.R., Jones, J.W., Smith, J.W., and Le Cuero, J. (1982). Efficacy of antibiotic prophylaxis in high risk gastroduodenal operations. *Am. J. Surg.*, **143**, 94–8.
43. Sjostedt, S., Levin, P., Malinborg, A.S., Bergman, U., and Kayer, L. (1989). Septic complications in relation to factors influencing the gastric microflora in patients undergoing gastric surgery. *J. Hosp. Infect.*, **13**, 191–7.
44. Cainzos, M., Alcade, J.A., Patel, J., and Puente, J.L. (1989). Anergy in patients with gastric cancer. *Hepatogastroenterology*, **36**, 36–9.
45. Garibaldi, R.A., Skolnick, D., and Maglio, S. (1986). Post-cholecystectomy wound infection. *Ann. Surg.*, **204**, 650–4.
46. Cahill, C.J., and Pain, J.A. (1988). Current practice in biliary surgery. *Br. J. Surg.*, **75**, 1169–72.
47. Cainzos, M., Patel, J., and Puente, J. (1989). Anergy in patients with biliary lithiasis. *Br. J. Surg.*, **76**, 169–72.
48. Wells, G.R., Taylor, E.W., Lindsay, G., and Morton, L. (1989). Relationship between bile colonisation, high risk factors and post-operative sepsis in patients undergoing biliary tract operations while receiving a prophylactic antibiotic. *Br. J. Surg.*, **76**, 374–7.
49. Morris, D.L., Jones, J.A., Harrison, J.D., Andrews, G.I., Phillips, R.J.M., and Slack, R.C.B. (1989). Randomised study of prophylactic parenteral sulbactam/ampicillin and cephazolin in biliary surgery: significant benefit in jaundiced patients. *J. Hosp. Infect.*, **13**, 261–6.
50. Mufti, M.E., Rakas, F.S., Glessa, A., *et al.* (1989). Ceftriaxone versus clavulanate potentiated amoxycillin for prophylaxis against post-operative sepsis in biliary surgery: a prospective randomised study in 200 patients. *Curr. Med. Res. Opin.*, **11**, 354–9.
51. Berne, T.V., Yellin, A.E., Appleman, M.D., Gill, M.A., Chenella, F.C., and Heseltine, P.R.N. (1990). Controlled comparison of cefmetazole with cefoxitin for prophylaxis in elective cholecystectomy. *Surg. Gynecol. Obstet.*, **170**, 137–40.
52. Rodriguez, J., Puiq, L.C.J., Arnau, C., Porta, M., and Vallue, C. (1989). Antibiotic prophylaxis with cefotaxime in gastroduodenal and biliary surgery. *Am. J. Surg.*, **158**, 428–33.
53. Thompson, J.E., Benman, R.S., and Dotz, J.E. (1990). Predictive factors for bactibilia in acute cholecystitis. *Arch. Surg.*, **125**, 261–4.
54. Lai, E.C.S., Tam, P.C., Paterson, I., *et al.* (1990). Emergency surgery for severe acute cholangitis. *Ann. Surg.*, **211**, 55–9.
55. Lewis, R.T., Goodall, R.G., Marien, B., Park, M., Lloyd-Smith, W., and Wiegard, F.M. (1990). Simple elective cholecystectomy: to drain or not to drain. *Am. J. Surg.*, **159**, 241–5.
56. Cahill, C.J. and Pain, J.A. (1988). Current practice in biliary surgery. *Br. J. Surg.*, **75**, 1169–72.
57. Leader. (1971). Sepsis after appendicectomy. *Lancet*, **ii**, 195.
58. Bauer, T., Vennits, B., Holm, B., *et al.* (1989). Antibiotic prophylaxis in acute non-perforated appendicitis. The Danish Multicentre Study. *Ann. Surg.*, **209**, 307–11.

59. Grant, C., Danso, T.K., and Worsonu, L. (1989). Prophylaxis against post-appendicectomy wound infection. *Int. Surg.*, **74**, 129–32.
60. Seco, J.L., Ojeda, E., Reguilon, C., *et al.* (1990). Combined topical and systemic antibiotic prophylaxis in acute appendicitis. *Am. J. Surg.*, **159**, 226–30.
61. Menaker, G.J. (1987). The use of antibiotics in surgical treatment of the colon. *Surg. Gynecol. Obstet.*, **164**, 581–96.
62. Johnston, D. (1987). Bowel preparation for colorectal surgery. *Br. J. Surg.*, **74**, 553–4.
63. Keighley, M.R B., Arabi, Y., Alexander Williams, J., Youngs, D., and Burdon, D.W. (1979). Comparison between systemic and oral prophylaxis in colorectal surgery. *Lancet*, **i**, 894–7.
64. Solla, J.A. and Rothenberger, D.A. (1990). Pre-operative bowel preparation. A survey of colon and rectal surgeons. *Dis. Colon Rectum*, **33**, 154–9.
65. Saadia, R. and Schein, M. (1989). The place of intra-operative antegrade colonic irrigation in emergency left sided colonic surgery. *Dis. Colon Rectum*, **32**, 78–81.
66. Banich, F.E. and Medak, S.J. (1989). Intra-operative colonic irrigation with povidone iodine. *Dis. Colon Rectum*, **32**, 219–22.
67. Clarke, J.S., Condon, R.E., Bartlett, J.G. (1977). Pre-operative oral antibiotics reduce septic complications of colon operations. *Ann. Surg.*, **186**, 251–9.
68. Kaiser, A.B., Herrington, J.L., Jacobs, J.K., Mulherin, J.L., Roach, A.C., and Sawyer, J.L. (1983). Cefoxitin versus erythromycin, neomycin and cefazolin in colorectal operations. *Ann. Surg.*, **198**, 525–30.
69. Coppa, G.F. and Eng, K. (1988). Factors involved in antibiotic selection in elective colon and rectal surgery. *Surgery*, **104**, 853–8.
70. Lau, W.Y., Chu, K.W., Poon, G.P., and Hok, K. (1988). Prophylactic antibiotics in elective colorectal surgery. *Br. J. Surg.*, **75**, 782–5.
71. Heritage, J., Dyke, G.W., Johnston, D., and Lacey, R.W. (1988). Selection of resistance to gentamicin in the faecal flora following prophylaxis for colorectal surgery. *J. Antimicrob. Chemother.*, **22**, 249–56.
72. Dionigi, R., Mozzilo, N., and Ventriliglia, L. (1989). Comparative multicentre study on efficacy and safety of aztreonam and gentamicin in prophylaxis of high risk colorectal surgery. *J. Chemother.*, **1**, Suppl 2, 22–7.
73. Menzies, D., Gilvert, J.M., Shepherd, M.J., and Rogers, T. (1989). A comparison between amoxycillin/clavulanate and mezlocillin in abdominal surgical prophylaxis. *J. Antimicrob. Chemother.*, **24**, Suppl B, 203–8.
74. Hall, C., Curran, F., Burdon, D.W., and Keighley, M.R.B. (1989). A randomised trial to compare amoxycillin clavulanate with metronidazole plus gentamicin in prophylaxis in elective colorectal surgery. *J. Antimicrob. Chemother.*, **24**, Suppl B, 195–207.
75. Hoffman, C.E.J., McDonald, P.J., and Watts, J.M. (1981). Use of pre-operative cefoxitin to prevent infection after colonic and rectal surgery. *Ann. Surg.*, **191**, 353–7.
76. Georgoulis, B., Papaioannou, N., Katrahoura, A., and Seitanides, B. (1983). Open randomised study of cefoxitin versus metronidazole in the prevention of infection after colorectal surgery. *Am. J. Proctology, Gastric., Colon and Rectal Surgery*, **1**, 10–2.
77. Rowe-Jones, D.C., Peel, A.L., Kingston, R.D., Shaw, J.F., Teasdale, C., and Cole, D.S. (1990). Single dose cefotaxime plus metronidazole versus three dose cefuroxime plus metronidazole as prophylaxis against wound infection in colorectal surgery: multicentre prospective randomised study. *Br. Med. J.*, **300**, 18–22.
78. Galandiuk, S., Polk, H.C., Jagelman, D.G., and Fazio, V.W. (1989). Re-emphasis of priorities in surgical antibiotic prophylaxis. *Surg. Gynecol. Obstet.*, **169**, 219–22.
79. Diamond, T., Mulholland, C.K., and Parks, T.G. (1988). A prospective randomised trial to compare triple dose mezlocillin with triple dose cefuroxime plus metronidazole as prophylaxis in colorectal surgery. *J. Hosp. Infect.*, **12**, 215–9.
80. Kager, L., Ljungdahl, I., Malmborg, A.S., Nord, C.E., Pieper, R., and Dahlgren, P. (1981). Antibiotic prophylaxis with cefoxitin in colorectal surgery. *Ann. Surg.*, **191**, 277–82.
81. Gruwez, J.A., Lerut, J., Cristiaerns, M.R., *et al.* (1988). Single dose prophylaxis with cefotetan in elective abdominal surgery. *Chemoterapia*, **7**, 218–22.
82. Morton, A.L., Taylor, E.W., Lindsay, G., Wells, G.R. (1989). A multicentre study to compare cefotetan alone with cefotetan and metronidazole as prophylaxis against infection in elective colorectal operations. *Surg. Gynecol. Obstet.*, **169**, 41–5.
83. Strachan, C.J.L. (1989). Problems related to regimens and duration of administration. When is one shot not enough? Royal Society of Medicine, *Round Table Series*, **14**, 36–41.
84. Polk, H.C. and Lopez-Mayor, J.F. (1969). Post-operative wound infection: a prospective study of determinant factors and prevention. *Surgery*, **66**, 97–103.
85. Haddock, G., Hansell, D.T., and McArdle, C.S. (1988). Survey of antibiotic prophylaxis in gastrointestinal surgery in Scotland: five years on. *J. Hosp. Infect.*, **11**, 286–9.

20

Gastrointestinal tract infection

JOHN A.R. SMITH

Introduction

In surgical practice gastrointestinal infection may be the reason that the patient presents or may be a complication of surgical management. When it occurs after surgery infection results in an increased mortality, morbidity, and in the cost of treatment. Not all infection requires urgent surgical intervention, and there have been significant advances over the last decade in the understanding of the pathogenesis, diagnosis and management of these conditions.

Peritonitis

Pathology/bacteriology

Peritonitis is a localized, or generalized, inflammation of the peritoneum resulting in a serous exudate which rapidly becomes purulent. The peritoneum itself becomes dull and congested and fibrinous adhesions form between the peritoneum and individual loops of bowel. This process may result in the infection being walled off, or generalized infection may occur if the process is incomplete.

In surgical practice the commonest source of peritonitis is perforation of the gastrointestinal tract. The severity of the inflammation is dependent on the substance leaking, the duration of contamination, and any resulting bacterial infection. It is usual to separate *chemical* peritonitis resulting from leak of sterile gastric juices, bile, urine, or pancreatitis from *septic* peritonitis where infected or faecal contents are released. The organisms involved also depend on the organ perforated especially as regards the incidence of anaerobic infection.

However, it is clear that with the passage of time most chemical peritonitis becomes infected. Penetrating wounds of the abdominal wall may introduce pathogenic bacteria, but direct trauma to the gastrointestinal tract (GIT) is a more potent source of infection.

In female patients, ascending infection from the genital tract is an important cause of peritonitis, particularly in parts of Africa (1). Haematogenous spread causing peritonitis has been implicated in infection which may complicate ascites, but is an unusual source. Primary peritonitis is now uncommon and is usually caused either by pneumococcal or streptococcal infection, the latter being the more common. The origin of infection is obscure. Happily modern antibiotics have improved prognosis significantly. Tuberculous peritonitis is uncommon in the western world but must be remembered in the immigrant population and in people who travel overseas frequently.

Non-bacterial peritonitis

The usual cause of peritonitis when it is not infected is leakage of gastric acid or bile into the peritoneal cavity. Meconium peritonitis may complicate intrauterine perforation of the GIT and can lead to ascites or neonatal obstruction. Granulomatous peritonitis may result from sarcoidosis or tubercular infection. Of greater concern in surgical practice is the problem of starch peritonitis, fortunately rare now that gloves are available which avoid the use of both talcum and starch.

Pathological consequences of peritonitis

When peritonitis occurs there is loss of plasma, water, and electrolytes into the inflamed peritoneal cavity, and loss of fluid into the distended small bowel loops as a consequence of the associated ileus. Local infection and systemic sepsis will risk further cardiovascular compromise and the absorption of bacteria and toxins is enhanced by the inflamed peritoneum. Cardiopulmonary function may be affected adversely by abdominal distension. There is an increased risk of loops of bowel becoming adherent and of adhesions forming, so that intestinal obstruction becomes more common.

Bacteriology

Where peritonitis is caused by perforation the infecting organisms will be mixed Gram-negative aerobic pathogens. The risk of anaerobic infection with *Bacteroides fragilis* increases in the distal ileum and large bowel (2). Ascending infection from the female genital tract also involves mixed organisms, coliforms, anaerobic cocci, streptococci and the bacteroides range all being implicated (3).

Streptococcus pyogenes, pneumococci, enterobacteriaceae, and gonococci have all been associated with primary peritonitis. Specific organisms such as *Mycobacterium tuberculosis* are self evident. Peritonitis in association with peritoneal dialysis involves a wide range of organisms including coagulase negative and positive staphylococci, diphtheroids, Gram-negative coliforms, and various yeasts (3, 4).

Conservative management

All patients with peritonitis require intravenous fluids to replace both the conventional daily requirement and the fluid lost. Monitoring by pulse, blood pressure, and hourly urine volume is essential and most patients will require central venous pressure monitoring or, if available, pulmonary wedge pressure measurements. Any degree of ileus will result in vomiting which is why nasogastric intubation and aspiration is recommended. Adequate analgesia is essential. Investigations should include an erect chest or lateral decubitus abdominal radiograph to identify free intraperitoneal gas. Blood tests will include serum amylase, blood culture, and baseline haematological and biochemical measurements. Severely ill patients will require arterial blood gas analysis.

Indications for antibiotic therapy

In theory antibiotics should be reserved for patients with bacterial peritonitis, those with a high risk of superimposed infection, and for those high-risk patients where the risk of infection would be a serious hazard. However, in practice, the risk of secondary infection is so high that the early administration of antibiotics is mandatory. The only exception is when an elevated serum amylase indicates the presence of acute pancreatitis.

Indications for surgery

Surgical treatment is important but there are contraindications, which may be absolute or temporal. Thus, no patient should be subjected to surgery until resuscitation has restored the systolic blood pressure to greater than 100 mmHg and the urine output to more than 40 ml/h (5). When dealing with faecal peritonitis these aims may not be achieved however, and surgery should not be delayed excessively in this group.

The indications for surgery are:

1. Peritonitis in the presence of a perforation of the alimentary tract. It should be remembered that no free air is detected on chest or abdominal radiographs in up to 25 per cent of patients with a perforated duodenal ulcer.
2. Peritonitis, or peritonism, which does not respond rapidly to the resuscitative measures outlined above.
3. Evidence of bacteraemia or septicaemia, when it becomes necessary to identify and remove the source of the infecting organisms.
4. Suspicion of faecal peritonitis.

Absolute contraindications to surgical intervention are a patient in whom the risks of surgery outweigh the potential benefits; for example, patients with advanced malignant disease, recent myocardial infarction, premortal presentation. A relative contraindication is the patient who has had insufficient resuscitation. A possible contraindication is pancreatitis if this diagnosis can be reached preoperatively, or primary peritonitis if peritoneal tapping allows a bacteriological diagnosis to be made. However, in practice it is usual for this diagnosis to be reached only when laparotomy has been undertaken for what is presumed to be one of the more common causes of secondary peritonitis.

Surgical principles

The mainstays of surgical treatment are thorough peritoneal debridement and attention to the underlying pathology. Debridement and peritoneal lavage with warm saline and water has been recommended for almost a century (6). The addition of tetracycline (1 g/L) to the lavage solution has produced incidences of wound infection and septic complications which are at least very impressive and at best very persuasive (7, 8).

There is some controversy about how radical the debridement should be. Radical removal of fibrinous plaques and thorough mechanical cleansing has been recommended with impressive results (9). However, the abdominal contents tend to be very friable in the presence of peritonitis and, therefore, both susceptible to trauma and difficult to repair with sutures. Where pus is present it is important to send specimens for bacteriological investigation, even when antibiotics have been administered. Any other debris, faecal matter etc., should be removed manually by sucker or by lavage. It is vital to ensure that the subphrenic, paracolic, subhepatic, and pelvic spaces are cleaned, and to remember that pus may collect between loops of bowel and in the mesentery.

When peritonitis occurs the small intestine is usually distended because of ileus. Because of the distension and friability it should be handled very carefully. Any fibrinous plaques that can be removed with ease should be dealt with but it is not necessary to compromise the integrity of the intestine to remove all such plaques. Careful retrograde evacuation of the small bowel contents into the stomach where they can be aspirated via the nasogastric tube appears to encourage recovery of function, relieve the diaphragmatic splinting and eases abdominal closure. Alternatively, decompression by intubation of the ileum can be used.

The surgery of the underlying pathology should be kept as simple as possible. In most circumstances, and particularly when dealing with peritonitis from anastomotic breakdown, the overriding principle is to avoid primary or reanastomosis (5). Alternative views will be considered in the appropriate sections. In general, the choice will lie between resecting the offending colonic pathology such as perforated diverticular disease, simple closure of an upper gastrointestinal perforation, or closure combined with a definitive procedure, for pathology such as a perforated chronic duodenal ulcer. Laparostomy may be valuable for a few conditions, such as abscess complicating pancreatitis (G. Glazer, pesonal communication, 1990), or secondary to a complex fistula (10). Post-operative peritoneal lavage has been recommended (11, 12) but there is no evidence that peri- or post-operative lavage are additive in their effect.

Intensive post-operative monitoring, maintenance of fluid and electrolyte balance, and continued antibiotic therapy is essential. A significant proportion of patients will require nursing in an intensive therapy unit and may need parenteral nutritional therapy. These patients are at risk of septicaemia and abscess formation post-operatively, in addition to adult respiratory distress syndrome, opportunistic infection and multiple organ failure.

Intraperitoneal abscess

Aetiology

An intra-abdominal abscess may develop where a diffuse peritonitis has been localized, as a complication of primary pathology, or as a consequence of surgery. Sixty per cent of intraperitoneal abscesses occur after an operation and are mostly due to an anastomotic leak (13). Perforation of any part of the GIT may result in abscess formation if it is localized, but perforations of the appendix, or of a colonic diverticulum are the most common causes.

Localization of a more diffuse peritonitis may be seen after perforated peptic ulcers. Abscess formation can complicate acute pancreatitis either because of infection in the region of the pancreatic necrosis or in a pseudocyst. The former tends to present within two to three weeks of the acute attack whereas the majority of pseudocysts present after six or more weeks (14, 15). (See Chapter 21.)

The possible sites of abscess formation are well-recognized.

1. A *pelvic abscess* is the usual site of a collection after acute appendicitis, but with the advent of modern methods of treating peritonitis, occurs in less than 3 per cent of patients. It may also result from leakage of a low anastomosis after an anterior restorative resection.
2. *Paracolic abscess* complicates localized perforation of the

colon, usually secondary to diverticular disease, less commonly to carcinoma. It must be stressed that the perforation, especially in acute diverticulitis, may be so small as to be unidentifiable (5). The major dangers associated with paracolic abscess are enlargement, fistula formation, localized peritonitis, or more seriously a generalized peritonitis, which may be either bacterial or faecal depending on the extent of the perforation. In patients with generalized peritonitis secondary to diverticular disease the risk of faecal contamination is 20 to 25 per cent (16).

3. *Subphrenic abscesses* have been complicated by attempts to subclassify them on an anatomical basis. It is more sensible to consider four areas—right and left subphrenic and right and left subhepatic (17). Jones has suggested a simple modification, namely anterior and posterior left subhepatic (5).
4. Other sites include *intramesenteric* and between *loops of bowel*, but these are seldom present in isolation, that is without the other classical sites being involved.

Diagnosis

The general concepts of identifying infection are covered in Chapter 10. The most important factor in detecting an abscess is a high index of suspicion, both at initial presentation and in the post-operative period. Diagnosis is easy if there is a palpable, tender mass or if the abscess is associated with signs of a fistula post-operatively. Other clues are an unexpected ileus, the failure to thrive after surgery or an unexplained pleural effusion.

Various methods of detection are available (Table 20.1) (18), but in practice ultrasound or computerized tomographic (CT) scans are the most widely used and effective investigations (19). Radio isotopic scans are favoured by some enthusiasts (20, 21) but have proved disappointing in the author's experience.

Table 20.1.

	Advantages	Disadvantages
Plain X-ray	Easy Repeatable Inexpensive	Non-specific Low sensitivity
Ultrasound scan	Cheap Repeatable Drainage possible Sensitive Specific	Difficult post-operation Confused by gas-filled bowel
CT scan	Sensitive Specific Drainage	Availability Problems with drains, clips, bowel gas High radiation dose
Isotope scan	? Valuable in difficult cases	Less specific

Supportive measures

Some patients will require no specific support. In all patients where there is toxicity, or evidence of septicaemia, measures as for the management of peritonitis will be required: intravenous fluids, oxygen by mask, monitoring of urinary output, careful management of fluid balance to avoid cardiac overload, and specific support of cardiac and respiratory function.

Indications for antibiotics

Antibiotics will not usually produce resolution of an abscess and patients are at risk of spreading infection and septicaemia. Some pelvic abscesses only present shortly before discharging spontaneously, or are amenable to digital drainage and decompression via the rectum. Unless the latter outcome is likely, all patients with proven intra-abdominal abscess, and patients with systemic disturbance and presumed abscess formation, should be given systemic antibiotic therapy.

However, the antibiotic given should be prescribed as part of a definite therapeutic policy based on the likely pathogens and local resistance patterns. A definite duration of treatment, usually a maximum of five days, should be selected with resort to surgical intervention if there is incomplete resolution at the end of this time.

Choice of antibiotics

Initial therapy is usually based on a 'best guess' policy. The majority of intra-peritoneal abscesses contain organisms from the GIT. Therefore the antibiotic regimen selected must be active against the anaerobic organisms, especially bacteroides, and the common aerobes especially the Gram-negative bacilli, *Strep. faecalis*, etc.

Metronidazole remains the agent of choice for anaerobic bacteria despite the newly available single agents which claim a broad spectrum of antibacterial activity. There are theoretical advantages to be gained from the use of the third-generation cephalosporins, the new carbapenem, or from the quinolones, but clinical experience suggests cefuroxime to be a satisfactory first-line agent against the aerobic bacteria.

It must be recognized that patients with intra-abdominal infection are at high risk of septicaemia, septic shock, and multiple organ failure.

Non-surgical management

It has been traditional teaching that all intraperitoneal abscesses should be drained surgically, preferably without encroaching on the peritoneal cavity. More recently such dogma has been questioned. Surgical drainage of appendix abscesses was associated with a higher morbidity than non-surgical management (23), and ultrasound-guided needle aspiration of subphrenic abscesses after total gastrectomy has been shown to be effective (23). In more general terms, percutaneous drainage is recommended either for treatment alone or prior to definitive surgery for intra-abdominal abscesses (24). Where an abscess forms as a complication of a necrotic tumour surgical drainage is likely to be required (25).

The possibility of non-surgical drainage depends upon the ability to make a diagnosis and to localize the collection accurately. Ultrasound and CT scanning have allowed these objectives to succeed in over 80 per cent of cases. The criteria to select patients for surgical or non-surgical intervention are less well defined. Sepsis scoring systems have been used but, as yet, with no clear conclusions. It is evident that mortality varies greatly between simple and complex abscesses to the extent that complex collections indicate the need for surgical intervention (26).

It is also vital to establish whether or not the abscess is in communication with the gastrointestinal tract, and if so either the degree of disruption of the anastomosis or of the disease process. Where the fistula is 'high', either in position in the alimentary tract or in output (greater than 500 ml per 24 h), spontaneous resolution is less likely.

Indications for surgery

The major indications for surgical drainage of intraperitoneal abscess are:

1. Development of septicaemia.
2. Failure to respond to non-surgical treatment within a defined time, e.g. five days.
3. Associated 'high' fistula.
4. Complex abscess.

Clearly, such advice must be tempered by consideration of the patient's general health and the extent of the underlying pathology.

Surgical principles

Such procedures are difficult and should not be delegated to junior surgical staff. Other viscera are often adherent to the abscess cavity, are friable, and must be separated with extreme caution and gentleness. The cavity should be drained and thorough peritoneal lavage performed after specimens have been obtained for urgent bacteriological investigation. Thorough lavage also helps to ensure that all areas are drained and irrigated, and that no undiagnosed collection remains undisturbed.

The role of drains is controversial. Thorough clearance of a cavity should make a drain unnecessary. However, the reality is that a raw, oozing area is often left with the cavity walled off by other viscera. There is no true lining tissue and the closed, or suction, drain allows both adequate drainage post-operatively and radiological evaluation of the progress of the cavity as it resolves.

Equally controversial is the management of the skin wound. Some authors recommend leaving the superficial layers open (27, 28). However, the combined use of thorough tetracycline lavage of the peritoneal cavity and systemic antibiotics allows primary wound closure with a wound infection rate of around five per cent, even where there has been a pericolic abscess (29).

Recurrent and complicated abscesses

The general principles of management are similar to those for primary abscesses. It is vital to assess the reason for the abscess recurring and in both groups to evaluate accurately the configuration of the collection and the underlying alimentary pathology. This will involve a combination of plain abdominal radiographs, ultrasound and CT scanning, and barium studies of the appropriate part of the GIT. Such abscesses are less likely to resolve without surgical intervention and there is an increased risk of mortality and morbidity following such procedures. Careful surgical drainage and treatment of the underlying pathology are the principals of successful treatment.

Laparostomy

The technique of leaving all layers of the anterior abdominal wall open has been attributed to Mickulicz (30). In modern times excellent results have been reported in the management of generalized peritonitis provided the wound was left open for not more than 72 h (31). More recently, leaving the wound to heal by secondary intention has become more common practice. Surprisingly the reported incidence of incisional hernia is only 50 per cent.

The technique of laparostomy allows frequent exploration, release of any infected collection, and adequate peritoneal lavage. Initial enthusiasm for this method has cooled and it is recommended now only for generalized faecal peritonitis and for haemorrhagic necrotizing pancreatitis, with or without septic complications (see Chapter 21).

Biliary infection

Range of pathology

It is important to differentiate 'biliary colic' and chronic cholecystitis from those conditions where there is a true element of infection. Even the diagnosis of acute cholecystitis often relates to the inflammatory changes seen in the wall on histological examination rather than to bacterial infection. The pathology to be considered in this section includes empyema of the gall-bladder, acute emphysematous cholecystitis, ascending cholangitis, biliary peritonitis, and hepatic abscess.

Aetiology

Under normal circumstances bile is sterile. Infection in the gall-bladder is implicated in the aetiology of mixed biliary calculi, and, in turn, stones in either the gall-bladder or the biliary tree encourage infection to develop secondary to stasis. Any other cause of obstructive jaundice has a similar effect but infection is more common with calculous disease. Stones in the gall-bladder are associated with infected bile in 30 per cent of cases, but stones in the common bile-duct produce bile infection in over 70 per cent of cases (32). It is important to remember that the T-tube in the common bile duct is a potential source of infection, and calcium bilirubinate stone formation is a recognized complication of T-tube drainage.

There are two conditions of particular importance—*empyema* of the gall-bladder and ascending cholangitis. In empyema, a stone impacted in Hartmann's pouch produces total obstruction and infection results in a gall-bladder full of pus. The reason some patients progress to an empyema and others have only an acute bacterial cholecystitis is not clear. The importance of empyema and cholangitis lies mainly in the increased risk of septicaemia and septic shock. Whilst empyema and ascending cholangitis are important in the developed world infestation with liver flukes is a specific type of cholangio-hepatitis occurring almost entirely in Chinese or others living along the coastline in south-east Asia.

Acute emphysematous cholecystitis is an uncommon condition seen most often in diabetic patients, but again cystic duct obstruction appears to be an important factor in aetiology. Acute acalculous cholecystitis is usually a complication of another illness, usually involving sepsis, e.g. burns (33).

Bacteriology

The widespread use of prophylactic antibiotics in clinical practice (34) has made it more difficult to obtain accurate data about the bacteriology of bile. In patients without biliary pathology bacteria can be identified occasionally but these have been described as contaminants by some workers (35). Bacteria are present in the bile of 30 to 56 per cent of patients with biliary disease and are more common in acute and chronic cholecystitis (37, 38) and when the cystic duct is occluded (36). Stones in the common bile-duct produce the highest incidence of infection (39) but in patients who have had multiple duct explorations the rate approaches 100 per cent (40).

The organisms most frequently isolated are the enterobacteriaceae, *E. coli*, *Klebsiella* spp., and streptococci (41). Anaerobic bacteria are less common. However, it has been suggested that this may be related to the difficulty in isolating anaerobic organisms and that the correct culture of infected bile will allow isolation of anaerobic bacteria in over 40 per cent of cases (42). *Bacteroides* and *Clostridia* spp. may be involved, but only in combination with aerobic organisms, and usually only after biliary-enteric anastomosis (43).

There is some debate about whether biliary infection ascends from the bowel or descends from the liver. Evidence exists to support both theories but favours excretion of live organisms from the liver where they are normally phagocytosed and destroyed by the Kupffer cells (44).

General management

In theory it is reasonable to differentiate infective and non-infective diseases of the biliary system, but in practice the management is similar with intravenous fluids, analgesics, and antiemetics. It is suggested that opiates such as morphine should not be used because of the risk of smooth muscle spasm, but in practice the adequacy of pain relief is more important. There is no indication for the routine use of antibiotics in managing biliary disease.

Specific management

The changes which have taken place in the management of biliary disease are due, in large part, to the availability of facilities which allow earlier diagnosis, most particularly ultrasound scanning. The specific indications for antibiotic therapy are systemic disturbance such as rigors, suggestive of ascending infection or of pus under pressure, evidence of septicaemia, or severe physical signs in association with pyrexia lasting more than 24 h.

Acute cholecystitis

The conventional management of acute cholecystitis (and biliary colic) is to allow the acute attack to settle on the above regimen and to proceed to elective cholecystectomy six weeks later. It is important to emphasize that clinical diagnosis alone is insufficient (45) as the diagnosis may be inaccurate in over 30 per cent of cases. However, there are other disadvantages of this traditional approach—readmission with another attack (13 per cent), failure of conservative management (13 per cent), and patient default (10 per cent) (46). *Emergency* cholecystectomy is seldom indicated but should be performed for imminent perforation or frank biliary peritonitis. It may also be performed when the diagnosis is made only at laparotomy for undiagnosed peritonitis.

However, *early* cholecystectomy within 72 h of presentation, is practised increasingly often. Early surgery has the advantage of reducing overall hospital stay and of avoiding the problems already described for the elective approach. When early surgery is performed under ideal circumstances, i.e. by an experienced surgeon and with full radiological facilities, there is no evidence of increased mortality or morbidity (47–50). It may be difficult to arrange to operate on such patients within 72 h because of busy theatre schedules and occasionally the inflammatory reaction is such that safe cholecystectomy cannot be achieved. Under these circumstances cholecystotomy is indicated (5).

The 1990s and beyond are likely to be the era of laparoscopic cholecystectomy. With increasing experience it would appear that more than 95 per cent of patients requiring cholecystectomy can be dealt with by the laparoscopic route. Infection remains the most common postoperative complication of endoscopic cholecystectomy but the incidence would appear to be very low—one per cent (110).

Empyema of the gall-bladder

Empyema complicates 2 to 3 per cent of patients with gall-bladder disease. Bacterial culture of the gall-bladder contents is positive in over 80 per cent of cases. Antibiotics effective against the enterobacteriaceae should be administered as therapy, and early cholecystectomy performed. Cholecystotomy, or even partial cholecystectomy, are valuable alternatives if there are technical difficulties (5, 46).

Jaundice or common bile-duct exploration

The bile is infected in over 75 per cent of patients when jaundice is due to calculous disease, but in under 10 per cent when the jaundice due to tumour (39, 48). Patients who have had multiple explorations of the duct are at highest risk of infection (41). Anaerobic bacteria are uncommon and usually are found in patients with an anastomosis between the biliary and intestinal systems (43). Thus, there is sufficient evidence for patients who are likely to require choledochotomy to have prophylactic antibiotics, but as yet there is no evidence that the newer cephalosporins give better results than the second generation agents (51).

In addition to infective complications, patients with obstructive jaundice are at increased risk of wound failure, haemorrhage, and renal failure. Therefore, it is important to take specific steps to reduce the incidence of these complications, by ensuring adequate hydration, perioperative diuresis, meticulous surgical technique, and by correcting any clotting defect pre-operatively with vitamin K_1 by injection.

Controversy persists about the use of pre-operative biliary drainage. External drainage procedures produce more problems than they prevent (52). However, endoscopic sphincterotomy has been advocated, especially in elderly patients (53, 54), either alone or as a preliminary to cholecystectomy (55).

Acute cholangitis

The management of cholangitis has been either conservative, with intravenous fluids, antibiotics and careful observation, or more aggressive with early surgical intervention following antibiotic therapy. Much of the argument supporting conservative management related to the high morbidity and mortality following surgery (56, 57), and it is clear that antibiotic therapy fails in up to 30 per cent of cases (58). Patients with underlying malignant pathology have a worse prognosis than those with calculous disease (59).

Significant improvements in the results of managing cholangitis have come from early endoscopic drainage combined with antibiotic therapy (60, 61). Indeed, it is now recommended that endoscopic retrograde cholangiography should be used in all patients with severe, acute cholangitis and that sphincterotomy may be performed in the presence of stones, in patients who are at high risk, and in those who have previously had a cholecystectomy performed (62). Where cholangitis is complicated by stricture formation surgical therapy will be required (62, 63).

Biliary peritonitis

The general management is as described in earlier for peritonitis. Experience after percutaneous cholangiography has demonstrated that bile in the peritoneal cavity does not always cause peritonitis, but infected bile invariably does. The commonest cause of biliary peritonitis is rupture of the gall-bladder due to gangrene or acute infection, but leakage after removal of a T-tube, used to drain the common bile-duct, is not uncommon (54, 64). Localized leaks can be managed conservatively but generalized peritonitis demands laparotomy, peritoneal lavage, and cholecystectomy. It is important to attempt to remove all calculi which have been discharged from the gall-bladder.

Hepatic abscess

Classically two types of liver abscess are described — pyogenic and amoebic. It is important to remember hydatid cysts in the differential diagnosis as treatment of this condition demands great care to avoid spillage of the cyst fluid which carries a risk of anaphylactic reaction and the spread of daughter cysts.

Pyogenic abscess

This condition is uncommon in Great Britain. Diagnosis is often delayed (65) and such delay is associated with an increased mortality (66). Despite the introduction of antibiotics the overall incidence of pyogenic liver abscesses has not changed in fifty years (67) but the pathogenesis has — appendicitis causing portal pyaemia is much less common, while biliary infection in the elderly is on the increase.

General causes of abscess are:

1. Biliary obstruction and ascending infection.
2. Portal pyaemia especially caused by complicated diverticular disease.
3. Direct spread from contiguous organs, e.g. peptic ulcer or cholecystitis.
4. Liver trauma or hepatic infarction.
5. Secondary to bacteraemia or septicaemia.
6. Complicating other hepatic pathology.

However, in almost 60 per cent of cases no cause is found (68).

The infecting organism is dictated by the underlying cause. The majority of organisms isolated are *E. coli* and anaerobes but where hepatic abscess complicates generalized septicaemia, staphylococci, and streptococci are more common. It is more common for the right lobe of the liver to be involved, followed by both lobes to be involved and least frequent is involvement of the left lobe alone. Abscesses may remain discreet or may coalesce to produce a large cavity.

The clinical features are superimposed on the underlying disease process so that a high index of suspicion is essential if early diagnosis is to be achieved. If not diagnosed, spread to adjacent anatomical spaces — the subphrenic space or pleural cavity, or to adjacent organs, particularly the lungs — may occur. Frank peritonitis is relatively uncommon.

Diagnosis Various associated features are reported — high ESR; leucocytosis; sympathetic pleural effusion or an air/fluid level in the liver itself (69). The most important investigation is ultrasound scanning, supplemented as necessary by CT or technetium scan.

Treatment Antibiotic therapy is essential, the choice depending on the likely cause. Where doubt exists a broad spectrum antibiotic, against Gram-positive and negative organisms as well as the anaerobic bacteria, should be given.

Drainage of abscesses under ultrasound control is increasingly popular and allows more rational prescription of antibiotics (65). Where this fails to produce resolution formal surgical drainage, by the transperitoneal route, is indicated (67). It is vital to diagnose and treat the underlying disease process, e.g. biliary obstruction or diverticular disease, if this has been identified.

Amoebic abscess

These abscesses are usually more painful and tender than the pyogenic variety. Liver involvement occurs in between 3 and 7 per cent of patients with amoebiasis (67). Rupture into the colon, lung, pericardium, and retroperitoneum has been reported. Serology is used to confirm the diagnosis once ultrasound scan has demonstrated the presence of abscess formation. Treatment is with metronidazole, but large abscesses may require formal drainage under antibiotic cover.

Diverticular disease

Pathology

Diverticular disease is common after the age of 45 but is asymptomatic in approximately 90 per cent of people (70). Seventy-five per cent of diverticulae are confined to the sigmoid colon and almost 90 per cent to the left colon, the rectum being spared. Infective complications occur because of stasis and because of superinfection with both aerobic and anaerobic gut organisms. Treatment is required for complications of the disease, these complications being classified according to Hinchey's staging (71):

(A) Fistula formation.

(B) Inflammation and perforation.
Stage I—sigmoid obstruction, intracolic or mesenteric abscess.
Stage II—localized pericolic abscess.
Stage III—generalized septic peritonitis.
Stage IV—faecal peritonitis.

Fistulae may involve other parts of the small or large intestine or the genitourinary system. Because of the thickness of their wall the ureter and uterus are rarely involved but the bladder and vagina are the more common sites. Where infective complications of diverticular disease result in, or are associated with, stricture formation it is often difficult to differentiate this from colorectal neoplasm.

Conservative management

Conservative therapy is the first choice in the management of an exacerbation of diverticular disease. It can be difficult to differentiate patients who have an infective complication from those with non-infected diverticular disease. Intravenous fluids are indicated and, unless it is quite clear that the complication is not infective, intravenous antibiotics active against aerobic and anaerobic gut organisms are required. Cefuroxime 1.5 g and metronidazole 500 mg three times daily is a popular and effective regimen although it has been suggested that cefotaxime, as a single agent, may have a sufficiently broad spectrum of activity to be of value.

Treatment should continue until the patient is apyrexial and until the localized abdominal tenderness has resolved, when a high residue diet is carefully introduced. At least 50 per cent of all acute admissions for diverticulitis will respond to this treatment (72) and, once recovered, investigation by barium enema and/or colonoscopy can be arranged.

More recently, a localized diverticular abscess would be treated without surgical intervention in some centres, at least in the early stages. The clinical signs of infection can be relieved by percutaneous drainage of the abscess (73) but it should be noted that all patients in this series underwent definitive surgery at a later stage. This approach is not recommended in the presence of a faecal fistula (74) and is only effective if a strict protocol is followed. This protocol involves ensuring catheter patency by regular irrigation, regular monitoring by sinography, replacement of blocked catheters, and maintenance of the other conservative measures already detailed.

Indications for surgery

There are three basic indications for surgery in the management of diverticulitis. Urgent laparotomy is required for generalized peritonitis and is recommended by some authorities for the management of a faecal fistula (74). Early surgery is indicated where conservative therapy has failed, and as a planned procedure where a pericolic abscess has been managed initially by percutaneous drainage (73, 74). A further indication for surgery is where there is doubt about a coexisting carcinoma, or where symptoms are recurrent and sufficiently troublesome to justify definitive therapy. Readmissions are frequent in this condition (72) and surgery is to be recommended, particularly in younger patients.

Diverticular abscess

The range of recommended surgical treatment for this condition is wide. Preliminary percutaneous drainage, intravenous fluid replacement, and antibiotic therapy followed by resection six weeks later means that a one stage procedure can be performed. The total hospital stay is less and the overall mortality and morbidity is not compromized. However, other surgeons would advocate laparotomy and drainage of the abscess, together with one of several options. Some surgeons would undertake no other procedure. Others would perform a defunctioning colostomy with or without delayed resection according to whether the patient develops a complication of the abscess, e.g. fistula or recurrence. The other alternative procedures are the same as for complications discussed elsewhere in this chapter.

Diverticular perforation

In addition to pericolic abscess and fistula formation, perforation can cause either purulent or faecal peritonitis. The 'traditional' approach was to drain the perforation and to defunction the colon as a first stage, followed by resection and finally by closure of the colostomy. Each of these stages carried a significant morbidity and the total hospital stay was long.

More recently, there has been a considerable debate about the relative merits of a Hartmann's procedure or a primary resection, with or without a protective stoma. Resection is safe, a mortality of two to three per cent being reported (75). More precise recommendations have been advanced (61)—a Hartmann's procedure for peritonitis and primary resection and anastomosis for those patients with less severe complications. Primary anastomosis carries an acceptable rate of mortality and morbidity as judged by wound infection (10 per cent) and clinical anastomotic leakage (7 per cent) (76). It has suggested that devices to protect the anastomosis may allow earlier, more radical surgery without compromizing the outcome (77), although as yet no controlled data are available. It is now clear that leaving a diseased segment increases the risk of post-operative fistula (78).

Fistulae secondary to diverticulitis

Despite radiological advances, barium enema remains more reliable than CT scanning (79), and where a vesico-colic fistula is suspected, cystoscopy is the next most important investigation. Attempts to treat fistulae conservatively have occasionally been successful but cannot be recommended on the evidence available. Palliative colostomy is commonly used but the fistula seldom closes (80).

The main controversy surrounds the use of primary anastomosis. Most authorities agree that the fistula should be resected with the diseased segment of the colon and the involved part of the other viscus. Primary anastomosis has been associated with a high incidence of anastomotic problems (81, 82) but this may relate to the experience of the surgeons performing the operation. Evidence from specialist units favours radical resection, primary anastomosis and no colostomy (83). Where expertise is available this is the treatment of choice. If not, resection and a Hartmann's procedure is safer and therefore to be recommended.

Bowel gangrene

Ischaemic colitis

This rare condition must be distinguished from ulcerative colitis. The severity depends on the extent of the ischaemic insult and upon whether it is reversible or proceeds to frank gangrene (84). In gangrene, the risks are of perforation, peritonitis, and clostridial infection (5). However, in all forms of ischaemia of the alimentary tract there is an increased risk of bacterial translocation and systemic endotoxinaemia. Treatment must include resuscitation, oxygen supplementation, and surgery where there is any hint of gangrene. Broad spectrum antibiotic therapy, effective against Gram-negative organisms, bacteroides, and *Clostridium perfringens* is required.

At operation the extent of the ischaemic change has to be identified clearly. It is usual to find bloodstained fluid in the peritoneal cavity and, because this may be contaminated with bacteria, peritoneal lavage with tetracycline and saline is required. Resection of the affected part is indicated but primary anastomosis should be avoided. Reanastomosis can proceed safely once the patient has recovered.

Small bowel ischaemia

Irreversible ischaemic change occurs after 4 to 6 h of obstruction of the arterial blood supply. The resultant stasis and increased permeability of the intestinal wall means that bacterial overgrowth and absorption is frequent. The problem has been well reviewed (85). Few patients present at a stage where cure is possible without some form of resection. Diagnosis is difficult and often delayed. The patients are usually old and in a high-risk category.

Clues to the diagnosis are the presence of atrial fibrillation, a past history of peripheral vascular disease or of recent myocardial infarction. Investigation may show a solitary loop of dilated small bowel on abdominal radiography, or the presence of a metabolic acidosis. With a suitable clinical picture these are important indicators that surgery is required for the diagnosis to be confirmed.

Resuscitation must include administration of an antibiotic regimen effective against a broad range of gut organisms. It is difficult to assess the full extent of ischaemic change so that antibiotic therapy should continue for at least five days.

Mesenteric embolectomy can be successful in a small proportion of selected patients, usually only those operated on early (85). Resection of all affected bowel is essential and, where there is any doubt about the viability of the remaining bowel, primary anastomosis should be avoided by the use of a stoma and a mucous fistula. It is valuable for a deliberate, second look procedure to be performed at 24 to 48 h to ensure that the ischaemic change has not extended. Furthermore, where extensive ischaemia is present, and resection at the time of the first operation would involve leaving insufficient proximal small intestine to sustain life, a second-look procedure at 24 h may allow a less radical resection to be performed. However the mortality from this condition is very high and a significant proportion of patients do not survive for the second procedure to be undertaken. Recruitment into a home parenteral nutrition programme may be required for long term survival in those patients who do survive massive resection.

Strangulated hernia

This produces a more localized clinical picture similar to that described above. Because the result of strangulation is a closed loop obstruction the risk of bacterial overgrowth (28) and of perforation of the closed loop is high. A similar situation develops in other causes of mechanical intestinal obstruction, and it is important to remember that the bacterial overgrowth may contribute to the later development of gangrene in the bowel wall (86). Furthermore the commonest cause of collapse in such patients is Gram-negative septicaemia (28).

In order to minimize the risk of collapse patients with obstruction due to strangulation of an internal or external hernia should have adequate resuscitation with intravenous fluids, oxygen by mask, and therapeutic antibiotics active against both aerobic and anaerobic gut bacteria, before surgery is contemplated. The only exception to this rule is the presence of generalized peritonitis. It is prudent to gain control of the closed loop, both proximally and distally, before the hernia is reduced surgically. The loop can then be resected with minimal risk of perforation and of release of bacteria or endotoxin into the systemic circulation.

Other intra-abdominal infection

Appendicitis and appendix abscess

The treatment of choice for appendicitis remains appendicectomy. Antibiotics with activity against bacteroides subspecies should be administered prophylactically. In patients who have a perforated or gangrenous appendicitis 'prophylaxis' is no longer applicable and a 5-day therapeutic course is indicated. Imipenem may be as effective as combination antimicrobial therapy but larger studies are required to answer this question. Controversy persists about whether any advantage is conferred by leaving the wound or subcutaneous tissue open (28) but no controlled data is available. The advantage of primary wound healing is clear.

In the management of appendix abscess non-surgical therapy, including percutaneous drainage, has a lower morbidity than surgical drainage (86). Interval appendicectomy is not always necessary but is usually advised unless there are significant medical contraindications to operation (87). Appendicectomy can be complicated by pelvic abscess (see above) but only in 3 to 4 per cent of patients. Abscess involving the invaginated appendix stump has been reported (88, 89) and may cause peritonitis. There is no evidence that failure to invaginate the appendix stump is dangerous (90, 91).

Meckel's diverticulum

Meckel's diverticulum has been reported to be present in two to three per cent of the population (92, 93) but acute inflammation occurs in only 20 per cent of cases. When laparotomy is performed for acute inflammation antibiotics should be given prophylactically as for acute appendicitis. Perforation of an acutely inflamed diverticulum is not uncommon, especially if a foreign body has penetrated the diverticulum (94).

The risks of excising an asymptomatic diverticulum are considerable (95) and therefore an asymptomatic diverticulum identified at surgery for another condition should not be resected.

Small bowel diverticulae

Solitary diverticulae are of no major import, but bacterial overgrowth in the static outpouches of multiple diverticulae of the small bowel can cause malabsorption. Radical resection is not possible but intermittent courses of such antibiotics as tetracycline can be very helpful.

Caecal diverticulae

Right sided diverticular disease is very much less common than disease in the sigmoid colon. Both true and false diverticulae can occur (96). Most are diagnosed at laparotomy for presumed appendicitis and, in most cases, a prophylactic antibiotic will already have been administered. Local resection and primary repair of the caecal wall should be done if possible. Rarely when local resection is not possible a limited right hemicolectomy is indicated (97, 98). There is no indication for surgical treatment of a solitary diverticulum of the caecum identified at barium enema.

Typhoid perforation

Typhoid fever is uncommon in Great Britain but in tropical countries, even in Europe, the disease is prevalent. Perforation is not uncommon but multiple perforations may be encountered in the five per cent of patients who do perforate. Surgery gives better results than conservative management (99, 100). After adequate resuscitation (101) careful laparotomy under antibiotic cover is required to identify all perforations. This is followed by thorough peritoneal debridement and lavage. If there are multiple perforations close together, resection and anastomosis is used (102, 103). For solitary perforations, or perforations separated anatomically, the choice is primary closure or excision followed by closure. Recent evidence has demonstrated a lower mortality when excision and suture is performed (104, 105). Overall mortality approaches 20 per cent (100).

Abdominal wall infection

Post-operative wound infection

After abdominal surgery the majority of wound infections are caused by endogenous organisms. Even when prophylactic antibiotics are used infection rates of between 5 and 10 per cent are reported depending on the operations performed, and on whether the procedure is performed electively or as an emergency. Wound dressings do not prevent post-operative infection (106).

The usual treatment of established infection is to lay the wound open and allow it to heal by granulation. Reclosure at four days under antibiotic cover with metronidazole and ampicillin has been recommended (107, 108), but, as the latter study included fewer than 50 patients, caution in acceptance of this regimen must be exercised.

Antibiotic therapy is classically indicated in the management of wound infection in patients who are toxic, have spreading cellulitis, and for those patients who are at high risk when infection develops, such as those with prosthetic implants, valvular heart disease, etc. Particular care must be exercised in patients with diabetes mellitus.

Peristomal infection

Peristomal infection is remarkably rare. It may occur as a complication of stomal retraction when the extent and urgency of treatment required depends on how far the stoma has retracted. Most serious is total retraction causing faecal peritonitis (see above). Debridement and resiting of the stoma are indicated where there is subcutaneous infection.

A mucocutaneous fistula may result when sutures used to close the abdominal wall are placed too deeply and penetrate the bowel, but more commonly infection secondary to a fistula complicates recurrent disease, most frequently inflammatory bowel disease of the Crohn's type. Local therapy or systemic antibiotics are seldom effective. Resiting of the stoma with resection of any recurrent disease is required.

Synergistic gangrene

The alternative term of progressive synergistic necrotising cellulitis is very descriptive from a clinico-pathological viewpoint. This condition is caused by a combined infection with a micro-aerophillic streptococcus and an aerobic organism, usually *Staph. aureus*. It usually follows an abscess or other wound infection but is a recognized complication of diabetes mellitus. (See Chapter 18.)

Treatment is urgent. Antibiotic therapy with benzyl penicillin, metronidazole and gentamicin or a cephalosporin, is the most popular combination. Oxygen by mask is administered but the cornerstone of management is wide excision of all the affected skin down to the deep fascia. Regular reinspection in the first 24 to 48 h is essential with further excision of any skin of dubious viability. Later split skin grafting produces an acceptable cosmetic result.

Actinomycosis

This rare, chronic infection may mimic appendix abscess or even caecal carcinoma. It usually complicates perforated appendicitis. Classically, adjacent muscle, skin and viscera are involved by the development of fistulae and sinuses. The organism can spread in the portal venous system to cause honeycombed liver (109). Treatment is by a prolonged course of benzyl penicillin and lincomycin.

References

1. de Muylder, X. (1987). The management of pelvic sepsis. *Proc. Assoc. Surg. E. Africa*, **10**, 24–6.
2. Collee J. G. (1989). Peritoneal microbiology. In *The peritoneum and peritoneal access* (ed. S Bengmark), pp. 60–73 John Wright, Bristol.
3. Houang, E.T. (1984). Aspects of the vaginal microbial flora. *Res. Clin. Forums*, **6**, 7–10.
4. Eisenberg, E.S., Leviton, I., and Soeiro, R. (1986). Fungal peritonitis in patients receiving peritoneal dialysis: experience with 11 patients and review of the literature. *Rev. Infect. Dis.*, **8**, 309–21.
5. Jones, P.F. (1987). *Emergency abdominal surgery* Blackwell Scientific Publications, Oxford.
6. Kennedy, J.W. (1905). Appendicitis: the earliest and complete removal of the appendix. *Surg. Gynecol. Obstet.*, **1**, 216–20.
7. Stewart, D.J. and Matheson, N.A. (1978). Peritoneal lavage in appendicular peritonitis. *Br. J. Surg.*, **65**, 54–6.
8. Krukowski, Z.H , Stewart, M.P.M., Alsayer, H.M., and Matheson, N.A. (1984). Infection after abdominal surgery. *Br. Med. J.*, **288**, 278–80.
9. Hudspeth, S. (1975). Radical surgical debridement in the treatment of advanced generalised peritonitis. *Arch. Surg.*, **110**, 1233–6.
10. Mughal, M.M., Bancewicz, J., Irving, M.H. (1986). Laparostomy: a technique for the management of intractable intra-abdominal sepsis. *Br. J. Surg.*, **73**, 253–9.
11. Fowler, R. (1975). A controlled trial of intraperitoneal cephaloridine administration in peritonitis. *J. Paediat. Surg.*, **10**, 43–50.
12. Stephen, M. and Loventhal, J. (1979). Continuing peritoneal lavage in high risk peritonitis. *Surgery*, **85**, 603–6.
13. Meyers, M.A. (1976). Intraperitoneal spread of infections. In *Dynamic radiology of the abdomen* (ed. M.A. Mayers). *Normal and pathologic anatomy*. Springer-Verlag, New York.
14. Bradley, E.L., Clements, J.L., and Gonzalez, A.C. (1979). The natural history of pancreatic pseudocysts: a unified concept of management. *Am. J. Surg.*, **137**, 135–41.
15. Keenan, D.J., McIlrath, E.M., Johnston, G.W., and Kennedy, T.L. (1980). Pseudocyst and abscess of the pancreas. *Ulster Med. J.*, **49**, 173–9.
16. Phels, M.T., Chapuis, P.H., Bokey, E.L., and Hayward, P. (1982). Diverticular disease: a retrospective study of surgical management 1970–1980. *Aust. NZ J. Surg.*, **52**, 53–6.
17. Mitchell, G.A.G. (1940). The spread of acute intraperitoneal effusions. *Br. J. Surg.*, **28**, 291–313.
18. Filly, R.A. (1979). Detection of abdominal abscesses—a combined approach employing ultrasonography: computed tomography and gallium-67 scanning. *J. Can. Assoc. Radiol.*, **30**, 202–10.
19. Knocher, J.Q., Kocher, P.R., Lee, T.G., and Welch, D.M. (1980). Diagnosis of abdominal abscesses with computed tomography ultrasound and in leucocyte scans. *Radiology*, **137**, 425–32.
20. Saverymuttu, S.H., Croxton, M.E., Peters, A.M., and Lavender, J.P. (1983). Indium III, tropolonate leucocyte scanning in the detection of intra-abdominal abscesses. *Clin. Radiol.*, **34**, 593–6.
21. Schulak, J.A., Corry, R.J. (1987). Surgical complications. In *Essentials of surgery* (ed. D.C. Sabiston). Saunders, Philadelphia, Penn.
22. Lewin, J., Fenyo, G., and Engstrom, L. (1988). Treatment of appendiceal abscess. *Acta Chir. Scand.*, **154**, 123–5.
23. Jahne, J., Meyer, J.J., Milbradt, H., and Pichlmayr, R. (1989) Conservative treatment of intra abdominal complications with interventional radiological techniques. *Surg. Endosc.*, **3**, 16–20.
24. Treutner, K.H., Truong, S., Klose, K., Schubert, T., Schumpelick, V. and Gunther, R.W. (1989). Intra-abdominal abscesses—precutaneous catheter drainage versus operative treatment. *Klin. Wochenschr.*, **67**, 486–90.
25. Mueller, P.R., White, E.M., Glass-Royal, M., *et al.* (1989). Infected abdominal tumours: percutaneous catheter drainage. *Radiology*, **173**, 627–9.
26. Malangoni, M.A., Shumate, C.R., Thomas, H.A., and Richardson, J.D. (1990). Factors influencing the treatment of intra abdominal abscesses. *Ann. Surg.*, **159**, 167–71.
27. Dudley, H.A.F. (1986). Laparotomy, wound management and drainage. In *Emergency surgery* (ed. H.A.F. Dudley), pp. 259–70. John Wright, Bristol.
28. Van der Werken, C., Stassen, L.P., and Van Vroonhoven, J.M. (1989). Post appendicectomy wound infection, a solved problem? *Neth. J. Surg.*, **41**, 100–3.
29. Krukowski, Z.H., Koruth, N.M., and Matheson, N.A. (1985). Evolving practice in acute diverticulitis. *Br. J. Surg.*, **72**, 684–6.
30. Korepanov, V.I. (1989). Open abdomen technique in the treatment of peritonitis. *Br. J. Surg.*, **76**, 471.
31. Steinberg, D. (1979). On leaving the peritoneal cavity open in acute generalised suppurative peritonitis. *Am. J. Surg.*, **137**, 216–20.
32. Taylor, T.V. (1985). The gall-bladder and bile ducts. In *Surgical gastroenterology*, pp. 153–94. Blackwell Scientific Publications, Oxford.
33 Slater, H. and Goldfarb, I.W. (1989). Acute septic cholecystitis in patients with burn injuries. *J. Burn Care Rehabil.*, **10**, 445–7.
34. Haddock, G., Hansell, D.T., and McArdle, C.S. (1988). Survey of antibiotic prophylaxis in gastrointestinal surgery in Scotland—5 years on. *J. Hosp. Infect.*, **11**, 286–9.
35. Nielsen, M.L., Justesen, T., and Asnaes, S. (1974). Anaerobic bacteriological study of the human liver—with a critical review of the literature. *Scand. J. Gastroenterol.*, **9**, 671–7.
36. Dye, M., MacDonald, A., and Smith, G. (1978). The bacteriological flora of the biliary tract and liver in man. *Br. J. Surg.*, **65**, 285–7.
37. Edlund, Y.A., Mollstedt, B.O., and Ouchterling, O. (1958).

Bacteriological investigation of the biliary system and liver in biliary tract disease correlated to clinical data and microstructure of the gall-bladder and liver. *Acta Chir. Scand.*, **116**, 461–76.

38. Flemma, R.J., Flint, L.M., Osterhout, S., Shingleton, W.W. (1967). Bacteriological studies of biliary tract infection. *Ann. Surg.*, **166**, 563–70.
39. Nielsen, M.L. and Sustesen, T. (1976). Anaerobic and aerobic bacteriological studies in biliary tract disease. *Scand. J. Gastroenterol.*, **11**, 437–46.
40. Jackaman, F.R., Hilson, G.R.F., and Lord Smith of Harlow. Bile bacteria in patients with benign bile duct stricture. *Br. J. Surg.*, **67**, 329–32.
41. Shorey, B.A. (1979). Systemic antibiotic prophylaxis in gastrointestinal surgery. In *Surgical sepsis* (ed. C.J.L. Strachan and P. Wise), pp. 83–92. Academic Press, London.
42. England, D.M. and Rosenblatt J.E. (1977). Anaerobes in human biliary tracts. *J. Clin. Microbiol.*, **6**, 494–8.
43. Bourgault, A.M., England, D.M., Rosenblatt, J.E., Forgacs, P., and Bieger C. (1979). Clinical characteristics of anaerobic bactibilia *Arch. Intern. Med.*, **139**, 1346–9.
44. Dooley, J.S. (1983). Biliary tract infection: the background to successful treatment. In *A clinical approach to progress in infectious diseases* (ed. W. Brumfitt and J.M.T. Hamilton Miller), pp. 46–64. Oxford University Press, Oxford.
45. Schofield, P.F., Hulton, N.R., Baildam, A.D. (1986). Is it acute cholecystitis? *Ann. R. Coll. Surg. Engl.*, **68**, 14–16.
46. Cuschieri, A., and Bouchier, A.D. (1988). The biliary tract. In *Essential surgical practice* (ed. A. Cushieri, G.R. Giles, and A.R. Moosa). pp. 1020–75 John Wright, Bristol.
47. Glenn, F. and Heller, G.J. (1946). The surgical treatment of acute cholecystitis. *Surg. Gynecol. Obstet.*, **83**, 50–4.
48. Järvinen, H.J. and Hästbacka, J. (1980). Early cholecystectomy for acute cholecystitis. A prospective randomised study. *Ann. Surg.*, **191**, 501–5.
49. Fowkes, F.G.R. and Gunn, A.A. (1980). The management of acute cholecystitis and its hospital cost. *Br. J. Surg.*, **67**, 613–17.
50. Sharp, K.W. (1988). Acute cholecystitis. *Surg. Clin. North Am.*, **68**, 269–74.
51. Fabian, T.C., Zellner, S.R., Gazzaniga, A., Hanna, C., Nicholas, R., and Waxman, K. (1988). Multicentre open trial of cefotetan and cefoxitin in elective biliary surgery. *Am. J. Surg.*, **155**, 77–80.
52. Sirinik, K.R. and Levine, B.A. (1989). Percutaneous transhepatic cholangiography and biliary decompression. Invasive, diagnostic and therapeutic procedures with too high a price? *Arch. Surg.*, **124**, 885–8.
53. Seifert, E. (1988). Long term follow up after endoscopic sphincterotomy. *Endoscopy*, **20**, 232–5.
54. Neoptolemos, J.P., Davidson, B.R., Shaw, D.E., Lloyd, D., Carr-Locke, D.L., and Fossard, D.P. (1987). Study of common bile duct exploration and endoscopic sphincterotomy in a consecutive series of 438 patients. *Br. J. Surg.*, **74**, 916–21.
55. Duron, J.J., Roux, J.M., Imbaud, P., Dumont, J.L., Dutet, D., and Validre, J. (1987). Biliary lithiasis in the over seventy-five age group: a new therapeutic strategy. *Br. J. Surg.*, **74**, 848–9.
56. Boey, J.H. and Way, L.W. (1980). Acute cholecystitis. *Ann. Surg.*, **191**, 264–70.
57. Lai, E.C.S., Tam, P.C., and Paterson, I.A. (1990). Emergency surgery for acute cholangitis: the high risk patients. *Ann. Surg.*, **211**, 55–9.
58. Leung, J.W.C., Chung, S.C.S., Sung, J.J.Y., Banez, V.P., and Li, A.K.C. (1989). Urgent endoscopic drainage for acute suppurative cholangitis. *Lancet*, **i**, 1307–9.
59. Gigot, J.F., Leese, T., Dereme, T., Coutinho, J., Castaing, D., and Bismuth, H. (1989). Acute cholangitis: Multivariate analysis of risk factors. *Ann. Surg.*, **209**, 435–8.
60. Leese, T., Neoptolemos, J.P., Baker, A.R., Carr-Locke, D.L. (1986). Management of acute cholangitis and the impact of endoscopic sphincterotomy. *Br. J. Surg.*, **73**, 988–92.
61. Lai, E.C.S., Paterson, I.A., Tam, P.C., Choi, T.K., Fan, S.T., and Wong, J. (1990). Severe acute cholangitis: the role of emergency nasobiliary drainage. *Surgery*, **107**, 268–72.
62. Lai, E.C.S. (1990). Management of severe acute cholangitis. *Br. J. Surg.*, **77**, 604–5.
63. Kashi, H., Lam, F.T., and Giles, G.R. (1989). Recurrent pyogenic cholangitis. *Ann. R. Coll. Surg. Engl.*, **71**, 387–9.
64. Horgan, P.G., Campbell, A.C., Gray, G.R., and Gillespie, G. (1989). Biliary leakage and peritonitis following removal of T tubes after bile duct exploration. *Br. J. Surg.*, **76**, 1296–7.
65. Leading article (1980). Pyogenic liver abscess. *Br. Med. J.*, **280**, 1155–6.
66. Sheinfeld, A.M., Steiner, A.E., and Rivkin, L.B. (1982). Transcutaneous drainage of abscesses of the liver guided by computed tomography scan. *Surg. Gynecol. Obstet.*, **155**, 662–6.
67. Pitt, H.A. (1983). Liver abscess. In *Surgery of the alimentary tract* (ed. R.T. Shackleford and G.D. Zuidema), Vol. 4, pp. 465–97. Saunders, Philadelphia, Penn.
68. Northover, J.M.A., Jones, B.J., Dawson, J.L., and Williams, R. (1982). Difficulties in the diagnosis and management of pyogenic liver abscess. *Br. J. Surg.*, **69**, 48–51.
69. Giles, G.R. (1988). The liver. In *Essential surgical practice* (ed. A. Cuschieri, G.R. Giles, and A.R. Moossa), pp. 998–1000. John Wright, Bristol.
70. Giles, G.R. (1988). The colon, rectum and anal canal. In *Essential surgical practice* (ed. A. Cuschieri, G.R. Giles, and A.R. Moosa), pp. 1193–231. John Wright, Bristol.
71. Hinchey, E.J., Schaal, P.G.H., Richards, G.K. (1978). Treatment of perforated diverticular disease. *Adv. Surg.*, **12**, 85–109.
72. Kourtesis, G.J., Williams, R.A., and Wilson, S.E. (1988). Surgical options in acute diverticulitis: value of sigmoid resection in dealing with the septic focus. *Aust. NZ J. Surg.*, **58**, 955–9.
73. Flancbaum, L., Nosher, J.L., and Brozin, R.E. (1990). Percutaneous catheter drainage of abdominal abscesses associated with perforated viscus. *Ann. Surg.*, **56**, 52–6.
74. Stabile, B.E., Puccio, E., and Van Sonnenburg, E. (1990). Preoperative percutaneous drainage of diverticular abscess. *Am. J. Surg.*, **159**, 99–104.
75. Levien, D.H., Mazier, W.P., Surell, J.A., and Raiman, P.J. (1989). Safe resection for diverticular disease of the colon. *Dis. Colon Rectum*, **32**, 30–2.
76. Mealy, K., Salman, A., and Arthur, G. (1988). Definitive one-stage emergency large bowel surgery. *Br. J. Surg.*, **75**, 1216–9.
77. Ravo, B., Mishrick, A., and Addei, K. (1987). The treatment of perforated diverticulitis by one stage intra-colonic bypass procedure. *Surgery*, **102**, 771–6.
78. Finlay, I.G. and Carter, D.C. (1987). A comparison of emergency resection and staged management in perforated diverticular disease. *Dis. Colon Rectum*, **30**, 929–33.
79. Johnson, C.D., Baker, M.E., Rice, R.P., Silverman, P., and Thompson, W.M. (1987). Diagnosis of acute colonic diverticulitis: comparison of barium enema and CT. *Am. J. Radiol.*, **148**, 541–6.
80. Pugh, J.I. (1964). On the pathology and behaviour of non-traumatic vesico intestinal fistula. *Br. J. Surg.*, **51**, 644–57.
81. Shatila, A.H. and Ackerman, N.B. (1976). Diagnosis and management of colovesical fistula. *Surg. Gynecol. Obstet.*, **143**, 71–4.
82. Morrison, P.D., and Addison, N.V. (1983). A study of col-

ovesical fistulae in a district hospital. *Ann. R. Coll. Surg. Engl.*, **65**, 221–3.

83. Rao, P.N., Knox, R., Barnard, R.J., and Schofield, P.F. (1987). Management of colovesical fistula. *Br. J. Surg.*, **74**, 362–3.
84. Marston, A. (1986). *Vascular disease of the gut*. Edward Arnold, London.
85. Ottinger, L.W. (1978). The surgical management of acute occlusion of the superior mesenteric artery. *Ann. Surg.*, **188**, 721–31.
86. Lewin, J., Fenyo, G., and Engstrom, L. (1988). Treatment of appendiceal abscess. *Acta Chir. Scand.*, **154**, 123–5.
87. Befeler, D. (1964). Recurrent appendicitis. *Arch. Surg.*, **89**, 666–8.
88. Mayo, C.W. (1934). *Appendicitis*. Proceedings of the Staff Meeting of the Mayo Clinic, Vol. 26, pp. 154–62.
89. Cleland, G. (1953). Caecocolic intussusception following appendicectomy. *Br. J. Surg.*, **41**, 108–9.
90. Kingsley, D.P. (1969) Some observations on appendicectomy with particular reference to technique. *Br. J. Surg.*, **56**, 491–6.
91. Sinha, A.P. (1977). Appendicectomy: an assessment of the advisability of stump invagination. *Br. J. Surg.*, **64**, 499–500.
92. Harbin, R.M. (1930). Meckel's diverticulum. *Surg. Gynecol. Obstet.* **51**, 863–8.
93. Soderlund, S. (1959). Meckel's diverticulum: a clinical and histological study. *Acta Chir. Scand.* (Suppl 248), 1–233.
94. Rosswick, R.P. (1965). Perforation of Meckel's diverticulum by foreign bodies, *Postgrad. Med. J.*, **51**, 105–7.
95. Leijonmarck, C.E., Bonman-Sanderlin, K., Frisell, J., and Räf, L. (1986). *Br. J. Surg.*, **73**, 146–9.
96. Peck, D.A., Labat, R., Waite, C.V. (1968). Diverticular disease of the right colon. *Dis. Colon Rectum*, **11**, 49–54.
97. Anscombe, A.R., Keddie, N.C., Schofield, D.F. (1967). Solitary ulcers and diverticulitis of the caecum. *Br. J. Surg.*, **54**, 553–7.
98. Gouge, T.H., Coppa, G.F., and Eng, K. (1983). Management of diverticulitis of ascending colon: 10 years experience. *Am. J. Surg.*, **145**, 387–91.
99. Keenan, J.P. and Hadley, G.P. (1984). The surgical management of typhoid perforation in children. *Br. J. Surg.* **71**, 928–9.
100. Maurya, S.D., Gupta, H.C., Tiwari, A., and Sharma, B.D. (1984). Typhoid bowel perforation: a review of 264 cases. *Int. Surg.*, **69**, 155–8.
101. Gibney, E.J. (1989). Typhoid perforation. *Br. J. Surg.*, **76**, 887–9.
102. Badejo, O.A. and Arigbabu, A.O. (1980). Operative treatment of typhoid perforation with peritoneal irrigation: a comparative study. *Gut*, **21**, 141–5.
103. Gibney, E.J. (1988). Typhoid enteric perforation in rural Ghana. *Journal of the Irish College of Physicians & Surgeons* **17**, 105.
104. Muckart, D.J. and Angorn, I.B. (1988). Surgical management of complicated typhoid fever. *S. Afr. J. Surg.*, **26**, 66–9.
105. Sitaram, V., Moses, B.V., Fenn, A.S., Khanduri, . (1990). Typhoid ileal perforations: a prospective study. *J. R. Coll. Surg. Engl.*, **72**, 347–9.
106. Chrintz, H., Vibits, H., Corditz, T.O., Harreby, J.S., Waadegaard, P., and Larson, S.O. (1989). Need for surgical wound dressing. *Br. J. Surg.*, **76**, 204–5.
107. Hermann, G.G., Bagi, P., and Christoffersen, I. (1988). Early secondary suture versus healing by second intention of incisional abscesses. *Surg. Gynecol. Obstet.*, **167**, 16–8.
108. Gottrup, F., Grode, P., Lundhus, F., Andrup, H., Holm, C.N., and Terpling, S. (1989). Management of severe incisional abscesses following laparotomy. Early closure under cover of metronidazole and ampicillin. *Arch. Surg.*, **124**, 702–4.
109. Cuschieri, A. (1988). The small intestine and vermiform appendix. In *Essential surgical practice* (ed. A. Cuschieri, G.R. Giles, and A.R. Moosa), pp. 1136–63. John Wright, Bristol.
110. The Southern Surgeons Club. (1991). A prospective analysis of 1518 laparoscopic cholecystectomies. *N. Engl. J. Med*, **324**, 1073–8.

21

Acute pancreatitis and pancreatic infection

MICHAEL J. McMAHON

Introduction

The human pancreas consists of secretory lobules, each approximately 5 mm in diameter, separated by fibrous septa. Pancreatic juice drains into intralobular ducts which in turn drain into interlobular ducts which lie in the fibrous septa. In acute pancreatitis caused by gallstones or alcohol, the two commonest causes, there is necrosis of peripancreatic parenchyma in the vicinity of the intra- and interlobular ducts. Polymorphs are found within the duct lumen indicating the presence of inflammation and necrosis of the duct wall may occur. Changes vary in severity from oedema and polymorph infiltration to large areas of necrosis of the gland and the peripancreatic tissues. Acute pancreatitis is characterized by a shock-like systemic illness during the first few days, from which the majority of patients recover. Formerly, as many as 20 per cent of patients died during this stage of the illness, but mortality rates have now fallen to between 5 and 10 per cent in most centres. Death during the early stages of the illness is usually associated with 'haemorrhagic' pancreatitis, so named because there is bruising and haemorrhagic infiltration of the pancreas and surrounding structures, and the accumulation of dark coloured fluid within the peritoneal cavity which is usually likened to 'prune juice'.

With improved methods of resuscitation many patients survive this early phase of the attack, but develop features of sepsis and progressive multiple organ failure in the ensuing days or weeks which is associated with necrosis in or around the pancreas. Infection frequently contributes to death in the later stages of the attack and constitutes one of the major challenges of therapy at the present time.

Infection and the aetiology of acute pancreatitis

Viral pancreatitis

The best known aetiological relationship between a viral infection and pancreatitis is that of mumps. There are numerous reports relating mumps to abdominal pain and raised levels of amylase, and conversely rising levels of antibodies to mumps virus have been reported in patients with acute pancreatitis. The extent of the actual association between the two diseases is confused by the fact that hyperamylasaemia of salivary origin occurs during mumps, and it remains unclear whether rising titres of antibodies during and after an attack of acute pancreatitis constitutes convincing evidence of infection by that virus. Acute pancreatitis has been associated with infections with enterovirus, Coxsackie and echovirus as well as with *Mycoplasma pneumoniae*, but only rarely has a putative association been proven by cultures. More recently, associations between acute pancreatitis and infection with hepatitis A and B, and HIV have been described.

Acute pancreatitis associated with viral and mycoplasmal infections is usually mild and self-limiting, hence the question of specific antiviral treatment is of great relevance. This is especially so because the association with the viral infection often becomes apparent only during the convalescent stage of the attack, and because it is probable that viral infections cause only a small minority of attacks of acute pancreatitis.

Bacteria and the cause of acute pancreatitis

Severe and fulminant pancreatitis results when staphylococcal toxin is injected into the pancreatic duct of dogs, and it has been suggested that haemorrhagic pancreatitis is a consequence of autodigestion of the pancreas by proteolytic enzymes derived from bacteria (4). Despite the fact that acute pancreatitis has been associated with specific infections such as *Legionella pneumophila*, *Yersinia*, *Salmonella typhi*, *Campylobacter*, and others, in isolated case reports, there is no evidence that infection plays a primary role in the causation of acute pancreatitis in the majority of patients. Bacteria can be isolated from the bile of most patients with gallstones, but there is little evidence that reflux of bile into the pancreatic duct occurs during the genesis of acute pancreatitis. It is most probable that a migrating gallstone causes transient obstruction of both biliary and pancreatic ducts and it is difficult to find evidence that bile-borne bacteria enter the pancreas. It is possible that infection within bile is one of the determinants of the severity of gallstone related acute pancreatitis, but strong evidence to incriminate bacteria is lacking. Even in the most severe degrees of haemorrhagic pancreatitis ascitic fluid is usually sterile. Before the role of bacteria is dismissed completely, it is important to remember that pancreatic enzymes themselves may have the capacity to digest and destroy organisms and hence the evidence of bacterial involvement in the initiation of the attack. Primary pyogenic cholangitis is complicated by acute pancreatitis in some patients. Even in this condition, however, it remains unclear whether infection is the causal link rather than obstruction of the pancreatic duct by the stones in the bile duct.

Table 21.1. Outline of treatment of acute pancreatitis.

MILD	SEVERE
• Analgesia (iv-im)	• Analgesia (iv)
• Intravenous crystalloid	• Intravenous: crystalloid colloid nutrition
• Clinical observation and input/output fluid chart	• Monitor central venous pressure, inotropes, urine output
• Monitor pulse and respiration	• Monitor pO_2, oxygen via mask, ventilation
• Nasogastric tube	• Nasogastric tube
	• Peritoneal lavage
	• Antibiotics
	• Percutaneous aspiration abdominal collections pleural effusion
	• Surgery (debridement)

It has been argued that it is not obstruction of the pancreatic duct which causes acute pancreatitis, but destruction of the normal barrier function of the ampulla which is rendered patulous and incompetent by the passage of a gallstone. This would clearly open the way for organisms in the duodenal lumen to enter the bile duct. Despite a careful search, Foulis was unable to find bacteria within the lumena of inflamed pancreatic ducts in patients who had died from acute pancreatitis (1).

Endotoxaemia in pancreatitis

Although it is rarely possible to culture organisms from the blood of patients with acute pancreatitis, endotoxaemia does occur. Foulis and his colleagues studied twenty-six attacks of acute pancreatitis and were able to detect Gram-negative endotoxin, as indicated by a positive limulas lysate assay, in thirteen of them. Although there was no significant relationship between severity of the attack and the presence of endotoxaemia, five of the eight patients classified as severe and three of the four patients who died were in the 'endotoxin positive' group (5). Rising titres of anti-enterobacterial common antigen have been described in patients with moderate and severe pancreatitis, although only one of the six patients who died in the acute stages of the attack exhibited increased antigen titres (6). In Leeds, the author has also found endotoxin in the plasma and peritoneal fluid of patients with severe pancreatitis.

It is possible that translocation of Gram-negative antigenic material from the gut to the plasma is the reason for endotoxaemia. The pancreas is intimately associated with the stomach, duodenum and the transverse colon, all of which become oedematous and inflamed in patients with pancreatitis, due to the proximity of the viscera to the inflammatory focus (Fig. 21.1). The breakdown in barrier function of the gut which is associated with inflammation may permit the translocation of Gram-negative material, particularly from the transverse colon. It is also possible that the potential for translocation is increased by starvation and therapy with antibiotics. Although

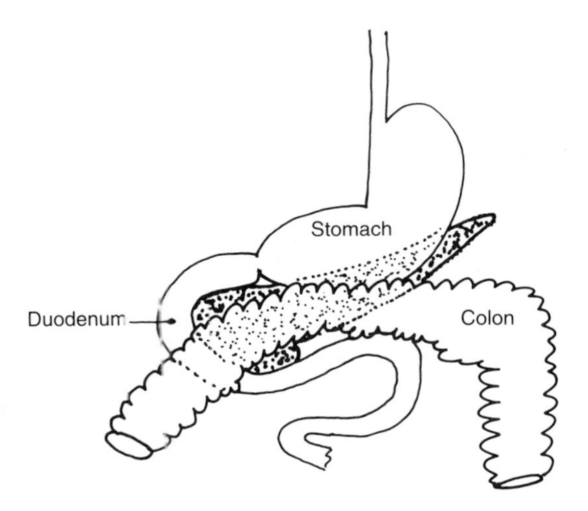

Fig. 21.1. Relationship of the pancreas to the stomach, duodenum and transverse colon. The position of the pancreas is indicated by the stippled area. When the pancreas becomes inflamed all the adjacent viscera may be involved, hence there is abundant opportunity for bacterial translocation from intestinal lumen to portal venous blood, particularly when the transverse colon is inflamed.

the induction of translocation and the role of Gram-negative endotoxin remains speculative and controversial in the pathogenesis of pancreatitis, they are potentially important.

The principal cause of death, and one of the greatest difficulties with the management of pancreatitis, is sepsis. Widespread endotoxaemia might contribute to the presence of a 'septic' state in the absence of specific evidence of pancreatic infection and in addition, translocation of live organisms might permit opportunistic secondary infection of necrotic areas within and around the pancreas. In the author's view the theories relating to these mechanisms do not provide a rationale for the use of antibiotics in the early stages of the attack.

The immune system in acute pancreatitis

When patients with acute pancreatitis develop infection recovery is usually a slow and gradual process, even when the infected focus is drained surgically. Moreover, wound healing is often poor and patients frequently exhibit a markedly cachectic response. In some patients there is progressive deterioration with the development of multiple organ failure despite all that therapy can offer. It is probable that there is considerable impairment of immune competence, and it has been shown that patients with severe pancreatitis develop an anergic state to routine skin-test antigens (7). Whether immune depression is, or is not, an important aspect of the pathogenesis of acute pancreatitis in man is unresolved, but there is experimental work to suggest that survival from induced pancreatitis can be improved by immuno-stimulation.

The situation in patients is confusing. On the one hand it has been argued that excessive stimulation of leukocytes permits loss of lysosomal secretions during rapid phagocytosis with consequent toxic effects upon the host (8). Other studies, however, show depression of phagocytosis in patients with severe pancreatitis. These observations are not necessarily contradictory because excessive stimulus secretion coupling may occur early in the course of the attack and may be followed by later depression of an overwhelmed phagocytic system. These aspects of severe acute pancreatitis warrant further study because they may open up potential avenues for therapy in a disease which has hitherto proved itself to be resistant to specific treatment despite the numerous avenues for therapy which exist according to our theoretical knowledge.

One type of 'phagocyte assist' therapy which has been employed during severe acute pancreatitis is plasmapheresis. Pilot studies suggest that there may be benefits (9) but much more work is required before this expensive and invasive treatment can be considered to have a role in the management of acute pancreatitis.

Treatment of the initial phase of the attack

General measures

There is no specific pharmacological treatment of acute pancreatitis which has been able to endure the critical scrutiny of a randomized clinical trial, although few treatments have been subject to a clinical trial of adequate power to provide a worthwhile contribution to factual knowledge. The mainstay of treatment is appropriate physiological support for the patient in order that he can survive the initial acute illness and the subsequent systemic and local complications. Patients with the most mild degrees of pancreatitis need little if any treatment, whereas those with a severe and fulminant attack may need intensive support with fluids, colloids, inotropes, and ventilation, and may even then succumb to the acute illness. It is routine for all patients in whom a diagnosis of acute pancreatitis is made to receive intravenous fluids and nasogastric aspiration which are continued for as long as appears to be necessary, using the criteria applied to other acute illnesses. Careful monitoring and surveillance are necessary, because about a quarter of the patients whose attack appears to be of moderate or mild severity at the time of admission will develop evidence of greater severity during the ensuing 48 h.

Nevertheless, patients who appear to have a very mild attack, as indicated by abdominal pain which settles rapidly, relatively minor degrees of abdominal tenderness, and little in the way of systemic disturbance, are unlikely to develop a worsening anamnesis or a collection in or around the pancreas. At the other extreme, patients who appear to have a clinically severe attack at the time of admission should be treated intensively with the expectation that complications will occur. The repeated assessment of recognized indices of severity, such as the APACHE II score, may help to assess the patient's progress, to predict impending severity, and to keep the clinician alert to the possibility that a turn for the worse may ensue (10).

In most respects, monitoring the course of the attack implies a careful observation of pulse, respiration, and temperature. It is important that adequate analgesia is provided to keep the patient comfortable, and this usually means intravenous or intramuscular opiates. Traditionally, morphine has been avoided because it can cause increased tone of the sphincter of

Oddi with hyperamylasaemia, and pethidine is usually used. In practice, omnopon is probably a suitable analgesic for many patients. Although the measurement of pO_2 is not necessary in patients with a mild attack, who have no evidence of respiratory embarrassment, it is important in more severely ill patients and low levels of arterial pO_2 should be treated by oxygen delivered by a face mask, with follow-up measurements of blood gases to ensure that adequate oxygenation is achieved. In the more severely ill patients ventilation may be necessary and it is probably better to resort to it sooner rather than later. In the patient with a severe attack measurement of central venous pressure and a careful record of urine output combined with pulse, blood pressure and the difference between core and peripheral temperature are guides to the requirements for crystaloids and colloids. In the fulminant attack it may be possible to obtain adequate cardiac output and peripheral perfusion only if excessive quantities of fluid are given. It may be necessary to strike a compromise between perfusion and pulmonary oedema, and such patients are extremely difficult to manage. The objective of treatment in the severely ill patient is to maintain physiological function of organ systems and to stave off the failure of organ systems until such time as complications in and around the pancreas can be identified precisely and treated.

The role of antibiotic therapy

From the foregoing, the routine use of antibiotics in the initial stages of acute pancreatitis would not seem logical because there is no evidence that infection plays a primary role in the genesis of the attack in the great majority of patients. Nevertheless, a proportion of clinicians routinely include antibiotics in the treatment of the attack. There have been four randomized trials of antibiotic therapy in patients with acute pancreatitis (3 of ampicillin, 1 of cephalothin) (11, 12, 13, 14). None of the drugs were shown to influence significantly the course of the attack and, in particular, the frequency of septic complications. However, none of the trials was of sufficient power to eliminate the possibility that the antibiotics had a significant influence upon the course of the attack. In view of the lack of a clear rationale for antibiotic therapy, and the results of these studies, it would seem reasonable to conclude that there is no justification for the routine use of antibiotics, and not unreasonable to speculate that their use might increase bacterial translocation from the gastrointestinal tract and give rise to overgrowth of resistant organisms.

If a specific infection such as pneumonia or pancreatic abscess emerges during the course of acute pancreatitis, antibiotics are logical. Where possible, the use of antibiotics should be based upon culture of the responsible organisms, but, as is often the case in severe septic illnesses, this is not always possible.

Biliary infection

The gall-bladder becomes inflamed in some patients who suffer from acute pancreatitis secondary to gallstones. It remains unclear whether this is a primary bacterial or biochemical inflammation and there is no clear indication of either the place of antibiotics nor the importance of the inflamed gall-bladder to the development of the attack. In a small proportion of elderly patients, who usually present with mild pancreatitis due to gallstones, acute cholangitis can supervene and cause deterioration in the patient's condition. In the author's view, the use of antibiotics for biliary complications of acute pancreatitis (or of the stone which causes the pancreatitis) is not justified unless cholangitis occurs.

Peritoneal lavage

It is the author's practice to perform peritoneal lavage using 1 litre of normal saline in patients with clinically severe acute pancreatitis. The principal reason for doing so is to confirm that acute pancreatitis is indeed the diagnosis, rather than another condition such as perforated peptic ulcer or a perforation of the biliary tract masquerading as pancreatitis. If bacteria, or animal or vegetable fibres, are recovered from the peritoneal return fluid, or from free ascitic fluid aspirated from the peritoneal catheter after its introduction, not only are antibiotics warranted, but the diagnosis of acute pancreatitis is probably incorrect. In such circumstances a laparotomy is justified.

Infective complications of acute pancreatitis

Development of complications

Although both may exist together, it is convenient to consider two categories of complications of acute pancreatitis. The first category consists of complications such as pulmonary oedema, renal failure, pneumothorax, flank staining, etc., which occur during the initial, acute, shock-like illness. The second category comprises complications which are more or less local to the pancreas, and includes pancreatic necrosis, abscess and pseudocyst, peripancreatic necrosis, pancreatic ascites, pancreaticopleural fistula, etc. It is these local complications which have become so important in recent years, because the success with which they can be treated is so often a determinant of death or survival from the attack.

The pathogenesis of local complications has not been precisely elucidated, but it is probable that necrosis plays a key part in development. In experimental animals, the blood supply to the pancreas may fall rapidly within a few minutes of the induction of acute pancreatitis, partly because of vascular occlusion by the pressure of oedema fluid and perhaps partly by arteriolar spasm. Even in patients with a relatively mild acute pancreatitis, small areas of necrosis are frequently present within the gland and these are larger and more confluent in patients with more severe attacks. Macroscopically visible pancreatic necrosis inevitably involves destruction of small ducts. When pancreatic juice is produced by the acini draining into these ducts it will enter the necrotic area and can potentially form a small 'lake' of pancreatic juice, which may rapidly become activated by substances within the necrotic tissue. This can lead to the formation of an enlarging area of necrosis which may contain partially digested tissue debris. Necrosis can also occur in peripancreatic fatty tissue. It is believed that enzymes exude from the surface of the gland into the surrounding tissue during the early stages of pancreatitis, and that a combination of phospholipase and co-lipase is able to digest the cell membrane of the fat cell and then the fat within it. Necrotic foci, within or outside the pancreas, usually resolve spontaneously, leaving nothing but a small area of scar to indicate their existence. Larger areas of necrosis do not heal so readily and may give rise to four types of local complication.

1. *Pancreatic necrosis* (Fig. 21.2)
   This is an area of fluid and necrotic tissue within the pancreas in which dead tissue is the major component.
2. *Extrapancreatic necrosis*
   Necrosis of the fat around the pancreas can coexist with an almost intact gland. In other patients it is associated with large necrotic areas within the pancreas itself.

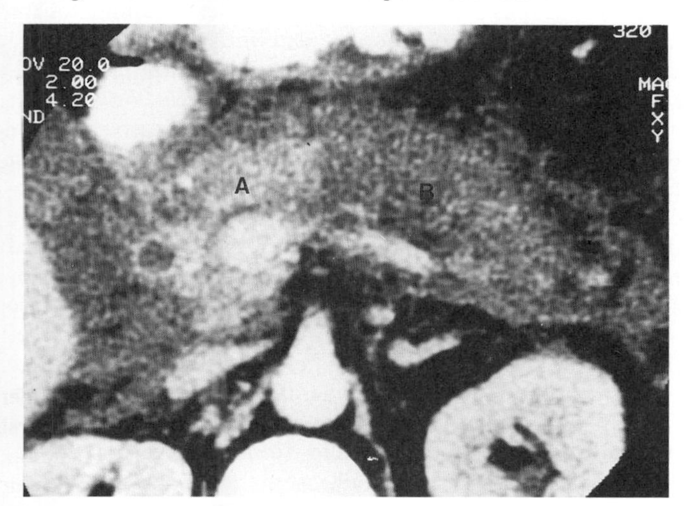

Fig. 21.2. Details from CT scan showing uninfected pancreatic necrosis. Intravenous contrast has been injected and the head of the pancreas has enhanced (A) but there is poor enhancement of the body and tail of the gland (B). (Courtesy of Dr A. G. Chalmers.)

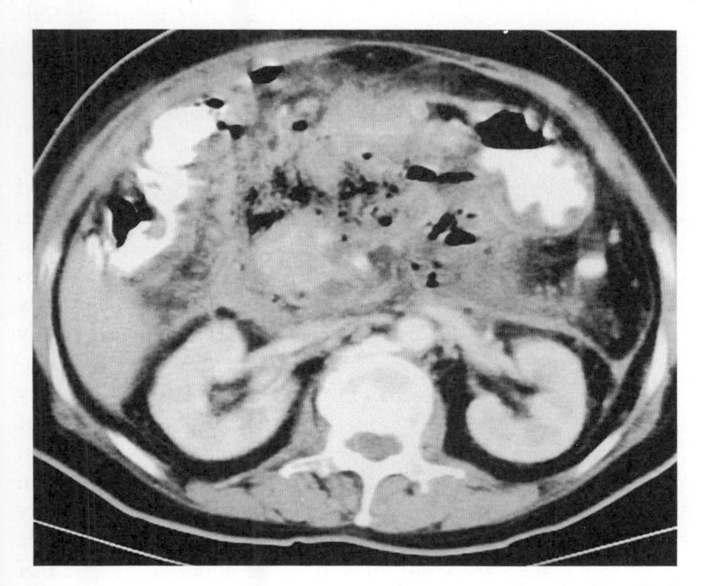

Fig. 21.3. CT scan showing pseudocyst in the body of the pancreas. (Courtesy of Dr A G Chalmers.)

3. *Pancreatic pseudocyst* (Fig. 21.3) A pseudocyst is a collection of pancreatic fluid within a cavity which is not lined by epithelium. It may lie within or adjacent to the pancreas and pseudocysts are occasionally apparently remote from it. A pseudocyst is a result of an area of necrosis involving a major duct upstream of which there is considerable pancreatic juice production. Accumulation of the juice in an area of softened and necrotic pancreas adjacent to the ductal system may cause occlusion of the downstream part of the duct which prevents the juice from draining into the duodenum along the duct itself.

This can cause a vicious cycle whereby the greater the degree of fluid accumulation the more pressure there is on the duct and the less easily the fluid can drain away. Not surprisingly, a pseudocyst can reach a large size and may occasionally decompress spontaneously by erosion into an adjacent viscus such as the duodenum or stomach. The existence of a pseudocyst may remain occult for many months and give rise to symptoms of post-prandial epigastric pain and weight loss, not dissimilar to those of an upper gastrointestinal malignancy. Occasionally, a pseudocyst can rupture into the peritoneal cavity and give rise to pancreatic ascites.

4. *Pancreatic abscess*
   This is an area of infected pus and necrotic tissue within or adjacent to the pancreas. Pus is the major component, debris and pieces of skeletalized tissue with the resemblance of fragments of grey blotting paper may be present within the cavity.

Sterile and infected collections

Patients with evidence of a fluid collection related to the pancreas or evidence of pancreatic or peripancreatic necrosis can pursue a very benign course, leading to spontaneous resolution of the complication or the opportunity to carry out an 'elective' surgical intervention with a high prospect of success. More usually, the patient exhibits 'toxic' symptoms which may be of such severity that death due to fulminant sepsis and multiple organ failure cannot be averted. It is often unclear whether the patient with a 'septic' pancreas has an infective cause of the sepsis, or whether the patient's clinical condition is due to a combination of necrotic tissue and activated pancreatic enzymes. It is common experience that an extremely 'septic' clinical picture can arise from a pancreatic collection from which organisms cannot be cultured. Nevertheless, it is important to identify patients with infected pancreatic necrosis, because they may develop a sudden deterioration with the rapid onset of multiple organ failure. In a large study from Ulm in Germany, over half the patients with infective necrosis were found to have pulmonary failure (15). Pulmonary failure is found in a small proportion of patients with uninfective necrosis, or with pancreatic abscess. Overall, 40 per cent of patients of 114 patients who underwent operation for established pancreatic necrosis were found to have infective necrotic tissue (16). Of great interest was the fact that the frequency of infection increased up to the third week, but was lower in operations carried out at a later stage (Fig. 21.4). A relation-

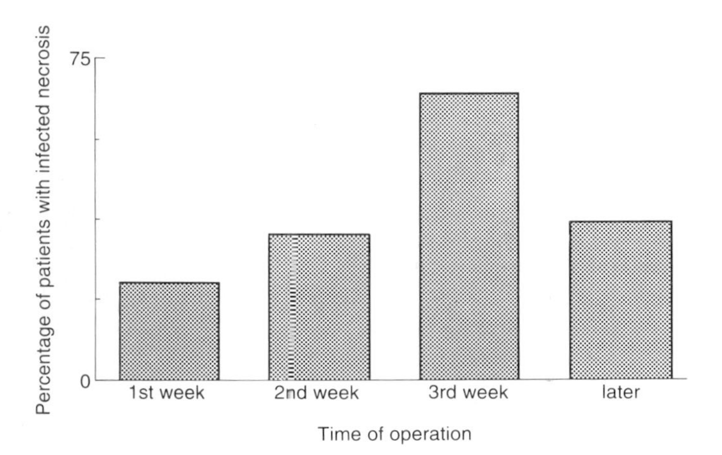

Fig. 21.4. Percentage incidence of infection in necrotic pancreatic and peripancreatic tissue compared with timing of the operation to remove it. [Drawn from data of Beger, H.G. *et al*, (16)].

ship between the volume of necrotic tissue and the frequency of infection was also observed.

This data is consistent with the concept that pancreatic necrosis is usually sterile during the early stages of acute pancreatitis, but becomes infected later during the attack. The infection is probably opportunistic, and translocation of intestinal bacteria may be an important element in its initiation because Gram-negative intestinal organisms are commonly responsible. The relationship between infection and the volume of necrotic tissue is also consistent with an opportunistic mechanism (see Abacterial sepsis syndrome, p. 115 in Chapter 13).

Diagnosis of the complications of acute pancreatitis

Diagnosis of pancreatic collections

When a patient suffers a severe or protracted attack of acute pancreatitis, two questions in particular need to be answered. Is there is a collection in or around the pancreas, and if so is it infected?

Ultrasound may be of value, particularly if there is a pseudocyst with relatively little involvement (and hence dilatation) of adjacent hollow viscera. However, in the ill patient with acute pancreatitis, ultrasound is not a reliable imaging technique for the pancreas, and patients should undergo CT scan if there is any question that a collection exists. CT scan carried out before and after a rapid intravenous injection of contrast medium is a highly sensitive technique to detect necrosis of the pancreas or adjacent tissues (17). This is not to say that all patients with acute pancreatitis need be screened by CT, because it has poor discriminatory power for the differentiation of patients who will develop a necrosis from those who will not if used as a routine procedure during the first day or two of the attack. However, after a few more days have elapsed and it is possible clinically to differentiate patients who have a rapidly resolving attack from those with more severe and protracted pancreatitis, a contrast-enhanced CT scan becomes highly precise. Non-specific markers of severity or inflammation such as the APACHE II sepsis score or C-reactive protein, may be of value for the selection of patients who need to be imaged if CT facilities are scarce or distant (10, 18). The urgency with which the investigation should be carried out depends upon the patient's clinical status. In the author's own practice, where a policy of delayed operative intervention is used, it is only necessary to request a CT scan within the first week of the attack when it appears that the patient is sufficiently ill that imminent operative intervention or percutaneous drainage might be needed.

The diagnosis of infection is thought to be important because there is a widespread view that infective necrosis needs surgical intervention. Certainly, patients with infective collections are usually more severely ill than those with sterile necrosis and thus more likely to be considered candidates for urgent operative intervention. If deterioration of the clinical condition of the patient is the prime indication to operate, rather than the appearances of the pancreas on contrast enhanced CT, it can be argued that it does not matter whether the presence of infection is confirmed or not. However, if it can be shown that a 'wait and see' policy is more likely to be successful in the patient with sterile necrosis and progressive deterioration, more usually the case in patients with infected necrosis, then a knowledge of the bacterial status of the pancreas might help the surgeon predict the course of the disease and hence make the decision to operate at the correct time. Sometimes, infection is only too apparent from the presence of gas bubbles in the peripancreatic tissues on CT scan (Fig. 21.5). In most cases gas pockets are not evident, and percutaneous aspiration of fluid from the necrotic collections is possible with CT or ultrasonic guidance and gives a reliable indication of the presence or absence of infection (19, 20, 21).

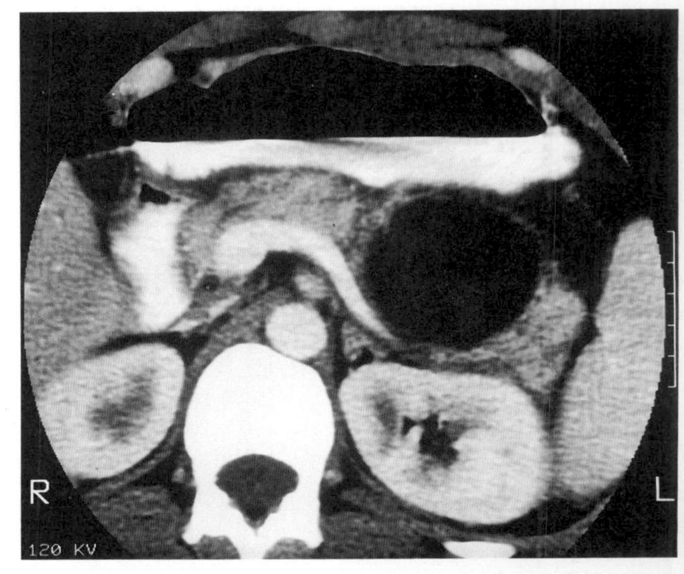

Fig. 21.5. CT scan showing infected necrosis in and around the pancreas. Gas shadows can be seen in the tissue in front of the pancreas. (Courtesy of Dr AG Chalmers.)

Management of the 'septic' pancreas

General measures

Although it is convenient from a conceptual point of view to discriminate between the acute, shock-like illness and the later complications of acute pancreatitis, in practice both are often superimposed. Although some patients with a relatively severe early component to the illness appear to make a progressive recovery and then relapse some days later due to pancreatic or peripancreatic necrosis, it is more usual for the patient with severe symptoms or a fulminant course during the initial stages of the attack to remain extremely ill until it becomes apparent that a large area of necrosis is present. Thus, the management of the severe illness usually blends imperceptibly with the management of the local complication in the pancreas.

The broad policy of management advocated by many surgeons is to treat the attack conservatively until it settles, or for as long as possible, before resorting to surgical intervention. Early surgery, by formal pancreatectomy or debridement, during the initial few days of the attack has become a less popular option. There is little doubt that the later operations are associated with a better outcome, but part of the reason for this may be the fact that the most severely ill patients demand earlier surgery. Nevertheless, it is better to avoid operation during the first ten or so days of the attack because a high mortality rate may be anticipated during this time (22). The onus thus falls upon the clinician pursuing conservative management to enable surgery to be delayed for as long as possible whilst preventing the onset of multiple organ failure. An operation carried out once multiple organ failure is established is unlikely to be successful.

The principal planks of conservative management are careful attention to fluid and electrolyte balance, respiratory care, and nutritional support. The author generally advocates intravenous nutrition, and it is commenced about five days after admission to hospital when it is clear that the attack of pancreatitis is severe. Because glucose intolerance is especially likely to occur in patients with acute pancreatitis, a relatively modest total calorie provision is used (about 1600 kcal per day in the average patient) and about half the calories are given as lipid emulsion, the other half as glucose. Care is needed to monitor blood glucose levels and insulin should be given if hyperglycaemia occurs. Patients with acute pancreatitis are particularly liable develop infective complications associated with the central venous catheter and great care must be used to prevent infection. There should be constant vigilance for the onset of pulmonary or respiratory failure, and occasionally, measures such as plasmapheresis or plasmafiltration may help to offset decline into multiple organ failure (9).

Antibiotic policy

Although most patients with pancreatic sepsis receive antibiotics from time to time, there is no evidence that the use of antibiotics can delay the onset of infected necrosis nor effectively treat it. Logically, it might seem appropriate to use an antibiotic which can penetrate pancreatic tissue and juice (23), but the infection is usually centred in necrotic tissue and it is not certain that antibiotics adequately reach the contents of pancreatic collections. If infection is proven by percutaneous aspiration or surgery, it is logical to use an antibiotic which is effective against the organisms which are cultured. The author usually withholds antibiotics until the time of surgery in the hope that they will be maximally effective, but the advent of respiratory complications frequently indicates the need for antibiotic treatment before operation is undertaken for a pancreatic complication. The cephalosporins are favoured and caution should be exercised in the use of aminoglycosides. The combination of acute pancreatitis and aminoglycoside therapy may make the patient more likely to develop renal failure.

Percutaneous aspiration

If fluid is a major component of a pancreatic collection, percutaneous aspiration, guided by ultrasound or CT, undoubtedly has a role in management, and also gives the opportunity to determine whether bacterial infection is present (Fig. 21.6). Aspiration of the collection through a needle which is withdrawn when the fluid has been removed is less liable to lead to infection than the insertion of an indwelling (pigtail) catheter, but in the author's experience fluid re-collects rapidly in most patients. Moreover, the infection which is introduced through an indwelling catheter does not usually lead to overwhelming local sepsis. A catheter can be left on free drainage but flushed daily under strictly aseptic conditions. Even if there is eventually reaccumulation of fluid and the development of a pseudocyst or abscess, this is a relatively small price to pay to avoid an urgent operation in the early stages of an attack of acute pancreatitis. Good imaging is necessary for the accurate and precise placement of percutaneous drains and the radiologist should be encouraged to place them in the flanks if possible in order that drainage can occur under the influence of gravity. Percutaneous drainage is generally unsuccessful if the major component of the collection is necrotic tissue rather than pancreatic juice or pus.

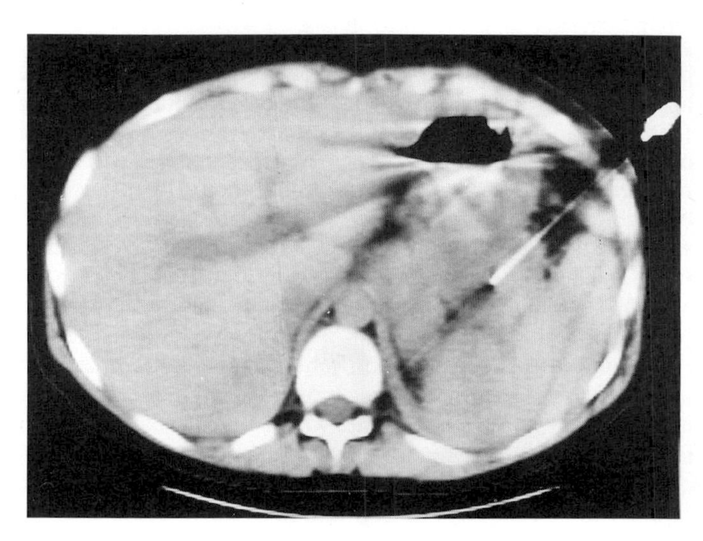

Fig. 21.6. Percutaneous aspiration of a pancreatic collection. The CT scan shows the aspiration needle *in situ* in a pancreatic pseudocyst after aspiration of its contents. (Courtesy of Dr AG Chalmers.)

Surgical debridement

The principal role of surgery during the first month or six weeks after acute pancreatitis is to remove necrotic tissue which is preventing recovery from the attack. At later stages, surgery may also be needed to treat a pseudocyst or abscess of the pancreas. Generally speaking, surgery is best avoided in patients with severe pancreatitis because of the magnitude of the septic illness and the probability that impaired immunity will be present. In practice, less than 10 per cent of patients who develop pancreatitis need surgery to debride necrotic tissue. The operation should be delayed as long as possible in the hope that the attack may eventually settle to the extent that it can be carried out, if needed, as an 'elective' procedure many weeks after the initial admission to hospital. Nevertheless, it is important that, if surgery is undertaken, the operation is performed before the onset of multiple organ failure. It is useful to consider that the patient may well be no better, or even a little worse, for 48 or 72 h after pancreatic debridement, probably because endotoxaemia occurs massively during the operative procedure.

The timing of operation is based entirely upon the clinical progress of the patient, but a contrast-enhanced CT scan is extremely important in order to decide what operation to perform and where to look for necrotic tissue. The surgeon cannot judge the viability of the pancreas at the time of operation (24).

If there is no alternative but to operate, for fear that the patient will die if conservative treatment is continued, and necrotic pancreatic or peripancreatic tissue has been identified by contrast enhanced CT, then it is generally agreed that debridement of necrotic tissue is the procedure of choice. Access may be through the gastrocolic omentum, or directly to the necrotic area by inserting a finger through the root of the transverse mesocolon. Digital dissection is used to remove the slimy peripancreatic necrotic tissue or the rather dry blotting paper-like necrotic pancreas, and the CT scan is placed on the radiograph viewing box in the operating theatre in order to be sure exactly where the necrotic tissue lies and how best to get at it. Surprisingly, bleeding is not usually a problem. If peripancreatic necrosis is the principal abnormality, or if there are extensive and wide-ranging necrotic cavities extending from the pancreas it is probably better to open the gastrocolic omentum. If the majority of the necrosis is centred within the pancreas then the approach through the root of the transverse mesocolon has attractions (25, 26). The problems really begin when the debridement has taken place. Scooping out necrotic tissue inevitably leaves segments of the pancreas which have become separated from the normal drainage ducts. Pancreatic juice oozes into the cavity from which the necrotic tissue was removed and this is activated by blood and the remnants of necrotic tissue. If this fluid accumulates in the operated area it rapidly digests the tissue planes which have been used to gain access and the most horrible septic mess results which frequently causes the death of the patient.

There are essentially two techniques to obviate this distressing complication. First, drains can be inserted so that the cavity can be irrigated and secretions and irrigation fluid flushed away, if possible under the influence of gravity (Fig. 21.7). Large amounts of irrigating fluid are needed and it may be several weeks before drains can be removed from the abdomen. There is an argument for the inclusion of an antiprotease solution in the fluid used to irrigate the drains, but its value has not been proved. In order to facilitate drainage under gravity when the patient is supine place the drains into the necrotic cavity as posteriorly as possible. The most consistent drain is one which goes into the tail of the pancreas behind the splenic flexure of the colon (Fig. 21.8) and in some patients there is an additional drain into the head of the gland. These drains are brought out into the flank area and secured by a

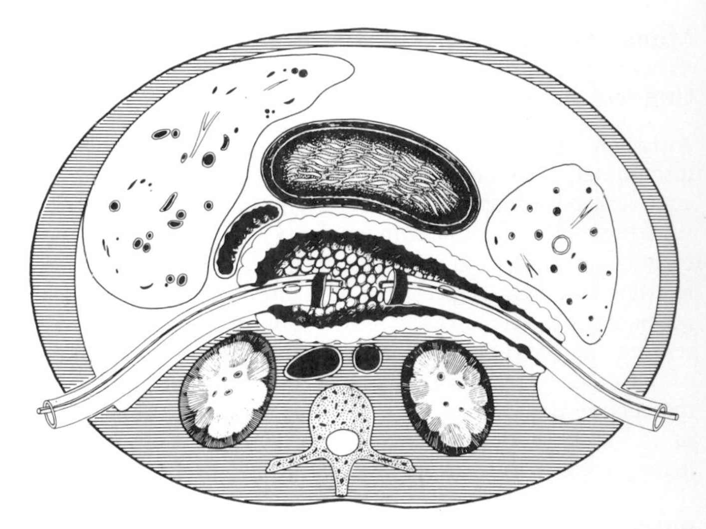

Fig. 21.7. Cross-section of abdomen, showing irrigating drains placed in the civity from which necrotic pancreas has been removed. The drains are brought out in a posterior position so that gravity can aid drainage. (From Larvin, M. *et al.* (25), with permission.)

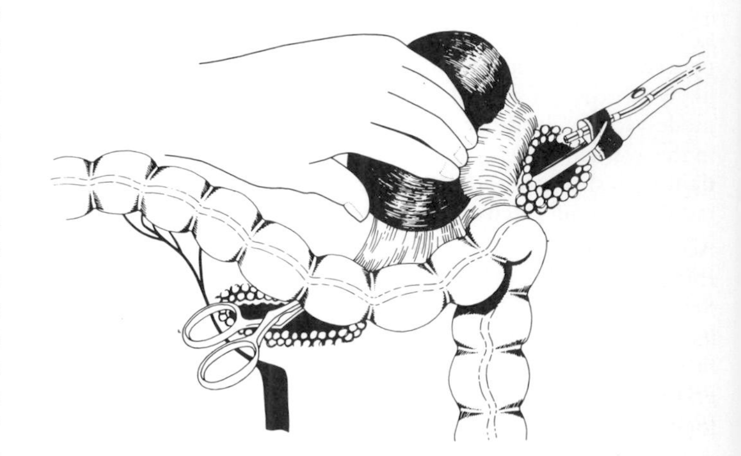

Fig. 21.8. Drainage of a cavity in the body and tail of the pancreas. Access to the cavity has been gained through the transverse mesocolon and a finger has been passed from the cavity into the upper part of the left paracolic gutter behind the spleen just above the splenic flexure of the colon. The drain, which has been brought through the abdominal wall, is pulled into the pancreatic cavity using forceps. Alternatively, a large Hegars dilator can be used to pass the drain through the abdominal wall and into the pancreatic cavity. (From Larvin, M. *et al.* (25), with permission.)

large disc to minimize discomfort to the patient. The drains are withdrawn as the cavity shrinks, which is determined from sinograms carried out at weekly intervals. The other technique to manage the cavity after debridement is to pack it with gauze which acts somewhat like a wick to soak up the secreted enzymes. The wick, of course, becomes saturated and for this reason it is necessary to change the gauze daily. When the gauze is changed the cavity is carefully inspected and any further necrotic tissue removed. Daily re-laparotomy is a very laborious and time-consuming procedure which usually necessitates continued ventilation of the patient until the cavity is granulating well and the procedure is more straightforward.

The author has used both procedures, but favours the closed cavity irrigation and drainage for intrapancreatic necrosis, and the packing technique for extensive extrapancreatic necrosis. Even when using the latter, an irrigating drain is placed at the time of the initial laparotomy in order that the patient can be converted to tube drainage as soon as a clean granulating cavity exists. Whichever method of drainage is used, these patients present a difficult challenge to the surgeon. Great care is needed in the performance of the operations because it there is damage to a bowel loop, the duodenum or the transverse colon, a fatal outcome is much more likely. Careful and precise post-operative management is necessary to anticipate, prevent and, if necessary, treat the numerous complications which can occur. These include recurrent sepsis (sometimes due to the fact that the drain has become blocked) and bleeding. The latter is a surprisingly infrequent problem when the extent of intra-abdominal digestion is considered, and usually responds to a judiciously placed pack. If tube drainage appears to be problematic, it is possible to introduce an endoscope through the drain in order to extract fragments of necrotic material.

Many patients are in hospital for two or three months after pancreatic debridement, but the constant light at the end of the tunnel is that if the patient survives this most severe and debilitating illness, he is likely to make a fairly full recovery and lead a relatively normal life. Even with extensive necrosis of the pancreas, diabetes can usually be controlled by dietary means alone and the chronic need for insulin is unusual.

Summary

Acute pancreatitis and its management remain enigmatic. The role of infection remains unclear but it is probably an opportunistic secondary phenomenon and needs to be treated on its merits. The identification and management of pancreatic necrosis pose a continuing challenge to the therapist, although gratifying results can be achieved by adherence to physiological principles and details of management.

References

1. Foulis, A. K. (1980). Histological evidence of initiating factors in acute necrotising pancreatitis in man. *J. Clin. Pathol.*, **33**, 1125–31.
2. Reuner, I. G., Savage, W. T., Pantoja, J. L., and Renner, V. J. (1985). Death due to acute pancreatitis. A retrospective analysis of 405 autopsy cases. *Dig. Dis. Sci.*, **30**, 1005–18.
3. Thal, A. and Molestina, J. E. (1985). Studies on pancreatitis. III: Fulminating haemorrhagic pancreatic necrosis produced by means of staphylococcal toxin. *Arch. Pathol. Lab. Med.*, **60**, 212–20.
4. Keynes, W. M. (1980). A non-pancreatic source of the proteolytic enzyme amidase and bacteriology in experimental pancreatitis. *Ann. Surg.*, **191**, 187–99.
5. Foulis, A. K., Murray, W. R., Galloway, D., *et al.* (1982). Endotoxaemia and complement activation in acute pancreatitis in man. *Gut*, **23**, 656–61.
6. Kivilaakso, E., Valtonen, V. V., Malkamaki, M., *et al.* (1984). Endotoxaemia and acute pancreatitis: Correlations between the severity of the disease and the anti-enteral bacterial common antigen–antibody titre. *Gut*, **25**, 1065–70.
7. Garcia-Sabrido, J. L., Valdecantose, E., Bastida, E., and Tellado, J. M. (1989). The anergic state as a predictor of pancreatic sepsis. *Zent. GI Chir.*, **114**, 114–20.
8. Rinderknecht, H. (1983). Fatal pancreatitis, a consequence of excessive leukocyte stimulation? *Int. J. Pancreatol*,. **3**, 105–12.
9. Larvin, M., Lansdown, M. R. J., McMahon, M. J., Chalmers, A. G., Turney, J. H., and Brownjohn, A. M. (1988). Plasmapheresis: a rational treatment for fulminant acute pancreatitis. *Br. Med. J.*, **297**, 593–4.
10. Larvin, M. and McMahon, M. J. (1989). APACHE-II score for assessment and monitoring of acute pancreatitis. *Lancet*, **ii**, 201–5.
11. Craig, R. M., Dordal, E., and Myles, L. (1975). The use of ampicillin in acute pancreatitis. *Ann. Intern. Med.*, **83**, 831–2.
12. Finch, W. T., Sawyers, J. L., and Schenker, S. (1976). A prospective study to determine the efficacy of antibiotics in acute pancreatitis. *Ann. Surg.*, **183**, 667–70.
13. Howes, R., Zuidema, G. D., and Cameron, J. L. (1975). Evaluation of prophylactic antibiotics in acute pancreatitis. *J. Surg. Res.*, **18**, 197–200.
14. Stone, H. M. and Fabian, T. C. (1980). Peritoneal analysis in the treatment of acute alcoholic pancreatitis. *Surg. Gynecol. Obstet.*, **150**, 878–82.
15. Bittner, R., Block, S., Buchler, M., and Beger, H. G. (1987). Pancreatic abscess and infected pancreatic necrosis. Different local and septic complications in acute pancreatitis. *Dig. Dis. Sci.*, **32**, 1082–7.
16. Beger, H. G., Bittner, R., Block, S., and Buchler, M. (1986). Bacterial contamination of pancreatic necrosis. A prospective clinical study. *Gastroenterology*, **91**, 433–8.
17. Larvin, M., McMahon, M. J., Chalmers, A. G. (1990). Dynamic contrast-enhanced CT: Precise identification and localisation of pancreatic necrosis complicating acute pancreatitis. *Br. Med. J.*, **330**, 1425–8.
18. Mayer, A. D., Bowen, M., Cooper, E. H., and McMahon, M. J. (1984). C-reactive protein: an aid to assessment and monitoring of acute pancreatitis. *J. Clin. Pathol.*, **37**, 207–11.
19. Hiatt, J. R., Fink, A. S., King, W., and Pitt, H. A. (1987). Percutaneous aspiration of peripancreatic fluid collections: a safe method to detect infection. *Surgery*, **101**, 523–30.
20. Gerzof, S. G., Banks, P. A., Robbins, A. H., *et al.* (1987). Early diagnosis of pancreatic infection by computed tomography-guided aspiration. *Gastroenterology*, **93**, 1315–20.
21. Banks, P. A., Gerzof, S. G., Chong, F. K., *et al.* (1990). Bacteriologic status of necrotic tissue in necrotizing pancreatitis. *Pancreas*, **5**, 330–3.
22. Smadja, C. and Bismuth, H. (1986). Pancreatic debridement in acute necrotizing pancreatitis: an obsolete procedure? *Br. J. Surg.*, **73**, 408–10.
23. Bradley, E. L. (1989). Antibiotics in acute pancreatitis. *Am. J. Surg.*, **158**, 472–7.
24. Nordback, I., Pessi, T., Auvinen, O. and Autio, V. (1985). Determination of necrosis in necrotizing pancreatitis. *Br. J. Surg.*, **72**, 225–7.

25. Larvin, M., McMahon, M. J., Chalmers, A. G., and Robisnon, P. J. (1989). Debridement and closed cavity drainage of the necrotic pancreas. *Br. J. Surg.*, **76**, 465–71.
26. Shi, E. C. P., Yeo, B. W., and Ham, J. M. (1984). Pancreatic abscess. *Br. J. Surg.*, **71**, 689–91.
27. Beger, H. G., Buchler, M., Bittner, R., Block, S., Nevalainen, T., and Roscher, R. (1988). Necrosectomy and post- operative local lavage in necrotizing pancreatitis. *Br. J. Surg.*, **75**, 207–12.
28. Bradley, E. L. (1987). Management of infected pancreatic necrosis by open drainage. *Ann. Surg.*, **206**, 542–50.
29. Pemberton, J. H., Becker, J. M., Dozois, R. R., Nagorney, D. M. Ilstrup, D., and Remine, W. H. (1986). Controlled open lesser sac drainage for pancreatic abscess. *Ann. Surg.*, **203**, 600–13.

22

Breast surgery

J. MICHAEL DIXON

Introduction

Breast anatomy

The breast is composed of fat, lobules, ducts, and connective tissue. Although the breast is said to be composed of a number of lobes, no tissue planes exist between these. There are fifteen to twenty major ducts connecting breast lobules to the nipple. A lobule with its terminal draining ductule is the functioning unit of the breast (Fig. 22.1). Each major duct drains between ten and one hundred terminal duct lobular units. Major breast ducts expand into a lactiferous sinus prior to narrowing down into a major collecting duct before opening onto the nipple.

Lymphatic drainage of the breast is from superficial to deep rather than toward the centre. The lymph then drains to the nearest regional nodes, either in the axilla or in the internal mammary chain. To a lesser extent lymph also drains by intercostal routes. The lymph node groups do not drain specific zones of the breast.

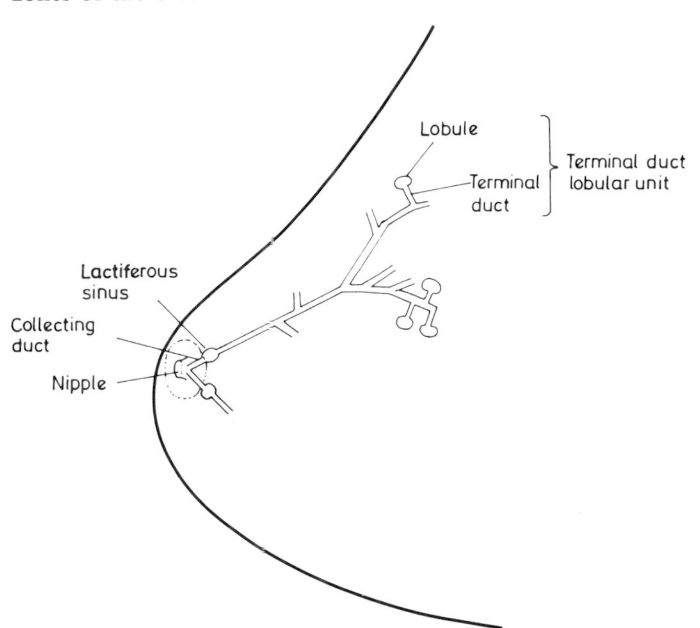

Fig. 22.1. The ductal and lobular system of the breast.

Changes in the breast during pregnancy

With the onset of lactation the breast lobules become distended with secretions which fill out the ductal systems. The secretion in the first 24 h is colostrum and milk follows on the second day of breast feeding.

Breast involution

Involution begins as soon as lactation ceases but also occurs at a much slower rate in association with age. Duct dilatation occurs as part of normal breast involution.

Anatomical site of breast infection

Infection of the nipple occurs in primary syphilis and herpes. Major duct infection presents as periductal mastitis, whereas mastitis neonatorum, lactational abscesses, granulomatous lobular mastitis, tuberculosis, and secondary syphilis affect the terminal duct lobular unit.

Mastitis neonatorum

Aetiology and pathogenesis

Continued enlargement of the breast bud in the first week or two of life occurs in about 60 per cent of normal newborn babies and the gland may reach several centimetres before regressing. Enlargement may be asymmetrical and is frequently associated with secretion of a colostrum-like substance known as Witch's milk. Involution over several weeks usually occurs but enlargement may persist for several months in breast fed babies. The enlargement is thought to be due to stimulation by maternal hormones.

Bacteriology

Staphylococcus aureus or rarely *Escherichia coli* are the organisms responsible for mastitis neonatorum.

Clinical features

Neonatal breast buds are commonly red and somewhat tender, but infection is uncommon. Occasionally, however, they do become infected and the breast bud becomes hard, tender, and erythematous. This infection usually occurs at the end of the first week of life and is as common in males as in females. Abscess formation can follow and this is characterized by thin, shiny, red skin overlying a fluctuant mass and fever. Some infants with breast abscesses are severely ill.

Management

In the early stage antibiotics may control the infection. As *Staph. aureus* is the most common organism then flucloxacillin or erythromycin are the antibiotics of choice. Where an abscess has developed, incision and drainage should be performed, combined with intravenous antibiotics in severely ill patients. The incision should be as peripheral as possible to avoid damage to the breast bud and nipple. Scar formation after incision may distort the nipple and impair the secretory activity of the gland in later life.

Lactating breast abscess

Puerperal mastitis and lactating breast abscess are now less common in developed countries, but are still a frequent problem in many parts of the world. The likely reasons for the decrease in frequency are better maternal and infant hygiene, changes in breast-feeding patterns, and earlier treatment by General Practitioners with appropriate antibiotics (1).

Aetiology and pathogenesis

It remains uncertain whether the organisms responsible for lactating breast infection are derived from the skin of the patient herself or from the mouth of her suckling child. Once the organisms have gained entry then milk is an excellent bacterial culture medium. When infection is present, the involved portion of the breast is often engorged with milk and drainage into the major ducts is poor. Whether problems with milk drainage result from blockage of a major breast duct or occur as a consequence of infection is unknown.

Bacteriology

Staph. aureus is the organism responsible for most breast infections in lactating women. *Staph. epidermidis* and streptococci have also been isolated.

Clinical features

Infection associated with breast feeding is most common in the first month after delivery. Some women do develop infection associated with weaning. During this period the breasts can be engorged and the baby has usually developed teeth, which can cause damage to the skin of the breast or nipple. Lactating breast infection presents with pain, swelling, and tenderness (Fig. 22.2). In the later stages a fluctuant mass with overlying shiny, red skin develops. Axillary lymphadenitis is not usually a feature of lactating breast infection. Patients can be toxic with pyrexia, tachycardia and leucocytosis. Bacteraemia, but rarely septicaemia, can follow lactating breast infection.

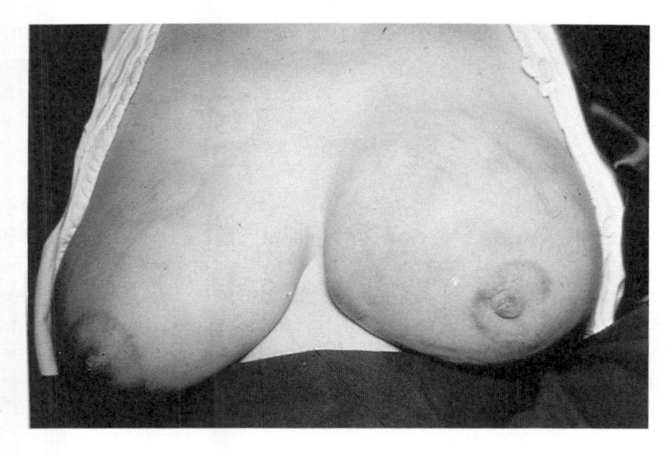

Fig. 22.2. Puerperal mastitis of the left breast. Note the erythema and oedema and obvious signs of inflammation in the left breast, particularly medially. (See plate section.)

Management

It is the general view that antibiotics administered early in infection associated with breast feeding can abort abscess formation. It is likely that earlier recognition and treatment of breast infection in lactating women is the most important factor in the reduction in the incidence of lactating breast abscess (1). As over 50 per cent of staphylococci are resistant to penicillin, the appropriate antibiotics are flucloxacillin 500 mg four times a day, or in patients with penicillin sensitivity, erythromycin 500 mg four times a day. Breast feeding should be continued as this will promote drainage of the engorged segment and help to resolve the infection (2).

Fluctuation may be a late sign of abscess formation and patients whose condition does not improve rapidly on antibiotic therapy should have needle aspiration performed with a 19-gauge needle over the point of maximum tenderness. This will avoid unnecessary surgical intervention in patients without pus formation. It also provides material for bacteriological culture and, in patients where there is a suspicion of an underlying carcinoma, material for cytological examination.

There are a number of options available for the management of women with lactating breast abscesses, when these are either clinically evident or diagnosed on aspiration.

1. Where the skin overlying the abscess is normal then aspiration of the pus, combined with antibiotic therapy has been shown to be effective (3). The aspiration is repeated every two to three days until no further pus is obtained. In countries where large numbers of breast abscesses are still seen, this treatment is considered appropriate in half of all patients with lactating breast abscesses. It avoids the need for a general anaesthetic. An argument against its use is that breast abscesses may be multilocular but the effectiveness of this treatment suggests that most breast abscesses are probably unilocular.

2. Incision and drainage should be performed in patients where the skin overlying the abscess is obviously abnormal and necrotic. Incision should be performed through the area of abnormal skin or over the point of maximum fluctuation. Some authors routinely take biopsies of the abscess wall to ensure an underlying carcinoma is not missed, but this is probably unnecessary. It has been common practice to drain these abscesses with a dependent drain through a separate stab incision. This is no longer considered necessary. The abscess cavity can be left open or obliterated with deep mattress sutures (4). If the wound is to be left open, then it is not necessary to pack the abscess cavity tightly with swabs or gauze unless there are problems with haemostasis. Packing the wound, particularly if done tightly, is painful for the patient and there is some evidence that prolonged daily packing, particularly with hypochlorite containing solutions, may delay healing. The initial use (48 to 72 h) of an antibiotic cream such as Fucidin Caviject, which is a cream containing sodium fucidate, is less painful and appears as effective as packing.

It is the authors' practice to discontinue antibiotic therapy if the abscess is incised, drained, and the cavity left open. If the cavity is sutured, appropriate antistaphylococcal antibiotics are given at the time of surgery and continued for five to seven days (1). The first dose is given intravenously and subsequent doses are taken orally.

Patients who have incision and drainage of their breast abscess usually have to stop breast feeding, whereas patients treated by aspiration and antibiotics are more likely to continue to breast feed. Bacteria and flucloxacillin or erythromycin within the milk do the child no harm (2). A number of antibiotics are contraindicated during lactation including tetracycline, ciprofloxacin and chloramphenicol, as they enter the breast milk and will do the child harm. Patients being treated with these antibiotics should NOT continue to breast feed. If breast feeding is discontinued, suppression of lactation by hormonal means is not usually necessary, but if considered appropriate, bromocriptine 2.5 mg twice a day for 14 days is the most effective agent for stopping the production of breast milk (2).

Periductal mastitis

Periductal mastitis is a benign condition affecting the major subareolar breast-ducts. It is poorly understood and it has been given a variety of terms by different authors. It is probably a separate condition from duct ectasia and affects predominantly young women with a mean age of 32 years (5). The predominant cell in the periductal inflammation is usually the plasma cell which explains why *plasma cell mastitis* is one of the terms which have been used for this condition. Whether this periductal inflammation leads to destruction of the supporting elastic lamina of the duct and subsequently results in duct dilatation, or so-called *duct ectasia*, is not known (5). It is unfortunate that the most common term for this condition is, in fact, duct ectasia, as patients who have active periductal inflammation have little evidence of ectatic or dilated ducts and therefore, periductal mastitis is the preferred term for this condition.

The clinical syndrome of periductal mastitis is now well recognized and characterized by non-cyclical mastalgia, nipple discharge, nipple retraction, periareolar inflammation, non-lactating breast abscess, and mammillary fistula (5).

Microscopically, the major breast-ducts themselves show little or no sign of dilatation but are surrounded by a variety of inflammatory cells which can include polymorphs, plasma cells, lymphocytes, giant cells, and not infrequently, granulomata. (Fig. 22.3).

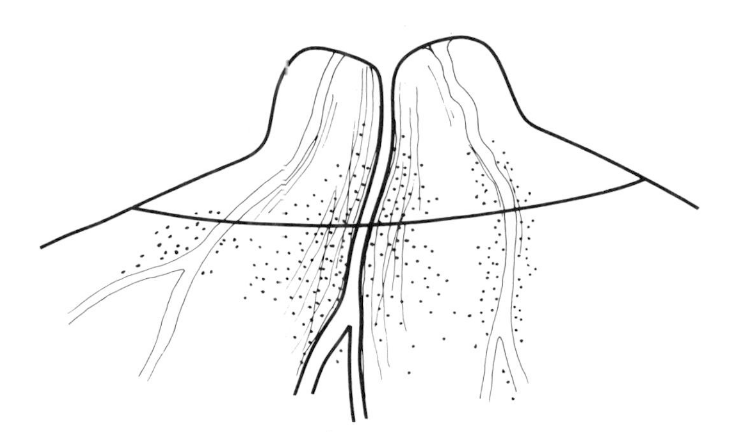

Fig. 22.3. A schematic diagram of periductal mastitis. The diseased duct is seen centrally, its walls are slightly thickened, there is evidence of early nipple retraction at the site of the involved duct. Black dots represent an increased inflammatory infiltrate.

Aetiology and pathogenesis

It has long been suspected that bacteria may have a role in the aetiology of periductal mastitis. Early studies suggested that the lesions were sterile but there is now an overwhelming body of evidence to indicate that bacteria play some part in this condition (5). Organisms, particularly anaerobic organisms, have been isolated from nipple discharge, periareolar breast abscesses and mammillary fistulae of patients with periductal mastitis. It is also of interest that breast biopsy performed in patients with periductal mastitis, is associated with an increased frequency of wound infection. The organisms responsible for infection are the same as those isolated from patients with other symptoms and complications of periductal mastitis (5). Therefore, bacteria play some role in the aetiology of this condition but it is unlikely that they are the sole causative agents.

Bacteriology

The organisms isolated from the lesions of periductal mastitis include enterococci, anaerobic streptococci, *Bacteroides* spp. and staphylococci. Although *Staph. aureus* is frequently isolated, anaerobic organisms, particularly bacteroides are more common, especially when an abscess has developed.

Clinical syndrome of periductal mastitis

Breast pain

Clinical features

The breast pain associated with periductal mastitis is non-cyclical. The pain may precede the appearance of the inflammatory mass or be an isolated symptom. The frequency with which periductal mastitis causes breast pain is unknown, since few patients with pain as their only symptom undergo biopsy.

Management

Pain occurs in association with periductal inflammation and this inflammation appears to be related to specific bacteria. Therefore antibiotics with a spectrum of activity against the range of organisms isolated from this condition, such as flucloxacillin or cephradine combined with metronidazole, or co-amoxyclav alone may be useful.

Periareolar inflammatory mass

This accounts for between 3 and 4 per cent of all benign breast masses (5).

Clinical features

These most commonly affect women between the age of 25 and 40 years. The masses are usually present at the periareolar margin and are associated with overlying skin erythema and the masses themselves are tender. There is usually some alteration in the nipple, with retraction at the site of the involved duct.

Management

The treatment of a periareolar inflammatory mass associated with periductal mastitis is unsatisfactory. Broad-spectrum antibiotics have been reported to be ineffective and surgical intervention can be complicated by wound infection and mammillary fistula. Although resolution without specific treatment does occur, if left untreated an abscess or a mammillary fistula can develop. If there is clinical doubt about the diagnosis then a fine needle aspirate of the inflammatory mass should be performed and this allows a definitive diagnosis.

Recent studies have suggested that co-amoxyclav, 375 mg three times a day, or metronidazole 200 mg three times a day combined with flucloxacillin 500 mg four times a day or cephradine 500 mg four times a day, are effective in resolving periareolar inflammation in this condition (5). However, periareolar inflammatory masses have a tendency to recur and it remains to be seen whether antibiotic therapy modifies the natural history of these lesions.

Patients whose inflammation does recur require excision of the involved ductal system. This is performed through a circumareolar incision. The duct involved can be identified because of nipple retraction at the site of the diseased duct. Removal of 2 to 3 cm of the involved duct under appropriate antibiotic cover is all that is required.

Nipple discharge

Nipple discharge is present in 15 to 20 per cent of patients with periductal mastitis (5). It can vary in colour and consistency, it is usually less viscid than the discharge seen in older patients with so called 'duct ectasia'. The discharge may be unilateral or bilateral.

Management

Patients over the age of 35 should have mammography. Persistent single-duct dicharge, and single-duct discharge which contains blood on testing can be treated by microdochectomy. Troublesome discharge from multiple ducts is treated by total duct excision (6). Patients whose discharge is not troublesome and in whom investigation has failed to show any evidence of malignancy, can be reassured and discharged.

Nipple retraction

Nipple retraction occurs early in periductal mastitis and is present in up to 75 per cent of patients who present with periareolar inflammation (7). The degree of retraction early in the disease is slight and can be missed if not carefully looked for. Marked retraction or nipple inversion occurs much later in the disease (5).

Management

Fine needle aspiration cytology should be performed if nipple retraction is associated with a breast mass and, if no specific diagnosis is made, biopsy must follow. Patients over the age of 35 should have mammography. In patients without either a mass or mammographic suspicion of cancer, observation with repeated clinical examination is all that is required.

Non-lactating periareolar breast abscess

Non-lactating periareolar breast abscesses are related to periductal mastitis and are now more common in the U.K. than those occurring during the puerperium (4). Breast abscesses due to periductal mastitis occur in the periareolar region, the average age of patients being 35 years. Patients may present with a fully developed abscess (Fig. 22.4) or present initially with periareolar inflammation that later becomes fluctuant.

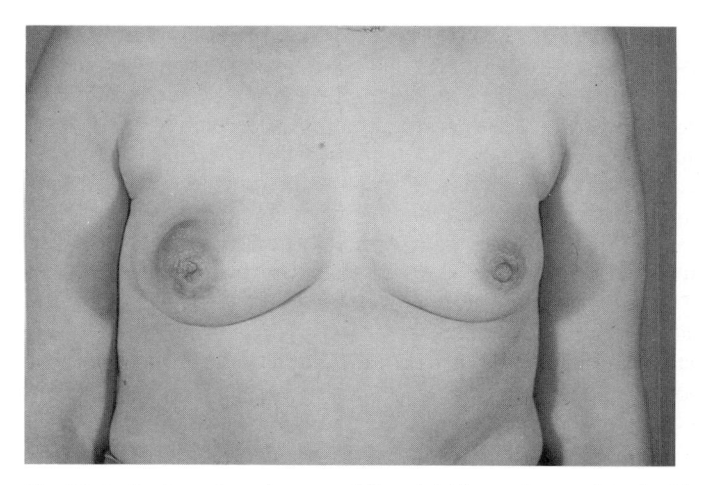

Fig. 22.4. Periareolar abscess of the right breast associated with periductal mastitis. The right nipple is retracted towards the site of infection and an obvious abscess is evident pointing at the areolar margin. (See plate section.)

Management

As in breast abscesses which occur during lactation the presence of pus is not always clinically evident and in patients who have a periareolar inflammatory mass that does not resolve on antibiotic therapy, or where there is strong clinical evidence of an abscess, aspiration with a 19-gauge needle should be performed. If pus is not aspirated, the material in the needle should be sent for bacteriological culture and cytology to exclude an inflammatory carcinoma.

The standard treatment for non-lactating breast abscess is incision and drainage. However, this treatment is frequently associated with recurrence and mammillary fistula formation. This is because the underlying condition, that of periductal mastitis, remains. If incision is performed it should be over the point of maximum fluctuation, which is nearly always at the areolar margin. A biopsy of the cavity should be performed to exclude an underlying carcinoma. A non-lactating breast abscess can occasionally be the presentation of a carcinoma, often a comedocarcinoma, where there is associated necrosis. Dependent drainage, and packing of the wound is not necessary. Suture of the wound with obliteration of the abscess cavity combined with appropriate antibiotic treatment has been reported to be effective (4). Recently in patients where the skin overlying the abscess is normal, repeated aspiration combined with antibiotic therapy has proved successful. This latter treatment may have the advantage of reducing the incidence of subsequent mammillary fistula.

Patients with recurrent periareolar abscess formation should have the underlying diseased duct excised, under antibiotic cover, as a separate procedure through a circumareolar incision once the inflammation and infection has settled (5).

Mammillary fistula

A mammillary fistula is a communication between the skin, usually in the periareolar region, and a major subareolar breast duct (Fig. 22.5). The term mammillary fistula was introduced by Atkins in 1955 to describe this condition, although it was first reported by Zuska in 1951 (5). Early reports suggested that these fistulae occurred as a result of duct obstruction or were related to the presence of squamous epithelium lining the subareolar breast ducts, this epithelium being present as a congenital abnormality. The association between a mammillary fistula and periductal mastitis was first recognized in the 1960s (8). It is the current view that periductal mastitis is the underlying cause of the majority of mammillary fistulae. The squamous epithelium lining the fistula tract is now considered to be a metaplastic response to chronic inflammation and not a congenital abnormality, and duct obstruction is no longer thought to be a major aetiological factor (5).

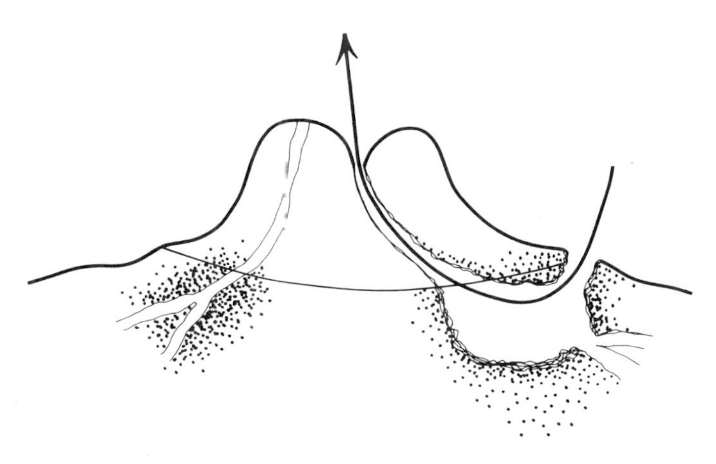

Fig. 22.5. A schematic diagram of a mammillary fistula. At one side of the diagram a duct can be seen surrounded by numbers of black dots which represent periareolar inflammation. A biopsy of this area, incision and drainage if an abscess develops at this site, or spontaneous discharge usually at the areaolar margin, results in a mammillary fistula, seen on the other side of the diagram. Note the retracted nipple at the site of the involved duct.

Clinical features

Women with mammillary fistula have a median age of 35 years. The fistula may develop spontaneously, due to discharge of a periareolar inflammatory mass through the skin, it may occur after a biopsy of an area of periductal mastitis or, in up to a third of patients with non-lactating breast abscess, it follows incision and drainage (9). The opening onto the surface of the skin is usually at the periareolar margin. Retraction of the nipple at the site of the involved duct is present in almost all patients. Occasionally, there can be more than one opening at the areolar margin from a single involved duct (Fig. 22.6).

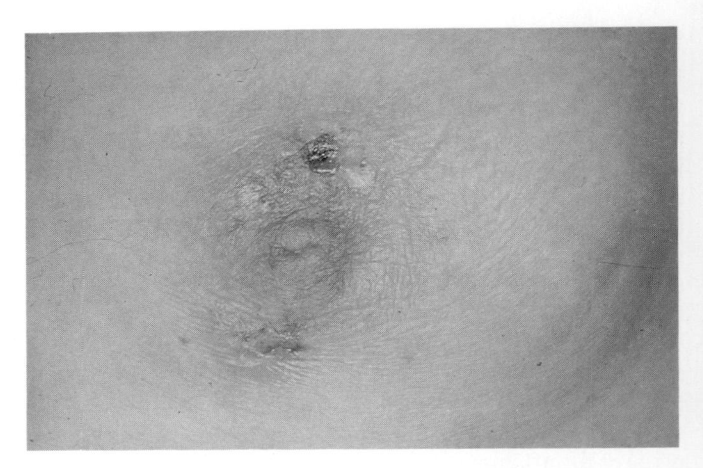

Fig. 22.6. Mammillary fistula with two external openings from a single diseased duct. Note the slit-like central retraction of the nipple at the site of the diseased duct. (See plate section.)

The pathology in mammillary fistula in the early stages is active periductal inflammation with acute and chronic inflammatory cells, with or without granulomata. In the later stages the inflammation is less active and fibrosis is the dominant feature.

Management

The optimal method of surgical treatment of mammillary fistulae is uncertain. Atkins placed a probe through the fistula and then cut down onto the probe to open up the fistula tract (Fig. 22.7). Although this is effective, it produces an ugly scar right across the areolar and nipple. Simple excision of the fistula and primary closure of the wound without antibiotic cover has a high recurrence and infection rate (9). Excision of the fistula and primary closure under antibiotic cover with flucloxacillin, or cephradine combined with metronidazole, or co-amoxyclav alone is now considered the optimal surgical approach to this condition (9). Excision of all subareolar breast ducts is sometimes necessary to evert the nipple and produce a satisfactory cosmetic result. This has been reported to produce a loss of nipple sensation in some patients, but has the

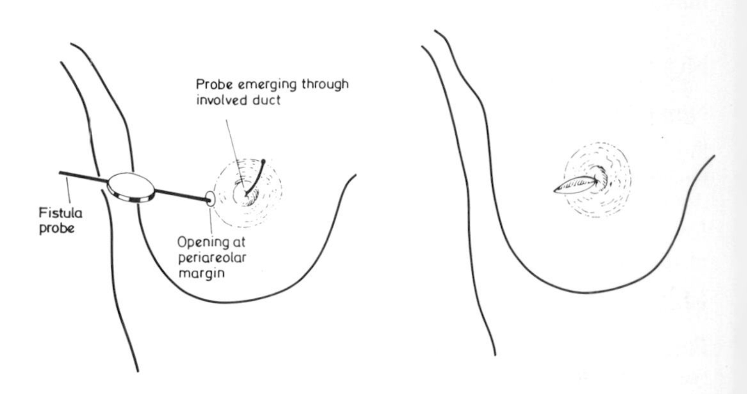

Fig. 22.7. Operative technique for mammillary fistula. A probe is placed through the fistula (a) and the tissue over the probe excised with all inflammatory tissue being excised (b). The wound is left open for healing.

advantage of preventing further episodes of periductal mastitis and fistula formation (6).

Tuberculosis

Tuberculosis of the breast was first described by Astley Cooper. It can be primary or secondary but secondary tuberculosis is much more common. In secondary tuberculosis, infection usually reaches the breast by lymphatic spread from axillary, mediastinal, or cervical nodes or directly from underlying structures such as rib, costochondral junction, or pleura (10). Haematogenous spread from a primary focus in the lung is very uncommon.

Clinical features

Tuberculosis of the breast predominantly affects women in the latter part of the childbearing period and because it is now rare in developed countries, the diagnosis is difficult to make clinically. Clues to the diagnosis are a history of costal, sternal, or axillary tuberculosis and the presence of a breast or axillary sinus, which is present in 50 per cent of patients (Fig. 22.8). In the early stages there is an ill-defined mobile swelling, but later caseation occurs and an abscess or sinus develops. As the disease progresses and fibrosis becomes the predominant feature, a hard, non-tender mass develops which can mimic breast cancer by producing overlying skin tethering and nipple inversion. The commonest presentation of tuberculosis now is acute abscess formation due to secondary infection of an area of tuberculosis by acute pyogenic organisms.

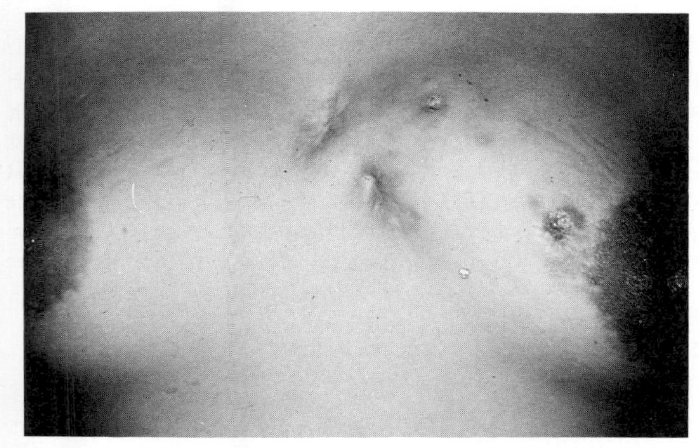

Fig. 22.8. Left breast involved by tuberculosis with multiple sinuses. (See plate section.)

Management

Diagnosis is often difficult to establish. Any patient presenting with a breast mass, or possible breast abscess, should have fine needle aspiration performed and a sample sent for cytology and bacteriological culture. An open biopsy is frequently required to establish the diagnosis of tuberculosis. Where tuberculosis is suspected, part of the biopsy should be sent for tuberculosis culture, as well as for histology as many other conditions produce a microscopic picture indistinguishable from tuberculosis. These conditions include sarcoidosis, mycotic infections (cryptococcosis, histoplasmosis, blastomycosis), metazoal infections (hydatid, cysticercosis), periductal mastitis, Wegener's granulomatosis, and granulomatous lobular mastitis (11). It is also important to recognize that tuberculosis and breast cancer can coexist.

Treatment

Treatment is with appropriate antituberculous chemotherapy, based if possible on the results of laboratory sensitivity testing. Surgery is also frequently required. When the lesion is small, chemotherapy is combined with local excision. Where there is obvious widespread disease within the breast, then mastectomy may be indicated.

Granulomatous lobular mastitis

This condition is classified separately from periductal mastitis although it is likely to be a variant of this condition. It is characterized by non-caseating granulomata and micro-abscesses which are confined to the breast lobule (12).

Bacteriology

Although bacteria may play some role in this condition, organisms have not been isolated consistently from the lesions of granulomatous lobular mastitis (12). It is an uncommon condition and studies are at present ongoing to determine the aetiology of this condition.

Clinical features

Young parous women are most frequently affected and they present with a tender extra-areolar breast lump which can have the clinical features of malignancy. Surgical intervention is frequently followed by wound infection and mammillary fistula and there is a strong tendency for this condition to persist or recur despite surgery (Fig. 22.9).

Management

The diagnosis can be established on fine needle aspiration cytology or on excision biopsy. It is the author's practice to perform fine needle aspiration cytology on all patients presenting with a breast mass; this allows diagnosis of this condition without recourse to open surgery. There is no specific treatment and the condition usually resolves spontaneously. The same antibiotics used in periductal mastitis have been tried without much success and corticosteroids have been advocated by some (12).

Peripheral non-lactating breast abscess

Peripheral breast abscesses are less common than periareolar abscesses associated with periductal mastitis. They may be

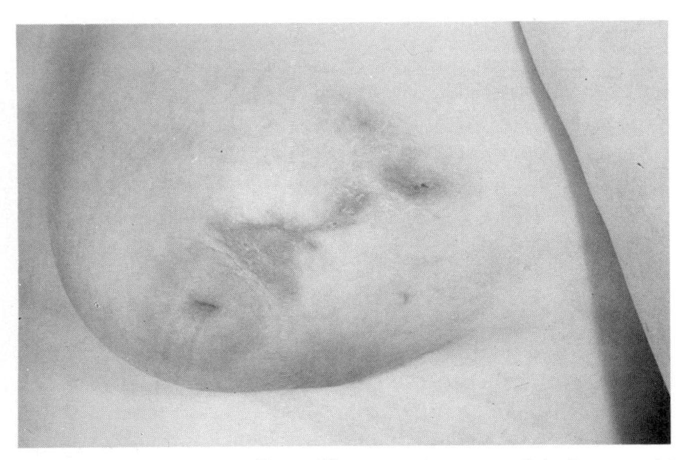

Fig. 22.9. Left breast affected by granulomatous lobular mastitis with evidence of multiple scars, sinuses and nipple retraction. (See plate section.)

associated with other diseases such as diabetes, rheumatoid arthritis, steroid treatment, and trauma (13) and can be associated with sebaceous cysts within the skin of the breast. However, the majority, develop in the absence of any predisposing factor. Pilonidal abscesses in sheep shearers and barbers affecting the breast have been reported (2).

Bacteriology

Staph. aureus is usually the causative organism, but some abscesses do contain anaerobic organisms, such as *Bacteroides melaninogenicus*, *B. bivius*, and *Peptostreptococcus* spp. (13).

Clinical features

These abscesses are more common in premenopausal than in postmenopausal women with a ratio of 3:1. Characteristically the patient presents with a lump which is tender and may be associated with inflammatory changes in the overlying skin with accompanying oedema of the breast. Systemic evidence of malaise or fever are usually absent. There may be a history of an underlying disease process and if the abscess is secondary to a sebaceous cyst then a punctum may be identified.

Management

A needle should be introduced into a suspected peripheral abscess to confirm the diagnosis. If the lesion does contain pus, a sample can be sent for bacteriology culture and if the lesion is solid, the fine needle aspirate can be sent for cytology to exclude an underlying malignancy. If frank pus is not aspirated and the lesion is considered to be infected, treatment with a combination of flucloxacillin and metronidazole or co-amoxyclav will abort abscess formation in a number of patients. The same treatment options as described for lactating breast abscesses can be used in peripheral abscesses, that is recurrent aspiration with antibiotics, or incision and drainage with biopsy of the abscess cavity combined in some instances with closure by obliterative sutures (1, 13).

Syphilis

This is now exceedingly rare. A primary chancre develops usually on the nipple or areola from kissing or from nursing an infected child.

Clinical features

In the initial stages, single or multiple painless ulcers are present, and organisms can be detected in the serous discharge from the ulcer on dark ground microscopy. Axillary lymphadenopathy is also present in the majority of patients with chancres. Secondary syphilis rarely involves the breast but when it does, it produces signs of mild acute mastitis. Occasionally, a gumma can affect the breast and present as a hard painless circumscribed mass, frequently involving the overlying skin, which may be ulcerated. Serology is positive only in the secondary and tertiary stages.

Management

It is important to establish the diagnosis by sending the serous discharge from painless ulcers for dark ground microscopy, and performing fine needle aspiration cytology, or biopsy, of discrete breast masses. Treatment is with appropriate antibiotics.

Other rare infections

Bacterial infections

Actinomycosis

Primary actinomycosis of the breast rarely occurs and secondary spread from pulmonary actinomycosis is also exceedingly uncommon. When the disease spreads from the lungs, it involves pleura, ribs, and pectoral muscle and extends through them to the breast (13).

Clinically, it presents as an indurated mass with sinus formation and excretion of sulphur granules.

Management

Penicillin is the treatment of choice.

Mycotic infections

Blastomycosis and pityrosporum have been reported but are rare. Three patients with fungal infection after breast augmentation have also been reported.

Helminthic and other infections

Filaria is common in the Far East, most reports eminating from south-east Asia, although infected patients have been recorded in France. It usually presents as a mass which contain granulomata on histological examination. The adult worm may also appear at the nipple.

Hydatid disease rarely affects the breast but in areas where hydatid disease is common, less than 0.5 per cent of patients with hydatid disease get breast involvement. They present with a mass which is usually cystic and the diagnosis can usually be made on aspiration. Treatment is by injection of hypertonic saline into the cyst, or by excision.

Two patients with leishmaniasis of the nipple have been reported. These were thought to be direct infections. Cysts due to cysticercosis and guinea worm infections also rarely occur (2, 11).

Viral infections

Mumps

Mastitis has been reported as a complication of mumps and in one review of an epidemic outbreak of mumps, 15 per cent of patients were reported to have mastitis. The incidence was 31 per cent in women over the age of 15 years (2). However, it is important to appreciate that females in this age group frequently experience breast pain and discomfort and no patient with this problem has ever presented to the author's Unit.

Herpes

Herpetic ulceration of the nipple has been reported but is exceedingly rare. When it does occur it is difficult to distinguish from eczema of the nipple, or from Paget's disease. Swabs for virology and a biopsy may be necessary to establish the diagnosis and exclude other causes.

Infection following breast surgery

Breast biopsy

Infection occurs in approximately four per cent of wounds following breast biopsy (5). The incidence of wound infection varies with the nature of the underlying condition. In patients with periductal mastitis/duct ectasia the infection rate is five times greater than in patients with other conditions. The organisms responsible for infection are the same as those isolated from the nipple discharge of patients with periductal mastitis, and from the complications of periductal mastitis. The infection rate is highest in those patients with periductal inflammation without evidence of duct dilatation, and in those patients presenting with a periareolar inflammatory mass (5).

Infection following other procedures

There is increasing use of tissue expanders and breast implants for breast reconstruction and augmentation. Any infection present in association with these foreign materials is difficult, if not impossible, to eradicate and usually means that the expander or prosthesis has to be removed. The organisms responsible for infection are usually *Staph. epidermidis* or *Staph. aureus* and occasionally streptococcus. Therefore, attempts should be made to prevent infection by administrating appropriate antibiotic prophylaxis.

Antibiotic prophylaxis in breast surgery

Minor surgical procedures

If a patient is suspected of having periductal mastitis and surgery is to be undertaken, antibiotic treatment should be given peri- and post-operatively. Strictly, this might not be considered to be antibiotic prophylaxis as organisms are known present in the majority of these lesions. The appropriate antibiotics are cephradine or flucloxacillin combined with metronidazole or co-amoxiclav alone. The first dose should be given intravenously and the doses are flucloxacillin 500 mg, or cephradine 500 mg and metronidazole 500 mg, or co-amoxyclav 1.2 g. Antibiotics are continued orally for five days, the doses being flucloxacillin and cephradine 500 mg four times a day, metronidazole 200 mg three times a day, and co-amoxyclav 375 mg three times a day.

Antibiotic prophylaxis in patients having prosthetic material implanted

Due to the risk of infection in these patients antibiotic prophylaxis is indicated. The organisms responsible for infection in these patients are usually staphylococci and occasionally streptococci. Appropriate prophylaxis is, therefore, provided by penicillin and flucloxacillin, unless there is a penicillin allergy, when erythromycin should be given. For patients having a tissue expander inserted, either immediately at the time of mastectomy or as a delayed procedure, antibiotics should be started intra-operatively and continued until all drains are removed. The initial dose of antibiotic is benzyl penicillin 1.2 g and flucloxacillin 1 g given intravenously. There is a significant rate of infection in patients having tissue expanders inserted at the time of mastectomy. One of the reasons is that the injection port is placed immediately adjacent to the axillary wound drain. Patients who have an axillary clearance require drainage for sometime. The drain entry site frequently becomes inflamed and infected. Most infections after mastectomy now occur secondary to infection of the drain site. In order to reduce the chance of infection caused by bacteria passing via the drain site to the area around the injection port of a tissue expander, it is the authors practice to continue antibiotics until all drains have been removed. Antibiotics are administered intravenously for 24 h and thereafter given orally, the doses being penicillin V 250 mg four times a day and flucloxacillin 500 mg four times a day. Patients who have tissue expanders inserted as a delayed procedure, usually do not require a drain and so a single dose of antibiotics is all that is required.

Patients having prostheses inserted for breast augmentation, at the time of mastectomy, or having tissue expanders removed and replaced with prostheses, have a lower reported incidence of infection. The prosthesis is usually inserted beneath the muscle in a separate compartment and a single prophylactic dose of antibiotics is probably sufficient for all patients having these prostheses inserted.

Most non-implant breast operations are considered 'clean' procedures and it has been traditional teaching that prophylactic antibiotics are not indicated in 'clean' operations. However this teaching has rarely been tested in a clinical trial. A recent study of 1218 patients undergoing hernia repair ($n = 612$) or breast surgery ($n = 606$) indicated wound infection rates could be halved in these 'clean' operations using a perioperative second generation cephalosporin (14). Therefore routine perioperative antibiotic prophylaxis in breast surgery may be of value.

References

1. Benson, E. A. (1989). Management of breast abscesses. *World J. Surg.*, **13**, 753–6.
2. Hughes, L. E., Mansel, R. E., and Webster, D. J. T. (1989). *Benign disorders and diseases of the breast. Concepts and clinical management*, pp. 143–50. Ballière Tindall, London.
3. Dixon, J. M. (1988). Repeated aspiration of breast abscesses in lactating women. *Br. Med. J.*, **297**, 1517–8.
4. Benson, E. A. and Goodman, M. A. (1970). Incision with primary suture in the treatment of acute puerperal breast abscess. *Br. J. Surg.*, **57**, 55–8.
5. Dixon, J. M. (1989). Periductal mastitis/duct ectasia. *World J. Surg*, **13**, 715–20.
6. Hadfield, G. J. (1989). Noncosmetic operations for benign breast disease. *World J. Surg.*, **13**, 757–60.
7. Rees, B. I., Gravelle, I. H., and Hughes, L. E. (1977). Nipple retraction in duct ectasia. *Br. J. Surg.*, **64**, 577–80.
8. Sandison, A. T. and Walker, J. C. (1963). Inflammatory mastitis, mammary duct ectasia and mammillary fistula. *Br. J. Surg.*, **50**, 57–64.
9. Bundred, N. J., Dixon, J. M., Chetty, U., and Forrest, A. P. M. (1987). Mammillary fistula. *Br. J. Surg.*, **74**, 466–8.
10. Apps, M. C. P., Harrison, N. K., and Blauth, C. I A. (1984). Tuberculosis of the breast. *Br. Med. J.*, **288**, 1874–5.
11. Symmers, W. S. T. (1966). The breasts. In: *Systemic pathology*. (ed. G. Payling Wright), pp. 953–5. John Wright, Bristol.
12. Going, J. J., Anderson, T. J., Wilkinson, S., and Chetty, U. (1987). Granulomatous lobular mastitis. *J. Clin. Pathol.*, **40**, 535–40.
13. Rogers, K. (1990). Breast abscess and problems with lactation. In *Benign breast disease*. (ed. J. Smallwood and I. Taylor), pp. 96–108. Edward Arnold, London.
14. Platt, R., Zaleznik, D. F., Hopkins, C. C., *et al.* (1990). Perioperative antibiotic prophylaxis for herniorrhaphy and breast surgery. *N. Engl. J. Med.*, **322**, 153–60.

23

Infection in vascular surgery

COLIN J.L. STRACHAN

Introduction

To the practising vascular surgeon the development of a post-operative infection is stressful, regardless of site. If the infection involves a prosthetic graft, patch or suture line it becomes a nightmare. Unlike the dramatic catastrophe of acute, uncontrollable haemorrhage from a suture line in the immediate post-operative period, prosthetic graft infection (PGI) is characterized by a more chronic, indeterminate malaise which often leads to loss of limb, or life itself, after some months. It is one of the most expensive forms of hospital-acquired or nosocomial infection.

Hospital-acquired infections are usually preventable; therefore the peripheral vascular surgeon must at all times maintain a careful audit of his infection rate. In the UK this will be required for the Confidential Enquiry into Perioperative Deaths (CEPOD), for peer review within his hospital, and for national comparative audit. Infection occurring after clean surgery has become one of the top three reasons for medico-legal pursuit in both North America and Europe in the last five years. As the number of prosthetic reconstructions increases every year, and the quality of cardiovascular care improves, life expectancy extends into and beyond the eighth decade. Graft infections may occur many years after the implantation, they are likely to increase in number as more prosthetic implant procedures are performed and will account for an increasing fraction of the £110 million currently spent in the UK alone on hospital acquired infection.

For medical students and post-graduates, particularly those with an interest in training as vascular surgeons, this chapter provides background information on microbiology, incidence, diagnosis, management and prevention of infection in peripheral vascular surgery.

Incidence of infection

Occlusive disease

The term occlusive disease includes several histopathologies, from atheroma to Takayasus' disease. Atheroma, or atherosclerotic narrowing and occlusion, is the commonest cause of critical limb ischaemia. It occurs in 80 to 90 per cent of all those who present with an ischaemic leg in northern Europe or America. Diabetic distal disease accounts for most of the remainder. Of the patients with atheromatous disease only 5 to 10 per cent will present at primary referral with an infected lesion secondary to ischaemia, whereas 80 per cent of diabetic patients will have a lesion with a positive microbiological culture at the time of referral. The diabetic physician usually waits until first-line anti-infective measures have failed before seeking a surgical opinion. The establishment of diabetic foot clinics with regular Doppler ankle/brachial pressure index assessment should allow earlier referral of patients for reconstructive surgery rather than the ablative surgery which is so often inevitable.

The incidence of infection in the other occlusive pathologies depends upon whether the lesion affects the large vessels or the supply vessels: entrapment syndromes, Takayasus' disease, intimal hyperplasia, Buerger's disease, cystic adventitial disease, etc., or a combination of either, with microcirculatory disturbance such as the variants of collagen disease based, autoimmune arteritis. The incidence also depends upon the patient's host defence mechanisms (see Chapter 4). Apart from diabetic patients only those with low serum transferrin levels have an increased rate of infection. As a general rule, the more peripheral the ischaemic lesion, the more frequently skin ulceration will occur permitting bacterial colonization.

Occlusive disease can, of course, affect the smallest diameter vessels, thus an embolus may arise from a cardiac source, or atheromatous trash from an ulcerated plaque major vessel. The final common pathway compromized is the capillary. Infection may lead to *in situ* thrombosis of digital vessels, secondary to activation of leucocytes and platelet aggregation. Infection causes activation of leucocytes, generates free radicals, enzymes and leukotrienes, and increases endothelial cell injury and vascular permeability. This provides an ideal medium for streptococcal and anaerobic infection leading to cellulitis and lymphangitis. Deep infection follows, and amputation is the inevitable and unavoidable sequel.

Aneurysmal disease

Atheromatous aneurysms

Abdominal aortic aneurysm (AAA) repair is performed with increasing frequency. The prevalence of AAA is 6 per cent in 75-year-old males, in both ultrasound and autopsy studies, and 6 per cent in 85-year-old females. Until the early 1970s, elective operations on aortic, femoral, and popliteal aneurysms were considered clean, non-contaminated procedures. Many papers since then have shown that the aneurysm wall or fibrin contained within the aneurysm, if cultured at operation, yields bacteria in 15 to 20 per cent of elective cold operations and in 30 per cent of tender or ruptured aneurysms (1, 2). Improved culture techniques have shown that coagulase-negative staphylococci (CNS) are the principal infecting agent. The importance of this finding in graft infection is discussed later.

Inflammatory aneurysms

Approximately five per cent of all aortic aneurysms are inflammatory. Despite the name, bacteria are not present in the dense, thickened fibrotic wall of this subtype of aneurysm. The aetiology is probably linked with retroperitoneal fibrosis, and is thought to be due to an allergic reaction to the leak of insoluble lipid (ceroid) from atheromatous plaques through a thinned arterial wall.

Mycotic aneurysm

This term is used for infective aneurysms, of whatever cause, and they usually present as a pyrexia of unknown origin until the tender mass is found in an acute abdomen, often only by ultrasound. Mycotic aneurysms can develop in up to 15 per cent of patients with bacterial endocarditis. They develop insidiously from the infective damage, often long after the septicaemic episode. Staphylococci, salmonellae, and even bacteroides have been described in the aetiology. The high incidence of gut flora involved suggests that translocation of bacteria through the bowel wall leads to microemboli seeding the aortic wall during episodes of bacteraemia. Percutaneous damage and inoculation during angiographic procedures through poorly prepared skin, or in a compromized host, is a minute risk within the reported complication rate of 0.1 per cent.

Thus operations on aneurysms are potentially contaminated and require appropriate prophylactic antibiotic precautions. Despite great care current mortality rates are still 30 per cent for elective or emergency operations on mycotic aneurysms.

False or pseudoaneurysms

False aneurysms occur after external trauma by needle, knife, or external violence. They are wholly outside the arterial wall and surrounded by fibrosis. Although initially sterile, the blood or liquefied clot contained within them can be infected subsequently. Pseudoaneurysm is a favourite term for leaks which occur at the anastomosis between prosthetic grafts and the arterial wall, and are now regarded as the end product of suture or prosthetic fabric infection. These commonly occur in the groin.

Audit of infection

Morbidity and mortality

The first report of a large series of vascular graft implants was by Hoffert *et al.* in 1965 (3). They reported a 2.2 per cent incidence of infection after aorto iliac/femoral bypass grafting. In 1972 Szilagyi *et al.* reported on 3397 patients with 40 infections (1.2 per cent) showing that grafts wholly within the abdomen had a low incidence of infection at 0.7 per cent, whereas prosthetic grafts inserted into, or commencing in, the groin had 1.6 to 3 per cent incidence of infection (4). If a vein was used for femoro-popliteal grafting the rate dropped to 0.4 per cent. The mortality rate was 33 per cent overall, with infection of the aortic stump and body of the graft being almost synonymous with death in early reports.

More recently, in carefully selected cases, *in situ* regrafting has been successful with both survival and long term patency appearing to be better than after extra anatomic reconstruction. The pros and cons will be discussed later. Septicaemia, peripheral infected emboli, and multiple anaesthetics required for flap amputations, graft extirpation, wound packing, and redressing etc. lead to death due to multiple organ failure.

Recent reports have been only marginally better with O'Hara *et al.* reporting an incidence of infection of 0.4 per cent for aorto-iliac reconstruction and 1.3 per cent for aorto-femoral grafts (5). Also in 1986 Dunham *et al.* reported 1.3 per cent infection in patients after prosthetic femoro-popliteal grafting (6). However, the more recent reports have been more accurate and have included infection by CNS which, in the seventies, were regarded as unimportant skin commensals. The classification of infection, which is described in detail in the next section, has also been improved.

In North American reports of large numbers of procedures, the overall rate of infection, which includes wound infection, is not always given. In a report from Canada, Walker *et al.* reported 26 per cent total infection in 1984 (7), and Earnshaw *et al.* 19 per cent in Nottingham in 1988 (8).

There is a great need for further well-controlled, prospective audit clearly stating the pathogens, culture methods, graft and suture materials, site of infection, and whether the infection occurred early or late.

Early infection

Infection is generally regarded as 'early' if it presents within three to four months of the primary graft procedure. The early presentation may be as a groin infection with a tender lump in the groin due to perigraft pus, a pyrexia, and leucocytosis. Wound infection is the most obvious sign of early infection, often following a lymphatic leak from the groin wound which is the commonest site of early prosthetic infection. *Staphylococcus aureus* is the commonest organism. Fresh bleeding often ensues after a few days of serosanguinous discharge.

Intra-abdominal infection. Aorto-enteric infection usually presents later. The first sign may be a prolonged post-operative ileus, particularly if the duodenum has been thinned and attenuated over a large aneurysm sac and the perigraft haematoma then becomes infected. Mechanical obstruction may occur if small bowel loops adhere to the infected limb of a bifurcated graft.

Late infection

Femoro-popliteal grafts

Ischaemic limb pain, either acute or chronic, due to thrombosis or infected occlusion of a femoro-popliteal graft may present several years after operation. Sometimes the graft remains patent and the only sign of infection is an indolent red swelling at either end of the graft with limb swelling due to lymphatic spread, or occasionally concomitant venous thrombosis.

Aortic grafts

Straight grafts rarely become infected but perigraft infection is the form of presentation in 60 to 70 per cent of infected bifurcated grafts to the groin. They may become infected following repair of a pseudoaneurysm of the groin, or sinus excision. The remaining 20 to 30 per cent present as graft enteric erosion or fistula formation, the latter adhere to an anastomotic suture line and often present with a small herald bleed or a slow melaena—only a few have a torrential haemorrhage.

Classification of infection

Pre-operative

Gangrene and digital necrosis

The end stage of ischaemia is gangrene and this is classically described as dry or wet. If dry there is much less risk of infection either locally, systemically, or after ablative surgery. It is rarely worth sending material from a mummified digit for microbiological culture. If the gangrene is moist and has the smell of putrefaction, heavy anaerobic infection is likely with *Clostridia* spp., anaerobic streptococci, *Pseudomonas* spp., *Proteus* spp. and coliforms, especially in aged, incontinent patients. Eighty per cent of lower limb amputees are over 70 years of age and 50 per cent over 80. Infection has to be tackled urgently to prevent septicaemic death from multiple organ failure, and to save as much functional and viable limb as possible. Antibiotic therapy is of secondary importance to excision of dead tissue before gas gangrene spreads rapidly along tissue planes (see Chapter 18).

Primary aorto-duodenal fistula

The primary aorto-duodenal fistula was first described by Sir Astley Cooper in 1830 (9). It is thought that the duodenum becomes densely adherent and thins over the expanding aneurysm, becomes ischaemic, and then subsequently erodes and a fistula develops. The patho-physiology of a secondary fistula is relatively similar. An aorto-caval fistula is one of the few presentations of an aortic aneurysm which does not carry an infective risk—unless the large arterio-venous shunt and cardiac decompensation is associated with oedema and streptococcal cellulitis of the lower limb. Fistulae into the ureter or renal pelvis are rare. Fever and a high white cell count may follow left sided ischaemic colitis from inferior mesenteric artery occlusion when this is associated with occlusive disease of the superior mesenteric artery or the coeliac axis.

Post-operative

Amputation stump infection

Below knee amputation (BKA) is prone to infection, skin necrosis, and wound breakdown. In some centres 20 to 25 per cent of all BKAs require reamputation at a higher level (10). Failure to heal is more common if there has been an incision for bypass surgery distal to the knee. Whilst most stumps fail to heal because of persisting ischaemia which then develop secondary infection, there is no doubt that in diabetic amputees the presence of gross contamination distally may compromise the chosen level.

There are few good studies which have monitored the role of infection in the primary healing of amputations (11). Prediction of the optimum level for amputation by skin blood flow and other methods may be helpful, but a scoring system is needed which includes infection risk factors such as the presence of gangrene, previous bacteraemia, cellulitis, lymphangitis, or multiple resistant organisms. Berridge *et al.* found 30 per cent of patients had pre-operative infection, mainly *Staph. aureus* and *Klebsiella* spp., and 40 per cent developed post-operative infection despite using five days of penicillin with or without metronidazole in diabetic patients (11). They felt this confirmed the need for prophylaxis with a broad spectrum antibiotic.

Classification of infection after vascular reconstruction

In 1972 Szilagyi *et al.* defined three basic grades of infection (4) (Table 23.1). This grading recognized the clinicopathological significance of the infection and became the bench mark for reporting morbidity and mortality, hospital stay and cost implications of each grade.

Table 23.1. Grades of infection after vascular surgery.

Grade	
I Dermal	confined to skin margins of wounds, superficial pustules (Fig. 23.1)
II Subcutaneous	involving the subcutaneous fat and lymphatics with infected seroma or lymph discharges (Fig. 23.2)
III Prosthetic fabric infection	any part of the graft involved in infection (Fig. 23.3)

Adapted from Szilagyi *et al.* (4)

The clinical appearance of each type of infection is seen in Figs 23.1 to 23.3, and the wide variety of possible sequelae of graft infection is illustrated in Fig. 23.4. Despite the value of this classification it became clear that Grade III infection had

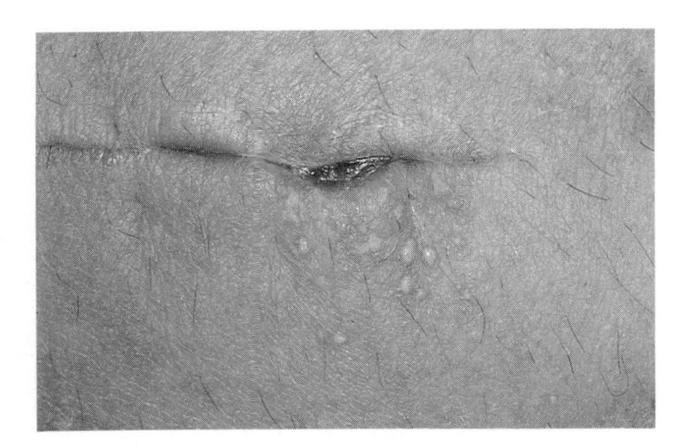

Fig. 23.1. Superficial skin infection. (See plate section.)

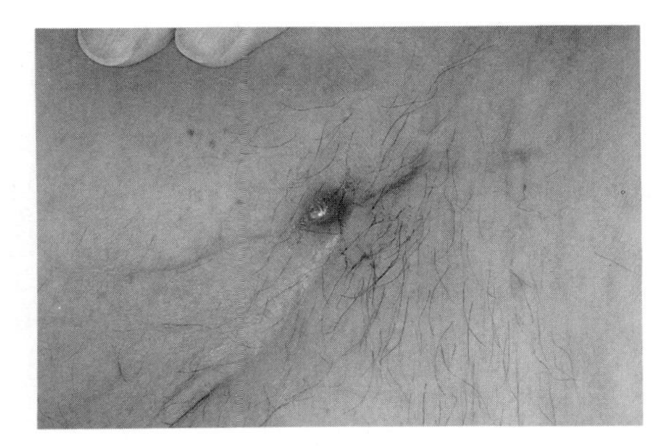

Fig. 23.2. Infection of subcutaneous tissues. (See plate section.)

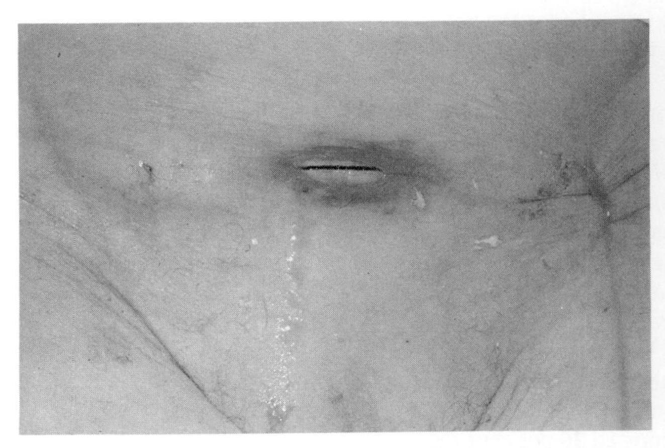

Fig. 23.3. Graft exposed in the wound. (See plate section.)

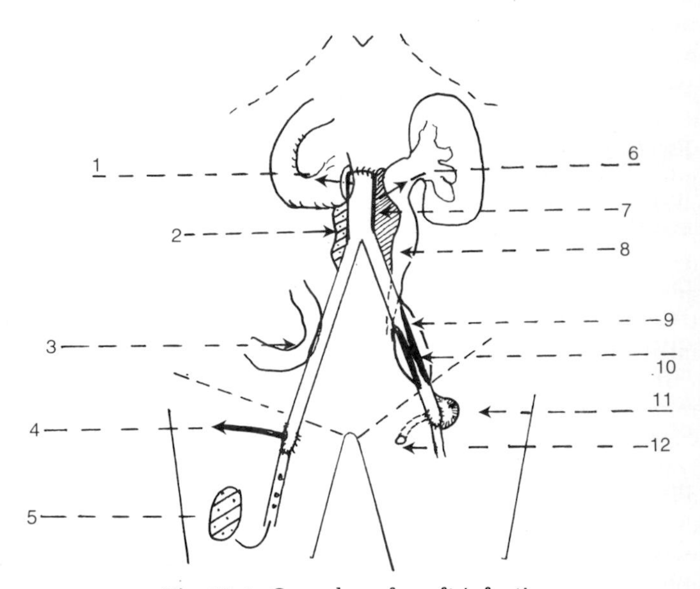

Fig. 23.4. Sequelae of graft infection.

1. Secondary aorto-duodenal fistula (GEF)
2. Perigraft pus (PGI)
3. Graft-enteric erosion (GEE)
4. Secondary haemorrhage
5. Septic emboli → high abscess
6. Ureteric fistula
7. Perigraft haematoma
8. Hydronephrosis
9. Perigraft 'sterile' fluid
10. Graft thrombosis
11. Pseudoaneurysm
12. Infected sinus

a great variety of subtypes, and that there was too great a range in the probability of death. For instance death only occurs in 10 per cent of patients where one limb of a graft involving the groin is infected whereas 60 to 70 per cent of patients with aortic stump infections die.

To overcome this, in 1983 Bunt proposed four subtypes of Grade III infection (12):

IIIa: Graft infection (PGI).

IIIb: Graft enteric erosion (GEE).

IIIc: Graft enteric fistula (GEF).

IIId: Aortic stump infection.

To improve the correlation between the incidence of infection and the outcome he insisted that the following information be recorded: type of graft material used, infecting organism cultured, which end of the graft was involved (distal or proximal), and the systemic severity of the infection.

The second modification of Szilagyi's classification came from Veith's group (13). They subdivided Grade III and created Groups IV and V as follows:

Group III: Infections involving the body of the graft but not an anastomosis.

Group IV: Infections surrounding an exposed anastomosis without bacteraemia or anastomotic bleeding.

Group V: Infections involving graft/artery anastomosis with septicaemia and/or anastomotic bleeding at the time of presentation.

Groin discharges and infections

Primary healing of an incised groin wound produces little or no fluid discharge. When the wound produces more than a few drops of pale yellow serum per day this is termed as serous discharge. When does a serous discharge become a wound infection? If the discharge contains blood infection is more likely to occur. Contamination by the resident or transient flora of the groin is possible and may lead to infection. If the organisms cultured are slime-producing CNS then it should be audited as an infection, even if there is no morbidity at the time. A correlation should be made subsequently with late infection.

If there is skin damage during operation by diathermy, retractors or poor suture technique ischaemia of the wound edge may result in skin edge necrosis. If there is damage to lymphatics or groin lymph nodes, particularly during femoral aneurysm surgery or revision procedures, lymphatic leaks may occur. These present with an increasing volume of clear to turbid milky discharge 7 to 10 days post-operatively, often at the time of suture removal. Wet dressings left unchanged are then colonized and the wound can become colonized from perianal faecal flora. If resuturing fails to stem the flow a chronic lymphatic fistula may develop. If the skin heals but lymph leakage continues, a lymphocoele forms. This must not be mistaken for a haematoma or approached with a needle, seeking resolution. The former may give a 'red face' and the latter lead to colonization of a sterile collection or promote a chronic fistula. Chronic sinus formation with a purulent discharge may occur when the skin over the upper end of a femoro-popliteal bypass graft develops erythema and a limited, and usually localized, late suture line infection appears.

Secondary fistulae

Graft enteric fistulae (GEF). In 1953 Brock *et al.* described a patient with a secondary aorto-enteric fistula as a complication one year after a homograft aortic replacement (14). In 1956, Claytor *et al.* reported the first prosthetic fistula (15) and two years later McKenzie recorded the first successful repair (16). The average time of presentation is two to three years after operation and they can involve any part of the bowel from the third part of the duodenum to the rectosigmoid colon. Secondary aorto-colonic fistulae are very rare and may be associated with a neoplasm. They occur less frequently now that vascular surgeons understand the importance of interposing viable tissue such as aortic wall, omentum, or retroperitoneal tissue between bowel and the graft.

Although the strict definition of a fistula requires the two lumens to be in direct communication, it is usually accepted that there need not be a 'hole' between the two but frequently a loss of mucosa with the prosthesis eroding through the defect. Some may communicate through a pseudoaneurysm and this may spare the body of the graft from periprosthetic pus. Bowel organisms naturally predominate on microbiological culture. The herald bleed is more dramatic and the mortality rate is much higher (50 per cent) than in erosions.

Graft enteric erosions (GEE)

This complication, where the mucosa remains intact between graft and bowel lumen, has been recognized since the early 1960s and the adherence/mechanical erosion theory is conventionally applied. They are reported as a late occurrence, averaging two years after operation, although the appearance earlier has been reported. The author has seen an inflamed appendix adhere to a prosthetic graft, peritonitis occurred and led to a secondary adherence of small bowel. Since there is no direct exposure of graft to the bowel lumen there is usually time for investigative workup and the reported mortality rate of 16 per cent is much lower than that for intra-abdominal vascular graft infections (12).

Aortic stump infection

Very few patients have survived this condition. It is difficult to achieve a secure closure of the aorta if the original graft was sutured immediately distal to the renal arteries. The sutures cut through and an aortic blow-out is the most frequent mode of death.

Cost of infection

The cost of hospital-acquired infection (HAI) in the UK in 1985 was approximately £115 million per annum (17). If a 50 per cent reduction in the incidence of HAI could be achieved by better infection control and integrated audit systems as much as £50 million could be saved. On average an extra four days hospitalization are required for any nosocomial infection. Infection after vascular surgery is one of the most expensive forms of HAI with weeks rather than days of extra hospital care required as well as extra hours spent in the operating theatre and intensive therapy units.

One simple way to reduce expenditure is to reduce excessive and prolonged prescription of antibiotics. Antibiotic prophylaxis is of value and in 1983 Kaiser *et al.* confirmed the cost–benefit analysis of antibiotic prophylaxis in vascular surgery (18). In that study the cost of infection was scored according to the Szilagyi grade of infection. In 1982 a Grade I infection cost an additional $3600, Grade II $4000 and Grade III $6200, and it should be remembered that Grade III patients are surviving longer in the last eight years, and cost more. Translating these figures into the inflationary age of the early

1990s in the UK a Grade III infection now costs £3000 per week, with an average additional cost of £10 000 per graft infection.

The additional burden of recovery from vascular infection on community costs has yet to be assessed. Instead of returning to work, or regaining an independent life, these patients need greatly increased medical and nursing attendance, particularly if amputation has been the price of recovery.

Polk has warned of the increasing medico-legal costs of unanticipated wound infection in clean surgery (19). In 1985 he noted that it was the second commonest cause of malpractice action in the USA. For this, if for no other reason, the vascular surgeon must know his infection rates. In the best centres a 1 to 2 per cent overall infection rate is quoted. The law demands that any risk above the 1 per cent level is the threshold for informed consent.

Identification of site of infection

Scanning techniques

Ultrasound

Perigraft fluid is easier to identify since the advent of Duplex scanning. Needle aspirate under ultrasound control allows microbiological culture of the organism responsible. This technique is best suited to the groin and lower limb where the differential diagnosis of pseudoaneurysm from other pulsatile masses can be made. Portable machines make bedside diagnosis possible in the very sick. B-mode ultrasound can show the length of the infected tunnel, particularly if leucocyte scanning is not readily available. Ultrasonography is less valuable for the detection of abdominal PGI because of overlying intra-abdominal gas.

Computerized tomographic scanning

Computerized tomography (CT) is widely used in the assessment of AAA to determine the relationship to the renal arteries, the thickness of the wall, the extent of the fibrin clot within the sac and the probable site of rupture. Its further application to the diagnosis and management of PEI, GEF, and GEE infections is invaluable. Cunat *et al.* have described the small pockets of gas in and around aortic grafts, produced by gas-forming organisms (20). CT-guided aspiration has been used since 1978 enabling the clinician to differentiate old haematoma from perigraft pus. This can but time especially if a CNS infection is present with septicaemia, when intravenous vancomycin can be given to halt the blood borne spread. CT is much less dependent on the skill of the operator than ultrasound and is quicker than gallium scanning. It is invaluable in late post-operative infections and can identify other retroperitoneal causes of prolonged gastroduodenal ileus such as pancreatitis and perigraft haemorrhage.

Radionucloide scanning

Conventional gallium-67 scanning has the disadvantage of the delay between injection and imaging, nomally 72 h because of the slow uptake into inflammatory cells. Now that labelled leucocyte scanning is available this has become the preferred imaging technique. These techniques are less specific in the early post-operative period, with some false-positives due to haematoma. False-negatives are rare, and they may, as an additional benefit, show other foci of infection responsible for the clinical signs and symptoms. In Brighton the author has found commercially available ^{99m}Tc-Exametazine (Ceretec T. M.) leucocyte scatigraphy highly sensitive but has no experience of 111-Indium-labelled immunoglobulin G scans, which avoid contact with patients' blood, but will probably be no more accurate.

Magnetic resonance imaging

MRI has not yet shown itself to be superior to CT scanning with contrast, but does avoid intravenous injection of contrast. Calcification in the arterial wall is a problem, as is the ferrous content of the needle when attempting needle aspirate. Because of the cost of the equipment it is unlikely that MRI will challenge CT scan as a diagnostic tool for PGI for some years.

Contrast radiology

In certain situations radiology still has a valuable role.

Sinograms

Sinograms of openings in the groin are not frequently performed because of the risk of bacteraemia and septicaemia. They may still be invaluable in the groin to show the relationship of contaminated tissue to uncontaminated extra anatomic routes for revascularisation, e.g. the obturator foramen.

Arteriography

Like sinography, arteriography helps to plan the re-routing of grafts rather than to diagnose infection. Digital subtraction angiography may provide unexpected information about junctional pseudoaneurysms in failing or occluded grafts. They also show whether there are suitable inflow and outflow vessels for reconstruction.

Barium studies

Although the ribs of dacron grafts involved in GEE or GEF have been described coated with barium after upper gastrointestinal tract barium studies, these are requested less frequently nowadays because of false-negatives in GEE and barium interference with subsequent CT scanning.

Endoscopy

The ability to visualize the bile stain on the graft surface at duodenoscopy provides more accurate data than barium appearances. More often there is haemorrhagic mucosa, punctate ulceration, or extrinsic pulsatile compression. Microbiology cultures from these areas are rarely helpful. In addition oesophago-gastroscopy is of value in excluding bleeding from a peptic ulcer or from varices in a patient who also has an aneurysm.

Microbiological identification

The septicaemic patient with obvious early graft infection has a heavy bacterial innoculum, and in 80 per cent of patients the organism is easily isolated by standard techniques. Twenty per cent will have a 'sterile pus' report, either at surgery or from prior diagnostic aspiration, particularly if potent broad spectrum antibiotic therapy has been given. Late graft infection will remain a microbiological mystery in 80 per cent of cases if the search ends at routine culture and Gram stain. Bandyk *et al.* have shown that more sensitive culture techniques of the graft fabric, using ultrasonic loosening, allowed maximum recovery of CNS for subsequent growth on special trypticase broth and other agar media (21, 22). He isolated the CNS, *Staph. epidermidis*, in this way from 60 per cent of late PGI. The inability to identify CNS, and the erroneous labelling of the 'sterile fluid' as an autoimmune foreign body reaction, is a big problem in western Europe.

Coagulase-negative staphylococci (CNS) are distributed unevenly on the body surface but are the commonest of the resident flora. *Staph. epidermidis* predominates on the head and trunk, and the older the patient the greater the number of species and biotypes found. The groin provides a moist warm environment and on admission for aortic surgery the groin or perineal skin was found to be colonized in 70 per cent of patients (25). One-third of these isolates had multiple resistance to five or more antibiotics. Following prophylaxis with three doses of antibiotic the post-operative incidence of resistance had doubled. This phenomenon was first described after antibiotic prophylaxis of longer duration for cardiac surgery by Archer and Armstrong who concluded that antibiotic prophylaxis perpetuates a hospital reservoir of resistant CNS which can be transferred from patient to staff and vice versa (24).

Although persistence is a problem, the biggest difficulty in eradicating CNS from implanted prostheses is the ability of some strains to form extracellular polysaccharide slime from the glycocalyx. Bayston and Penny discovered this substance in 1972 (25). It promotes adherence and once the prosthesis is colonized by CNS within the biofilm, the host defence mechanisms are impotent and even the antimicrobials most active against CNS, vancomycin, and teicoplanin, fail to penetrate.

Another virulent organism isolated from infections after lower limb bypass grafting is *Pseudomonas aeruginosa*. This species releases an endotoxin which leads to anastomotic dehiscence, graft thrombosis and spreads rapidly along the graft (26). Failure to treat quickly infection by this organism can often result in a high thigh amputation.

Prevention of infection

Vascular surgeons are very interested in new methods of diagnosing and treating established infection, but rarely read papers on the perioperative measures that can and should be taken to prevent infection. Most publications relating to the control of hospital infection appear in microbiological journals and relate to asepsis, antisepsis, and antibiotics given pre-operatively during surgery and pre-operatively.

Exogenous or airborne contamination can occur pre-operatively as well as during the operation. Colonization by multiresistant CNS may occur on a prior admission for arteriography when the patient is placed in a bed next to a patient with an aortic graft who already harbours resistant strains, which are then hand transmitted by ward or medical staff. This ecosystem may be even more dangerous if there are patients with stomata or burns in a mixed general surgical ward. In addition, resistant strains are readily produced in the community by repeat prescriptions of antibiotics for cellulitis or ulcers.

Systemic spread of infection can be initiated by poor aseptic techniques. Poor skin cleaning can permit CNS systemic access during arterial or venous puncture, or they may enter subsequently by colonizing a central venous line. Systemic spread from urethral catheters infected with CNS again endorses the need for both asepsis and antisepsis when implanting temporary indwelling devices, or subsequently when caring from the meatus or site of skin entry.

It is unwise to extrapolate the effects of shaving and of antiseptic bathing from large series of general surgical operations to preparation for vascular surgical procedures. Brandberg *et al.* reported an infection rate of 17.5 per cent after vascular surgery which was reduced to 8 per cent by the introduction of between three and eight pre-operative chlorhexidine showers (27). There is no doubt that pre-operative cleansing with chlorhexidine gluconate 4 per cent will reduce the frequency of colonization by multiply resistant CNS in the groin up to seven days post-operatively, compared with povidone–iodine or controls (23). There may be value in continuing skin antisepsis post-operatively. The author's current regimen is to ensure that the patient has a full bath with chlorhexidine 25 ml, as well as a hair wash 24 h pre-operatively. Early on the morning of surgery a clipper shave is followed by a repeat bath and a third bath is provided five days after operation.

Contamination of the graft by personnel is most likely to occur during the operation. Prosthetic contamination occurs at the time of handling and insertion. Wooster *et al.* demonstrated a 56 per cent incidence of contamination of knitted grafts, predominantly by CNS, but lowered this to 35 per cent by changing gloves prior to preclotting the graft (28). The role of glove puncture and adhesive skin drapes are discussed in earlier chapters.

Adherence of CNS to the graft depends on the physical and biochemical nature of the fabric. In general the looser the weave of the graft fabric, e.g. knitted dacron, the more the slime penetrates, and infection may persist because of the limited access to host defence mechanisms. Adherence of CNS to dacron is 100-fold greater than to expanded PTFE (22). It is possible that dacron, coated with collagen, gelatin, or albumin may prevent adherence of CNS to the fabric, or that any contaminating CNS may be shed as the soluble coatings dissolve.

Antibiotic prophylaxis

There are many studies which have shown that wound infection after vascular surgery can be reduced by administering antibiotic prophylaxis. By reporting only the few graft infections which occur in the short period of each study the assumption is made that prophylaxis reduces the rate of graft infection, but this takes no account of the graft infections

Table 23.2. Management options for infected prosthetic grafts.

Site of Infection	Contamination	Options
Aortic graft	Heavy	No excision (rare, systolic blood pressure less than 50 mmHg)
		Excision and immediate extra-anatomic bypass graft (axillo-femoral) pre-excision of the infected graft is preferred, post-excision may be necessary.
		Excision and *in situ* replacement with antibiotic bonded gelatin coated dacron graft and irrigation with antiseptic or antibiotic and antibiotic beads and autogenous vein/artery and homologous vein graft
Isolated limb of graft	Light	Excision and extra-anatomic femoro-femoral crossover graft via the obturator canal.
Pseudoaneurysm or		Part excision and replacement with a fresh prosthesis, muscle cover is important.
Lower limb graft		Autologous vein patch or autologous vein tube may be used as an alternative.
		No excision—*in situ* irrigation with antiseptic or antibiotic

which present late. Some authors propose that antibiotics should be continued beyond the operation until all major lines, catheters, nasogastric tubes, etc., have been removed, i.e. at least three days (29). This surely risks the development and perpetuation of multiple resistant CNS. Standard practice in the UK is to give three doses of cefuroxime to cover the 18 h with an added dose on the operating table if more than two units of blood are lost. In North America, cefazolin, with a short half-life, is still favoured.

The antibiotic should be active against both types of staphylococci (aureus and epidermidis) and *E. coli*, cefuroxime 1.5 g IV on induction of anaesthesia would seem adequate. Of the newer agents ceftriaxone, with a much longer half-life, appears to be the best. If the patient is allergic to penicillin, is undergoing revision surgery, or an infected graft is to be removed, vancomycin provides the best antibiotic cover.

Concurrent surgery. Inguinal or femoral hernia repair is often performed with aortic surgery, particularly if it is close to a groin incision. Cholecystectomy *en passant*, for asymptomatic gallstones first discovered at laparotomy, is probably meddlesome but some authors advocate cholecystectomy on asymptomatic patients if there is a low risk of common bile-duct stones or bactibilia (30). Other problems involving clean-contaminated operations have to be judged on their individual risk–benefit ratio.

Treatment of infection

Principles of *in situ* management

The earlier methods of managing infection by graft excision alone, or by excision followed by revascularization *in situ*, had mortality rates of 74 per cent and 61 per cent respectively (12), and have lost favour. Alternative management stratagems are listed in Table 23.2. Of these sequential management by remote revascularization followed by graft removal was popular until recent studies of staged removal with a time interval of three to five days between, reported a lower mortality (31). More conservative *in situ* replacement, or non-excisional methods, are gaining ground. Irrigation systems have been devised which use antibiotics or antiseptic fluids and different types of polymethyl methacrylate beads incorporating antibiotics are available – from commercially available gentamicin beads to hand rolled vancomycin beads (32). Whilst they are locally effective in the groin (33) they are painful to remove and require a further anaesthetic. Collagen felt containing gentamicin has recently been evaluated and may prove to be a more acceptable alternative (34).

The use of autogenous artery is advocated in staged removal using occluded iliac or femoral vessels after endarterectomy (28). Another method of providing short-term conduits is the temporary use of homologous veins covered by immunosuppressive drugs – but this appears an extreme and relatively untried method.

The use of tissue wedges of omentum or muscle interspersed between fresh grafts and surrounding contamination is a valuable adjunct in the retroperitoneum or groin. The details of the wide variety of possible procedures are listed briefly in Table 23.2 but for further details, the reader is referred to the collation of articles by Bandyk (35). In 1991 the first antibiotic (rifampicin) bonded grafts have been inserted in the UK by the author and appear to be the most promising new development.

References

1. Fielding, J. W. L., Black, J., Ashton, F., and Slaney, G. (1981). Diagnosis and management of 528 abdominal aortic aneurysms. *Br. Med. J.*, **283**, 355–9.
2. MacBeth, G. A., Rubin, J. R., McIntyre, K. E., Goldstone, J., and Malone, J. M. (1984). The relevance of arterial wall micro-

biology to the treatment of prosthetic graft infections vs arterial infection. *J. Vasc. Surg.*, **1**, 750–6.
3. Hoffert, P.W., Gensler, S., and Haimovici, H. (1965). Infection complicating arterial grafts. *Arch. Surg.*, **90**, 427–35.
4. Szilagyi, D.E., Smith, R.F., Elliott, J.P., and Vrandecic, M.P. (1972). Infection in arterial reconstruction with synthetic grafts. *Ann. Surg.*, **176**, 321–33.
5. O'Hara, P.J., Hertzer, N.R., and Beven, E.G. (1986). Surgical management of infected abdominal aortic grafts: review of a 25 year experience. *J. Vasc. Surg.*, **3**, 725–31.
6. Durham, J.R. Rubin, J.R., and Malone, J.M. (1986). Management of infected infra inguinal bypass grafts. In *Re-operative arterial surgery* (ed. J.J. Bergan and J.S.T. Yao), pp. 359–77. Grune & Stratton, Philadelphia.
7. Walker, M., Litherland, H.K., Murphy, J., and Smith, J.A. (1984). Comparison of prophylactic antibiotic regimens in patients undergoing vascular surgery. *J. Hosp. Infect.*, **5**, Suppl. A, 101–6.
8. Earnshaw, J.J., Slack, R.C.B., Hopkinson, B.R., and Makin, G.S. (1988). Risk factors in vascular surgical sepsis. *Ann. R. Coll. Surg. Engl.*, **70**, 139–43.
9. Cooper, A.P. (1830). *Lectures on the principles and practice of surgery*, p. 156. Westley, London.
10. Haynes, I.G. and Middleton, M.D. (1981). Amputation for peripheral vascular disease: experience of a district general hospital. *Ann. R. Coll. Surg. Engl.*, **63**, 342–3.
11. Berridge, D.C., Slack, R.C.B., Hopkinson, B.R., and Makin, G.S. (1989). A bacteriological survey of amputation wound sepsis. *J. Hosp. Infect.*, **13**, 167–72.
12. Bunt, T.J. (1983). Synthetic vascular graft infections. I: Graft Infections. *Surgery*, **93**, 733–46.
13. Samson, R.H., Veith, F.J., Janko, G.S., Gupta, S.K., and Scher, L.A. (1988). A modified classification and approach to the management of infections involving peripheral arterial prosthetic grafts. *J. Vasc. Surg.*, **8**, 147–53.
14. Brock, R.C., Rob, C.G., and Forty, F. (1953). Reconstructive arterial Surgery. *Proc. R. Soc. Med.*, **46**, 115–30.
15. Claytor, H., Birch, L., Cardwell, E.S., Zimmerman, S.L. (1956). Suture line rupture of a nylon aortic bifurcation graft into the small bowel. *Arch. Surg.*, **73**, 947–50.
16. Cunningham, C. and Goldstone, J. (1990). Quoted in: Management of aorto-enteric and aorto-caval fistulae. In *The cause and management of aneurysms* (ed: R.M. Greenhalgh, J.A. Mannick, and J.T. Powell), p. 461. W.B. Saunders, London.
17. Currie, E. and Maynard, A. (1989). Economic aspects of hospital acquired infections. Discussion paper 54, Department of Health Economic University of York, pp. 1–17.
18. Kaiser, A.B., Roach, A.C., Mulherin, J.L., Clayson, K.R., Allen, T.R., Edwards, W.H., *et al.* (1983). The cost effectiveness of antimicrobial prophylaxis in clean vascular surgery. *J. Infect. Dis.*, **147**, 1103–4.
19. Polk, H. (1985). Pre-operative skin preparation for surgery (when and how?). In *State of the art of surgery* (ed. T.P. Ruedi), p. 9. Proceedings of 31st Congress Societe Internationale Chirurgicae.
20. Cunat, J.S., Haaga, J.R., Rhodes, R., Bekeny, J., El Yousef, S. (1982). Periaortic fluid aspiration for recognition of infected graft. *Am. J. Roentgenol.*, **139**, 251–3.
21. Bandyk, D.F., Berni, G.A., Thiele, B.L., and Towne, J.B. (1984). Aorto-femoral graft infection due to Staphylococcus epidermidis. *Arch. Surg.*, **119**, 102–8.
22. Schmitt, D.D., Bandyk, D.F., Pequet, A.J., Malangoni, M.A., and Towne, J.B. (1986). Mucin production by Staphylococcus epidermidis. *Arch. Surg.*, **121**, 89–94.
23. Mannion, P.T., Thom, B.T., Reynolds, C.S., and Strachan, C.J.L. (1989). The acquisition of antibiotic resistant coagulase-negative staphylococci by aortic graft recipients, *J. Hosp. Infect.*, **14**, 313–23.
24. Archer, G.L. and Armstrong, B.C. (1983). Alteration of staphylococcal flora in cardiac surgery patients receiving antibiotic prophylaxis. *J. Infect. Dis.*, **147**, 642–9.
25. Bayston, R. and Penny, S.R. (1972). Excessive production of mucoid substance in Staphylococcus SIIA: a possible factor in colonization of Holter shunts. *Developmental Medicine and Child Neurology*, **27**, (suppl.) 25–8.
26. Rotschafer, J.C. and Shikuma, L.R. (1986). Pseudomonas aeruginosa susceptibility in a University hospital: recognition and treatment. *Drug. Intell. Clin. Pharm.*, **20**, 575–81.
27. Brandberg. A., Holm, J., Hammersten, J., and Schersten, T. (1979). Post-operative wound infections in vascular surgery. In *Effect of pre-operative whole body disinfection by shower bath with chlorhexidine soap in skin microbiology: relevance to infection* (ed. H. Maibaeh and R. Aly), pp. 98–102. Springer-Verlag, New York.
28. Wooster, D.L., Louch, R.E., and Krajden, S. (1985). Intraoperative bacterial contamination of vascular grafts: a prospective study. *Can. J. Surg.*, **28**, 407–9.
29. Moore, W.S. (1982). Pathogenesis of vascular graft sepsis. In *Extraanatomic and secondary arterial reconstruction* (ed. R.M. Greenhalgh), pp. 1–11. Pitman, London.
30. Tennant, W.G. and Baird, R.N. (1990). Secondary intra-abdominal pathology: concomitant or sequential surgery. In *The cause and management of aneurysms* (ed. R.M. Greenhalgh, J.A. Mannick, and J.T. Powell), pp. 322–3. W.B. Saunders, London.
31. Stoney, R.J. and Reilly, L.M. (1986). How should we treat infected grafts? In *Vascular surgery: issues in current practice* (ed. R.M. Greenhalgh, C.W. Jamieson, and A.N. Nicolaides), pp. 309–14. Grune & Stratton, London.
32. Calhoun, J.H., Mader, J.T. (1989). Antibiotic beads in the management of surgical infections. *Am. J. Surg.*, **157**, 443–9.
33. Bailey, I.S., Bundred, N.J., Pearson, H.J., and Bell, P.R.F. (1987). Successful treatment of an infected graft with gentamicin beads. *Eur. J. Vasc. Surg.*, **1**, 143–4.
34. Jorgansen, L.G., Sorensen, T.S., and Lorentzen, J.E. (1991). Clinical and pharmacological evaluation of gentamicin containing collagen in groin wound infections after vascular reconstruction. *Eur. J. Vasc. Surg*, **5**, 87–91.
35. Bandyk, D.K. (1990). Graft infections. In *Seminars in vascular surgery*, Vol. 3 (ed. R.B. Rutherford), pp. 77–80.

24

Urology

PATRICK J. O'BOYLE and SIMON HARRISON

Introduction

Urinary tract infection (UTI) continues to present a fascinating challenge to modern urological practice. The development of specific microbiological diagnostic techniques and potent antibiotics means that, with appropriate selection and administration, the surgeon may reasonably expect success in overcoming the threat of bacterial invasion.

The role of the surgeon is to ensure that this powerful armamentarium may be used effectively to strengthen the hosts resistance against the virulence of the infecting organism. An important task for the urologist is to identify predisposing factors which may lead to the development and persistence of infection. Thus a logical policy of antibiotic prophylaxis can be adopted.

At the other end of the spectrum of UTI, treatment of life-threatening conditions requires close attention to the basic surgical principles of relief of obstruction or other complicating factors which may inhibit the efficiency of antibiotic therapy. At the same time, the provision of adequate multi-system support, commensurate with the individual patient's needs, must be considered and continuously evaluated.

It seems likely that the vast majority of UTIs are effectively dealt with by the body's natural defence mechanisms assisted by the simple instruction to the patient to ensure adequate hydration and to void regularly. In a recent study in the author's unit 30 per cent of patients who had bacteriologically proven UTI had eliminated the organism spontaneously within 48 h, without antibiotic administration. Alternatively we have seen patients treated for days with powerful antibiotics to minimal effect, who have been shown subsequently to have associated urinary tract obstruction demonstrated, for example, by simple ultrasound examination.

Therefore, the purpose of this chapter is to emphasize the need for attention to basic surgical principles in the treatment of infection, and to review the management of specific conditions which are encountered in routine urological practice.

Diagnosis of infection

In clinical medicine the interpretation of laboratory findings must be considered in conjunction with the symptoms and signs elicited by careful examination of the patient. Typical symptom complexes and physical signs usually indicate a provisional diagnosis and permit the selection of appropriate confirmatory investigations.

The standard 'clean catch' mid-stream specimen of urine (MSSU) is fundamental to the initial diagnosis of UTI, but requires careful attention to detail of collection, storage, transport, microscopy, and selection of appropriate culture technique to ensure reliable microbiological evaluation.

In the collection of an MSSU it is important that the patient understands exactly what is required to ensure a suitable 'clean catch' specimen. Basic instruction in preparatory cleansing and the collection of a true mid stream specimen is usually delegated to the nursing staff and it is essential that the responsibility for ensuring the collection of adequate specimens is appreciated.

Ideally the sample should be transferred immediately to the

laboratory. If this is not practical, refrigeration at 4 °C or the addition of boric acid to the sterile container will inhibit bacterial proliferation. Alternatively, dip slides, which have selective medium on one side and nutrient agar on the other, may be immersed in the specimen and subsequently posted in their container to the laboratory for assessment.

More specialized urine specimens may be obtained, where specifically indicated, from the bladder by suprapubic needle puncture and aspiration or by urethral catheterization, from the ureter by selective ureteric catheterization and from the renal pelvis by fine needle percutaneous aspiration.

It is essential to indicate clearly to the laboratory, on the accompanying referral form, what information is required and why the investigation has been ordered. Furthermore the degree of urgency and the importance which will be attached to the results should be emphasized.

If possible, an indication of the type of pathogen suspected will help the microbiologist choose appropriate culture media for anaerobic or for acid-fast bacilli, and details of any current antibiotic therapy which may interfere with routine culture techniques should be indicated.

Laboratory examination of the urine is by microscopy and bacteriological culture. Microscopy will show the presence of red blood cells (RBCs), white blood cells (WBCs), casts, organisms, and ova. The finding of significant numbers of RBCs, or microscopic haematuria, is important since this can be the earliest sign of transitional cell carcinoma and further investigation by intravenous urography, endoscopy, and exfoliative cytology are mandatory.

The presence of WBCs in the urine indicates inflammation. Sterile pyuria normally indicates significant renal tract pathology. Classically this finding used to indicate tuberculosis, but in the UK concurrent consumption of antibiotic, which suppresses the culture of bacteria, is usually responsible. Other inflammatory and neoplastic conditions, urinary tract calculi, recent urinary tract instrumentation, analgesic abuse, and papillary necrosis should also be considered.

The results of urine culture are expressed quantitatively, a concentration of greater than 10^5 organisms/ml urine in pure culture being regarded as highly suggestive of infection (1). Lesser concentrations may be significant, particularly in states of high fluid output or in patients on antibiotic treatment, and should be interpreted with caution. Mixed bacterial cultures commonly indicate contamination, particularly in the absence of WBCs, and should be repeated unless the clinical picture suggests that action is urgently required. An indwelling catheter may be responsible but intestinal fistula formation, and intravesical neoplasia should be excluded. A synopsis of some common combinations of results is shown in Table 24.1.

Microbiology of urinary tract infection

Gram-negative bacilli, particularly *Escherichia coli*, are the commonest urinary pathogens. The large bowel acts as a reservoir for the bacteria from which certain strains seem particularly prone to invade the urinary tract. They can be classified according to the somatic or O antigen which may be useful when investigating recurrent or relapsing infection. The bacteria have fimbriae or pili (small hair-like extrusions from the bacterial cell wall), which form a bond with tissue cell receptors, a complicated phenomenon involving ligands and adhesins known as bacterial adherence. Other coliforms which cause urinary infection include *Klebsiella* and *Pseudomonas* species. These organisms are prone to develop antibiotic resistance and are seen particularly in hospital acquired infections. *Proteus* species have particular significance in the urinary tract due to their ability to produce urea splitting enzymes which liberate ammonia, and alkalinize the urine. This environment encourages stone formation with the deposition of matrix, a viscous substance which calcifies to form the classical staghorn calculus as a cast of the pelvi-calyceal system.

Infection may also occur with Gram-positive cocci. *Staphylococci saphrophyticus* are seen especially in young women

Table 24.1. Interpretation of urinary laboratory findings on microscopy and culture.

Specimen	Organisms	WBCs	RBCs	Comments and recommended action
MSSU	$>10^5$/ml	+	±	Probable UTI
MSSU	10^3–10^4/ml	+	±	Probable UTI (?high fluid intake)
MSSU	10^5/ml	–	–	Possible UTI or contaminant—repeat
MSSU	Mixed culture	±	±	?Contaminant. Indwelling catheter, vesico-colic fistula possible causes—repeat
MSSU	–	+	–	Possible treated UTI, recent instrumentation, calculus, tumour, or tuberculosis
MSSU	–	–	+	Possible urinary tract tumour, IVU and cystoscopy essential
Suprobubic aspiration	Any	±	±	Probable UTI (except low counts of skin flora)
Catheter specimen (*not* indwelling catheter)	$>10^3$/ml	±	±	Probable UTI

while enterococci, such as *Streptococcus faecalis*, are seen in hospital acquired infections. Pathogenic strains of *Staph. epidermidis* (coagulase-negative staphylococci) are commonly implicated in infection of prostheses and implants.

Anaerobic organisms are unusual but may be seen in association with indwelling catheters or enteric fistulae. Gas forming organisms can ferment sugar in the urine of diabetic patients and give rise to a classical sign, the 'gas pyelogram' which may readily be seen on a plain abdominal film.

Fungal infections are also unusual, but may be important to remember, particularly in diabetic or immunocompromised patients or following prolonged antibiotic therapy.

Genito-urinary tuberculosis, now rare in the UK, is common in Third World countries and hence in immigrant populations. The common presentation of frequency, nocturia (TB can also mean 'tiny bladder'!), haematuria, weight loss, lassitude, and pyrexia, suggest the diagnosis. The possibility must be transmitted to the laboratory since special staining techniques, such as Zeihl–Neelson staining for *A*cid and *A*lcohol *F*ast *B*acillus (AAFB), together with specific slope cultures and guinea pig innoculation will be necessary to confirm or refute the diagnosis.

Schistosomiasis is of enormous importance on a global scale, but rare in UK practice. The diagnosis usually involves demonstration of the characteristic ova on urine microscopy.

Chlamydia trachomatis is the commonest sexually transmitted infection in the UK, and a source of much misery. It is important to remember to treat both partners. Identification of the organism, which is neither a virus nor bacterium, by cell culture is laborious and expensive. Anti-chlamydial antibody detection may be useful, particularly to exclude the diagnosis. A 'trial by therapy' using oxytetracycline may be a more practical way of making the diagnosis, by inference rather than by positive identification.

Factors influencing the incidence of infection

Host resistance

Regular voiding, elimination of residual urine, adequate hydration, and avoiding constipation are attractive concepts and of considerable importance. However, urinary infections may develop despite attention to these simple parameters. In the female there are formidable immunological defence mechanisms provided by cervico-vaginal antibodies and by specific secretory IgA (sIgA) which not only produce agglutination, but also prevent bacterial adherence. In the male, specific antibacterial factors in the prostatic secretions together with the anatomical length of the urethra are clearly important.

In both sexes the bladder is defended by the tight junctions of the characteristic umbrella cells of transitional epithelium whilst, at the same time, the mucosa produces an antibacterial mucus layer. This enhances mucosal resistance by preventing bacterial adherence and a bacteria-engulfing slime assists in the elimination of organisms by voiding.

Prostheses

Susceptibility to infection is a balance between host resistance and bacterial virulence. The presence of foreign material in the urinary tract may affect this equilibrium. Some organisms, such as pathogenic strains of *Staph. epidermidis* and *Pseudomonas aeruginosa*, —which are commonly implicated in infection of prostheses—can produce a complex carbohydrate mucoid slime layer or glycocalyx. This may enhance virulence by interfering with the penetration of antibody, complement, phagocytes, or antibiotics. A bacterium which adheres to a prosthesis may have a protective coating of glycocalyx which impedes effective antibacterial control and may require removal of the infected prosthesis to ensure elimination. In urinary tract prostheses coagulase-negative staphylococci predominate suggesting that this organism, which normally is of low virulence, may demonstrate particular characteristics such as slime production. This may enhance its virulence in the presence of the prosthesis (2).

Antibiotic selection

Each antibiotic has specific characteristics which must be evaluated in the management of the individual patient. Choosing an appropriate antibiotic involves cooperation with the local microbiologist and hospital pharmacist. Each has specialist

Table 24.2. Antibiotic prophylaxis regimens.

Patient group/procedures	Antibiotic regimen
Lower urinary tract procedures urethrotomy, etc. Stone surgery, ESWL (selected cases)	Gentamicin 120 mg IV or Netilmicin 150 mg IV or Cefotaxime 1 g IV ± Ampicillin 500 mg IV } on induction of anaesthesia Repeat dose prior to removal of catheter
Transrectal prostatic biopsy	Gentamicin 80 mg IV + Metronidazole 1 g pr
Prior to implantation of urological implants	Ciprofloxacin 500 mg pre-operatively and for 48 h Cefuroxime 750 mg pre-operatively and for 48 h
Patients with valvular heart disease	Amoxycillin 1 g + Gentamicin 120 mg IV 15 min prior to surgery. Repeat dose 6 h post-operatively and prior to catheter removal

Table 24.3. Suitable antibiotics for the treatment of urinary tract infections.

Condition	Antibiotic	Dose	Duration	Comments
Cystitis	Trimethoprim	200 mg bd	3–5 days	
	Nitrofurantoin	100 mg qds	3–5 days	As macrocyrstals.
	Amoxycillin	250 mg tds	3–5 days	Resistant *E. coli* are common in hospitals.
	Co-amoxyclav	250 mg tds	3–5 days	If organism resistant to above. (NB: 10 to 14-day courses advisable for men).
	Ciprofloxacin	250 mg bd	3–5 days	
Serious upper tract infection and bacteraemia	Gentamicin	80 mg tds*	–	*Serum levels should be monitored and the dose adjusted accordingly.
	Netilmicin	100 mg tds*	–	
	Cefuroxime	750 mg–1.5 g tds	–	Add ampicillin 500 mg qds in severe cases.
	Cefotaxime	1–2 g tds	–	
Prostatitis	Trimethoprim	200 mg bd	4–6 weeks	
	Ciprofloxacin	500 mg bd	4–6 weeks	
Epididymo-orchitis	Oxytetracycline	500 mg qds	2 weeks	If *Chlamydia* suspected.
	Trimethoprim	200 mg bd	2 weeks	If presumed non-sexually transmitted pathogen.
	Ciprofloxacin	500 mg bd	2 weeks	
Genito-urinary tuberculosis	Rifampicin	450 mg	3 months	Always use at least 3 agents to avoid bacterial resistance.
	Isoniazid	300 mg		
	Ethambutol	800 mg		
	followed by			
	Rifampicin	450 mg	3 months	Pyrazinamide may also be added.
	Isoniazid	300 mg		

knowledge to contribute. The clinical microbiologist will know the prevalence of pathogenic organisms in the hospital environment, together with sensitivity and resistance patterns and will aid in the selection of the most effective antibiotic. The pharmacist may modify the choice after considering interrelated drug reactions which may be influenced by the patient's other medication, and by advice on cost-effective management.

Many hospitals now produce a 'best buy' guide for choice of antibiotic prophylaxis and treatment of common infections. This should be continually updated to take account of prevailing local factors.

Guide-lines for the administration and dosage of specific antibiotics are given in Tables 24.2 and 24.3, but these are examples of what is thought to be effective treatment at this time in the author's practice and will vary with local resistance patterns, etc.

Antibiotic prophylaxis

Endoscopic surgery

Operative urology has been revolutionized by developments, particularly in optical technology, which now permit the urologist access to virtually the entire urinary tract using appropriate endoscopic equipment. This has resulted in the development of the concept of minimally invasive surgery, which may mean a safer and less traumatic operative procedure for the patient with consequently faster recuperation and shorter hospital stay. Complications are infrequent and consist mainly of haemorrhage and infection. Significant haemorrhage can usually be avoided by meticulous operative technique and careful patient selection. Every effort should be made to anticipate and to forestall the development of infection and thus antibiotic prophylaxis has received considerable attention.

The use of routine prophylactic antibiotics remains controversial, but it seems logical to advocate this policy in situations which are known to provoke the release of potentially lethal organisms into the systemic circulation. Procedures that carry a significant risk of bacteraemia include urethral dilatation, urethrotomy, endoscopic bladder and prostatic surgery, litholapaxy, ureteroscopy, percutaneous stone surgery, and transrectal prostatic biopsy. The authors routinely administer antibiotics in these situations, usually a single dose at the induction of anaesthesia to ensure adequate circulating levels during surgery. In those patients known to have infected urine pre-operatively a full course of antibiotics, given according to the sensitivity of the cultured organism, is more suitable treatment.

Extracorporeal shock wave lithotripsy (ESWL)

The majority of renal tract calculi can now be safely treated by a combination of ESWL and percutaneous or endoscopic approaches using adjuvant electrohydraulic, ultrasonic, or pulse dye laser techniques to disintegrate the stone. During stone fragmentation bacteria can be liberated and the associated urothelial trauma permits ready access to the circulation. Although some centres give all patients prophylactic antibiotic, this may represent over treatment.

However, patients who have large or staghorn calculi, infected urine, valvular heart disease, or any form of surgical prosthesis should undoubtedly receive antibiotic cover. Appropriate regimens are indicated in Table 24.2.

Urological implants

The use of inert foreign material to correct urinary tract disorders, particularly in surgery for incontinence and impotence, has increased significantly in recent years. Insertion of artificial urinary sphincters, colposuspension operations using buttresses of extraneous materials, and injection of Teflon to tighten an incompetent bladder neck or urethra are common operations used to combat incontinence. Semi-rigid mechanical and inflatable hydrokinetic penile prostheses may help resolve the problems of impotence. Silastic testicular prostheses may relieve psychological trauma following loss of a testis. Surgery to relieve urinary obstruction may involve the use of long term bypass indwelling conduits such as the double J ureteric stent. Urethral and prostatic obstruction may be overcome by the insertion of permanent tubular prostheses or indwelling stents.

Extreme care must be taken in the pre-operative evaluation of the patient to eradicate active or chronic foci of infection, and meticulous attention paid to the principles of aseptic surgical technique in order to ensure a successful outcome. An infected prosthesis is a disaster which may leave the patient much worse off than before operation.

Prophylactic antibiotics are mandatory when undertaking any implant procedure and any evidence of early infection must be dealt with promptly using full bacteriological investigative facilities together with the expertise of the microbiologist if any hope of salvage is to be entertained.

Vesico-ureteric reflux

Some children are born with incompetent uretero-vesical valves which may permit reflux of urine into the upper renal tracts. This is frequently associated with an abnormality of the renal papilla which allows entry of the refluxing urine into the renal parenchyma. If the urine is infected this may result in renal scarring and the development of chronic infected foci in the kidney which may be difficult to eradicate.

Anti-reflux to surgery to increase the length of the intramural ureter was once commonplace, but has now been superceded in many centres by submucous injection of Teflon, a minimally invasive procedure. It is now also apparent that the use of long-term low-dosage antibiotic administration can prevent further damage to the kidney and may buy time to allow nature to correct the defect as the child grows and the trigone matures. Nitrofurantoin and trimethoprim have been shown to be effective in preventing re-infection, usually in doses of 1–2 mg/kg/day, given usually as a nightly bolus (3).

Treatment of urinary infection

Upper urinary tract infection

Acute upper UTI frequently results in a dramatically ill patient with high fever, severe loin pain and tenderness and associated frequency, nocturia, urgency, and dysuria. A precise diagnosis is required urgently since a combination of infection and obstruction will rapidly lead to irreversible renal damage. The important differential diagnosis is between acute pyelonephritis and pyonephrosis—an infected and obstructed kidney.

Careful clinical examination, urine microscopy, plain abdominal film, and urinary tract ultrasound will usually confirm the diagnosis and indicate the need for emergency decompression of an obstructed system. This is usually achieved by percutaneous nephrostomy, a relatively atraumatic procedure, which deals effectively with the crisis and provides a specimen for proper bacteriological evaluation. Antibiotics should be given parenterally to ensure rapid and adequate absorption to achieve effective tissue levels, and the patient carefully monitored. Suitable initial regimens, are indicated in Table 24.3. When the infection has been controlled further investigation to determine the precise nature of the obstruction may proceed using intravenous urography or renography so that planned surgical correction can be arranged if indicated.

Another acute presentation is the development of a perinephric abscess, which usually arises from a chronically infected kidney, associated with stone disease or from persistent obstruction. There may be a large, tender loin mass, and once again emergency decompression is reqired, usually by means of surgical drainage under full antibiotic cover. Infection will persist, or rapidly recur, unless the underlying abnormality is corrected. However, effective early treatment will permit a subsequent elective operation to be planned when renal function has been adequately evaluated; unfortunately nephrectomy is often the only reasonable option.

The renal carbuncle, usually a staphylococcal, metastatic haematogenous infection, is rarely seen nowadays presumably because anti-staphylococcal antibiotics are now so effective and because of the overall improved state of nutrition and hygiene in our present society. When a renal carbuncle is encountered underlying factors such as diabetes, chest infection, or possibly, and more commonly nowadays, drug addiction should be remembered. Ultrasound-guided aspiration of the abscess will confirm the diagnosis, provide drainage and allow installation of antibiotic into the abscess cavity. Carbuncles are, however, frequently multilocular and may ultimately require formal surgical attention.

Chronic and relapsing upper UTI may present a much greater diagnostic and surgical challenge involving the use of long-term, low-dose antibiotic therapy, possibly for years, combined with corrective surgical procedures to eliminate pockets of poor tissue perfusion and resistant infection.

Lower urinary tract infection

It is important to distinguish between lower urinary tract colonization and infection. Many patients, particularly the elderly, seem to tolerate a heavily contaminated lower urinary tract without any apparent morbidity. It may be inappropriate, or even positively harmful, to attempt to influence this relationship by antibiotic administration or by surgical intervention. The importance of recognizing colonization is to ensure that no significant treatable underlying pathology, such as a neoplasm or chronic stone disease, is overlooked.

Symptomatic lower UTI and acute infective episodes are usually heralded by the development of bladder irritative symptoms; frequency, nocturia, urgency, and incontinence. These symptoms require full investigation and treatment since infection causes much misery and may indicate serious associated pathology.

Cystitis

The diagnosis of acute bacterial cystitis rarely proves difficult since urinary culture will reveal the pathogen, usually *E. coli*. In the young, sexually active female, a single high dose of an oral antibiotic will frequently eliminate the offending organism. Relapsing infection should be managed by a full course of antibiotic, but if this is not successful, other predisposing factors should be sought by urinary flow studies and ultrasound screening of the renal tract, together with intravenous urography and endoscopy if symptoms persist. Frequently, no urinary tract abnormality can be found, even after careful screening, and long-term low-dose antibiotic therapy for three or six months is then indicated. Bacterial UTI in the male is uncommon in the absence of readily apparent predisposing factors. In this context it is surprising how often phimosis is overlooked. More than one infection should always lead to a full urological investigation including urinary flow studies which will frequently reveal unsuspected lower urinary tract obstruction. Corrective surgery may then be undertaken, with appropriate antibiotic prophylaxis.

Prostatitis

Acute bacterial prostatitis is uncommon but unmistakable. A pyrexial patient who has severe perineal pain radiating to the thighs and penis, frequency and a poor urinary stream, and an exquisitely tender prostate on rectal examination, requires urgent antibiotic therapy. *Escherichia coli* and *Strep. faecalis* are the usual pathogens and should be treated by antibiotics which are known to penetrate prostatic tissue: erythromycin, trimethoprim, or ciprofloxacin. If rapid relief of symptoms is not achieved, rectal examination should (very gently!) be repeated, when a characteristic fluctuant mass may be easily palpated. This will require endoscopic incision and drainage which presents a dramatic visual appearance to the surgeon as pus pours out and the thin-walled prostatic abscess cavity collapses. Antibiotics should be continued for a six-week course to ensure elimination of the organism.

Chronic bacterial prostatitis may result from inadequately treated acute prostatitis or from unsuspected urinary tract obstruction. A urinary flow rate and ultrasound estimation of residual urine volume are helpful. Some patients are prone to prostatic calcification, a poorly understood but common finding, which requires screening for diabetes and tuberculosis. Chronic prostatitis usually occurs in middle age and has an intermittent relapsing course. Typically, the patient complains of hypogastric, perineal and penile pain radiating to the thighs, accompanied by symptoms of bladder base irritation and frequently the complaint of poor sexual function. Rectal examination usually elicits vague tenderness and gentle methodical prostatic massage should be performed in an attempt to obtain a specimen of expressed prostatic secretion (EPS). If successful, a drop of the EPS should be examined microscopically for WBCs and to exclude trichomonas, and the remainder of the EPS collected by saturating a culture swab which is sent in transport medium to the microbiology laboratory. Best guess antibiotics are a six week course of ciprofloxacin, or tetracycline if *Chlamydia* is suspected.

All too often the attempt to establish a causative organism fails despite examination of fractionated urine specimens before and after prostatic massage (4). The frustrated surgeon and equally frustrated patient then find themselves in the grey area of diagnosing non-bacterial prostatitis or prostatodynia, a condition refractory to treatment and thought to be due to psychosomatic illness. Medication then becomes somewhat empirical, relying on a combination of long-term antibiotics, antiprostaglandin anti-inflammatory agents and mild sedation.

Epididymo-orchitis

Accurate diagnosis of the cause of an acutely painful swollen testis is a surgical emergency. Torsion of the testis must be excluded since this is readily amenable to surgical correction if diagnosed early, i.e. within 6 h of onset. When treating a child or young adult the most important question for the surgeon to ask is: 'Why am I *not* exploring this testis?'

The onset of puberty and subsequent sexual activity may complicate the picture. A history of exposure to mumps and involvement of the body of the testis may suggest a viral aetiology. Usually, this is unilateral and may result in dramatic swelling and pain. Unfortunately the tough fibrous tunica albuginea does not readily permit inflammatory swelling of the testicular parenchyma and the resulting relative ischaemia will lead to testicular atrophy. The Leydig cells are more resistant to damage than the seminiferous tubules so hormone production may be preserved.

Ultrasound examination of the scrotum can be helpful and will usually demonstrate abscess formation or localized epididymal swelling if present. It will also help to exclude the rare presentation of testicular tumour which should never be overlooked. If the inflammatory process is confined to the testis, the examination is made easier by performing a local anaesthetic spermatic cord block which can produce dramatic relief of pain. If scrotal examination reveals a swollen tender epididymis with little tenderness of the body of the testis and a normal spermatic cord the likely diagnosis is epididymitis.

Erythromycin or ciprofloxacin give good tissue penetration and oxytetracycline is a reasonable choice to treat epididymitis in the sexually active, to deal with *Chlamydia*. In severe infection an aminoglycoside plus amoxycillin will eliminate most serious pathogens and inhibit spread of infection.

In the older age-group epididymo-orchitis is most commonly seen after urethral instrumentation or transurethral prostatectomy. The use of prophylactic antibiotics has virtually eliminated this complication in the immediate post-operative period, and routine bilateral vasectomy is no longer practised. More usually the very anxious patient will be admitted two to three weeks after surgery with an alarming swelling of the scrotum. Trimethoprim may be given while awaiting urine culture and sensitivity and, if appropriate, continued for four weeks in full dosage. In severe infection an aminoglycoside is indicated. If rapid improvement does not ensue, scrotal abscess or testicular infarction should be suspected in which case orchidectomy will be indicated. If a conservative policy is pursued, the patient must be warned that resolution may take up to three months.

Tuberculosis is rarely seen nowadays, but must always be considered in a persisting infection of the epididymis, particularly with sinus formation. The characteristic 'rosary' effect on the vas with nodularity of the epididymis due to caseating abscesses is unmistakeable, but fortunately is rare in the U.K. Tuberculosis elsewhere in the urinary tract should be sought and closely monitored during treatment, since epididymal involvement is normally by haematogenous spread, rather than by retrograde extension along the vas. An insidiously developing prostatic abscess, contracted bladder, ureteric stricture, or progressive renal destruction may require surgery to hasten the elimination of disease.

Treatment follows the usual lines with full anti-tuberculous chemotherapy and any surgery considered necessary should be undertaken at about six weeks after the start of antibiotic administration. It must be emphasized that antituberculous chemotherapy should be closely supervised by a specialist who is familiar with the complications which may occur with this potentially toxic regimen. Three drugs will usually be administered to prevent bacterial resistance. A suitable regimen comprises isoniazid, rifampicin, and ethambutol (5).

Catheter-associated infection

Urine cultures from patients with long-term indwelling catheters will invariably show bacterial growth. Treatment with antibiotics will not sterilize the urine whilst the catheter remains in position and is rarely indicated. The misconceived, continuing use of a variety of antibiotics will result in a population of antibiotic resistant organisms which may preclude alternative surgical treatment and may cause extremely serious problems if introduced into the hospital environment, particularly in surgical wards.

Recurrent, symptomatic, lower urinary tract infections usually indicate a poor fluid throughput and, although efforts to encourage increased oral intake may be disappointing or impractical, this is by far the best solution to an extremely difficult problem of management. A search should also be made for reservoirs of infection other than the catheter itself; for example, bladder calculi which may readily develop from the deposition of 'egg-shell' encrustations released when the catheter is changed.

The use of continuous irrigation by three way catheters or by regular bladder washout is expensive, time-consuming and should be reserved for carefully selected cases with significant symptomatic infection. The addition of antiseptics is rarely beneficial. Some patients suffer repeated, frequent blockage due to slime produced particularly by *Pseudomonas* and *Proteus* spp. If the patient is capable of performing bladder washout at home, either alone or with the assistance of a relative or friend, simple irrigation with boiled (and cooled!) water can be surprisingly effective. The patient should know how to deal with a blocked catheter and time spent helping them to understand fully the care of their catheter will be well-rewarded. Intermittent self-catheterization is another tried and tested technique which may be effective in the correct circumstances.

Sometimes recurring symptomatic infection and catheter blockage may force the surgeon to reconsider the prospect of surgical intervention, usually to relieve obstruction or to deal with incontinence. In this situation, in particular, the surgeon will not wish to encounter a population of antibiotic resistant organisms! Finally, an alternative form of urinary diversion may be the only procedure which can be realistically entertained to improve the situation in these extremely difficult cases.

Infected implants

Infection following the insertion of a urological prosthesis is potentially a surgical disaster. Treatment regimens designed to salvage the prosthesis are rarely successful so an early decision to remove the implant is essential.

Local signs and symptoms such as tenderness, erythema, and discomfort are more common when infection occurs than systemic signs. A low grade pyrexia and persistent leucocytosis should not be dismissed. Systemic antibiotics should be given, but if resolution of the signs of infection do not occur rapidly the device must be removed before the overlying tissues are eroded. Once healing has occurred a further attempt at prosthesis insertion may be undertaken some months later (2).

Urinary tract infection in special circumstances

Pregnancy

The same range of pathogens are encountered during pregnancy as in the non-pregnant female, with *E. coli* predominating. Increased susceptibility to infection may result from urinary stasis due to the progesterone effect, particularly evident in the ureter, or from mechanical obstruction due to the enlarging gravid uterus. Significant asymptomatic bacteriuria should be treated since 40 per cent of these will go on to develop UTI which carries some risk to the fetus (6).

In pregnancy the choice of antibiotic therapy is limited by the possible danger to the fetus, and short courses are desirable, carefully monitored by regular urine culture. Combinations of a beta-lactam/antibiotic with a beta-lactamase inhibitor are usually effective, co-amoxiclav being a reasonable choice. Other antibiotics which may be safely used in pregnancy are, amoxycillin, cephalexin, and nitrofurantoin.

In general radiation is best avoided during pregnancy, but if complicating factors are suspected and ultrasound studies are equivocal, a single-shot intravenous urogram film 20 min after the injection of contrast will usually demonstrate the site of any obstructive lesion.

The elderly

The management of UTI in the elderly poses particular problems, mainly due to deteriorating renal function. Some antibiotics are best avoided, in particular the tetracyclines which may aggravate renal insufficiency by combined salt depleting and anti-anabolic effects, and nitrofurantoin which may give rise to irreversible peripheral neuropathy. Aminoglycosides should, likewise, be used with caution and serum levels carefully monitored if renal deterioration or the complication of vestibular ototoxicity are to be avoided.

The mainstay of treatment, however, is to ensure adequate hydration, regular voiding, and to avoid constipation, by no means easy in a population who may have fixed ideas in these matters (7)!

Children

Except in the newborn, urinary infection is more common in girls than boys. It is a major bacterial infection of childhood and can damage the urinary tract, or prevent proper development, if left untreated. The urine for culture may need to be collected by a sterile technique such as urethral or suprapubic catheterization. Investigation of the young child with urinary infection should exclude developmental abnormality of the urinary tract and, in infants, a combination of ultrasound and micturating cystourethrography is required to exclude obstruction and vesico-ureteric reflux. In older children ultrasound and a plain abdominal film will usually provide the necessary information, with more invasive investigations reserved for recurrent infection. The investigation and management of the more complex problems should be conducted in a specialist paediatric unit.

References

1. Kass, E.H. (1956). Asymptomatic infection of the urinary tract. *Trans. Assoc. Am. Phys.*, **69**, 56–63.
2. Carson, C.C. (1989). Infections in Genitourinary prostheses. *Urol. Clin. North Am.*, **16**, 139–47.
3. Verrier Jones, K. (1990). Antimicrobial treatment for urinary tract infections. *Arch. Dis. Childhood*, **65**, 327–30.
4. Meares, E.M., Jr. and Stamey, T.A. (1968). Bacteriologic localisation patterns in bacterial prostatitis and urethritis. *Investigative Urology*, **5**, 492–6.
5. O'Boyle, P.J. and Gow, J.G. (1976). Genito-urinary tuberculosis: Study of 20 patients. *Br. Med. J.*, **1**, 141–3.
6. Tan, J.S. and File, T.M. (1990). Urinary tract infections in obstetrics and gynaecology. *J. Reproductive Med.*, **35**, 339–42.
7. Bendall, M.J. (1984). A review of urinary tract infection in the elderly. *J. Antimicrob. Chemother.*, **13**, Suppl. B, 69–78.

Further reading

Lock, S. (ed). (1978). Diseases of the urinary system. In *Today's treatment 3*. British Medical Journal Publications, Devonshire Press, England.

Hindmarsh, J.R. (1987). Urinary tract infection. In *The scientific basis of urology* (ed. A.R. Mundy), pp. 183–201. Churchill Livingstone, Edinburgh.

Fowler, J.E. Jr. (1989). *Urinary tract infection and inflammation*. Year Book Medical Publishers, Chicago.

Pfau, A. (1990). Urinary tract infections. In *The scientific foundations of urology* (ed. G.D. Chisholm and W.R. Fair), pp. 131–42. Heinemann, Oxford.

25

Plastic surgery

ARTHUR McG. MORRIS

Introduction

There are many opportunities for infection to occur in the wide range of procedures performed in plastic surgery. The traditional methods of soft tissue reconstruction using skin flaps and grafts to treat the results of trauma or cancer ablation are vital in the prevention of infection, but the procedures are themselves vulnerable to infection. A major part of plastic surgery is the treatment of chronic open skin defects and complications that are referred from other specialties. The wounds in these patients are often infected at the time of referral. The performance of more complicated and prolonged invasive procedures, frequently involving teamwork with other specialties has increased the opportunities for infection.

In addition, the development of prosthetic implants in breast, hand, and aesthetic surgery has opened up a new dimension of infection risk. In many wounds infection can be controlled easily with a successful result, but infections associated with implants almost invariably require the removal of the implant and result in failure of the procedure. In such elective surgery everything possible should be done to minimize any risk of complication.

Predisposing factors for infection

Vulnerability of the skin

Forming the outer covering of the body, the skin is vulnerable to injury from many different physical agents: blunt and sharp trauma, heat, cold, chemicals, and radiation. The outer keratinized layer is specially toughened to resist mild injury but once breached, micro-organisms can gain entry into the vulnerable underlying dermis and soft tissue. In addition, the skin is colonized by resident micro-organisms such as staphylococci on the surface, in sweat glands and hair follicles. If the skin is devitalized or damaged they can gain entry and may cause infection.

Pathogenic organisms

Many organisms can cause skin and soft tissue infection. The common ones are *Staphylococcus aureus*, *Streptococcus pyogenes*, *Pseudomonas aeruginosa*, *Proteus*, and coliforms. Skin healing can usually proceed in the presence of mild infection but when *Strep. pyogenes*, and to a lesser extent, *Ps. aeruginosa* are present wound healing is impaired and grafts can be lost.

Wound factors

Several factors influence the incidence of infection of a wound.

Mechanism of injury

Clean 'tidy' wounds inflicted with a sharp instrument are much less likely to become infected than an 'untidy' contused wound. An injury from a blunt instrument or a crush is more likely to damage or devitalize the surrounding tissue predisposing to infection. The presence of dead tissue, debris, foreign body, and haematoma, particularly when large tissue planes are opened up also makes infection more likely.

Time of injury

Recently inflicted wounds are less likely to become infected. After 8 hours without treatment the risk is significantly greater and after 24 h most wounds are infected. The quality of first-aid treatment with early closure of an open wound with a clean dressing will help to minimize the risk of infection. This variation of contamination, depending on the time before treatment is commenced, means that treatment must be modified to minimize the risk of infection. Primary closure is permissible in early clean wounds but delayed primary or secondary closure is indicated for older, contaminated, or crush injuries. Prophylactic antibiotics will not usually be required in clean wounds treated early but are essential in wounds seen and treated late, or in contaminated untidy injuries.

Time of surgery

Prolonged operations with exposure of soft tissues, for example the complex microsurgical procedures involved in replantation of an amputated limb, or major cranio-facial surgery increase the risk of infection and antibiotic prophylaxis is essential.

Burns

Burns give rise to a risk of infection in two principle ways: the local effect of the burn and the systemic effect. Bacterial infection of the wound is a severe problem in the treatment of burn patients. The large raw surface area of the wound, kept warm by the body heat, covered in exposed soft tissue, necrotic debris, and exudates is ideally suited as a culture medium for micro-organisms. Surface contamination is almost inevitable but does not necessarily lead to infection.

The severe systemic effect of larger burns gives rise to a decrease in body resistance which predisposes to infection. The breaching of the body surface with infection can cause systemic effects by septicaemia or by the release of toxins as in toxic shock syndrome. Major injury and shock predisposes to toxaemia and septicaemia as a result of the effects on the intestinal tract (see Chapter 13).

Tissue blood supply

If the skin blood supply is inadequate the devitalized tissue is vulnerable to infection and defence mechanisms such as hyperaemia are impaired. This occurs easily in the degloving type of injury where large areas of skin and soft tissue are lifted, disrupting the blood supply. There may also be an open wound allowing contamination. Infection is a common result if the tissues are not treated correctly (Fig. 25.1).

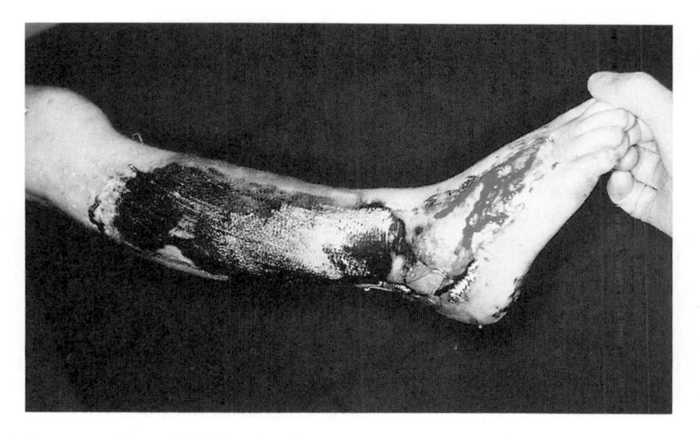

Fig. 25.1. Result following incorrect treatment by primary suture of an extensive degloving injury. The devitalized flap has necrosed and become infected. (See plate section.)

In pressure sores the tissue viability is impaired by ischaemia as a result of pressure, particularly over a bony prominence. Some pressure areas present as a deep seated abscess because the subcutaneous fat, with its poorer blood supply, is more vulnerable to ischaemia and infection. Slough in a wound encourages the growth of micro-organisms.

Tissue transfer

Reconstructing soft tissue and skin cover is an ideal way of preventing further entry of micro-organisms into an open wound and in some circumstances helps to clear infection. However, during the steps of reconstruction the transferred tissues are vulnerable to infection and the best results are obtained by ensuring that conditions are favourable prior to treatment. Reconstructive operations must be avoided in the presence of acute infection.

Grafts

Free grafts are completely detached from their blood supply before application to a new site. Success depends on the graft establishing a new blood supply from the graft bed and, until this happens, the graft is vulnerable to infection. All living grafts are vulnerable but bone grafts, especially in large pieces—or composite grafts—are at greatest risk of failure from infection.

The graft bed must be clean and free of debris before a graft is applied. A swab should be taken so that the wound culture is known before operation if an open wound is to be repaired. The presence of beta haemolytic streptococci of groups A, B, C, and G are an absolute contraindication to free skin graft transfer as the graft may be completely destroyed and liquified. *Pseudomonas aeruginosa* has similar but less marked effects. Pus acts as a mechanical barrier to graft take and the skin graft must be incised to release infected blisters.

Flap transfer

A flap carries its own blood supply at all times and, if well-designed with a good blood supply, is as resistant to infection as normal tissue. Muscle and musculo-cutaneous flaps are particularly robust and, by introducing a new blood supply, can be used to cover defects such as exposed bone, tendon, and joints even in the presence of chronic infection. Under a flap there is considerable dead space which, if filled with haematoma or seroma, is vulnerable to infection. Closed suction drainage should be used to reduce the risk of infection. Antibiotic treatment will be required in salvage situations where there is chronic infection and the choice of antibiotic will depend on the preoperative wound swab results.

If the flap has been raised with an inadequate blood supply, far from improving the wound healing process, the ischaemic tissue will itself be more vulnerable to infection.

Free tissue transfer

The free flap is detached in the same manner as a free graft but the blood supply is re-united by micro-vascular anastomosis to local blood vessels. Therefore, it has the ability to introduce new revascularised tissue into an area and thus has the same advantages as the traditional flap in assisting wound healing and thereby preventing infection. The ability to have the flap on a long vascular pedicle allows the anastomoses to be performed some distance away from the defect, and this is particularly helpful in defects where previous radiotherapy has been used and has caused fibrosis and impairment of blood supply, predisposing to infection.

However, the free flap is very vulnerable to ischaemia if the vascular anastomoses are compromised. The use of leeches to aid venous drainage and decrease swelling in an effort to resuscitate an ailing flap has recently been reintroduced. A complication of leech therapy in the presence of vascular insufficiency is infection by *Aeromonas hydrophyla*, a common resident organism on leeches.

Implants

An implant, which is an inert, space filling device, can cause infection by acting as a foreign body. Once established, infection is more difficult to eradicate in the presence of a foreign body. A study of infected breast prostheses by Courtiss *et al.* (1) showed that haematoma was a common problem prior to infection developing.

Chronic wounds, including pressure sores

An open defect in the body surface predisposes to wound infection by allowing easy access to the more vulnerable underlying tissues. A distinction must be drawn between contamination and infection. For example, even though a wound swab may show a positive growth of a pathogenic micro-organism this does not necessarily mean that there is infection. Clinical signs such as erythema or cellulitis of the surrounding area, lymphadenopathy, or systemic effects such as pyrexia, are required for the diagnosis of infection. Infection alone is rarely the cause of a chronic ulcer but prolonged infection may delay healing.

The great majority of chronic ulcers are below the waist level (96 per cent of pressure sores are below the umbilicus), and most varicose ulcers are near the level of the ankle. This predisposes to infection, as contamination by faecal flora is more common. Also the wound healing potential is frequently impaired in these patients by general illness and debility, continuing pressure, and poor blood supply, particularly in the lower limb where arterial impairment may be present in addition to venous insufficiency.

Burn management

General care

Burn injuries are a common cause of death and disability, with both local and systemic effects. In the initial acute phase, when the treatment and prevention of shock is vital for survival in burns of a large percentage of body surface, it is easy to neglect the management of the burn wound. Yet infection of the wound can itself contribute to the systemic effect of the injury.

Infection is the most important threat to survival in successfully resuscitated patients, as the burn wound interferes with the protective function of the skin and respiratory tract. Thermal injury leads to the depression of immunity, exacerbating infection. There is also a hypermetabolic response and part of the cause of this response is thought to be the breakdown of the intestinal mucosal barrier releasing endotoxin and bacteria into the circulation. It has been observed that early oral feeding markedly attenuates the hypermetabolic response.

Prevention of infection is the mainstay of treatment of the burn wound and superficial burns will heal spontaneously in about ten to fourteen days. If infection occurs, healing will be delayed and a superficial burn may be rendered deeper and subsequently require skin grafting. Deeper burns, of the deep dermal and full thickness variety, take much longer to heal spontaneously and are thus more likely to become infected. Wound care with aseptic technique, antimicrobial agents, and cross-infection control are the mainstay of prevention of infection.

It is vital at the outset to establish basic parameters by examination of the patient and taking a history: time of injury, causative agent, percentage of body surface burned, depth of burn, general fitness of patient prior to injury, and respiratory injury or evidence of smoke inhalation. If the burn surface area is greater than 15 per cent in an adult or greater than 10 per cent in a child, intravenous fluid resuscitation is required and a urinary catheter should be inserted, using aseptic technique to help monitor urine output. This must be done as a first priority as fluid loss starts at the time of the burn and is greatest in the first few hours.

For first aid, the burn surface must be kept as clean and uncontaminated as possible to prevent infection. Clean towels or sheets are an ideal temporary cover during the initial assessment and start of resuscitation. Large burns, requiring intravenous resuscitation, are best treated in a specialist burn unit with adequate facilities for isolation. Smaller burns do not usually require sophisticated facilities but if grafting is required care is needed to prevent infection spreading both to and from burn patients. Many small superficial burns can easily be treated in the out patient setting away from the risk of cross-infection.

Prevention of infection

Isolation

Isolation can be achieved for patients with large burns by treatment in specially designed facilities with individual cubicles and filtered air changes. At several stages in treatment of deep burns the patient will require surgery or other treatment, such as burn baths, and it is usually not possible to carry out the treatment in the cubicle. Therefore strict infection control measures by staff to prevent cross-infection are required in the operating room and therapy bath areas, and when it is not possible to admit a patient to a specialist treatment area.

Burns of smaller area can be isolated by covering with an occlusive dressing allowing out-patient treatment, if home conditions are suitable and help is available. This will reduce the risk of acquired infection with antibiotic resistant hospital pathogens.

Systemic treatment

Systemic treatment using prophylactic antibiotics has been recommended in the past to prevent streptococcal infection and against Gram-negative infection. However, the antibiotic cannot reach the avascular part of a burn wound, and exposure to antibiotics encourages the growth of resistant bacteria (2, 3). Prophylactic broad spectrum antibiotic also gives rise to the risk of fungal infection. When a burn patient presents late, contamination will already have occurred, the risk of infection is increased, and the burn may already be infected. Systemic antibiotic therapy is much more important in these patients, particularly when the burn involves the lower limb or perineal area. Tetanus prophylaxis should be initiated as appropriate.

Local treatment

It is not possible to sterilize a burn wound but the burn is usually relatively clean and uncontaminated by micro-organisms at the outset. The aim of treatment is to keep the wound clean and to prevent further contamination, thereby reducing the risk of infection and promoting healing. Initial cleaning is performed using a mild, non-alcohol-based antiseptic such as povidone iodine or aqueous chlorhexidine (Hibiscrub diluted 1:4 with saline), gently removing all loose devitalized tissue and debris using aseptic techniques. It is not necessary to deroof all blisters. Small flaccid ones can be left and larger ones should be incised or aspirated to release the blister fluid. The burn is then usually treated by exposure, dressings, or excision and grafting.

Exposure

Exposure of the burn is a specific treatment in which nothing touches the burn except air. The exudate from the burn evaporates to form a dry eschar which then protects the burn from further contamination. Until this happens isolation in a clean air environment is necessary. Exposure treatment is ideal for the face and burns of single surfaces only (Fig. 25.2). It is not recommended for large areas which cross joints as the dry eschar will crack allowing the entry of micro-organisms. Hair should be trimmed or tied back to help to prevent contamination of burns around the face and ears.

Burn dressing

The purpose of a dressing is to absorb exudate, prevent contamination, provide protection, and support the burn while allowing healing. There is a bewildering array of burn dressings available but all have drawbacks and the ideal dressing has yet to be developed. A major challenge for a burn wound dressing is absorption of the copious exudate which is released in the first 48 h.

The traditional dressing has an inner non-adherent layer, e.g. tulle gras, covered by a transmission layer of gauze and an absorbent layer of wool held in place by an outer conforming bandage. The dressing should be sufficiently thick and absorbent to prevent soakage to the surface which would allow entry for micro-organisms.

New synthetic dressings aim to keep the inner layer of the wound moist which theoretically enhances epithelialization. Semi-permeable films (for example, Opsite or Tegaderm) do not have the necessary absorbent properties and large collections of exudate can accumulate tending to lift it off t

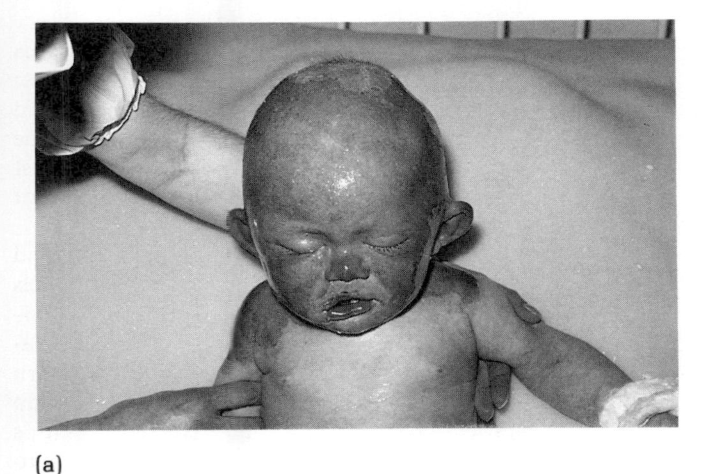

(a)

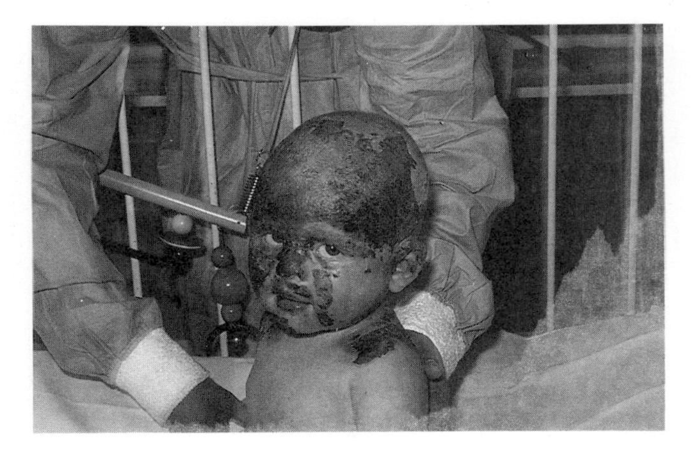

(b)

Fig. 25.2. (a) Superficial burns caused by a scald. Exposure treatment is ideal for burns of the face; (b) Result eight days later. The scabs separated easily after a bath. (See plate section.)

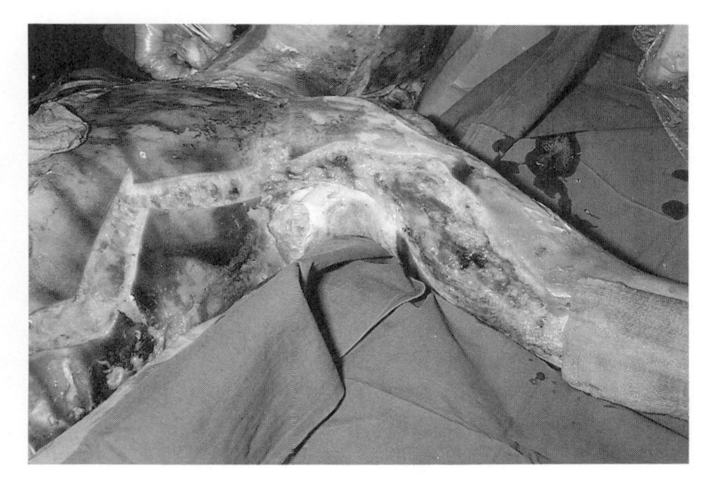

Fig. 25.3. Escarotomy used for emergency release of constricting escar in a circumferential flame burn of trunk and arm. Incision down to viable tissue increases the risk of infection and a Flamazine gauze dressing has been used. (See plate section.)

surrounding skin, breaking the seal and allowing contamination.

Semi-occlusive hydrogel dressings, such as Geliperm and Scherisorb, have a better absorptive capacity but keeping them on all but small wounds is difficult in practice and they are not easy to use in burns. Occlusive hydro-colloid dressings (for example, Granuflex) are composite layers of inner hydrogel for absorption with an outer elastomer and adhesive layer. They provide an easily applied self-adhesive occlusive dressing for smaller burns, but the large amounts of exudate can cause difficulty with large burns particularly over joints, leading to leakage.

Biological dressings, for example freeze-dried pig skin, are useful for some burns. Pig skin may help to limit exudate formation and provides a slightly flexible covering initially. Once dried it has the same disadvantages as an eschar formed by the exposure of a burn and any movement which causes cracks can allow the entry of micro-organisms. Human biological dressings such as amnion are difficult to obtain, and impossible to sterilize, and therefore carry the disadvantage of possible transmission of infections such as HIV.

Topical treatment

The application of suitable antibacterial agents are an aid in preventing infection. They may help to reduce the recontamination of the wound by micro-organisms from skin sweat glands and hair follicles. Topical antibiotics are not recommended and there is no place for the use of multiple antibiotic sprays. Topical neomycin can be absorbed from the burn wound causing deafness. Topical silver sulphadiazine 1 per cent cream (Flamazine) is a useful agent in the prevention of infection by *Ps. aeruginosa* and is usually applied on the inner layer of gauze in the wound dressing (Fig. 25.3).

Dressing changes are kept to a minimum as each time the dressing is changed the procedure is a considerable ordeal for the patient with large burns. If the burn is superficial the dressing should only be changed after at least seven days as early change of dressing can offer an opportunity for contamination and healing cannot be expected before then. If the inner layer of a dressing is adherent at the time of dressing change it should not necessarily be removed unless there is infection present. The dry inner-layer can be covered by a new light dressing and left for a few more days. A convenient method of dressing a hand burn is to use a polythene bag containing a small amount of antiseptic cream such as Flamazine secured with a bandage on the forearm (Fig. 25.4). It allows early mobilization while providing a protected environment. Burns of the hand and the lower limb should be treated by elevation of the affected part in the early stages to prevent oedema and stiffness.

Early excision and grafting

Early excision and grafting of the burn, removing the burned tissue and providing early cover by skin grafting, is the ideal

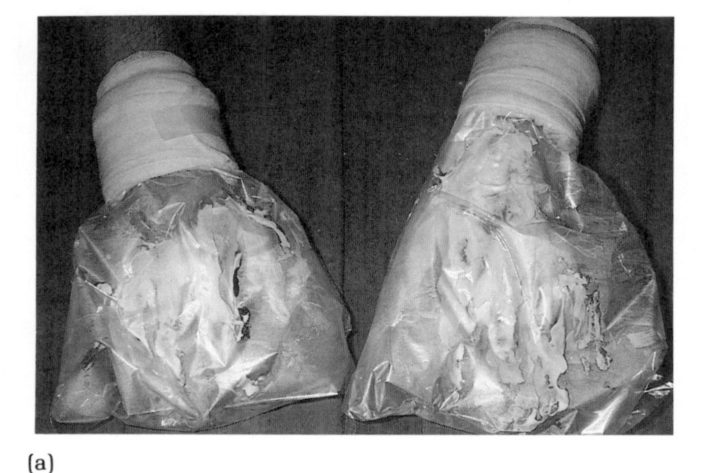

(a)

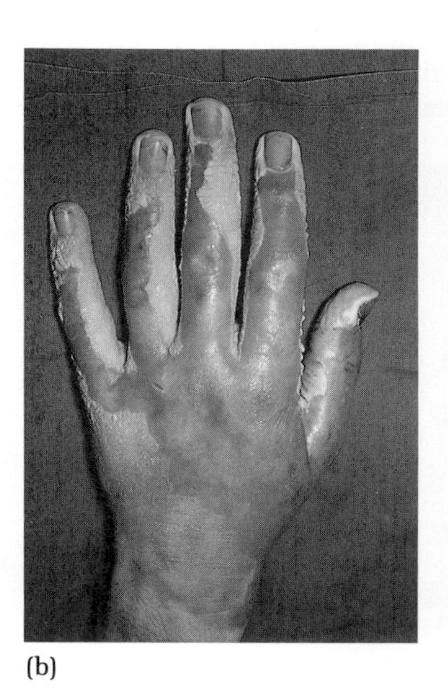

(b)

Fig. 25.4. (a) Polythene bags used for bilateral hand burns. The burn is smeared with Flamazine cream and the bag is changed daily; (b) Left hand completely healed at eight days. (See plate section.)

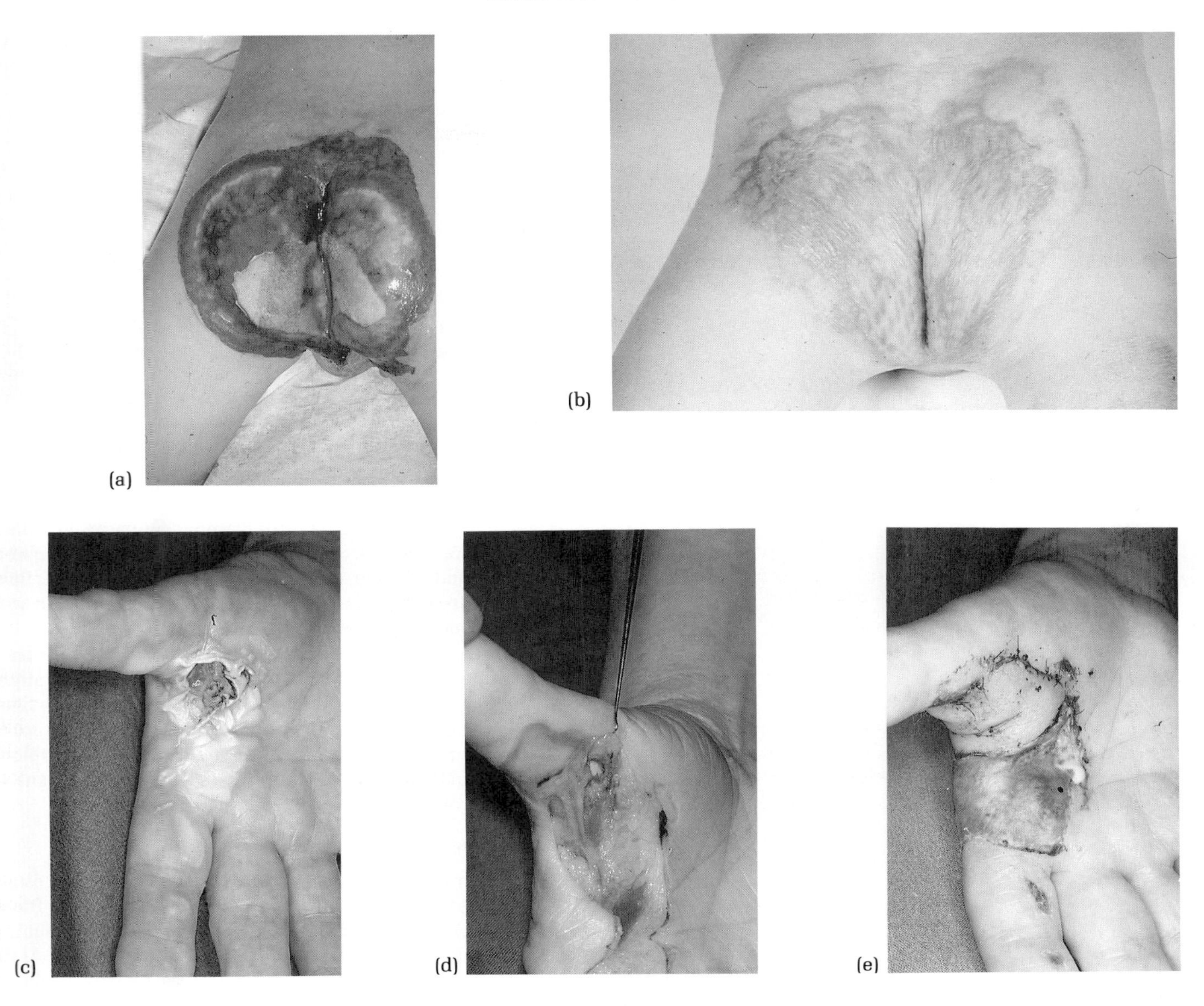

Fig. 25.5. Early excision of burns: (a) Deep burn of perineum treated by exposure for 48 h followed by excision and grafting. Mesh grafts were used to encourage take in a potentially contaminated area. Rapid healing took place; (b) Result at three months; (c) Deep electrical burn of the thumb; (d) Early excision and flap repair is essential to prevent infection. The metacarpo-phalangeal joint has been opened; (e) Local flap repair to the area of exposed joint and tendon, split skin graft to the area with a good vascular bed. The healed wound one week later. (See plate section.)

method of infection prophylaxis (Fig. 25.5). Early skin cover reduces the hypermetabolic response, helps to restore immunocompetence, and increases resistance to infection. It shortens treatment time thereby decreasing the risk of infection in an open wound, restores skin cover, and leads to better quality of scars.

If the patient is fit enough for an anaesthetic, early excision and grafting has become the recommended routine policy in most burn centres, for the treatment of deep dermal and deep burns. Burns extending up to 20 per cent of body surface can readily be treated but larger burns will need to be treated in stages because of the non-availability of donor sites and the blood loss entailed.

Treatment of infection

Diagnosis

The early diagnosis of burn wound infection is made difficult by the fact that fever and leucocytosis are components of the induced inflammatory response. Furthermore contamination of a wound and even the presence of a foul smelling dressing is not necessarily diagnostic of infection. Diagnosis depends on clinical findings initially (Fig. 25.6) and the infective organism is determined by laboratory testing.

High fever with rigors or shock suggest septicaemia, and blood cultures are essential. Dressings should be taken down to allow inspection of the wound. Surrounding cellulitis with

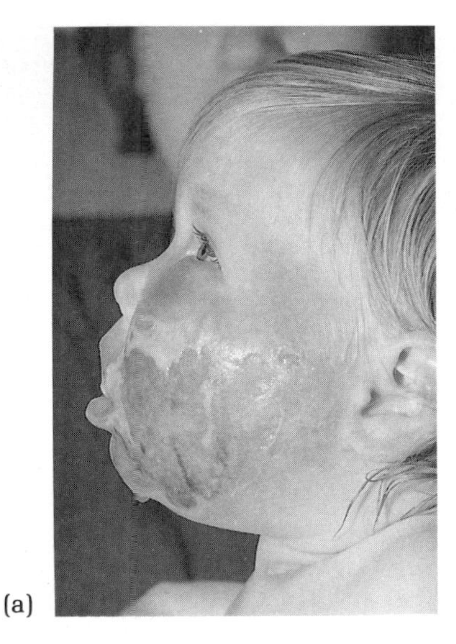

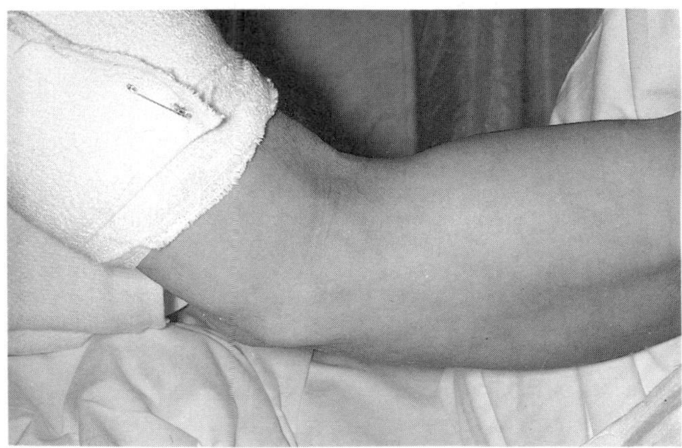

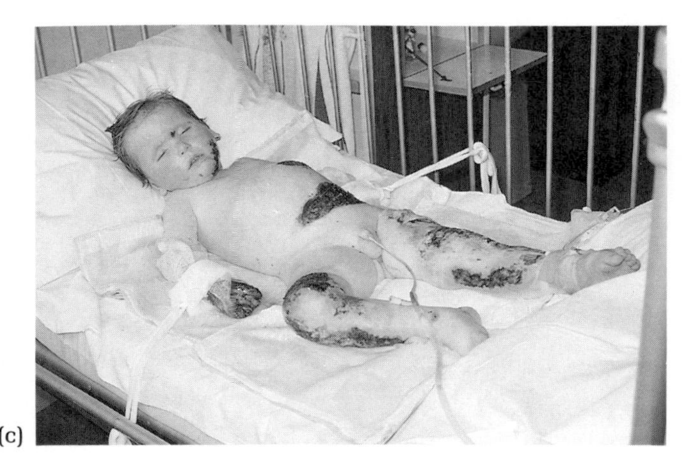

Fig. 25.6. Infected burns: (a) *Streptococcus pyogenes* infection in a 4-day-old contact burn. Note the surrounding erythema and the weeping exudate; (b) Erythema beyond the edge of this dressed burn and lymphangitis is diagnostic of infection; (c) Severe systemic infection in a child with flame burns. Blood culture grew *Pseudomonas aeruginosa*—as suggested by the green discoloration on the burn. The right hip is flexed and abducted and a joint aspirate grew *Staph. aureus*. (See plate section.)

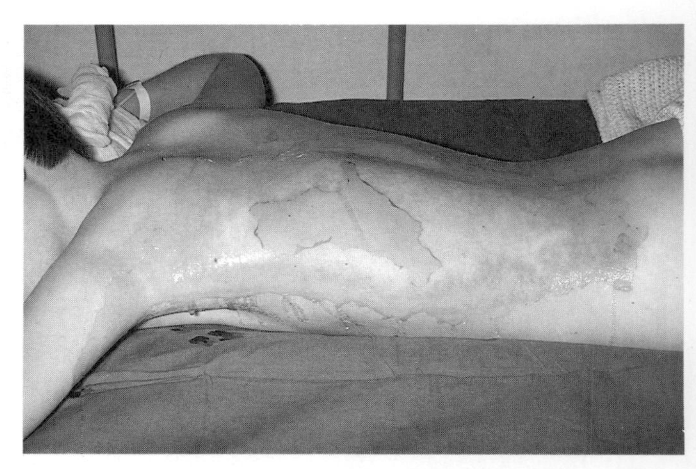

Fig. 25.7. The erythema at the edge of this flame burn signifies a superficial burn at the edge of a deeper burn, not infection. (See plate section.)

erythema or lymphangitis and lymphadenopathy are diagnostic of infection. Care is needed not to confuse the peripheral erythema and oedema which is an early sign of a superficial burn with local infection (Fig. 25.7). An increase in pain with throbbing suggests infection.

Wound swabs taken from the surface or culture of a piece of excised slough should be performed. Regular wound swabs should be taken for culture on all patients with burns at times of dressing changes and prior to surgery. However, culture of an organism is not necessarily an indication for antibiotic therapy which should only be initiated if there are signs or symptoms of infection.

Septicaemia

If septicaemia is suspected intravenous access should be established and the patient must be monitored carefully. Blood should be cultured to establish the causative organism but it is essential that intravenous antibiotic therapy is instituted. If the burn wound is infected and swab results are already available, a specific antibiotic can be commenced. Otherwise gentamicin 80 mg 8-hourly should be given initially, and subsequent doses monitored by measuring blood levels, plus co-amoxiclav 1 g 8-hourly, if the patient is not allergic to penicillin. This antibiotic regimen should be altered if necessary depending on the result of blood cultures.

Toxic shock syndrome is rarely caused by infection in burns but, if it occurs, urgent antibiotic therapy with flucloxacillin or erythromycin is indicated in addition to a fresh frozen plasma transfusion.

The infected burn wound

The object of treatment in an infected burn should be to clean the wound as soon as possible, to allow healing to proceed if the burn is superficial or to prepare a suitable bed to accept a skin graft if the burn is deep. Antibiotics, while effective in the treatment of infection in superficial burns, cellulitis and septicaemia, cannot get into avascular slough and have a supportive role only in the treatment of infected deep burns. Antibiotics should be used to treat invasive local infection causing cellulitis or lymphangitis.

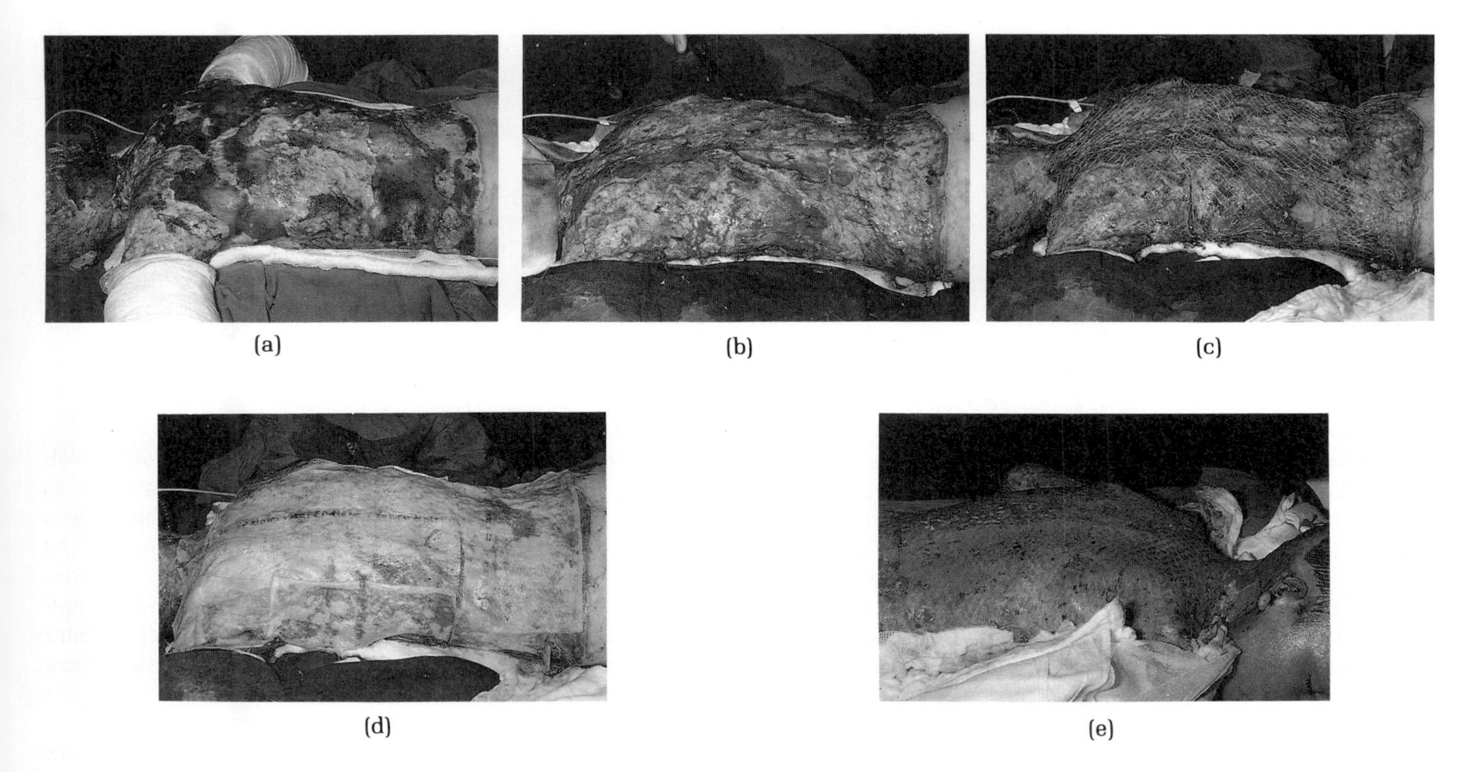

Fig. 25.8. Excision and grafting of a 60 per cent flame burn: (a) The slough on the back is still present two weeks after injury. The patient has been lying on a bed of Flamazine on a convential dressing while the burn of the front was excised and grafted; (b) There is no infection present but systemic antibiotic is essential during surgical debridement as a bacteraemia is inevitable; (c) Expanded mesh grafts are applied to the burn; (d) A layer of lyophilized pig skin is applied under the dressing to prevent dessication of the bed while the mesh heals; (e) Good take of the grafts three weeks later despite the patient having to lie on them for part of the time. (See plate section.)

Superficial burns will usually continue to heal spontaneously if the infection is controlled by topical antiseptic treatment, but infection by *Strep. pyogenes* can prove disastrous by destroying epithelial elements and may convert a superficial burn into a deep one. Treatment with oral flucloxacillin 250 mg 6-hourly or erythromycin 250 mg 6-hourly should be started immediately and continued until three consecutive clear swab results are obtained or the wound is healed. *Ps. aeruginosa* infection should also be treated by antibiotics if there is evidence of surrounding cellulitis or systemic effects. Ciprofloxacin 500 mg twice daily, orally is a suitable antibiotic.

In a deep burn, infected slough must be removed and surgical debridement is the most effective method to achieve this. It can be done gradually at the time of therapy baths or when dressings are changed by gently excising dead tissue. Chemical desloughing agents, for example Varidase or Aserbine, used as a dressing will help to soften and remove debris. The mechanical desloughing action of changing the dressing is probably more important than the precise substance used in the dressing. Topical desloughing agents used should not be painful and should only be applied to the wound, not to surrounding healed areas. Alternatively, the desloughing can be carried out at operation under general anaesthetic (Fig. 25.8).

Skin cover—graft or flap repair

Once a clean vascular bed is obtained the application of a skin graft in favourable circumstances allows healing. The usual method is to apply a split skin graft. A full thickness graft is not recommended in an infected burn because it will take less readily and could be lost. If chronic infection is still present, a mesh graft gives better results by preventing haematoma and seroma formation and allows pus to come to the surface (Fig. 25.8). If the bed has non-vascular areas, such as exposed bone, cartilage, tendon or joint, skin flap repair is essential (Fig. 25.5). Appropriate systemic antibiotic, determined by the results of swab cultures, should be used when a flap or graft is applied to a contaminated or infected wound. Grafting should not be performed in the acute phase of infection.

A positive bacterial culture is not a reason for postponing surgery, but if *Strep. pyogenes* is isolated no graft or flap procedure should be performed. The skin graft must be cut under aseptic conditions using clean surgical instruments at a site separate from the burn to try to prevent infection of the donor site. The graft can be applied directly to the wound or it can be stored at 4 °C in a sealed container wrapped in a saline soaked gauze to keep it moist and applied later as a dressing if there is excessive bleeding or oozing at the time of operation.

Implants

The development of silastic has produced a vast increase in the use of prostheses in surgical reconstruction. Other implant materials are also available in various metals, acrylic, and fabric. While in the normal course of events these implants can be accepted into the body with little or no tissue reaction, the development of infection is usually a serious risk to the implant, resulting in failure of treatment.

Factors predisposing to infection

Types of prosthesis

There are two basic types of prosthesis: the fixed volume preformed implant and the tissue expander. The preformed implant is inserted into the tissues to fill a defect of soft tissue, skeletal defect, or joint. Once in position it can be left undisturbed for many years. The greatest risk of infection is at the implantion stage and late infection is unusual. Composite implants made of more than one material such as a silastic implant covered in polyurethane foam are no more likely to become infected, but once infected are more difficult to treat.

In the last ten years tissue expanders have been developed. These prosthetic devices are inserted subcutaneously as part of a planned multistage procedure. After insertion the prosthesis is expanded by injection of fluid into the lumen of a specially toughened inflation port. Once the desired stretching of the skin has been achieved, the expander is removed and replaced by a permanent static prosthesis in the case of breast reconstruction, or removed completely and the excess skin advanced as a flap to cover a defect. The risk of infection is greater in expansion techniques as a result of the multistage procedure with increased opportunity for entry of infection.

Foreign body

The presence of a foreign body (the implant) in the wound predisposes to and exacerbates infection. If there is any contamination at the time of implantation, especially with haematoma formation, infection is likely to occur. All suture material used should be absorbable so as not to increase the amount of foreign body in the wound.

Wound closure

Any breach of the skin wound or overlying skin is a ready portal of entry for infection. If the insertion of an implant stretches the overlying skin unduly, pressure necrosis can occur with exposure of the implant. An exposed implant is certain to become infected. Later movement of an implant eroding skin or mucous membrane gives rise to contamination. Solid implants should have no sharp edges which could encourage erosion of the surrounding tissue.

Site

An implant in most parts of the body, placed subcutaneously with good skin cover, is generally unlikely to become infected. However, if the implant is placed to support the nasal bridge line and is inserted via a nasal mucosal incision the incidence of infection and loss of the implant is greatly increased.

Implants in the breast are potentially exposed to infection if the implant is placed subcutaneously, particularly after a subcutaneous mastectomy as the breast duct system is connected to the surface. Wound swabs taken from breast tissue grow a variety of organisms, the commonest being *Staph. epidermidis* or coagulase negative staphylococci. This may contribute to the development of capsular contracture but is rarely the cause of frank infection around a breast implant. Placing the prosthesis in a pocket beneath the muscle separates the implant from the breast tissue and reduces the incidence of capsular contracture.

Radiotherapy to the area of an implant, for example after the treatment of breast cancer, gives rise to greater fibrosis and poor blood supply so that wound healing is impaired and the skin cover is less elastic resulting in a greater risk of exposure and infection.

Prevention of infection

Technique

Precise surgical dissection, keeping to tissue planes and developing an accurate pocket with good quality skin cover is essential. Haemostasis must be meticulous and, if bleeding is encountered, closed suction drainage should be employed. The implant must be handled with care and inserted without contamination from the skin edge of the wound as far as possible. A swab moistened in povidone–iodine, placed at the edge of the wound, is useful to lubricate the implant so that it can be inserted more easily.

Healing of the insertion wound by primary intention is the aim and care should be taken not to traumatize the wound edge by rough handling. Fine sutures should be used and all buried sutures should be absorbable to minimize the risk of additional foreign body formation and infection. If skin cover is very tight the use of a skin flap or muscle flap to cover the implant should be considered. Subsequent wound dehiscence must be treated as a matter of urgency with resuture of the wound and antibiotic therapy if the implant is to be saved.

Prophylactic antibiotics

In general, the rate of infection in implants is low and many plastic surgeons do not use prophylactic antibiotics routinely (4). The need for antibiotic prophylaxis depends chiefly on the type of implant and the site of use. An injection of flucloxacillin or cefuroxime given as one dose intra-operatively and two subsequent doses is sufficient, if prophylaxis is required, in uncomplicated cases. Irrigation of the wound cavity with povidone–iodine has been shown to decrease capsule formation around breast implants but whether it prevents infection has not been proven (5).

Tissue expansion

Special considerations apply to the prevention of infection when tissue expanders are being used. The entry wound should, ideally, be in a site remote from the expander so that it is separated from the stresses of expansion which could stretch and burst the wound allowing the entry of bacteria. An incision aligned radially to the expansion forces is less likely to be disrupted. The expansion valve should be in a separate site under a good layer of subcutaneous tissue. Prophylactic antibiotics are advisable for twenty-four hours and suction drains should be used if there is likely to be seroma or haematoma formation. At each expansion treatment the injection of sterile saline should be performed under strict aseptic precautions.

It is essential that a tissue expander is not inserted in the presence of infection or with a pre-existing open wound in the vicinity of the operation site. To do so would court the risk of infection.

When the expander is removed at the final stage of breast reconstruction and is to be replaced by a permanent prosthesis, the same prophylactic measures of meticulous technique, prevention of haematoma formation and antibiotic cover should be instituted. In the original report by Radovan (6) of breast reconstruction by tissue expansion, 7 per cent of patients developed infection, all at the second stage of replacement of the expander by the permanent implant.

Treatment of the infected prosthesis

In the early stages after insertion of a prosthesis or expander it is difficult to determine whether infection is present. Pain, swelling, and the oedema and bruising from surgery may suggest the possibility of infection. If there is any doubt, systemic antibiotic treatment should be given in the hope that infection can be forestalled.

Unless the implant is solid, fine needle aspiration of the cavity around the implant to get a specimen for bacteriological examination is unwise as the implant can easily be damaged. It may be possible to obtain a culture from the insertion wound if there is a discharge and this may aid in the selection of a suitable antibiotic. Treatment in the early stages of infection should be by systemic antibiotic which may save the implant. If the entry wound alone is infected it may be possible to prevent infection spreading to the implant cavity by judicious removal of a few sutures to allow pus to escape and by starting systemic antibiotic therapy.

Once frank infection has developed the wound should be reopened to clean the cavity under systemic antibiotic cover. If the infection is low-grade the implant can be reinserted, or a new one inserted, in the hope that infection will subside. This must only be done if there is adequate soft tissue cover. The chances of an implant being saved by this manoeuvre are low.

A much more satisfactory solution is to remove the implant, curette the cavity and then allow the infection to subside for several months. When the infected implant is composite, covered by polyurethane foam, a total capsulectomy is needed to remove all the foam in addition to removal of the implant. Once all sign of infection has been eliminated for at last three months after the cessation of antibiotics a repeat operation can be planned and the implant reinserted.

An infected tissue expander being used as a preliminary to permanent implant insertion must be removed to allow the infection to settle before trying again later. If the expander is being used to provide a flap for skin cover, it may be possible to perform rapid injection over a few days, under antibiotic cover, if the final expansion is almost obtained. The implant can then be removed and the flap inserted into its final position.

In some instances, if the injection port site becomes infected without the whole expander being involved, it may be possible to exteriorize the valve and continue expansion. The exteriorized port is a recognized technique which is sometimes used in children to save them the pain of repeated injections, and expansion can still proceed satisfactorily without the risk of infection if the expander is being used for flap advancement.

References

1. Courtiss, E. H., Goldwyn, R. M., and Anastasi, G. W. (1979). The fate of breast implants with infection around them. *Plast. Reconstr. Surg.*, **63**, 812–6.
2. Timmons, M. J. (1983). Are systemic prophylactic antibiotics necessary in burns? *Ann. R. Coll. Surg. Engl.*, **65**, 80–2.
3. Gillet, P. (1985). Antibiotic prophylaxis and therapy in burns. *J. Hosp. Infect.*, **6**, Supplement B, 59–66.
4. Krizek, T. J., Gottlieb, L. J., Koss, N., and Robson, M. C. (1985). The use of prophylactic antibacterials in plastic surgery: A 1980's update. *Plast. Reconstr. Surg.*, **76**, 953–63.
5. Burkhardt, B. R., Dempsey, P. D., Schnur, P. L., and Tofield, J. J. (1986). Capsular contracture: a prospective study of the effect of local antibacterial agents. *Plast. Reconstr. Surg.*, **77**, 919–30.
6. Radovan, C. (1982). Breast reconstruction after mastectomy using the temporary expander. *Plast. Reconstr. Surg.*, **69**, 195–206.

Further reading

Morris, A. McG., Stevenson, J. H., and Watson, A. C. H. (1989). *Complications of plastic surgery*. Baillière Tindall, London.

Muir, I. F. K., Barclay, T. L., and Settle, J. A. D. (1987). *Burns and their treatment* (3rd edn). Butterworths, London.

26

Neurosurgery

HARRY R. INGHAM and PENELOPE R. SISSON

Introduction

The types of micro-organisms which are implicated in many commonly encountered infections are determined by the underlying disease process. This general maxim is well exemplified in infections seen in neurosurgical practice, although this has only latterly been recognized. In this chapter the pathogenesis of different neurosurgical infections will be considered in some detail to allow an understanding of the importance of the various organisms involved and the chemotherapeutic management employed.

Brain abscess

Pathogenesis and microbiology

The microbiology of parenchymal brain abscess is closely related to the source or type of the infection, which may be categorized as follows: post-surgical and post-traumatic, sinugenic, otogenic, odontogenic, metastatic, due to congenital cyanotic heart disease, or cryptogenic (1).

Post-surgical and post-traumatic

Brain abscess arising as a consequence of post-operative infections is most often due to *Staphylococcus aureus* although, if an infected cavity such as an air sinus has been opened inadvertently during the procedure, a mixture of organisms may be encountered. Less common organisms include *Propionibacterium acnes* and Gram-negative bacteria, such as the enterobacteriaceae.

Staph. aureus is the commonest organism to be encountered in post-traumatic abscesses, but other species of bacteria may be found, depending on the nature of the lesion, e.g. *Streptococcus pneumoniae* where there is a fracture of the base of the skull.

Sinugenic

The commonest organism isolated from sinugenic abscesses, which are usually found in the frontal lobe of the brain, is *Strep. milleri* Lancefield group F, an organism commonly found in the mouth. However other organisms including anaerobic bacteria may be present, especially if there is a pansinusitis, or if there is involvement of the maxillary sinus with its possible communications with the oral cavity via the roots of the upper teeth.

Otogenic

Otogenic brain abscess is almost exclusively a complication of chronic suppurative otitis media associated with a cholesteatoma (see Chapter 27). The cholesteatoma usually arises as a consequence of chronic serous otitis media in which the Eustachian tube is blocked, and there is invagination of the pars flaccida of the tympanic membrane. Accumulation of squamous epithelial cells and aural secretions within the sac thus formed constitutes the cholesteatoma, which acquires a bacterial flora which is faecal in nature. Otogenic abscesses are found either in the temporal lobe or in the cerebellum.

Odontogenic

Odontogenic abscesses may occur as a consequence of acute dental infection (2); however, they have also been reported in the presence of asymptomatic dental infection (3). The abscess appears in the frontal lobe of the brain; the source is indicated by the absence of sinus infection and the isolation of a mixture of facultative and obligate anaerobic organisms typical of the flora of the gingival crevice.

Congenital cyanotic heart disease

Brain abscess is a well recognized complication of congenital cyanotic heart disease (CCHD) and may even occur after surgical intervention in this condition. Cerebral hypoxia is prone to occur because of the impaired oxygenation and the compensatory polycythaemia, which causes thickening of the blood. Areas of the brain thus affected provide an appropriate milieu for the growth of micro-organisms which then gain access to the systemic circulation via the right to left shunt in this condition. A range of micro-organisms may be involved including *Staph. aureus*, *Strep. milleri*, and anaerobic bacteria of various types. For the same reasons brain abscess may also complicate pulmonary arterio-venous fistulae.

Metastatic

Brain abscesses secondary to the spread of infection from distal foci in the body, like those associated with CCHD, tend to occur in the distribution of the middle cerebral artery and are often multiple. The organisms involved clearly reflect those of the primary foci. Before the general use of antimicrobial agents the lung was a common primary focus, with *Staph. aureus* being the most frequent isolate. Latterly its occurrence has been reduced although not eliminated. A wide range of organisms, including enterobacteriaceae, anaerobes, and unusual bacteria such as *Listeria monocytogenes*, may be encountered.

Cryptogenic

This diagnosis indicates a failure to identify the primary focus of infection. A detailed study of the bacteriology of such abscesses, which may be very complex, can in many instances indicate the likely origin and this should always be pursued.

Brain abscess in children

Chronic middle ear disease features less frequently in the aetiology of brain abscess in children than adults. In some series CCHD has been a common predisposing factor.

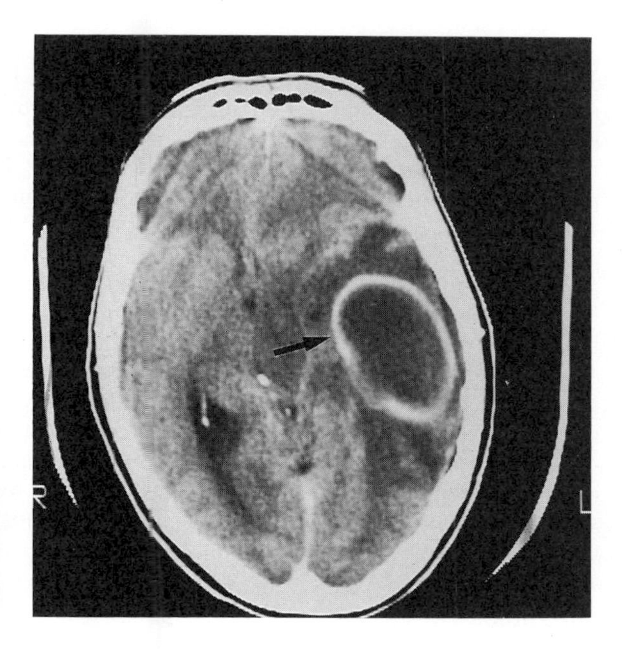

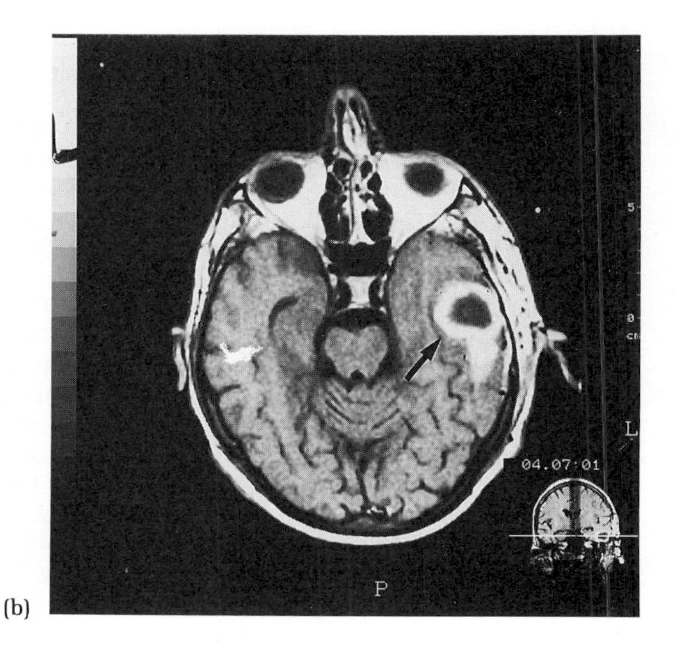

Fig. 26.1. Contrast-enhanced CT showing: (a) A left temporal lobe abscess (arrowed); (b) Axial gadolinium enhanced T1 weighted MRI scans showing a temporal lobe abscess (arrowed).

Meningitis, especially due to Gram-negative bacilli, may be the cause in this age group and an important example is *Citrobacter diversus*. In some instances such infections have occurred in clusters (4).

Diagnosis

Lumbar puncture is contraindicated in the investigation of suspected brain abscess because of the danger of brain stem herniation through the foramen magnum. Cerebro-spinal fluid (CSF) findings are varied and generally unhelpful.

Early diagnosis is essential and should be considered *in any patient presenting with headache and nausea or vomiting who is obtunded*. The absence of papilloedema and focal signs does not exclude the diagnosis. The diagnosis can be made by means of computerized tomography (CT) or magnetic resonance imaging (MRI) although in some instances the signs may be minimal and require the procedure to be repeated within 24 or 48 h (Fig. 26.1).

Management

Surgery

There have been a number of reports of the successful management of brain abscess, diagnosed at an early stage, with antimicrobial chemotherapy alone. In the majority of instances this will not suffice and early surgical intervention is indicated. It is generally accepted that total excision of the abscess is the surgical treatment of choice for cerebellar abscesses but few would now advocate this for other types of brain abscess. The procedure most frequently used today is burr-hole aspiration, which provides the option of further aspiration or excision if that ultimately becomes necessary.

Chemotherapy

Whichever surgical procedure is used it is essential that an adequate sample of pus be sent for bacteriological examination; until these results are available broad spectrum chemotherapy must be given. A suitable combination in an adult consists of ampicillin 1–2 g 6-hourly, metronidazole 500 mg 8-hourly and either gentamicin 80 mg 8-hourly or chloramphenicol 500 mg to 1 g 6-hourly. The same regimen applies to children with an appropriate reduction in dosage.

When results of culture become available the antibiotic regimen can, if necessary, be modified — for example, if *Staph. aureus* is present recourse would be made to flucloxacillin — 2 g 6-hourly possibly with the addition of either clindamycin 300 mg 6-hourly or fusidic acid 500 mg 8-hourly. In the authors' centre the accepted regimen is ampicillin, metronidazole, and gentamicin, usually given for a period of four to six weeks, with gentamicin levels being appropriately monitored. Steroids are often prescribed in the management of brain abscess but their value is uncertain. With the better knowledge that exists today of the bacteriology of brain abscess and the range of antimicrobial agents available, the once-common practice of instilling agents directly into the abscess cavity would seem to be redundant.

Outcome

Before the introduction of antimicrobials nearly all patients with brain abscess died and even the use of penicillin was associated with mortality rates of 30 to 40 per cent. With modern diagnostic and therapeutic techniques the mortality in brain abscess has been reduced to 10 per cent or less (5). A proportion of individuals who have recovered from brain abscess will have mild to moderate focal dysfunction whilst others will experience neurological deficits which are functionally incapacitating. Up to 70 per cent of patients who have had brain abscess will develop epilepsy.

Subdural and extradural infections

Pathogenesis and microbiology

The subdural space is a potential cavity between the arachnoid mater and dura mater. The latter adheres more firmly at the base of the skull than at the vault and, as a result, pus within the subdural space is usually located over the superior aspects of the cerebral hemispheres, sometimes involving the parafalcine space and the Sylvian fissures. Subdural empyema is less common than brain abscess but may account for up to 20 per cent of cases of intracranial suppuration (6). Although infections of the middle ear were once important causes of subdural empyema, most cases today are secondary to infections of the paranasal air sinuses. Less common causes are penetrating or compound wounds of the skull, operative infections, infected subdural haematomas, cranial osteomyelitis, meningitis, blood-borne spread, and extension of odontogenic or facial infections; rarely no source is apparent. The frontal air sinus is the commonest source and there may be concomitant cellulitis of the scalp (Pott's puffy tumour), epicranial abscess and extradural abscess. Small cortical or subcortical abscesses may coexist.

Although *Staph. aureus* may be implicated in subdural empyema unquestionably the commonest organism is *Strep. milleri*. The strains implicated commonly carry the group F antigen (7). Other important organisms implicated in subdural empyema include anaerobic bacteria (8, 9). This is a particularly common finding where there is pansinusitis or where otogenic or odontogenic sources are present. Subdural empyema secondary to surgery or trauma is usually due to *Staph. aureus*, less commonly Gram-negative organisms. Meningitis is a rare cause, the organisms involved being those associated with the common primary types of meningitis; *Strep. pneumoniae*, *Neisseria meningitidis*, and *Haemophilus influenzae*. Intracranial extradural abscess is usually a consequence of frontal sinusitis, craniotomy, or mastoiditis. Information on bacteriology is scanty but the mode of origin would suggest that the organisms most frequently cultured would be similar to those in subdural abscess, arising from otogenic or traumatic origins.

Diagnosis

Where the source of infection is the paranasal air sinuses there may be local pain, swelling, and erythema with or without

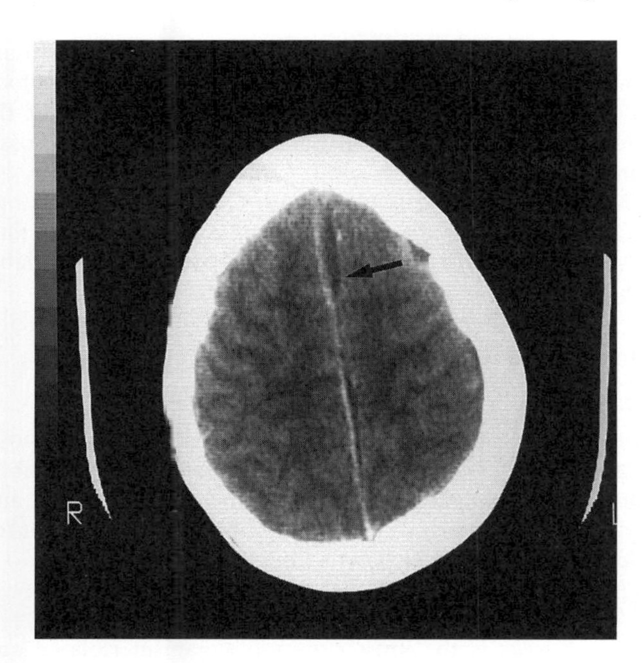

Fig. 26.2. Contrast-enhanced CT showing characteristic enhancement of a subdural empyema (arrowed).

periorbital oedema. The patient is usually febrile and there is a polymorphonuclear leucocytosis. Blood cultures may be positive. Intracranial pressure is frequently raised and epileptiform convulsions are common, with weakness or paralysis of the contralateral side. Meningeal irritation is frequently present but lumbar puncture is contraindicated because of the danger of brain-stem herniation. CSF findings may be normal or show a pleocytosis with a raised protein level.

Prompt diagnosis is essential to a favourable outcome. Either CT or MRI are the definitive investigations in this condition (Fig. 26.2).

Management

Surgery

Subdural empyema requires surgical drainage, both of the lesion itself and the underlying focus of infection. Opinion varies as to the relative merits of burr-hole drainage as opposed to craniotomy but whichever method is employed it is essential to ensure wide drainage. Where there are parafalcine collections it is probable that optimal drainage will be achieved by a small craniotomy.

Chemotherapy

The chemotherapeutic agents of choice in subdural empyema are penicillin G 1.2 g 4- to 6-hourly, supplemented with metronidazole and gentamicin, or chloramphenicol in full dosage, unless *Staph. aureus* is present, when flucloxacillin would be indicated. Steroids are thought to be of value where there is raised intracranial pressure. Progress should be monitored by regular scanning to detect reaccumulation of pus and care must be taken to exclude an associated parenchymal brain abscess.

Outcome

Before the availability of antibiotics the mortality in this condition was 100 per cent. With the introduction of penicillin the mortality rate fell dramatically but even with the newer antimicrobial agents available today 10 to 30 per cent of patients still die.

Spinal epidural abscess

Pathogenesis and microbiology

The epidural space, which lies between the spinal dura mater and the periosteum and ligaments lining the vertebral canal contains loose fat, areolar tissue, and a plexus of veins. The dorsal compartment is more commonly infected perhaps because of the greater abundance of dural fat; moreover, the ventral portion is more adherent to spinal ligaments and this tends to prevent extension of purulent material. Infections are infrequent in the cervical region possibly because the extradural space is only a potential space in the neck.

The effect of epidural abscesses on the spinal cord cannot always be explained in terms of pressure and it is thought that, in some instances, involvement of the vasculature of the cord results in ischaemia.

An epidural abscess may arise from direct extension from infected vertebral bodies, which themselves have become infected either by spread from a distal source via the bloodstream or by local spread. In the latter situation venous communications with Batson's plexus of veins may permit spread from abdominal and pelvic foci (10).

Common primary sources of infection which may be implicated are superficial skin infections, pelvic, abdominal, dental, and urinary tract infections, pharyngitis, and pneumonia. Epidural abscess may complicate lumbar puncture, infiltration of local anaesthetic, or the use of epidural catheters, and congenital dermal sinuses may also be involved. Predisposing factors include narcotic abuse, diabetes, decubitus, trauma, and surgery. Infections may be acute or chronic and the abscess may be mainly purulent or granulation tissue may predominate. The commonest organism isolated is *Staph. aureus*; others include *Strep. pyogenes*, other streptococci, including anaerobes, *Escherichia coli*, *Pseudomonas* spp., and mixtures of anaerobic and facultative anaerobic bacteria. Unusual organisms have been reported including *Salmonella* spp., *Aspergillus* spp., *Mycobacterium tuberculosis*, *Brucella* spp., *Nocardia* spp., and *Actinomyces* spp. Rarely, spinal abscess may be subdural in location.

Diagnosis

Spinal epidural abscess presents in the early stages with pain which may be associated with local tenderness to percussion. There is usually evidence of systemic infection. The condition may also present with meningitis. If there is a delay in diagnosis and treatment a neurological deficit may develop. The CSF white cell count may be moderately elevated with a mixed morphological picture, a raised protein but a normal glucose level unless there is associated meningitis. In the latter instance

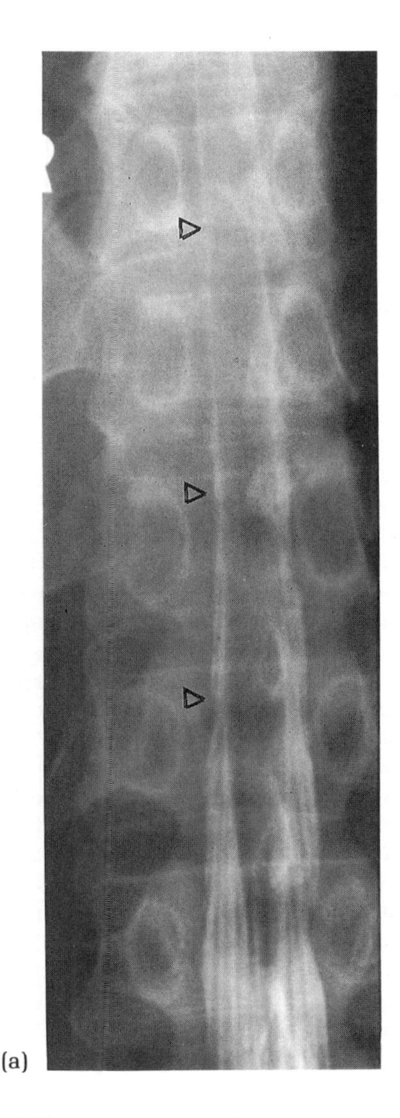

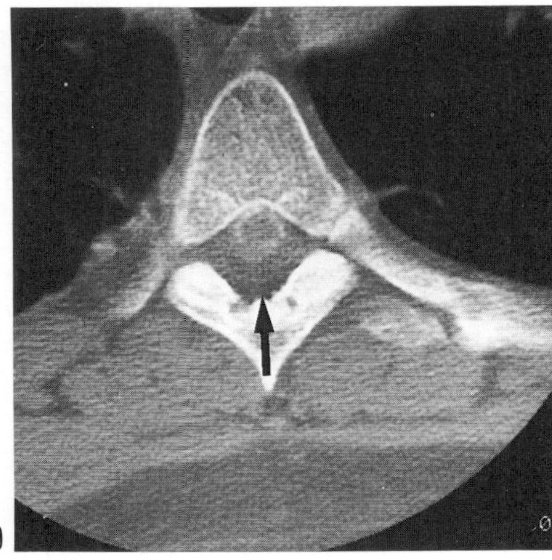

Fig. 26.3. (a) Myelogram showing an extensive spinal epidural abscess. Contrast is displaced away from the pedicles (arrows); (b) Spinal CT myelogram in the same patient showing a posterior situated epidural abscess (arrowed).

organisms may be present. With total spinal block Froin's syndrome occurs—yellow CSF with a high protein. Blood culture is often positive. In the more chronic form of the disease temperature and white cell count may not be grossly abnormal.

Myelography in conjunction with CT is the most accurate procedure for the diagnosis of epidural abscess but may be superceded when MRI becomes more readily available (Fig. 26.3).

Management

Surgery

The most important principle of management is early diagnosis as neurological sequelae, when they occur, may be irreversible. Surgical treatment consists of spinal cord decompression, and at operation a specimen of pus should be obtained and sent for microbiological examination and culture.

Chemotherapy

Staph. aureus is the most common organism isolated and initial chemotherapy should include flucloxacillin 2 g 6-hourly. Because of the relative frequency of streptococcal and Gram-negative bacillary infections, and the possible presence of anaerobic organisms ampicillin, gentamicin and metronidazole should also be given in standard dosage (see above). Chemotherapy can be adjusted when the results of bacterial culture are available. The role of steroids is unclear.

Outcome

Prognosis for neurological recovery will depend on the duration and severity of cord compression; the outlook being better with early decompression and in younger patients. In one large series (11) partial or complete recovery was observed in 65 per cent of individuals.

Infective venous sinus thrombosis

Pathogenesis and microbiology

Infections of the venous dural sinuses are now relatively rare compared with the pre-antimicrobial era, presumably in part reflecting the early use of antimicrobial chemotherapy for infections of the head and neck. The venous sinuses, which include the cavernous sinus, lateral or sigmoid sinus, and inferior and superior sagittal sinuses, are an intercommunicating network of valveless venous channels which accept blood from the brain, face, orbit, the para-nasal air sinuses, the ear, and the oro-pharynx (Fig. 26.4).

Cavernous sinus thrombosis

As shown in Fig. 26.4 the cavernous sinus has both afferent tributaries and efferent vessels. Spread of infection via the afferent vessels, is said to be associated with more rapid onset of disease. For example, this may occur from the face via the angular and facial veins through the anastomoses with the ophthalmic vein, otherwise known as the 'anterior route'. By

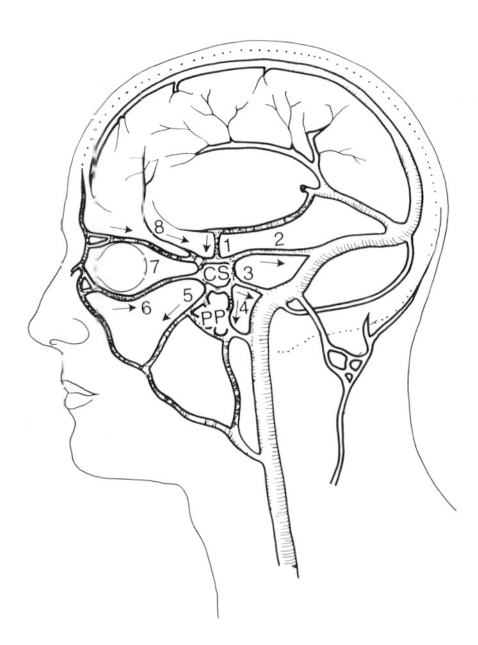

Fig. 26.4. Venous connections of the cavernous sinus. CS indicates cavernous sinus; PP, pterygoid plexus; 1, inferior cerebral vein; 2, superior petrosal sinus; 3, inferior petrosal sinus; 4 and 5, emissary veins to pterygoid plexus; 6, inferior ophthalmic vein; 7, superior ophthalmic vein; 8, sphenopariental sinus. Arrows indicate direction of venous flow. (Modified from Carpenter MB (1978) *Core text of neuroanatomy* (2nd edn) p 245. William & Wilkins, Baltimore.)

contrast, extension of infection through efferent vessels from the posterior mouth, pharynx, middle and inner ear via the inferior and superior petrosal sinuses, the pterygoid venous plexus, and the peri-carotid venous plexus, because it occurs against the normal direction of flow of the blood, is a slower, more insidious process.

Before the availability of antibiotics organisms most commonly implicated were *Staph. aureus* and *Strep. pyogenes* arising from infections involving the face, nose, and sinuses. These organisms are much less common today (12); of greater importance are mixed infections due to facultative and obligate anaerobic organisms in odontogenic infections. Other primary sources in this condition are the paranasal and sphenoid air sinuses, facial trauma, or surgery and tonsillar infections.

Cavernous sinus thrombosis may present as unilateral, retro-ocular pain later progressing to more clearcut signs such as proptosis and chemosis. In contrast to the more common condition of orbital cellulitis, there is more toxicity, eventual involvement of the other eye with pupillary abnormalities, visual loss and trigeminal nerve involvement due to the passage of involved nerves through the sinus. The once classical cause of cavernous sinus thrombosis, a staphylococcal infection of the nose or the adjacent area inferior to the eye, the so-called danger triangle, provided an overt pointer to the possible diagnosis. In the more indolent cases, where the primary focus is in the mouth or the deep structures of the neck, toxicity may be less obvious and signs are restricted to mild chemosis and proptosis in the early stages.

The polymorphonuclear leucocyte count is elevated and the CSF cellular and biochemical features suggest bacterial infection in about one-third of patients, blood cultures may be positive.

Infective lateral sinus thrombosis

This condition occurred most frequently in children with acute mastoiditis, less commonly secondary to meningitis or dental sepsis. Currently this clinical rarity is almost always secondary to chronic suppurative otitis media and may lead to widespread intracranial infection with involvement of the other venous sinuses and the internal jugular vein. Clinical features include fever, signs of raised intracranial pressure, sometimes unilateral VIth nerve palsy, with irritation of the Vth nerve. There is often mastoid tenderness and there may be discomfort in the neck due to spasm of the sternomastoid muscle. Pulmonary infiltrates due to emboli via the internal jugular vein may occur. Blood cultures may be positive. CSF findings are usually unremarkable. The principal organisms isolated in recent studies were *Proteus* spp., *Staph. aureus*, *E. coli*, and anaerobic bacteria reflecting the bacteriology of the original middle-ear disease.

Infective thrombosis of the sagittal and straight sinuses

Before the general availability of antimicrobials infective thrombosis of these sinuses complicated meningitis, which still accounts for half the cases currently encountered, infection probably reaching the sagittal sinuses via diploic veins. Other primary sources include the ethmoid, maxillary, and frontal air sinuses, lung infections, tonsillitis, dental and pelvic infection, and trauma. Infected thrombosis of the inferior sagittal and straight sinuses is very rare and is usually secondary to meningitis.

When meningitis is the primary cause, appropriate CSF changes are seen; with other primary sources the findings are less impressive. The organism most commonly implicated in infective thrombosis of the superior sagittal sinus is *Strep. pneumoniae*; less commonly reported organisms include *H. influenzae*, *Staph. aureus*, β-haemolytic streptococci, *Klebsiella* spp., *Pseudomonas* spp., and anaerobic streptococci. The most striking clinical features in this condition are severe headache, papilloedema, nausea, vomiting, and confusion. Convulsions and hemiplegia, or quadriplegia, are common and patients are usually febrile.

Diagnosis

Specific diagnosis is greatly facilitated by MRI but where this is not available CT is the radiographic investigation of first choice (Fig. 26.5).

Management

Surgical

Successful management of patients with sinus thrombosis requires early diagnosis, antimicrobial chemotherapy, extirpation of primary foci, and, where appropriate, surgical intervention. With lateral sinus thrombosis surgical decompression of the sinus is indicated together with mastoidectomy. Ligation

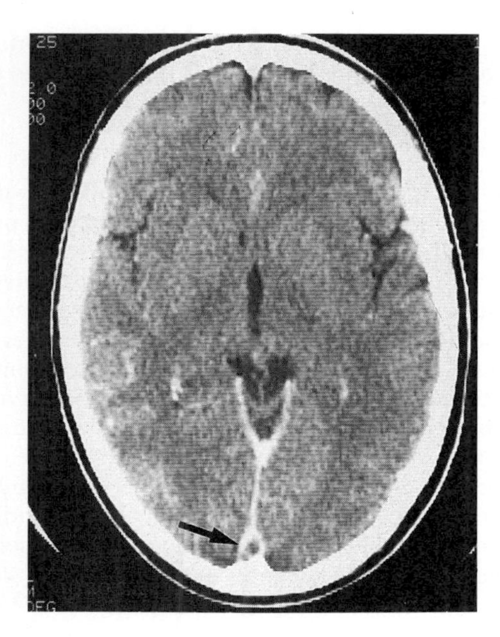

Fig. 26.5. Superior saggital sinus thrombosis. Contrast enhanced axial CT Scans showing the posterior end of the enhancing superior sagittal sinus with a filling defect in it due to thrombus (empty triangle sign arrowed).

of the internal jugular vein may rarely be used in patients not responding to initial surgery and chemotherapy in an attempt, probably belated, to prevent extension of the thrombus and metastatic infection.

It is generally accepted that surgical intervention, other than of the primary focus, has no role to play in infected thrombosis of the sagittal or cavernous sinuses.

Chemotherapy

Antimicrobial chemotherapy should be directed against the most likely organisms and should include ampicillin, metronidazole and either chloramphenicol or gentamicin in full dosage (see above). In those rare instances where staphylococcal infection is suspected, flucloxacillin, possibly with the addition of clindamycin or fusidic acid in standard dosage, should be employed.

The role of anticoagulants is uncertain, particularly as there is a danger of precipitating cerebral haemorrhage. Similar uncertainty surrounds the use of fibrinolytic agents. Corticosteroids may be of value if there is diffuse brain swelling due to the infection.

Outcome

Before the introduction of antibiotics the mortality of infective thrombosis varied from 30 to 100 per cent according to the type of sinus involved (13). More recent reviews (12) have reported lower but still significant mortalities.

Post-operative infections

Prevention

As post-operative infections of the central nervous system can be catastrophic every effort must be made to prevent them. Such measures will vary according to the procedures involved, which can be divided broadly into elective neurosurgery and insertion of foreign bodies.

The evidence for the adoption of prophylactic antibiotics in elective neurosurgery is still equivocal because only large scale, randomized clinical trials can provide the necessary data when the background infection rate may be as low as 1 per cent (19). However, many neurosurgeons prefer to cover such operations with antimicrobials. Some have employed a single intra-operative dose of vancomycin Ig IV and gentamicin or tobramycin 80 mg IV with streptomycin irrigating solution 50 mg/L (20). A one-day course of penicillin G 0.6 g 6-hourly has been shown to be a simple, effective regimen (21).

The prevention of shunt infections relies heavily on meticulous surgical technique and long-term follow-up. Careful attention to skin cleansing, irrigating the wound, valve, and catheter with antimicrobial agents such as gentamicin or vancomycin prior to insertion, and minimizing the handling of the shunt, are the most effective preventative measures.

Pathogenesis and microbiology

The bacteriology of post-operative infections in neurosurgery, as elsewhere, reflects that of the immediate environment, i.e. the patient's own flora and any airborne contamination of the operating theatre.

Three to four per cent of clean or clean-contaminated elective neurosurgical operations may become infected (14, 15). These infections are generally accepted to be theatre-acquired in most instances. The commonest micro-organism involved is *Staph. aureus* but a variety of others including *Proteus* species, *Klebsiella* species, and other Gram-negative facultative bacilli have been less commonly incriminated, along with typical skin flora such as *P. acnes* and *Staph. epidermidis*.

The implantation of foreign bodies such as cranioplasty plates and cerebrospinal fluid shunts is associated with high infection rates in some centres. Jennet and Miller (16) reported that 17 per cent of patients undergoing insertion of cranioplasty plates became infected, whereas infection rates for shunt procedures vary from 1 to 27 per cent (17, 18) with *Staph. epidermidis* accounting for 90 per cent of infections. Other organisms associated with these infections include diphtheroids, Gram-negative bacilli, *Staph. aureus*, and *Candida albicans*. The evidence suggests that CSF shunts become contaminated at insertion although overt infection may not be evident for several weeks or months. More rarely, organisms may enter the lower end of a shunt consequent upon bacteraemia.

Management

The management of patients with post-operative neurosurgical infections is dictated largely by the bacteria involved. As *Staph. aureus* is the most likely pathogen to cause infection following clean neurosurgery, initial antimicrobial chemotherapy must include flucloxacillin until definitive bacteriology is available. It may be prudent to include a broad-spectrum

Table 26.1. Dose of intrathecal antibiotics.

Author(s)	Antibiotic	Dose(s) in mg daily		
		Adult	Child	Infant (< 2 yr)
Garrod *et al.* (23)	Gentamicin	5	2.5	1
Donauer *et al.* (24)	Netilmicin	2–3 tds		0.4–0.5 bd
Bayston (personal communication)	Amikacin	20*	2–3	
Swayne *et al.* (25) / Bayston (26)	Vancomycin		20	10

* Block *et al.* (27) (one patient only).
From Ingham *et al.* (28).

regimen of ampicillin, metronidazole, and gentamicin until culture results are available.

Infections following the insertion of foreign bodies can be difficult to treat effectively whilst the foreign body remains *in situ*. Thus removal of the cranioplasty plate or CSF shunt is often required along with a course of systemic antimicrobial agents directed at the pathogens involved. Additional, intraventricular administration of antibiotics is favoured for some CSF shunt infections, particularly those caused by strains of *Staph. epidermidis* relatively resistant to antibiotics (Table 26.1). In such situations the additional systemic administration of rifampicin 300 mg 12-hourly may be beneficial.

Shunt infections due to *Candida* demand the immediate removal of the shunt and chemotherapy with amphotericin B and flucytosine under guidance from the microbiologists.

Post-traumatic infections

Prevention

The prevention of these infections rests largely upon definitive neurosurgery performed before infection can develop. In grossly contaminated wounds a broad-spectrum regimen of antimicrobials should be commenced on admission, e.g. ampicillin, metronidazole, and gentamicin, until definitive bacteriology is available. Less serious trauma carries a lower risk of infection but the consequence of it for an individual is severe. Adult patients with a CSF leak are usually commenced on prophylactic antibiotics such as penicillin 0.6 g 6-hourly IV, or phenoxymethyl penicillin orally 500 mg 6-hourly, and sulphadimidine 0.5–1 g 6-hourly IV, or by mouth whilst awaiting operative repair. Ampicillin and sulphonamide have been used successfully in compound depressed fractures of the skull (22).

Pathogenesis

Traumatic wounds of the skull may be grossly contaminated with debris such as soil or tarmac, or may become colonized with organisms constituting normal skin flora. Compound depressed fracture of the skull with disruption of the dura is associated with a ten per cent infection rate (22). The bacteria involved in such infections include *Staph. aureus*, *E. coli*, *Strep. pneumoniae*, and a wide variety of organisms usually associated with the environment depending on the circumstances of the injury. Patients with frontal-basal fractures and hence communication with the nasal sinuses or the oropharynx are particularly at risk of meningitis and brain abscess.

Management

The management of post-traumatic infections hinges on complete debridement of the wound, repair of torn dura and bony deficits where possible and the use of antimicrobial agents appropriate to likely infecting organisms. If meningitis is suspected therapy should be commenced with penicillin G 2 g every 2 h plus chloramphenicol 0.5–1 g 6-hourly; isolation of specific organisms will allow appropriate chemotherapy.

Summary

There are many causes of focal central nervous system infection and the bacteriology is complex but these two factors are closely related. Accurate bacteriology assists in management by suggesting the probable source of infection and allowing appropriate chemotherapy. Conversely, a knowledge of the primary focus will indicate the most likely organisms and permit early use of appropriate antimicrobials.

References

1. De Louvois, J., Gortvai, P., and Hurley, R. (1977). Bacteriology of abscesses of the central nervous system: a multicentre prospective study. *Br. Med. J.*, **ii**, 981–4.
2. Haymaker, W. (1945). Fatal infections of the central nervous system and meninges after tooth extraction. *Am. J. Orth. Oral. Surg.*, **31**, 117–88.
3. Ingham, H.R., High, A.S., Kalbag, R.M., Sengupta, R.P., Tharagonnet, D., and Selkon, J.B. (1978). Abscesses of the fron-

tal lobe of the brain secondary to covert dental sepsis. *Lancet*, **ii**, 497–9.

4. Graham, D. R. and Band, J. D. (1981). *Citrobacter diversus* brain abscess and meningitis in neonates. *J. Am. Med. Assoc.*, **245**, 1923–5.
5. Alderson, D., Strong, A. J., Ingham, H. R., and Selkon, J. B. (1981). Fifteen-year review of the mortality of brain abscess. *Neurosurgery*, **8**, 1–6.
6. Garfield, J. (1969). Management of supratentorial intracranial abscess: a review of 200 cases. *Br. Med. J.*, **i**, 7–11.
7. Parker, M. T. and Ball L. C. (1967). Streptococci and aerococci associated with systemic infection in man. *J. Med. Micro.*, **9**, 275–302.
8. Hitchcock, E. and Andreadis, A. (1964). Subdural empyema: a review of 29 cases. *J. Neuro. Neurosurg. Psych.*, **27**, 422–34.
9. Bannister, G., Williams, B., and Smith, S. (1981). Treatment of subdural empyema. *J. Neurosurg.*, **55**, 82–8.
10. Batson, O. V. (1940). The function of the vertebral veins and their role in the spread of metastases. *Ann. Surg.*, **112**, 138–49.
11. Danner, R. L. and Hartman, B. J. (1987). Update of spinal epidural abscess: 35 cases and review of the literature. *Rev. Infect. Dis.*, **9**, 265–74.
12. Southwick, F. S., Richardson, E. P., and Swartz, M. N. (1986). Septic thrombosis of the dural venous sinuses. *Medicine*, **65**, 82–106.
13. Meltzer, P. E. (1935) Treatment of thrombosis of the lateral sinus. *Arch. Otolaryngol.*, **22**, 131–42.
14. Savitz, M. H., Malis, L. I., and Meyers, B. R. (1974). Prophylactic antibiotics in neurosurgery. *Surg. Neurol.*, **2**, 95–100.
15. Geraghty, J. and Feely, M. (1984). Antibiotic prophylaxis in neurosurgery. *J. Neurosurg.*, **60**, 724–6.
16. Jennet, B. and Miller, J. D. (1972). Infection after depressed fracture of the skull. Implications for management of non-missile injuries. *J. Neurosurg.*, **36**, 333–9.
17. Bayston, R. (1975). Antibiotic prophylaxis in shunt surgery. *Rev. Med. Child Neurol.*, **17**, 535, 99–103.
18. Stromblad, L. G., Schalen, C., Steen, A., Sundbarg, G., and Kanime, C. (1987). Bacterial contamination in cerebrospinal fluid shunt surgery. *Scand. J. Infect. Dis.*, **19**, 211–4.
19. Haines, S. J. (1980). Systemic antibiotic prophylaxis in neurological surgery. *Neurosurgery*, **6**, 355–61.
20. Malis, L. I. (1979). Prevention of neurosurgical infection by intra-operative antibiotics. *Neurosurgery*, **5**, 339–43.
21. Cartmill, T. D. I., Al-Zahawi, M. F., Sisson, P. R., *et al.* (1989). Five days versus one day of penicillin as chemoprophylaxis in elective neurosurgical operations. *J. Hosp. Infect.*, **14**, 63–8.
22. Mendelow, A. D., Campbell, D., Tsementzis, S. A., *et al.* (1983). Prophylactic antimicrobial management of compound depressed skull fracture. *J. R. Coll. Surg. Edinb.*, **28**, 80–3.
23. Garrod, L. P., Lambert, H. P., and O'Grady, F. P. (1981). Meningitis. In *Antibiotic and chemotherapy* (ed. L. P., Garrod, H. P. Lambert, and F. P. O'Grady), p. 235. Churchill Livingstone, Edinburgh.
24. Donauer, E., Drumm, G., Moringlane, J., Ostertag, C., and Kivelitz, R. (1987). Intrathecal administration of netilmicin in gentamicin-resistant ventriculitis. *Acta Neurchir.*, **86**, 83–8.
25. Swayne, R., Rampling, A., and Newson, S. W. B. (1987). Intraventricular vancomycin for treatment of shunt-associated ventriculitis. *J. Antimicrob. Chemother.*, **19**, 249–53.
26. Bayston, R. (1988). CSF vancomycin concentrations. *J. Antimicrob. Chemother.*, **22**, 265.
27. Block, C. S., Cassels, R., Koonhoz, H. J., Robinson, R. G., and Laver-Allen, C. M. (1977). Klebsiella meningitis treated with intrathecal amikacin. *Lancet*, **1**, 1371–2.
28. Ingham, H. R., Kalbag, R. M., McAllister, V., Mendelow, A. D., and Sisson, P. R. (in press). Post-operative and post-traumatic infections. In *Pyogenic neurosurgical infections* (ed. H. R. Ingham, R. M. Kalbag, V. A. McAllister, A. D. Mendelow, and P. R. Sisson). Edward Arnold, London.

Further reading

Ingham, H. R., Kalbag, R. M., McAllister, V., Mendelow, A. D., and Sisson, P. R. (in press). In *Pyogenic neurosurgical infections* (ed. H. R. Ingham, R. M. Kalbag, V. A. McAllister, A. D. Mendelow, and P. R. Sisson). Edward Arnold, London.

27

Infection in ENT surgery

ANDREW C. SWIFT

Introduction

Infection accounts for much of the morbidity in disease of the ears, nose, and throat (ENT) and complications can be extremely serious. In this chapter the most common and important conditions seen in the UK will be presented rather than a comprehensive account of all possibilities. Thus diseases such as tuberculosis, scleroma, gangosa, or mycoses which are uncommon or seen in other parts of the world are not presented.

Several decades ago infective diseases were much more prevalent. The advent of antibiotics and improvements in both social conditions and medical care has lessened their incidence and severity. However, our understanding of common conditions continues to improve with information from current research.

Many ENT bacterial infections are polymicrobial and the combination of anaerobic and aerobic bacteria has been shown to be synergistic and much more destructive. The discovery of beta-lactamase production by bacteria such as staphylococci, *Haemophilus* spp. and *Bacteroides* spp. has lead to the concept of susceptible bacteria being protected by enzymes produced by other bacterial genera and probably explains why acute tonsillitis due to beta-haemolytic streptoccoci does not always respond to penicillin (1).

Head and neck surgery

Antibiotic prophylaxis

Wound infection after major head and neck surgery increases morbidity, prolongs hospital stay, and can lead to the demise of the patient. Operations which breach the mucosa of the mouth or pharynx are particularly at risk (Table 27.1). The effect may be minor dehiscence, fistula formation, or massive wound breakdown. The risk of wound infection is not significantly worse after conventional irradiation but is more likely with bad teeth: these should be removed prior to surgery (2).

Until recently there have been conflicting opinions about the need for chemoprophylaxis in head and neck surgery. A survey of Otolaryngologists in the UK showed little consistency amongst them in the use of antibiotics and the regimens used (3). However, wound infection rates without chemoprophylaxis may be as high as 87 per cent (4). Much of the confusion has arisen because trials have been poorly designed but the benefit of chemoprophylaxis has been clearly demonstrated (5).

Prophylaxis should be started intravenously early in the operation so that good tissue levels are present when the mucosa is opened. The antibiotic should be chosen to suite the most likely pathogens. Infections are often mixed and the commonest pathogens are streptococci, *Staphyloccocus aureus*, aerobic Gram-negative bacilli and anaerobes (6–8).

Intestinal Gram-negative aerobic bacilli (GNAB) are reported in 29–82 per cent of infected wounds but are seldom isolated before operation (9). Until recently they have been assumed to arise exogenously. However, an endogenous source from the stomach has been demonstrated and transfer to the neck is probably facilitated by the naso-gastric feeding tube (9). GNAB are invariably found in the mouth within a few days of operation yet many of these patients do not develop wound infection (10). This is because the wound is at most risk of bacterial contamination at the time of operation. Provided the pharyngeal repair is continent, the presence of GNAB within a few days will not lead to wound infection. However, these bacteria are potent pathogens if the internal suture line is dehiscent.

Antibiotics such as co-amoxyclav, cefazolin, erythromycin, clindamycin, and tinidazole are effective prophylactic agents (11, 12) and sometimes metronidazole is added (13). The spectrum of cover should include GNAB in patients with a previous tracheostomy or indwelling nasogastric tube. Short courses (less than 24 h) are effective; long courses will encourage bacterial resistance and select out pathogens in favour of the normal oral microflora.

General wound management

Wound infections after head and neck surgery normally cause varying degrees of dehiscence. Three-point junctions are particularly prone and care should be taken when planning incisions and raising flaps to prevent vascular impairment. Suction drainage should be used to prevent the collection of blood: if a haematoma or seroma does form then this should be aspirated or drained. Regular post-operative oral hygiene would seem advisable but is of unproven value.

Tracheostomy tubes should be changed aseptically. The patient should breathe humidified air and have regular airway suction. Established infections need intensive local toilet and more frequent tube changes. Chest physiotherapy should be administered because the ability to cough is lost and patients are prone to chest infections.

Established wound infections are treated by intensive local toilet, debridement, and local antiseptic dressings. Infection adjacent to the carotid artery can cause the vessel wall to necrose. Although unusual, the consequences are potentially lethal and the only hope of salvage is by local pressure control until the artery can be ligated or repaired in the operating theatre.

A fistula is a more frequent occurrence after wound infection. Treatment is by nasogastric feeding and local dressings. Most will close spontaneously given time although a small number will require surgery.

Salivary gland infection

Acute parotitis

The commonest infection of the parotid glands is mumps but several other viruses can also cause parotitis (14). Acute bacterial parotitis is uncommon but was not unusual several decades ago, especially in the elderly after abdominal surgery, and in the presence of dehydration or general debility. Parotitis was then often severe and incision and drainage formed part of the standard management. *Staph. aureus* used to be the commonest pathogen but now many organisms are implicated. Acute parotitis is, in general, a much milder disease than it was many years ago and presents equally in men and women, from adolescence to old age (15). There may be a history of similar episodes and a few may have Sjögren's syndrome. Most arise *de novo* but occasionally there is nearby infection such as tonsillitis, a quinsy, or dental abscess.

The gland is painful and swollen and pus can sometimes be expressed from the duct. A culture should be taken from the duct orifice and the patient started on antibiotics. Erythromycin is the agent of choice but amoxycillin or a cephalosporin may be suitable (15). Attention should be given to oral hygiene and a good fluid intake encouraged. A sialogram should be done after several weeks to identify correctable causes such as mucus plugs, calculi, or strictures.

In more serious infections a parotid abscess may develop. Needle aspiration or incision and drainage will then be necessary and the contents should be sent for aerobic and anaerobic culture (16). The antibiotic spectrum should be guided by the Gram stain but will probably need to include staphylococci and anaerobic organisms.

Recurrent sialadenitis

Recurrent sialadenitis is seen most commonly in the submandibular gland due to sialectasis, calculi, or duct stenosis. Acute parotitis becomes recurrent in a few patients possibly due to calculi, punctate sialectasia, or Sjögren's syndrome. Recurrent parotitis is seen at all ages, but in about a third symptoms start in childhood (17). The condition is unusual in children but tends to be self limiting, often resolving by early adulthood (18).

Recurrent inflammation may affect both parotid glands but, when unilateral, sialectasia may be present in the contralateral unaffected gland (17). Autoantibodies are sometimes detected but do not help to predict the clinical course. If Sjögren's syndrome is suspected a labial biopsy should be taken from the mucosal surface of the lower lip for histological confirmation.

Long-term follow-up shows that many patients improve spontaneously with time. Radiotherapy, steroids and parotid duct ligation have all been used but have been criticized in favour of observation, supportive therapy, and parotidectomy in selected patients (17). Some patients will develop intractable symptoms, disfiguring parotomegaly or a discrete parotid lump suggestive of a neoplasm. These patients should be offered a parotidectomy, and it may be necessary to remove the whole gland with preservation of the facial nerve.

Head and neck infections

The neck contains a large number of lymph nodes and potential fascial spaces, both of which may be associated with local infection. The nodes are widespread, arranged in groups and receive lymph from respective drainage zones (Fig. 27.1).

The structures in the neck are surrounded by layers of fascia between which lie potential spaces (Fig. 27.2). A basic knowledge of these spaces is needed to appreciate the site, likely direction of spread, and subsequent complications of local infection. The complications of neck space infections are potentially serious and sometimes fatal. They include airway obstruction from soft tissue swelling, mediastinitis, septicaemia, carotid artery haemorrhage, and jugular vein thrombosis. Attention should always be given to fluid balance since these patients will be pyrexial and may be unable to maintain an adequate fluid intake.

With the exception of a peritonsillar abscess neck space infections are uncommon and only the most important will be discussed.

Lymphadenitis

Typically, lymph nodes associated with infection are large and tender and their site is related to the primary source of infection. Confusion may arise with a large tender mass in the upper

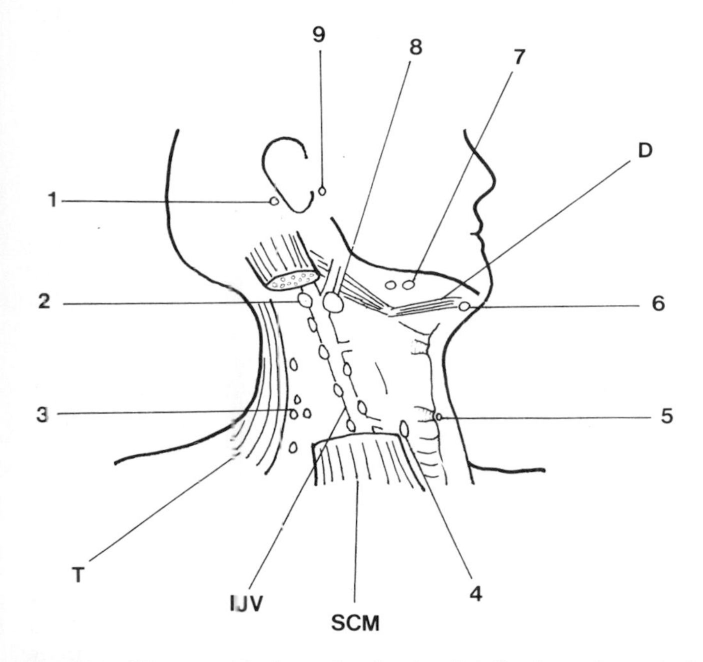

Fig. 27.1. Diagram to show the basic distribution of cervical lymph nodes. (T) trapezius muscle; (IJV) internal jugular vein; (SCM) sternocleidomastoid muscle; (D) digastric muscle. Nodes: (1) retro-auricular; (2) deep cervical chain; (3) posterior triangle nodes; (4) paratracheal; (5) prelaryngeal; (6) submental; (7) submandibular; (8) jugulo-digastric; (9) superficial parotid.

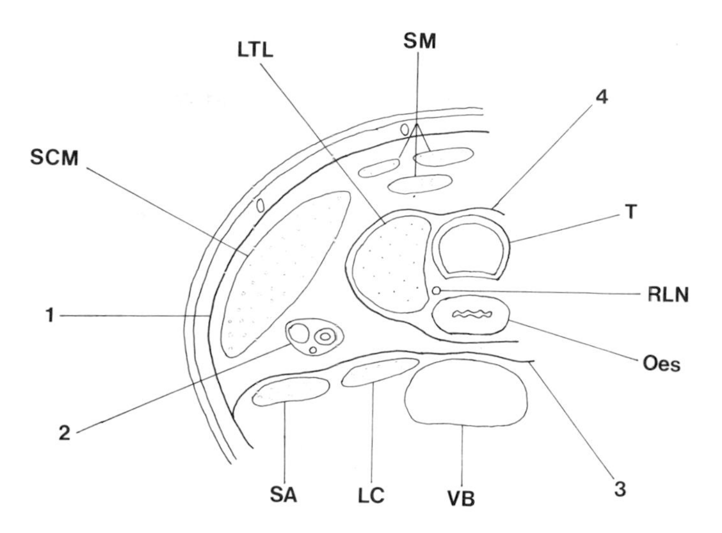

Fig. 27.2. Diagram of a transverse section of neck at the level of C6 to show the main fascial planes. (SCM) sternocleidomastoid muscle; (SA) scalenus anterior; (LC) longus colli; (VB) vertebral body C6; (Oes) oesophagus; (RLN) recurrent laryngeal nerve; (T) trachea; (SM) strap muscles; (LTL) left thyroid lobe. Fascia: (1) investing layer; (2) carotid sheath; (3) pre-vertebral fascia; (4) pretracheal fascia.

deep cervical region. This may be a confluent collection of nodes due to severe tonsillitis or a quinsy, but other alternatives include a parapharyngeal abscess or an infected branchial cyst. Infectious mononucleosis may present with massive bilateral lymphadenopathy and is confirmed by a Paul–Bunnell test.

In young children an acute viral illness can cause multiple, bilateral lymphadenopathy which may persist after the infection has resolved. This may give rise to concern, particularly if one lymph node is prominent. Careful follow-up is necessary and a blood dyscrasia should be excluded. Occasionally, excision biopsy may be required.

Less common causes for non-neoplastic lymphadenopathy include tuberculosis, sarcoidosis, toxoplasmosis, actinomycosis, and cat-scratch fever. HIV infection must also be considered.

Table 27.1. Classification for head and neck surgical procedures. The risk of wound infection is greatest in Classes III and IV.

Class I	Clean Radical neck dissection Parotidectomy/submandibular gland excision Thyroidectomy Excision of uninfected branchial cyst
Class II	Clean contaminated Laryngofissure Excision of laryngocele
Class III	Contaminated Total laryngectomy Laryngo-pharyngectomy Glossectomy Hemimandibulectomy
Class IV	Dirty Drainage of neck abscess

Peritonsillar abscess (quinsy)

A quinsy is an abscess between the fibrous tonsillar capsule and the pharyngeal superior constrictor muscle. The bacterial microflora is often β-haemolytic streptococci but may be mixed and include both aerobic and anaerobic bacteria. The infection is most commonly seen in young adults, is unilateral and lies adjacent to the upper pole of the tonsil. It often follows acute tonsillitis and there is frequently a history of recurrent tonsillitis. However, there are exceptions to all of these rules. The clinical features include general malaise, pyrexia, trismus, salivation, palatal swelling, and medial displacement of the tonsil. There will also be a large tender ipsilateral mass of upper deep cervical lymph nodes.

Treatment includes intravenous antibiotics, incision and drainage, or emergency abscess tonsillectomy. Penicillin or erythromycin are recommended but previous oral antibiotic treatment may modify this choice.

The distinction between peritonsillar cellulitis and an abscess is not always easy and judgement must be used. However, if an abscess has formed then immediate relief can be obtained by releasing the pus which is done by incising the soft palate above the tonsil under local anaesthesia. Abscess tonsillectomy is sometimes recommended as an alternative method of management but the author restricts this to patients who do not respond well to antibiotics and drainage.

Complications are potentially lethal and have led to the classical recommendation of tonsillectomy several weeks after a quinsy. Fortunately, with modern-day treatment these problems are rarely seen and if a tonsillectomy is not done only 20 per cent will develop a recurrent quinsy (19). Therefore it is the author's practice to offer tonsillectomy only to those who suffer from recurrent tonsillitis or who have had a previous quinsy.

Parapharyngeal abscess

A parapharyngeal abscess occurs in the lateral pharyngeal space which lies adjacent to the nasopharynx and oropharynx. It extends from the base of the skull to the submandibular gland and hyoid bone; the lateral wall is formed by the parotid gland and medial pterygoid muscle. The styloid structures divide the space into an anterior and posterior compartment. The carotid sheath runs through the posterior compartment; the latter communicates with the retropharyngeal space. The cause is often dental infection, severe tonsillitis, or quinsy; occasionally infection spreads from the parotid gland, petrous apex, or mastoid tip.

The clinical features depend on which compartment is infected but include a tender swelling in the upper part of the neck, trismus, fever, and pharyngeal bulging (20) (Fig. 27.3). Treatment is by intravenous antibiotics, incision, and drainage. Pus should be drained by a collar incision at the level of the hyoid. However, this is not without risk since intubation may be difficult and a period spent observing the response to antibiotics is advisable.

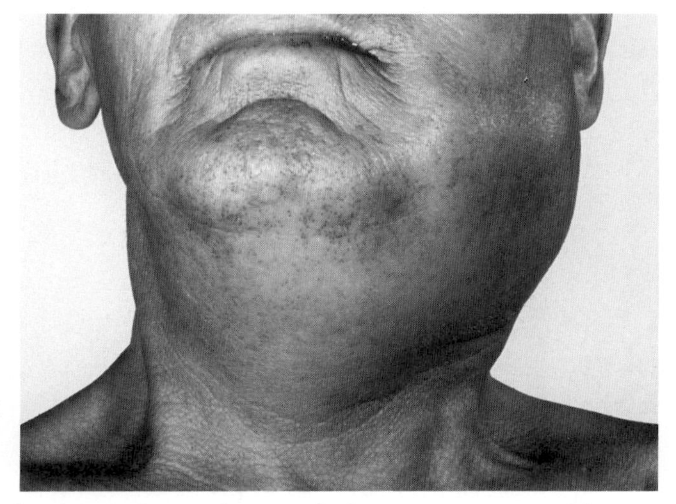

Fig. 27.3. Left parapharyngeal abscess in a 63-year-old man. (See plate section.)

Retropharyngeal abscess

A retropharyngeal abscess usually presents in infants from infection within local lymph nodes (nodes of Rouviere) after an upper respiratory tract infection. The infection is polymicrobial and includes anaerobic organisms as well as beta-lactamase producing bacteria (21). The child will be acutely ill, pyrexial, and the posterior pharyngeal wall will be swollen and may obstruct breathing. A lateral soft tissue radiograph of the neck may help to confirm the diagnosis (Fig. 27.4). Broad spectrum antibiotics should be given and the abscess drained with the child in the tonsillectomy position.

Retropharyngeal infection in adults is uncommon; it may follow local trauma or nearby infection in the ears, nose, throat, or teeth. The classical cause is tuberculosis of the cervical spine but non-tuberculous ostoemyelitis and immunosuppression should also be considered (20).

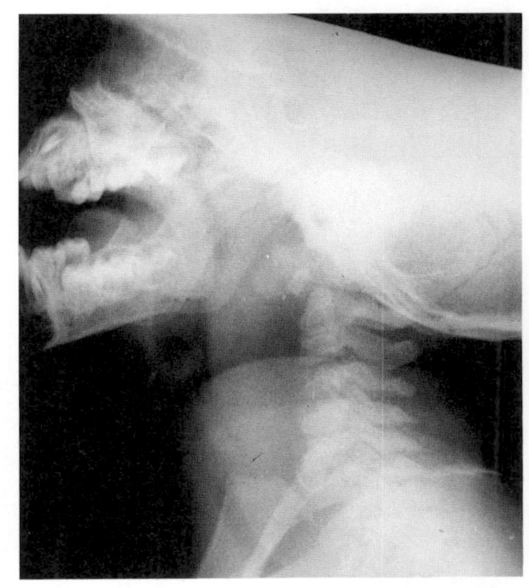

Fig. 27.4. Lateral radiograph of neck in a 12-month-old boy with a retropharyngeal abscess: note the increase in soft tissue thickness anterior to cervical spine.

Ludwig's angina

Ludwig's angina is a severe acute infection of the submandibular space and floor of mouth. The infection causes cellulitis with little or no pus but there is putrid infiltration and gangrene of the soft tissues. Clinically, there are painful brawny swellings of both suprahyoid regions and the floor of mouth. The latter displaces the tongue and this may obstruct the airway. Most cases arise in previously healthy adults and about 85 per cent have associated dental problems (23). A wide variety of micro-organisms have been isolated, the most common being streptococci, staphylococci, and bacteroides. In 50 per cent the bacterial flora is mixed.

Antibiotics are the mainstay of treatment since the infection is mainly cellulitic. Pathogens should be sought by culture of blood or tissue aspiration fluid. If no tissue fluid can be obtained 0.5 ml saline should be instilled, withdrawn, and cultured. Respiration should be closely monitored. Impending obstruction will cause rapid shallow breathing; stridor may be absent since the obstruction will usually be above the larynx. If obstruction is suspected a tracheostomy should be done—more safely performed under local anaesthesia since intubation will be difficult.

Surgical decompression used to be regarded as the optimum method of treatment before the advent of antibiotics and many techniques were described (24, 25). However, surgery should now be reserved for releasing pus under tension. The investing layer of deep fascia should be incised and the mylohyoid muscle divided.

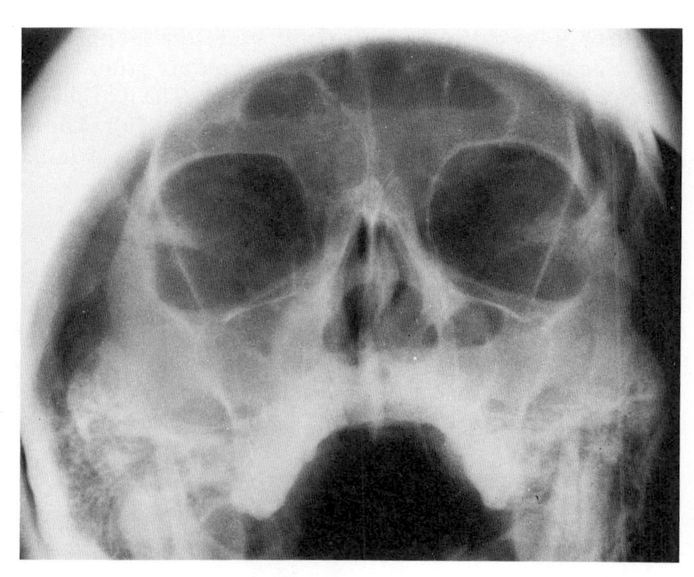

Fig. 27.5. Occipito-mental sinus radiograph to show changes associated with sinusitis. Note fluid levels in left antrum and both frontal sinuses. The right antrum displays gross mucosal thickening. (Courtesy of Dr H. Lewis-Jones, Consultant Radiologist, Walton Hospital, Liverpool.)

Infection of the nose and throat

Rhinosinusitis

There are three pairs of paranasal sinuses and a sphenoid sinus. Infection is most often seen in the maxillary antra or ethmoid sinuses, is less common in the frontal and rare in the sphenoid. When several sinuses are infected this is known as a pan-sinusitis.

Acute sinusitis

Acute sinusitis most commonly follows an upper respiratory tract viral infection. Common bacterial pathogens include *Streptococcus pneumoniae*, *Haemophilus influenzae*, and, in children, *Branhamella catarrhalis* (26, 27). Maxillary sinusitis may be secondary to a dental abscess and anaerobic organisms will invariably be present. The symptoms include facial pain, purulent rhinorrhoea, nasal obstruction, and tenderness over the affected sinus. Radiologically the affected sinus will be opaque, display marked mucosal thickening or there may be a fluid level (Fig. 27.5).

Treatment is by antibiotics and with systemic or topical decongestants. Antral washout is occasionally required if resolution does not occur. Unilateral nasal discharge in a child is most often due to a foreign body but unilateral choanal atresia is also a possibility.

Chronic rhino-sinusitis

The nasal mucosa is under autonomic neural control; in most people each side undergoes an alternating cycle of congestion and decongestion. Chronic congestion and stasis of excessive mucus may lead to infection, mucosal inflammation, ciliary immotility, and blockage of sinus ostia with subsequent sinusitis. Anaerobic bacteria are frequently isolated from infected sinuses and these may produce beta-lactamases (28, 29).

The anti-inflammatory effect of topical steroids is often beneficial. Systemic anti-histamines are given in allergic rhinitis and possible allergens should be avoided. Surgery is reserved for persistent disease. Functional endoscopic nasal operations are a recent advance in sinus surgery (30).

Nasal polyposis

Nasal polyps are grape-like swellings which usually arise from the ethmoid sinuses and middle meati on both sides of the nose. There is often a coexisting sinusitis of the ethmoid sinuses and maxillary antra and infection has been implicated in their pathogenesis, but this hypothesis is not universally accepted (31).

Complications of sinusitis

Infection can occasionally spread beyond the confines of an infected sinus. Acute ethmoiditis can extend across the thin lamina papyracea and lead to periorbital cellulitis, subperiosteal abscess, blindness or intracranial infection (32). Intracranial complications such as meningitis, subdural or intracerebral abscess formation or ostoemyelitis are seen more often with frontal sinusitis. Cavernous sinus thrombosis is a rare but life-threatening complication of sinus infection which causes bilateral proptosis and ophthalmoplegia (see Chapter 28).

Tonsillitis and pharyngitis

Sore throats are one of the most common problems which cause patients to consult their doctor. However, in spite of a wealth of knowledge there are still basic questions which remain unanswered such as why some people are prone to frequent recurrent tonsillitis and others are not. The part played by viruses in the pathogenesis of infection is not fully known but it is thought that bacterial tonsillitis often follows an initial viral infection.

Acute tonsillitis

Acute tonsillitis is most predominant in children. The clinical features include an acute sore throat, pyrexia, dysphagia, trismus, and cervical lymphadenopathy. On examination, the tonsils may be smooth, inflamed, and swollen or be covered by multiple patches of an exudate with pus exuding from the crypts (Fig 27.6).

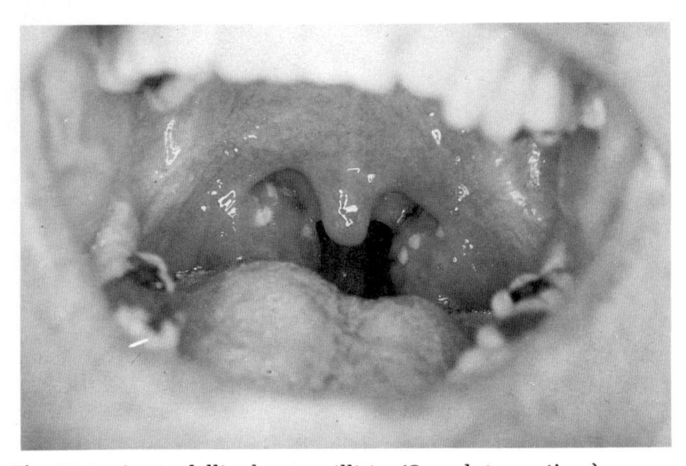

Fig. 27.6. Acute follicular tonsillitis. (See plate section.)

Although the main pathogen is Group A beta-haemolytic streptococcus, there are many commensals which are thought to become pathogenic in the presence of inflammation (33). Bacteria on the surface of the tonsil differ from those in the core limiting the usefulness of throat swab culture (34). The role of anaerobic bacteria is not fully known.

Treatment priorities include antibiotics, analgesics and maintaining an adequate fluid intake. Pencillin is the antibiotic of choice but is not always effective since infections may be polymicrobial and include beta lactamase-producing bacteria (35).

The decision to perform tonsillectomy is based on a history of frequent infections over several years (36). Large tonsils may contribute to upper airway obstruction as may the adenoids and this also may sway the decision toward surgery. Infectious mononucleosis may be clinically indistinguishable from acute tonsillitis but can be confirmed by a Paul–Bunnel test. In the presence of infectious mononucleosis ampicillin may cause a rash and may lead to litigation if used.

Pharyngitis

Acute pharyngitis is most often experienced as a sore throat with a common cold, but may become severe with bacterial superinfection. The lymphoid follicles on the posterior pharyngeal wall look prominent and hyperaemic and there may be cervical lymphadenopathy. Many of the causes of infective pharyngitis are listed in Table 27.2. Chronic pharyngitis is usually due to inflammation induced by irritants such as smoking, dust, or fumes. However, it may be secondary to infective foci such as poor dentition, sinusitis or a purulent cough.

Candida is a common oral commensal which may become pathogenic and cause multiple white patches over the oral mucosa and pharynx. Predisposing conditions include recent antibiotic use, radiotherapy, diabetes, or immunosuppression. Oral candidosis is often a presenting feature of HIV infection (37).

There are several causes of ulceration of the tonsil and these include a giant aphthous ulcer, acute streptococcal tonsillitis, infectious mononucleosis, Vincent's angina, tuberculosis, and syphilis. However, a tumour or haematological condition must be excluded.

Table 27.2. Causes of infective pharyngitis.

Viral infection	**Micro-organism**
Upper respiratory tract infection (common cold, influenza)	Rhinovirus Coronovirus Parainfluenza virus Influenza virus Adenovirus
Infectious mononucleosis	Epstein–Barr virus
Gingivitis, stomatitis	Herpes simplex virus
Herpangina	Coxsackie virus
Acquired immune deficiency syndrome	Human immunodeficiency virus
Bacterial infection	
Tonsillo-pharyngitis	Beta-haemolytic streptococcus
Peritonsillar cellulitis	Mixed aerobic/anaerobic bacteria
Vincent's angina	*Fusiform fusiformis.* Spirochaetes
Gonorrhoea	*Neisseria gonorrhoea*
Diphtheria	*Corynebacterium diphtheriae/ ulcerans*
Syphilis	*Treponema pallidum*

Laryngitis

Acute laryngitis is usually viral and causes a weak rough voice of variable pitch and strength associated with pain and soreness. The role of bacterial infection is not clear (38). Treatment should include vocal rest, steam inhalation, and analgesics. In contrast, chronic laryngitis is generally an inflammatory disorder related to local irritation such as smoking, fumes, dust, or vocal abuse. However, there is often a persistent source of infection in the sinuses or chest (39).

Laryngeal tuberculosis is uncommon but may affect all aspects of the larynx (40, 41). A biopsy should be taken to confirm the diagnosis and exclude malignancy. Treatment is by prolonged chemotherapy. Long term sequelae include laryngeal fibrosis and stenosis which may require surgery.

Laryngitis in children

Laryngeal infection in children is potentially dangerous because of the much smaller dimensions and greater airflow restrictions imposed by mucosal oedema, especially in the subglottis. Croup or laryngotracheobronchitis is a common cause of stridor in young children. The cause is viral but bacterial superinfection may occur. Features include a barking cough, pyrexia, and stridor which fluctuates and worsens gradually. Treatment includes humidity, reassurance, and observation. The place of antibiotics, steroids, oxygen, and nebulized adrenaline is controversial. Intubation, or less commonly tracheostomy, is sometimes necessary (42).

Acute epiglottitis is usually caused by *H. influenzae* Type B, and, in contrast, is much less common but more lethal. Typically, a 3-year-old child becomes acutely ill, sits drooling, and has increasing difficulty with breathing. The epiglottis will be cherry red but oral examination may precipitate sudden airway obstruction and should be avoided. Intravenous chloramphenicol (100 mg/kg body weight/24 h) is the antibiotic of choice (43), and early intubation is recommended (44).

Perichondritis

Perichondritis of the larynx is usually seen after radiotherapy and causes laryngeal pain, tenderness, and stridor. There may be persistent or recurrent malignant disease but a biopsy may give a misleading negative result and also exacerbate the perichondritis. Treatment includes antibiotics, steroids, and steam inhalation. If there is no improvement or progression then a total laryngectomy may be recommended in the absence of proven carcinoma. Laryngeal sections in such patients will often confirm the presence of tumour (45).

Infections of the ear

The external ear

Otitis externa

Infection of the external auditory canal is always painful and usually affects the whole of the canal skin. Less commonly a furuncle presents with exquisite pain due to infection of a hair follicle by *Staph. aureus*. Local trauma, swimming, or hot and humid conditions predispose to otitis externa. Recurrent or chronic infections are often bilateral, are associated with itchy canals in between episodes and there may be other skin conditions such as psoriasis or eczema. Chronic suppurative otitis media should be excluded.

Pulling the pinna or pushing the tragus is painful. The external canal will be swollen and in most cases there will be pus and/or wet soggy squamous debris. In chronic disease, the skin lining the canal may become very thick and there may be eczema of the conchal skin. An important aspect of treatment is thorough cleaning of the external canal. Topical applications such as glycerine and ichthammol, aluminium acetate or antibiotic/steroid preparations are then applied.

Malignant otitis externa

Malignant otitis externa is a painful, potentially fatal condition due to *Pseudomonas aeruginosa* which is more common in elderly, diabetic, and immunosuppressed patients. The onset is insidious; infection spreads rapidly throughout the temporal bone and surrounding tissues and may paralyse the facial nerve or the nerves passing through the jugular foramen.

Treatment includes aural toilet, surgical debridement, and high doses of an antipseudomonal antibiotic. Recent success has been described after several weeks of oral ciprofloxacin (46, 47).

The middle ear cleft

Acute otitis media

Acute otitis media (AOM) is an acute inflammation of the mucosa lining the middle-ear cleft. It is most common in young children, decreasing with age to become an uncommon problem in adults. Many patients have a preceding viral infection; although viruses may initiate the episode, AOM is generally considered to be a bacterial disease. *Streptococcus pneumoniae* and *H. influenzae* are both important pathogens (48). The most common features include otalgia and a red, opaque or bulging drum (49). In a few patients, the drum perforates and the ear discharges. In young children, pyrexia, diarrhoea, or vomiting is quite common.

Antibiotics are usually prescribed, particularly ampicillin, amoxycillin, or co-amoxyclav (49). However, there is controversy over both the duration of treatment and the need for antibiotics (49–51). Occasionally, myringotomy may be necessary should resolution be delayed. In recurrent AOM, consideration should be given to other sources of infection such as the adenoids or chronic sinusitis. Apart from persisting otitis media with effusion complications are rare. However, possibilities include acute mastoiditis, facial nerve paralysis, intracranial infection, labryrinthitis, and petrositis.

Acute mastoiditis

Although the mucosa lining the mastoid is invariably inflamed during AOM it is rare for this to progress to an acute mastoiditis. However, infection may occasionally persist as a latent or masked infection and cause otorrhoea and mastoid granulations.

Classical acute mastoiditis is usually seen in young children and presents with a short history of pain, pyrexia, malaise, and otorhoea. The tympanic membrane is almost always perforated and the pinna is displaced by a red tender swelling over the mastoid process.

Treatment is by intravenous antibiotics and post-aural drainage of the abscess by cortical mastoidectomy, although the timing of the latter is controversial (52).

Chronic otitis media

Chronic disease of the middle ear may be classified according to its anatomy: attico-antral or tubotympanic; or to its pathology: inactive chronic otitis media, active mucosal chronic otitis media, or active chronic otitis media with cholesteatoma.

Classically, tubo-tympanic disease was considered 'safe' in contrast to attico-antral disease which was considered 'dangerous' because of the likelihood of cholesteatoma and its associated complications. However, this simple concept is not entirely true (53). With inactive disease there may be a dry perforation or a clean posterior/superior retraction pocket. However, recurrent or persistent discharge, mucus, muco-pus, inflamed middle-ear mucosa, granulations, a polyp, or cholesteatoma means the disease is active.

Pathogens include Gram-negative aerobic bacteria, anaerobic bacteria, and staphylococci. Polybacterial culture is common and high bacterial counts are found (54). The presence of beta-lactamase producing microbes (1) and the synergism between anaerobic and aerobic bacteria have important implications in management.

Infection requires frequent aural toilet and topical application of antiseptics or antibiotic solutions. Theoretically there is a risk of cochlear damage with many topical preparations but persistent infection may also damage the inner ear. The effectiveness of systemic antibiotics is controversial (55, 56).

If a cholesteatoma is present then most patients will need mastoid surgery to delineate and eradicate the disease. After radical mastoid surgery a cavity is created which may be prone to infection. This usually responds to aural toilet although occasionally further surgical revision is required.

Potential complications of active chronic otitis media include intracranial abscesses, meningitis, sigmoid sinus thrombophlebitis, facial paralysis, and labyrinthitis.

The inner ear

Labyrinthitis

Labyrinthitis may be viral or bacterial. Viruses include herpes, mumps, influenza, and adenoviruses. The course is self-limiting but varying degrees of permanent damage may remain. Bacterial labyrinthitis is less common and is usually the result of middle ear suppuration. It is classified as serous or suppurative, the former being reversible and the latter causing permanent damage. Inflammation and infection may spread to the labyrinth across the round window but in chronic otitis media the portal of entry is more likely to be a labyrinthine fistula due to bony erosion by cholesteatoma.

References

1. Brook, I. (1989). The concept of indirect pathogenicity by β-lactamase production, especially in ear, nose and throat infection. *J. Antimicrob. Chemother.*, **24**, Suppl B, 63–72.
2. Raine, C. H. (1987). Chemoprophylaxis for head and neck cancer surgery. ChM Thesis. University of Liverpool.
3. Raine, C. H. and Swift, A. C. (1985). Antibiotic prophylaxis—a survey. *J. Laryngol. Otol.*, **99**, 183–5.
4. Becker, G. D. and Parell, G. J. (1979). Cefazolin prophylaxis in head and neck cancer surgery. *Ann. Otol.*, **88**, 183–6.
5. Raine, C. H., Bartzokas, C. A., Stell, P. M., Gallaway, A., and Corkill, J. E. (1984). Chemoprophylaxis in major head and neck surgery. *J.R. Soc. Med.*, **77**, 1006–9.
6. Bartzokas, C. A., Raine, C. H., Stell, P. M., Corkill, J. E., Withana, N., and Trafford-Jones G. M. (1984). Bacteriological assessment of patients undergoing head and neck surgery. *Clin. Otolaryngol.*, **9**, 99–103.
7. Brook, I. and Hirokawa, R. (1989). Microbiology of wound infection after head and neck cancer surgery. *Ann. Otol. Rhinol. Laryngol.*, **98**, 323–5.
8. Johnson, J. T. and Yu, V. L. (1989). Role of aerobic Gram-negative rods, anaerobes and fungi in wound infection after head and neck surgery: implications for antibiotic prophylaxis. *Head Neck*, **11**, 27–9.
9. Swift, A. C., Bartzokas, C. A., and Corkill, J. E. (1984). The gastro-oral pathway of intestinal bacteria after head and neck cancer surgery. *Clin. Otolaryngol.*, **1**, 263–9.
10. Swift, A. C., Bartzokas, C. A., and Corkill, J. E. (1987). The clinical significance of the gastro-oral pathway of intestinal bacteria after head and neck cancer surgery. *Clin. Otolaryngol.*, **12**, 455–9.
11. Johnson, J. T. (1987). Perioperative antibiotic treatment for contaminated head and neck surgery. In *Antibiotic therapy in head and neck surgery* (ed. J. T. Johnson) pp. 51–88. Marcel Dekker, New York.
12. Swift, A. C. (1988). Editorial. Wound sepsis, chemoprophylaxas and major head and neck surgery. *Clin. Otolaryngol.*, **13**, 81–83.
13. Sawyer, R. (1988). Clinical implications of metronidazole antianaerobic prophylaxis in major head and neck surgical procedures. *Ear Nose Throat J.*, **67**, 655–8.
14. Loughran, D. H. and Smith, L. G. (1988). Review: Infectious disorders of the parotid gland. *New Jersey Med.*, **85**, 311–14.
15. Lamey, P. J., Boyle, M. A., Macfarlane, T. W., and Samaranayake, L. P. (1987). Acute suppurative parotitis in outpatients: Microbiological and posttreatment sialographic findings. *Oral Surg. Oral Med. Pathol.*, **63**, 37–41.
16. Matlow, A., Korentager, R., Keystone, E., and Bohnen, J. (1988). Parotitis due to anaerobic bacteria. *Rev. Infect. Dis.*, **10**, 420–3.
17. Watkin, G. T. and Hobsley, M. (1986). Natural history of patients with recurrent parotitis and punctate sialectasis. *Br. J. Surg.*, **73**, 745–8.
18. Geterud, A., Lindvall, A. M., and Nylen, O. (1988). Follow-up study of recurrent parotitis in children. *Ann. Otol. Rhinol. Laryngol.*, **97**, 341–6.
19. Herbild, O. and Bunding, P. (1981). Peritonsillar abscess. Recurrence rate and treatment. *Arch. Otolaryngol.*, **107**, 540–2.
20. Dzyak, W. R. and Zide, M. F. (1984). Diagnosis and treatment of lateral pharyngeal space infections. *J. Oral Maxillofac. Surg.*, **42**, 243–9.
21. Brook, I. (1987). Microbiology of retropharyngeal abscesses in children. *Am. J. Dis. Child.*, **141**, 202–4.
22. Barratt, G. E., Koopmann, C. F., and Coulthard, S. W. (1984). Retropharyngeal abscess—a ten year experience. *Laryngoscope*, **84**, 455–63.
23. Moreland, L. W., Corey, J., and McKenzie, R. (1988). Ludwig's angina. Report of a case and a review of the literature. *Arch. Intern. Med.*, **148**, 461–6.
24. Lindner, H. H. (1986). The anatomy of the fasciae of the face and neck with particular reference to the spread and treatment of intraoral infections (Ludwig's) that have progressed into adjacent fascial spaces. *Ann. Surg.*, **204**, 705–14.
25. Weisengreen, H. H. (1986). Ludwig's Angina: Historical review and reflections. *Ear Nose Throat J.*, **65**, 457–61.
26. Gwaltney, J. M. (1990). Sinusitis. In *Principles and practice of infectious diseases* (3rd edn.) (ed. G. L. Mandell, G. Douglas, and J. E. Bennet), Chapter 47, pp. 510–14. Churchill Livingstone, Edinburgh.
27. Wald, E. R., Milmoe, G. J., Bowen, A., Ledesma-Medina, J., Salamon, N., and Bluestone, C. D. (1981). Acute maxillary sinusitis in children. *N. Engl. J. Med.*, **304**, 749–54.
28. Brook, I. (1989). Bacteriology of chronic maxillary sinusitis in adults. *Ann. Otol. Rhinol. Laryngol.*, **98**, 426–8.
29. Frederick, J. and Braude, A. I. (1974). Anaerobic infection of the paranasal sinuses. *N. Engl. J. Med.*, **290**, 135–7.
30. Stammberger, H. (1985). Endoscopic surgery for mycotic and

chronic recurring sinusitis. *Ann. Otol. Rhinol. Laryngol.*, **94**, Suppl **119**, 1–11.
31. Dawes, P., Bates, G., Watson, D., Lewis, D., Lowe, D., and Drake-Lee, A.B. (1989). The role of bacterial infection of the maxillary sinus in nasal polyps. *Clin. Otolaryngol.*, **14**, 447–50.
32. Swift, A.C. and Charlton, G. (1990). Sinusitis and the acute orbit in children. *J. Laryngol. Otol.*, **104**, 213–6.
33. Brodsky, L. (1989). Modern assessment of tonsils and adenoids. *Ped. Clin. North Am.*, **36**, 1551–69.
34. Surow, J.B., Handler, S.D., Telian, S.A., Fleisher, G.R., and Baranak, C.C. (1989). Bacteriology of tonsil surface and core in children. *Laryngoscope*, **99**, 261–6.
35. Brook, I. (1989). Treatment of patients with acute recurrent tonsillitis due to group A β-haemolytic streptococci: a prospective randomized study comparing penicillin and amoxycillin/clavulanate potassium. *J. Antimicrob. Chemother.* **24**, 227–33.
36. Tucker, A.G. (1982). The current status of tonsillectomy—a survey of otolaryngologists. *Clin. Otolaryngol.*, **7**, 367–72.
37. Editorial. (1989). Oral Candidosis in HIV Infection. *Lancet*, **30**, 1491–2.
38. Gwaltney, J.M. (1990). Acute laryngitis. In *Principles and practice of infectious diseases* (3rd edn) (ed. G.L. Mandell, G. Douglas, and J.E. Bennet), Chapter 44, p. 449. Churchill Livingstone, Edinburgh.
39. Stell, P.M. and McLoughlin, M.P. (1976). The aetiology of chronic laryngitis. *Clin. Otolaryngol.*, **1**, 265–9.
40. Smallman, L.A., Clark, D.R., Raine, C.H., Proops, D.W., and Shenoi, P.M. (1987). The presentation of laryngeal tuberculosis. *Clin. Otolaryngol.*, **12**, 221–5.
41. Soda, A, Robio H., Salarar, E, Ganem, J., Berlanga, D., and Sanchez A. (1989). Tuberculosis of the larynx: Clinical aspects in 19 patients. *Laryngoscope*, **99**, 1147–50.
42. Swift, A.C. and Rogers, J.H. (1987). The changing indications for tracheostomy in children. *J. Laryngol. Otol.*, **101**, 1258–62.
43. Freeland, A.P. (1987). Acute laryngeal infections in childhood. In *Scott-Brown's otolaryngology* (ed. A.G. Kerr), Vol. 6 *Paediatric otolaryngology* (ed. J.N.G. Evans) p. 449–65. Butterworths, Tunbridge Wells.
44. Burns, J.E. and Hendley, J.O. (1990). Epiglottitis. In *Principles and practice of infectious diseases* (3rd edn) (ed. G.L. Mandell, R.G. Douglas, and J.E. Bennet), Chapter 48, pp. 514–16. Churchill Livingstone, Edinburgh.
45. Stell, P.M. and Bowdler, (1988). The T3 glottic cancer. Diagnosis and management. In *Dilemmas in otorhinlaryngology* (ed. D.F.N. Harrison), pp. 272–5. Churchill Livingstone.
46. Hickey, S.A., Ford, G.R., Fitzgerald O'Connor, Eykyn, S.J., and Sonksen, P.H. (1989). Treating malignant otitis with oral ciprofloxacin. *Br Med. J.*, **299**, 550–1.
47. Sade, J., Lang, R., Goshen, S., and Kitzes-Cohen, R. (1989). Ciprofloxacin treatment of malignant external otitis. *Am. J. Med.*, **30**, 1388–416.
48. Bluestone, C.D. and Klein, J.O. (1988). Microbiology. In *Otitis media in infants and children*, Chapter 5, p. 45. Saunders, Philadelphia.
49. Froom, J., Culpepper, L., Grob, P., *et al.* (1990). Diagnosis and antibiotic treatment of acute otitis media: report from International Primary Care Network. *Br. Med. J.*, **300**, 582–6.
50. Bain, J. (1990). Justification for antibiotic use in general practice. *Br. Med. J.*, **300**, 1006–7.
51. Browning, G. (1990). Childhood otalgia: acute otitis media. *Br. Med. J.*, **300**, 1005–6.
52. Faye-Lunde, H. (1989). Acute and latent mastoiditis. *J. Laryngol. Otol.*, **103**, 1158–60.
53. Browning, G.G. (1984). The unsafeness of 'safe' ears. *J. Laryngol. Otol.*, **98**, 23–6.
54. Sweeney, G., Picozzi, G.L., Browning, G.G. (1982). A quantitative study of aerobic and anaerobic bacteria in chronic suppurative otitis media. *J. Infect.*, **5**, 47–55.
55. Browning, G.G., Picozzi, G.L., Calder, I.T., and Sweeney, G. (1983). Controlled trial of medical treatment of active chronic otitis media. *Br. Med. J.*, **287**, 1024.
56. Papastavros, T., Giamarellou, H., and Varlejides, S. (1989). Preoperative therapeutic considerations in chronic otitis media. *Laryngoscope*, **99**, 655–9.

Further reading

Bluestone, C.D. and Klein, J.O. (1988). *Otitis media in infants and children*. Saunders, Philadephia, Penn.

Brook, I. (1988). The swollen neck. Cervical lymphadenitis, parotitis, thyroiditis, and infected cysts. *Infect. Dis. Clin. North Am.*, **2**, 221–36.

Johnson, J.T. (ed.) (1987). *Antibiotic therapy in head and neck surgery*. Marcel Dekker, New York.

Kerr, A.G. (ed.) (1987). *Scott-Brown's otolaryngology* (5th edn), Vols 3–6. Butterworths, Tunbridge Wells.

Lusk, R.P., Lazar, R.H., and Muntz H.R. (1989). The diagnosis and treatment of recurrent and chronic sinusitis in children. *Pediatr. Clin. North Am.*, **36**, 1411–21.

Mandell, G.L., Douglas, R.G., and Bennett J.E. (ed.) (1990). *Principles and practice of infectious diseases*. Churchill Livingstone, Edinburgh.

Ramsey, P.G. and Weymuller, E.A. (1985). Complications of bacterial infection of the ears, paranasal sinuses, and oropharynx in adults. *Emerg. Med. Clin. North Am.*, **3**, 143–60.

28

Infection in ocular surgery

D. FRANK P. LARKIN and DAVID L. EASTY

Introduction

The functional disturbance caused by post-operative intraocular infection (endophthalmitis) is devastating compared with infection occurring in other body tissues because of the remarkable anatomical and physiological properties of the eye, such as perfect transparency of the cornea and ocular fluids, and the close physical proximity of intraocular structures that have different specialized functions. The thick scleral coat limits infection to the eye: extraocular spread and bacteraemia are not features of post-operative intraocular infection.

Extraocular orbital infection rarely follows surgical procedures, but does pose a threat to the general condition of the patient. The spectre of posterior spread and cavernous sinus thrombosis prompts intensive therapy in all such patients.

Surgery on the eye may be categorized as intraocular: cataract extraction with intraocular lens implantation, glaucoma fistulating surgery, and vitreous surgery; or extraocular: strabismus surgery and retinal detachment repair. Cataract surgery with prosthetic lens implantation is one of the most frequently performed of all surgical procedures in the developed world. Surgical infection associated with intraocular lenses is very infrequently seen compared with prostheses used in other surgical specialties. Silicone explants are applied to the external surface of the sclera in retinal detachment repair and these occasionally are associated with late extraocular infection and explant extrusion.

In this chapter, consideration will be given to

- prevention of infection in intraocular surgery;
- post-operative endophthalmitis and its management;
- infection following penetrating trauma.

Prevention of infection in intraocular surgery

The interior of the eye is sterile. The lids, conjunctiva, and tear film of normal individuals are colonized by commensal bacteria, usually coagulase-negative staphylococci (CNS), corynebacteria, or micrococci (1). Normal external eye flora are the predominant source of infecting bacteria and measures to prevent post-operative intraocular infection are fully justified. These include the pre-operative investigation, and use of topical antibiotic prophylaxis, appropriate surgical preparation, and technique.

Pre-operative investigation

The history and examination will identify some of the risk factors which might lead to intraocular infection. Atopic subjects have colonization of the eyelid skin by *Staphylococcus aureus* (2), a bacterium of comparatively greater pathogenicity in the eye than *Staph. epidermidis*. Similarly, patients with a history of infective blepharitis, or nasolacrimal duct obstruction are at higher risk of having pathogenic bacteria present. Every patient must be examined for active infection of the lid margin, conjunctiva, or lacrimal sac.

Culture for bacteria is indicated only in patients in whom infection is suspected. Surgery on patients with external eye infection should be postponed to allow adequate treatment. This may include drainage of the lacrimal sac if there is obstruction and regurgitation.

Antibiotic prophylaxis

The influence of antibiotics given prior to intraocular surgery on the incidence of endophthalmitis is uncertain because it has not been demonstrated in a controlled prospective trial. Such a trial, with a large number of patients and controls, is needed to obtain a statistically significant effect on the incidence of endophthalmitis (3).

There is a wide variation in use of pre- and post-operative antibiotics among ophthalmologists. Unresolved issues include the most effective agent, the dose, and duration of prophylaxis prior to surgery, and even the necessity for prophylactic antibiotics at all. Compared with untreated control eyes, topical antibiotic therapy reduces, but rarely eliminates the commensal flora. Gentamicin 0.3 per cent drops given prior to surgery and continued post-operatively decreased bacterial counts more effectively than chloramphenicol 0.5 per cent in a randomized controlled study by Burns and Oden (4). In another study, intensive topical administration of fusidic acid for two days was found to be as effective as gentamicin in reducing commensal flora (5).

In contrast, Dallison *et al.*, in a double-blind study, found that neither fusidic acid 1.0 per cent nor chloramphenicol produced a statistically significant reduction in the ocular microflora (6). This result was interpreted to indicate that the effect of topical antibiotic in clinical infection cannot be extrapolated to the effect on commensal flora, at least in terms of short-term prophylactic use. On the basis of the study by Burns and Oden (4), and irrespective of other factors such as cost, gentamicin appears to be the antibiotic of choice for the reduction of the external commensal flora. However, as with a number of other antibiotics which quantitatively reduce the external flora, its use as a prophylactic agent has not been shown to prevent intraocular infection.

Subconjunctival antibiotic, given immediately before surgery or after closing the eye, was shown by Kolker *et al.* to be superior to no prophylaxis (7). This observation was based on a lower incidence of endophthalmitis clinically diagnosed, but not confirmed bacteriologically. The antibiotics injected were a combination of penicillin G and streptomycin, no longer in general use; subconjunctival injection was not compared with topical prophylaxis.

In criticism of this route of therapy, Aronstam suggested that subconjunctival antibiotics, administered intra-operatively, might lead to higher incidence of delayed infection presenting at a time when the patient would no longer be under close supervision by an ophthalmologist (8).

Intra-operative intraocular administration is yet another reported route of administration of antibiotic prophylaxis, with similarly questionable conclusions. In cataract surgery camps in India, Peyman *et al.* injected gentamicin 50 μg into the anterior chamber at the end of surgery, and found that a lower rate of endophthalmitis resulted than in those patients treated with combined oral and topical chloramphenicol (9). Antibiotic toxicity to the corneal endothelium is a possible hazard of this route of administration and it was suggested by Peyman *et al.* that its use should be limited to areas of the world where there is a high risk of infection.

Surgical preparation and technique

Immediately prior to surgery, most ophthalmologists prepare the external eye and lid skin with disinfectant solution. The solution most widely used is povidone–iodine 5 per cent (diluted from 10 per cent stock solution with normal saline). This is a broad spectrum disinfectant which is effective in reducing the conjunctival bacterial flora (10). It has not been associated with corneal or ocular toxicity when applied in a single dose to the intact ocular surface (11, 12).

Use of a sterile plastic surgical drape to cover the eyelid margins when the eye is widely opened can isolate the potentially infective lid margins from the surgical field. This prevents inoculation of surgical instruments, sutures and intraocular lens implants with commensal bacteria.

As in general surgery, aseptic technique is used at all times. Particular risk of bacterial contamination attends contact between the intraocular lens implant and the conjunctiva or cornea (13): the prosthetic lens must be transferred directly from its sterile container into the eye.

Post-operative endophthalmitis and its management

Endophthalmitis following cataract, glaucoma or penetrating corneal surgery has steadily decreased in incidence this century. With advances is aseptic technique, antimicrobial agents, suture materials and wound closure generally, the incidence of endophthalmitis following cataract surgery has been variably reported as one per cent or less (14). Infection is bacterial in most cases, with *Staph. epidermidis*, *Staph. aureus*, and *Pseudomonas aeruginosa* being isolated most commonly (15, 16). Fungal infection is very rare and tends to present at a longer interval after surgery.

Acute post-operative endophthalmitis

The clinical presentation of post-operative bacterial endophthalmitis is characteristic, and early diagnosis is imperative as prognosis rapidly worsens with any delay.

Endophthalmitis caused by *Staph. aureus*, streptococci, or Gram-negative bacteria usually presents on the first or second day following surgery. CNS infection may not present until the third or fourth day. Pain is characteristic of endophthalmitis. It is accompanied by poor vision and severe anterior chamber inflammation, manifest as fibrin strands in the aqueous and frequently hypopyon (Fig. 28.1). Lid and conjunctival oedema are usually seen and this degree of inflammation is far in excess of that usually encountered in the days following surgery. No view of the vitreous or retina is possible once infection is established. Ultrasonography may show vitreous opacities; the presence of an afferent, or relative afferent, pupil defect indicates severe posterior segment damage.

Such marked inflammation following surgery is strongly suggestive of bacterial infection, but may be caused by a sterile inflammatory response to lens cortex remnants or to vitreous in the anterior chamber. Accordingly, bacteriological study of intraocular fluids at the earliest possible time is imperative. It is known that vitreous humour has a higher bacterial culture yield than aqueous (17). An aqueous sample is aspirated with a 27-gauge needle through the peripheral cornea. Vitreous is obtained through the pars plana either by needle paracentesis

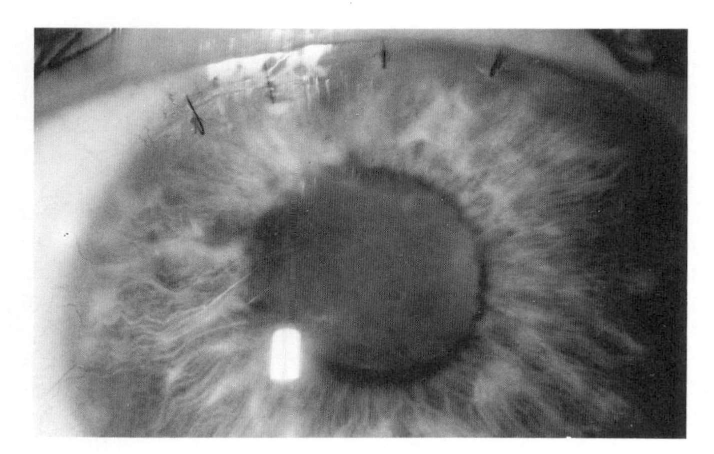

Fig. 28.1. Fibrinous membrane in the pupil, anterior to the intraocular lens implant, in a patient on the second day following surgery. The patient had pain and diminished visual acuity. *Staph.epidermidis* was cultured from aqueous and vitreous humour. (See plate section.)

or by an automated vitrectomy instrument. Glass slides are inoculated for Gram stain, and media for culture of aerobic and anaerobic bacteria and fungi.

Intravitreal antibiotics may be injected at the time of sample collection. This route of administration has become established since experimental data have become available on intraocular antibiotic levels and toxicity (18–20). At the present time, the authors recommend gentamicin 0.1 mg in 0.05 ml and vancomycin 2.0 mg in 0.1 ml normal saline. Based on the Gram stain, treatment also comprises intravenous, subconjunctival, and intensive topical antibiotic therapy. Gram-positive infections are treated with vancomycin or cephalosporin; Gram-negative infections are treated with gentamicin; those patients with no bacteria seen on Gram stain in whom bacterial infection is suspected are treated with a combination. Current experience is limited, but the indications are that the quinolone antibiotics, such as ciprofloxacin, may become established in therapy (21). In addition to antibacterial agents, topical mydriatic and hourly topical dexamethasone are given to dilate the pupil and to reduce inflammation respectively.

Vitrectomy has assumed a major role in the management of endophthalmitis, particularly if severe at presentation or not responding to antimicrobial therapy after 2–4 days. Rowsey has suggested vitrectomy in patients where vitreous inflammation prevents retinal visualization (22); Diamond has advocated vitrectomy if ultrasound demonstrates vitreous abscess formation (23). In addition to providing vitreous for culture, vitrectomy allows removal of infected vitreous, administration of antibiotics, clearance of the visual axis, and an opportunity to deal with complications associated with endophthalmitis such as pupillary inflammatory membranes and elevated intraocular pressure. The view of the fundus is often limited by inflammatory tissue in the anterior segment and by poor pupil dilatation, and only that vitreous which can be visualized can be cleared.

Delayed post-operative endophthalmitis

When the presentation of endophthalmitis is delayed, other infectious agents should be considered. Anaerobic endophthalmitis caused by *Propionibacterium acnes* characteristically presents as recurrent inflammation, partially responsive to steroid, at least three months after anterior segment surgery (24, 25). Fungal endophthalmitis, more commonly seen in immunocompromised patients and intravenous drug abusers, may cause post-operative endophthalmitis. It is characterized by an indolent course with mild symptoms and 'snowball' opacities in the vitreous.

Endophthalmitis complicating trabeculectomy may present many years after apparently successful glaucoma surgery, yet has acute onset, rapid progression and a poor visual prognosis (26). The common pathogens in this group are *Streptococcus* spp. and *Haemophilus influenzae* (27).

Different culture media are used to investigate delayed endophthalmitis. In general, close liaison with the microbiologists is helpful as many of the suspected organisms are fastidious and require long incubation times. Thioglycolate broth and anaerobic solid media are used for culture of *P. acnes*, Sabouraud agar for fungi, and chocolate agar for *H. influenzae*.

Vancomycin is the antibiotic of choice for chronic bacterial infections, including *P. acnes*. In endophthalmitis caused by fungi or complicating trabeculectomy, therapeutic vitrectomy is important. In fungal infection this is followed by sustained antimycotic treatment with amphotericin B or imidazole derivatives.

If instituted early, the results of treatment of post-operative endophthalmitis may be good, with recovery of good visual acuity. This is particularly so with the less virulent organisms such as *P. acnes*, fungi, and *Staph. epidermidis* infection in some cases (16). However, even with eradication of infection, many eyes with acute post-operative endophthalmitis do not obtain good vision and, in a number, phthisis bulbi results.

Infection following penetrating trauma

Following a penetrating eye injury, the priorities are: repair of the penetrating wound, removal of any intraocular foreign body (IOFB), repair of associated intraocular damage such as uveal prolapse or retinal detachment, and, possibly, administration of intraocular antibiotics. As in non-ocular penetrating injury, tetanus prophylaxis must be given at presentation: a booster or full course of tetanus toxoid to those within six hours of injury, and in addition, human tetanus immunoglobulin if the patient is not immunized.

Endophthalmitis is a possible complication of penetrating injury, but particularly if there is an IOFB. Endophthalmitis was reported by Barr to occur in only 4 of 22 eyes with penetrating injury where there was no IOFB (28). However, Williams *et al.* reported culture-positive endophthalmitis in 14 of 105 eyes with IOFBs (29).

In comparison with post-operative endophthalmitis, the striking features of traumatic infection are the high proportion of *Bacillus* and fungal infections, and the poorer visual prognosis. As in post-operative endophthalmitis, *Staph. epidermidis* is a commonly isolated pathogen. Brinton *et al.* isolated *Staph. epidermidis* in 7, and *Bacillus* species in 5 of 18 traumatic endophthalmitis cases (30). The series of 27 cases reported by Affeldt *et al.* included *Bacillus* infection in 8 and *Staph. epidermidis* in 6 patients (31). Injuries involving soil-contaminated IOFBs or vegetative matter have a higher incidence of *Bacillus* (30, 32) and fungal infection (31). The elaboration of toxins by *Bacillus* species (33) probably accounts for the rapidly worsening course of this infection and destruction of retinal tissue (15, 30–32).

In eyes without suspected endophthalmitis, prophylactic subconjunctival and topical antibiotics are usually given following surgical repair. Intraocular antibiotics are administered only in those patients in whom infection is suspected and vitreous aspirated for laboratory diagnosis. Taking into consideration the high incidence of *Bacillus* endophthalmitis, intraocular treatment should comprise vancomycin 1 mg and an aminoglycoside such as gentamicin 0.1 mg. If fungal infection is suggested by a history of trauma by vegetative material, amphotericin B 0.005 mg in 0.1 ml normal saline should be added. These agents are continued by intravenous, periocular and topical routes for at least five days according to clinical response. Vitrectomy, at the time of primary repair or after an interval, may enhance antibiotic effectiveness in addition to allowing IOFB removal and any other necessary surgical treatment.

In general, results of treatment of post-traumatic endophthalmitis have improved since the advent of vitrectomy techniques and intraocular antimicrobial agent injection (29). Prior to these advances, in many cases phthisis bulbi and loss of the eye resulted from injury. Nevertheless endophthalmitis following trauma has a much worse prognosis than that following surgery: this is particularly because of associated ocular injury, such as retinal detachment, and *Bacillus* infection.

References

1. Larkin, D.F.P. and Leeming, J.P. (1991). Alterations in the external eye bacteria in contact lens wear. *Eye*, **5**, 70–4.
2. Foster, C.S. and Calonge, M. (1990). Atopic keratoconjunctivitis. *Ophthalmology*, **97**, 992–1000.
3. Starr, M.B. (1983). Prophylactic antibiotics for ophthalmic surgery. *Surv. Ophthalmol.*, **27**, 353–73.
4. Burns, R.P. and Oden, M. (1972). Antibiotic prophylaxis in cataract surgery. *Trans. Am. Ophthalmol. Soc.*, **70**, 43–57.
5. Taylor, P.B., Tabbara, K.H., and Burd, E.M. (1988). Effect of pre-operative fusidic acid on the normal eyelid and conjunctival bacterial flora. *Br. J. Ophthalmol.*, **72**, 206–9.
6. Dallison, I.W., Simpson, A.J., Keenan, J.I., Clemett, R.S., and Allardyce, R.A. (1989). Topical antibiotic prophylaxis for cataract surgery: a controlled trial of fusidic acid and chloramphenicol. *Aust. NZ J. Ophthalmol.*, **17**, 289–93.
7. Kolker, A.E., Freeman, M.I., and Pettit, T.H. (1967). Prophylactic antibiotics and post-operative endophthalmitis. *Am. J. Ophthalmol.*, **63**, 434–9.
8. Aronstam, R.H. (1964). Pitfalls of prophylaxis. Alteration of post-operative infection by penicillin-streptomycin. *Am. J. Ophthalmol.*, **57**, 312–5.
9. Peyman, G.A., Sathur, M.L., and May, D.R. (1977). Intraocular gentamicin as intra-operative prophylaxis in South India eye camps. *Br. J. Ophthalmol.*, **61**, 260–2.
10. Isenberg, S.J., Apt, L., Yoshimori, R., and Khwarg, S. (1985). Chemical preparation of the eye in ophthalmic surgery: IV. Comparison of povidone–iodine on the conjunctiva with a prophylactic antibiotic. *Arch. Ophthalmol.*, **103**, 1340–2.
11. MacRae, S.M., Brown, B., and Edelhauser, H.F. (1984). The corneal toxicity of presurgical skin antiseptics. *Am. J. Ophthalmol.*, **97**, 221–232.
12. Wille H. (1982). Assessment of possible toxic effects of polyvinylpyrrolidone–iodine upon the human eye in conjunction with cataract extraction. *Acta Ophthalmol.*, **60**, 955–60.
13. Vafidis, G.C., Marsh, R.J., and Stacey, A.R. (1984). Bacterial contamination of intraocular lens surgery. *Br. J. Ophthalmol.*, **68**, 520–3.
14. Allen, H.F. (1978). Symposium: post-operative endophthalmitis. Introduction: incidence and aetiology. *Ophthalmology*, **85**, 317–19.
15. Puliafito, C.A., Baker, A.S., Haat, J., and Foster, C.S. (1982). Infectious endophthalmitis. Review of 36 cases. *Ophthalmology*, **89**, 921–9.
16. Olson, J.C., Flynn, H.W., Forster, R.K., and Culbertson, W.W. (1983). Results in the treatment of post-operative endophthalmitis. *Ophthalmology*, **90**, 692–9.
17. Forster, R.K., Abbott, R.L., and Gelender, H. (1980). Management of infectious endophthalmitis. *Ophthalmology*, **87**, 313–9.
18. Baum, J.L., Peyman, G.A., and Barza, M. (1982). Intravitreal administration of antibiotic in the treatment of bacterial endophthalmitis. III. Consensus. *Surv. Ophthalmol.*, **26**, 204–6.
19. Axelrod, J.L., Newton, J.C., Sarakhun, C., Lester, R.D., *et al.* (1985). Ceftriaxone: a new cephalosporin with aqueous humor levels effective against enterobacteriaceae. *Arch. Ophthalmol.*, **103**, 71–2.
20. Oum, B.S., D'Amico, D.J., and Wong, K.W. (1989). Intravitreal antibiotic therapy with vancomycin and aminoglycoside. An experimental study of combination and repetitive injections. *Arch. Ophthalmol.*, **107**, 1055–60.
21. Bron, A., Delbosc, B., Kaya, G., *et al.* (1988). Intérêt des quinolones en ophtalmologie, approche rationelle du traitment systèmique des endophtalmies bacteriennes. *Ophtalmologie*, **2**, 107–9.
22. Rowsey, J.J., Newsom, D.L., Sexton, D.J., and Harms, W.K. (1982). Endophthalmitis. Current approaches. *Ophthalmology*, **89**, 1055–66.
23. Diamond, J.G. (1981). Intraocular management of endophthalmitis. A systematic approach. *Arch. Ophthalmol.*, **99**, 96–9.
24. Roussel, T.J., Culbertson, W.W., and Jaffe, N.S. (1987). Chronic post-operative endophthalmitis associated with *Propionibacterium acnes*. *Arch. Ophthalmol.*, **105**, 1199–201.
25. Friberg, T.R. and Kuzma, P.M. (1990). *Propionibacterium acnes* endophthalmitis two years after extracapsular cataract extraction. *Am. J. Ophthalmol.*, **109**, 609–10.
26. Mandelbaum, S., Forster, R.K., Gelender, H., and Culbertson, W. (1985). Late onset endophthalmitis associated with filtering blebs. *Ophthalmology*, **92**, 964–72.
27. Flynn, H.W., Pflugfelder, S.C., Culbertson, W.W., and Davis, J.L. (1989). Recognition, treatment, and prevention of endophthalmitis. *Semin. Ophthalmol.*, **4**, 69–83.
28. Barr, C.C. (1983). Prognostic factors in corneoscleral lacerations. *Arch. Ophthalmol.*, **101**, 919–24.
29. Williams, D.F., Mieler, W.F., Abrams, G.W., and Lewis, H. (1988). Results and prognostic factors in penetrating ocular injuries with retained intraocular foreign bodies. *Ophthalmology*, **95**, 911–6.

30. Brinton, G.S., Topping, T.M., Hyndiuk, R.A., *et al.* (1984). Posttraumatic endophthalmitis. *Arch. Ophthalmol.*, **102**, 547–50.
31. Affeldt, J.C., Flynn, H.W., Forster, R.K., *et al.* (1987). Microbial endophthalmitis resulting from ocular trauma. *Ophthalmology*, **94**, 407–13.
32. O'Day, D.M., Smith, R.S., Gregg, C.R., *et al.* (1981). The problem of *Bacillus* species infection with special emphasis on the virulence of *Bacillus cereus*. *Ophthalmology*, **88**, 833–8.
33. Turnbull, P.C.B. and Kramer, J.M. (1983). Non-gastrointestinal *Bacillus cereus* infections: an analysis of exotoxin produced by strains isolated over a two year period. *J. Clin. Pathol.*, **36**, 1091–6.

29

Cardiothoracic surgery

DAVID P. TAGGART, A. CHRISTINE McCARTNEY, and DAVID J. WHEATLEY

Introduction

Infection is a significant cause of post-operative morbidity and mortality in patients undergoing cardiothoracic surgery. In addition to the general factors which predispose to infection, such as poor surgical technique, lengthy operations, increasing age, and malnutrition, the use of cardiopulmonary bypass and a period in an intensive care unit further predispose cardiac patients to infection. In patients undergoing pulmonary and oesophageal resections, lung infection is a common problem.

Cardiac surgery

Cardiac surgery has traditionally been regarded as 'clean' surgery in the absence of obvious sources of bacterial contamination. The most important infections are endocarditis in patients undergoing valve replacement and sternal wound infections in any patient following a median sternotomy. Cardiac surgical patients are particularly prone to infection because of certain requirements for open-heart surgery:

(a) The need for intensive invasive monitoring (which routinely requires central venous and radial artery cannulation, urinary catheters and occasionally Swan–Ganz catheters).

(b) Systemic activation of inflammatory mediators, such as complement, in the extracorporeal circuit produces 'whole-body inflammation' and widespread impairment of the immune system (1, 2) and a non-infective pyrexia for a few days following surgery.

(c) Exposure of a wide operative field and return of spilled blood in the chest to the pump ('cardiotomy suction') (3).

(d) The large number of medical and paramedical theatre staff necessary for cardiac surgery.

(e) The occasional requirement for mechanical support devices resulting in potential portals of entry for micro-organisms.

(f) The use of immunosuppressive drugs in transplant patients.

Thoracic surgery

In addition to the attendant risks of any major surgical procedure, patients requiring thoracic surgical procedures are more susceptible to infection through the general debilitation associated with cachexia of bronchial and oesophageal malignancies or chronic lung infection. Lung infection is an invariable component of bronchiectasis and also frequently accompanies bronchial neoplasms due to airways obstruction and oesophageal malignancies due to 'overspill'. Pre-operative physiotherapy reduces post-operative pulmonary complications in patients undergoing upper abdominal surgery (4), and is likely to be of even greater benefit in patients having pulmonary operations where there is pre-existing lung infection.

Empyema complicates approximately 1 per cent of pneumonias and can be suspected by aspiration of pleural fluid with a pH less than 7.0, lowered glucose, and elevated lactate dehydrogenase. Empyema can occur after any open chest procedure or instrumental perforation and is more common where underlying malignancy, chronic pulmonary problems and alcohol or drug addiction exist. While an 'acute' empyema can usually be managed by a combination of thoracocentesis (with or without tube thoracostomy) and antibiotics, the chronic empyema usually requires more diligent surgical intervention and obliteration of the pleural space.

Lung abscess may be secondary to any oesophageal condition which predisposes to 'overspill', including acute intoxication with alcohol or drugs, or may occur in association with malignancies, infarction or inadequate treatment of a pneumonia. Treatment, which includes diagnostic and therapeutic bronchoscopy, is aimed at the underlying disease process. Antibiotics are directed towards the organisms responsible, which are usually a combination of anaerobic (*Bacteroides* sp., *Fusobacterium* sp., and streptococci) and aerobic (staphylococci and Gram-negative bacilli) organisms. Antibiotic treatment should be continued for six to eight weeks and is most likely to succeed in younger patients with a clinical history of less than two months duration, a cavity of less than 3 cm diameter and no underlying bronchial disease.

Intensive care

In general, the risks of infection in a specialized cardiac intensive care unit (ICU) are fewer than in a general ICU; in the former few patients will have primary infections compared with the latter. One study which compared total infection rates in different ICUs within one hospital reported a 1 per cent incidence in the cardiac surgery ICU compared with 23.5 per cent in the general ICU; furthermore the incidence of acquired infection was 0.8 per cent in the cardiac ICU compared with 11.2 per cent in the general ICU (5). The majority of cardiac surgery patients stay in ICU for less than 24 h and most problems are those of acquired infection in long-stay patients. It was previously believed that most ICU-acquired infections were exogenous from other patients, the staff, and the environment, but it is increasingly recognized that most acquired infections are endogenous from the oropharynx or other parts of the gastrointestinal tract (6). Primary infection with endogenous organisms usually arises within three days of prolonged ventilation and is due to bacteria such as *Streptococcus pneumoniae*, *Haemophilus influenzae*, *Branhamella catarrhalis*, *Staphylococcus aureus*, and *Escherichia coli* which are present in the oropharynx or other parts of the gastrointestinal tract in otherwise healthy patients; in contrast secondary infection usually occurs in patients ventilated for more than seven days and is due to bacteria such as *Enterobacter* sp. and *Pseudomonas* sp. (7).

Heart–lung transplantation

As well as facing the standard risks of infection of cardiac surgery, transplant patients are additionally susceptible because of immunosuppressive therapy. Infection and rejection remain the main clinical problems associated with transplantation and may be clinically difficult to distinguish as they give rise to similar clinical features and may occur simultaneously. Infection accounts for up to half of early post-transplant deaths and may arise from blood transfusion, from the allograft, from nosocomial or environmental sources, from endogenous microbial flora, or from latent infection (8). The rate of infectious complications is related to the dose of immunosuppressive therapy but may be less with current regimens of cyclosporine, azathioprine, and steroids than with previous regimens. A recent review (8) of infectious complications of transplantation demonstrates that all classes of micro-organisms including bacteria (staphylococci, Gram-negative enteric bacteria and *Nocardia* sp.), fungi (*Aspergillus* sp., *Candida* sp., *Cryptococcus* sp.), viruses (cytomegalovirus, herpes simplex, herpes zoster), and protozoa (*Pneumocystis carinii*, *Toxoplasma gondii*) can infect recipients.

The threshold for suspecting infection in a transplant recipient should be very low at all times; while blood, urine, and sputum are being cultured it is usually prudent to perform simultaneous endomyocardial biopsy to exclude rejection. One simple precaution to reduce the risk of transmission of infection is to avoid the transplantation of organs from donors with serological evidence of cytomegalovirus or toxoplasmosis to sero-negative recipients. Recipients should also be screened for infection as re-activation can occur.

All transplant patients are prone to respiratory infections which emphasises the importance of early extubation and the need to avoid re-intubation.

Associated risks

The associated risks which predispose to infection are the same as those which apply in other areas of medicine and include poor surgical techniques, indiscriminate use of antibiotics, old age, and diabetes mellitus. Immunosuppression is a particular risk for transplant patients (see Chapter 4).

Antibiotic prophylaxis in cardiothoracic surgery

The principles of antibiotic prophylaxis are the same in cardiothoracic surgery as for any other surgical procedure. Prophylactic antibiotics are not a substitute for good surgical technique and should be used in a discriminating fashion to minimize the risk of bacterial overgrowth. Two questions remain to be resolved regarding antibiotic prophylaxis: broad versus narrow spectrum prophylaxis, and the optimal duration of treatment.

Coronary artery surgery

The predominant infective risk in coronary artery bypass graft (CABG) surgery is the development of deep sternal wound infection which is a catastrophic complication requiring prolonged hospital treatment and which can be fatal. The reported incidence varies from 0.5 to 4.5 per cent (9). The role of antibiotic prophylaxis in coronary artery surgery was unresolved until 1979. Fong *et al.* (10) in the first prospective double-blind study of drug (methicillin) versus placebo, in 105 patients, showed a reduction in sternotomy infections from 21 per cent in the placebo group to 0 per cent in the antibiotic group. In 1985 a repeat antibiotic versus placebo study was abandoned because 12 of 22 patients in the placebo group developed sternal wound infections compared with 1 of 16 patients treated with cephradine (11). However, Sutherland's prospective randomized trial of 904 patients (12) failed to show any benefit of prophylaxis in sternal wound infections with an infection rate of 1.1 per cent in the prophylactic group which was not significantly different from 1.76 per cent in the placebo group.

The predominant organism in wound infections is *Staph. aureus*. Coagulase-negative staphylococci (CNS) and diphtheroids are also commonly isolated from leaking sternal wounds and, although traditionally regarded as contaminants, they have more recently been incriminated in poor wound healing. The suggestion by Wells *et al.* (13) that saphenous vein transferred from the leg to the chest may be contaminated with Gram-negative bacteria thereby resulting in a 'clean-contaminated' operation, has subsequently been confirmed (14).

There is still controversy about the optimal antibiotic prophylaxis and the duration for which it should be given. Prophylactic antibiotics should have good activity against *Staph. aureus* and preferably also against CNS and diphtheroids. Most centres use either flucloxacillin alone, a cephalosporin alone, or a combination of flucloxacillin and an aminoglycoside (15).

It is increasingly apparent that there is no evidence to support continuation of prophylaxis beyond the early post-operative period (16) as effective prophylaxis depends on adequate serum and tissue concentrations of antibiotics *during* the operative period. Soteriou *et al.* demonstrated no difference in infection rates with antibiotic prophylaxis for four days or two days and subsequently reported that prophylaxis with a single pre-operative dose of ceftriaxone 2 g was as effective as four 0.5 g doses administered over 24 h (17).

Valve surgery

Post-operative endocarditis is usually referred to as 'early' or 'late'. Early endocarditis, arbitrarily described as occurring within two months post-operatively, might reasonably be considered perioperative infection and thus be amenable to prophylactic antibiotic therapy. Antibiotic prophylaxis for valve replacement was introduced by Starr's group in the early 1960s (18) after noting a high incidence of staphylococcal prosthetic heart valve endocarditis (PVE). The incidence of prosthetic endocarditis has fallen since then, though it is uncertain how much prophylactic antibiotics have contributed to this fall since there has also been steady improvement in surgical practice and equipment. A study of over 2000 patients having valve replacement between 1975 and 1982 showed an incidence of early prosthetic endocarditis of 1.45 per cent, 3.1 per cent at 1 year and 5.7 per cent at 5 years (19).

There has been no prospective randomized study to demonstrate the efficacy of antibiotic prophylaxis for valve replacement. An attempt by Goodman *et al.* at a prospective, randomized, double-blind trial to compare antibiotics with placebo in valve surgery was abandoned when two patients in the placebo group developed pneumococcal endocarditis (20). It would now be considered unethical to compare antibiotic and placebo in this setting. The only uncertainty at present is the optimal prophylactic regimen. With the current low incidence of PVE it would be difficult to prove the superiority of any one regimen over another. Opinions differ between those favouring broad spectrum (cephalosporins) to those favouring narrow spectrum flucloxacillin alone on the basis that *Staph. aureus* is the most likely organism.

Thoracic surgery

Antibiotic prophylaxis is widely employed for thoracic surgical procedures. Two prospective, randomized, double-blind studies have reported that cephalosporin prophylaxis significantly reduces wound infections but, although pulmonary infections were reduced, the differences between control and test groups did not reach statistical significance (21, 22).

The role of antibiotic prophylaxis in oesophageal surgery has not been clearly elucidated in the absence of large numbers of patients undergoing oesophageal resections. The normal oesophageal microflora consists of a mixture of aerobic and anaerobic organisms probably derived from the mouth (23) which proliferate in the obstructed oesophagus (24) and which are similar to those found in empyema (25). The most appropriate antibiotic prophylaxis therefore requires broad spectrum activity and Finlay *et al.* (24) have recommended the use of ampicillin or penicillin in combination with metronidazole and gentamicin. In a blind, randomized study, single-dose cefamandole has been reported to reduce wound infection following oesophageal resections for carcinoma (26).

Infective endocarditis

Infective endocarditis is an infection of the heart valves, and sometimes of the endocardium around congenital defects. Infective endocarditis was formerly known as subacute bacterial endocarditis but the nomenclature has changed with recognition that fungi, rickettsia, and chlamydia can also cause endocarditis. Before the advent of antibiotics, infective endocarditis had a mortality of 100 per cent. It still has a mortality of about 30 per cent despite improvements in antimicrobial agents and in surgical techniques and materials. The optimal management of infective endocarditis requires a team approach involving the cardiologist, microbiologist, cardiothoracic surgeon, and dentist. If surgical intervention is indicated, the cardiothoracic surgeon should be familiar with the patient's progress during medical treatment.

Pathophysiology and presentation

Infective endocarditis usually occurs at the site of a predisposing heart lesion or defect where a high velocity jet of blood leads to increased turbulence and damage to the endocardial surface. On such surfaces a platelet-fibrin clot is deposited and this clot, initially sterile, acts as a nidus for any micro-organisms released into the bloodstream from dental or other sources. Thereafter, the clot is an 'infected vegetation' which is relatively avascular. It is poorly understood, however, why some micro-organisms have a greater propensity for causing endocarditis than others, or how previously normal valves may become infected. For a detailed review of the pathogenesis of infective endocarditis see Freedman (27).

In the pre-antibiotic era subacute bacterial endocarditis commonly presented as a low grade febrile illness, usually in patients with rheumatic heart disease. Clinical examination revealed classical signs of endocarditis such as splinter haemorrhages, Osler nodes, Roth spots, and Janeway lesions (28, 29), which it is now known are due to formation of immune complexes. As infection progressed, patients died of cardiac failure or from a major embolic episode. Nowadays the presenting clinical features are more subtle, usually with rigors, fever, and often anorexia and malaise (30). There are several reasons for this and not least is the changing pattern of infective endocarditis; rheumatic fever is now less common while degenerative valve disease is more common, in an increasingly elderly population. There is also a greater prevalence of prosthetic heart valves, an increasing number of intravenous drug abusers, and an increased use of intravascular catheters, as well as the introduction of more effective antimicrobial agents. Coincident with this there has been a change in the causative micro-organisms. Classically, the predominant group of causative micro-organisms were the streptococci, but now staphylococci, both *Staph. aureus* and CNS, and other organisms are found.

In Table 29.1 the causative micro-organisms from 69 episodes of infective endocarditis in Glasgow Royal Infirmary during 1984–1989 are presented. In our series, there are equal numbers of *Staph. aureus* and streptococci. This may be related in part to the increase in *Staph. aureus* endocarditis in intravenous drug abusers and also to the fact that, as a tertiary referral centre, we do not see many of the patients with streptococcal endocarditis treated medically with success in other hospitals.

Table 29.1. Glasgow Royal Infirmary—Infective endocarditis, September 1984–August 1989. Organisms causing endocarditis in 69 episodes of infection.

Organism	Episodes
Staphylococcus aureus	25
Streptococci	25
Coagulase-negative staphylococci	10
Yeast	4
Coxiella burneti	1
Culture-negative	4
	69

Management

The clinician should always consider infective endocarditis in patients with fever, malaise, anorexia, and weight loss. The 'at risk' groups of patients include those with prosthetic valves or congenital heart defects as well as intravenous drug abusers. However, individuals with no previous underlying cardiac abnormality also constitute a significant number of patients with infective endocarditis (31). Table 29.2 details the predisposing factors in 69 episodes of infective endocarditis in our centre. The patients with no previously suspected heart disease, excepting intravenous drug abusers, are second in number to patients with prosthetic valve infective endocarditis.

Table 29.2. Infective endocarditis—Glasgow Royal Infirmary September 1984–August 1989. Predisposing cardiac conditions in 69 episodes of infective endocarditis.

Condition	Episodes
None previously suspected	31*
Prosthetic valve	24
Congenital heart disease	10
Rheumatic heart disease	4
	69

* 15 intravenous drug abusers

Blood cultures are the cornerstone of diagnosis of infective endocarditis and must be taken wherever clinical suspicion of endocarditis arises, and before antibiotics are commenced. The bacteraemia of endocarditis is consistent and low grade (32). Three blood cultures should be collected within 12–24 hours of the suspected diagnosis and usually the causative organism is isolated in the first two sets of cultures. Antibiotic therapy should not, however, be delayed until the results of blood cultures are available in patients with a definite clinical diagnosis of endocarditis. A combination of benzyl penicillin, 12 mega-units daily in 4-hourly doses, with gentamicin 80 mg is recommended (33). However, in patients with a history of intravenous drug abuse, recent cardiac surgery, or with skin infection, flucloxacillin is recommended in addition to penicillin and gentamicin. When the results of blood cultures are available, the antibiotic therapy may be adjusted accordingly. Recommendations for treatment of streptococcal and staphylococcal endocarditis have been made by the Endocarditis Working Party of the British Society for Antimicrobial Chemotherapy (BSAC) (33). In some patients with a clinical diagnosis of endocarditis, blood cultures may be negative. Often there is a history of prior administration of antibiotics, but usually these patients respond to therapy with penicillin and gentamicin. In medical patients with negative blood cultures the most frequent non-bacterial cause is *Coxiella burneti* and Q-fever endocarditis is diagnosed by detection of phase 1 and phase 2 antibodies to this organism by serum complement fixation test.

The microbiological diagnosis of infective endocarditis is essential for optimal antimicrobial therapy. The microbiology laboratory is not only responsible for isolation of the causative micro-organism but also in guiding therapy from the results of antimicrobial sensitivity tests. The minimum inhibitory concentration (often abbreviated to MIC) and minimum bactericidal concentration (often abbreviated to MBC) tests are necessary to guide dosage and ensure adequate serum antibiotic levels. It is recommended that frequent assays of aminoglycosides and vancomycin serum levels are performed in patients during therapy to minimize the development of toxicity.

The serum bactericidal test is widely used to assess the response to therapy but there is little evidence to date that this test is of prognostic value (34). However, there would appear to be a correlation between post-dose bactericidal titres of greater than 1 in 8 and bacteriological cure (35). There is evidence that measurements of C-reactive protein concentrations in patients with infective endocarditis are useful in monitoring the response to treatment and also to detect other infections and complications (36).

Of all the cardiological investigations in patients with infective endocarditis, echocardiography is particularly helpful. Echocardiography can detect vegetations and also assess haemodynamic status. Diagnostic sensitivity of echocardiography varies from 20 to 80 per cent depending on both the size of the vegetation and also when the echo is performed. It is important to realize that a negative finding on echo does not exclude the diagnosis of infective endocarditis. A large vegetation on the tricuspid value of an intravenous drug abuser is shown in the echocardiograph in Fig. 29.1

Antimicrobial therapy alone is usually adequate for treatment of infective endocarditis with the viridans groups of streptococci. Failure of medical treatment is often due to the presence of large vegetations, aneurysms, abscesses, especially of the aortic root, and particularly resistant micro-organisms, such as *Staph. aureus* or fungal endocarditis. We have recently had experience of five unusual cases of endocarditis with *Streptococcus agalactiae* (Group B streptococcus) and we advocate early surgery in such endocarditis because of the florid nature of the infection (37).

Valve replacement has had a major influence in reducing mortality and morbidity in patients with infective endocarditis and surgery has significantly reduced the mortality in patients with heart failure (38). Indications for surgical intervention include failure to control the infection with antimicrobial agents alone, haemodynamic deterioration, systemic embolization, echocardiographic changes, pericardial effusions, tamponade, or conduction defects.

Often the nature of the causative micro-organism itself can indicate early surgery, e.g. *Staph. aureus*, yeast, or CNS in early prosthetic valve endocarditis. The duration of antibiotic therapy has little influence on the timing of surgery with the main indications being deteriorating haemodynamic status, uncontrolled infection and embolic episodes.

Prosthetic valve endocarditis

The incidence of early PVE (occurring within two months of surgery) is generally less than 1 per cent but, when it does occur, is associated with a mortality rate of 70 per cent. The main causative micro-organisms are *Staph. aureus* and coagulase-negative staphylococci (Table 29.3). The potential sources of the infection are numerous and include the prosthesis itself, the intravascular lines, pacing wires, and urinary catheters. Such devices are readily colonized by skin commensals, namely the staphylococci and diphtheroids which are derived from staff or from the skin of patients themselves. When such an infection occurs it is often extremely difficult to identify the source. Early PVE can be minimized by good

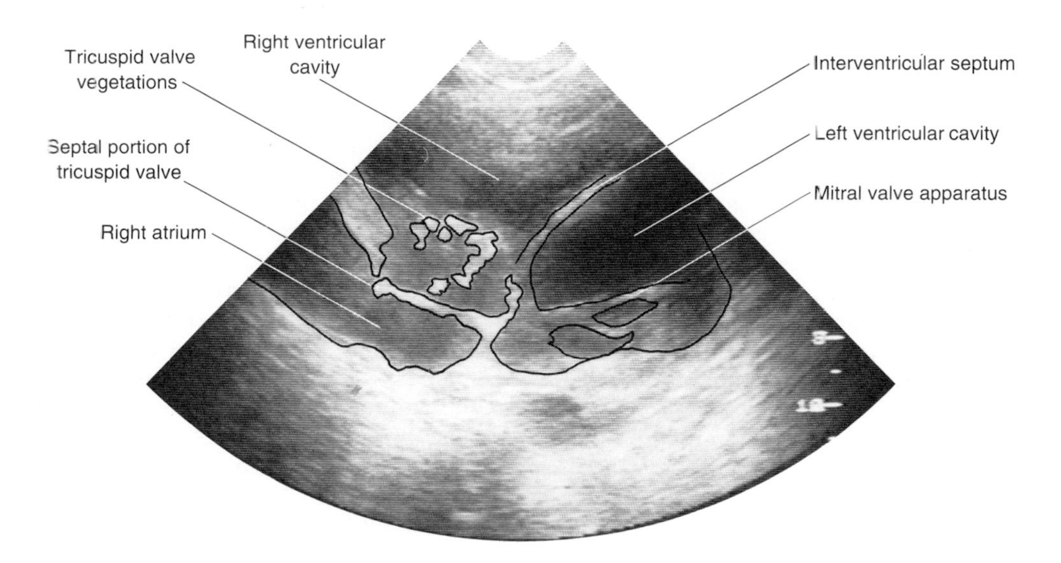

Fig. 29.1. A two-dimensional echocardiogram showing a large vegetation on the tricuspid valve. [Reproduced by kind permission of Dr D. A. S. Marshall, Department of Medical Cardiology, Glasgow Royal Infirmary.]

Table 29.3. Causative organisms in prosthetic valve endocarditis.

Causative organism	Percentage of isolates			
	Karchmer (39) (n = 125)	Mayer and Schoenbaum (40) (n = 462)	Calderwood *et al.* (19) (n = 116)	McCartney *et al.* (n = 26) (unpub.)
Coagulase-negative staphylococci	47	28	44	48
Staph. aureus	10	14	9	20
Streptococci	19	25	16	20
Aerobic Gram-negative bacilli	2	15	4	–
Diphtheroids	9	7	4	–
Fastidious Gram-negative coccobacilli	6	–	7	–
Fungi	2	9	4	12

surgical technique, strict attention to asepsis in theatre, and appropriate perioperative antibiotic prophylaxis (see above).

The causative micro-organisms of late PVE (occurring any time more than two months after surgery) are most often viridans streptococci as for native valve endocarditis. Consequently efforts in preventing late PVE have been directed towards minimizing bacteraemia from dental procedures. This involves appropriate dentistry prior to valve surgery, good dental hygiene, and antibiotic prophylaxis for dental procedures after surgery. Procedures which may be associated with bacteraemia should also be covered by prophylactic antibiotics. These would include urinary tract interventions, colonic surgery, or surgery for infective problems.

PVE nearly always requires a longer period of antibiotic therapy than native valve endocarditis. We recommend six weeks' therapy for early PVE and it is not uncommon to require early surgery (41). Triple therapy of vancomycin, rifampicin, and an aminoglycoside for two weeks followed by a further four weeks of vancomycin and rifampicin is recommended for early PVE with CNS (42).

Management of related surgical infections

Septicaemia is the most serious of all surgical infections following cardiothoracic surgery. Micro-organisms may invade the bloodstream from sternotomy wounds, chest infections, infection of the urinary tract, and colonized or infected central lines.

In the immediate post-operative period such infections may have dire implications. For example, a Gram-negative septicaemia may give rise to cardiovascular complications which may affect cardiac function and seriously compromise the patient. Any micro-organisms which enter into the bloodstream of a patient with a prosthetic valve may potentially cause PVE.

Post-operative management of cardiac patients must involve awareness of such sepsis. It is important that blood cultures are taken when a patient develops a sudden pyrexia and rigors. In the absence of a definite infective source it is prudent to provide broad spectrum antibiotic cover with a combination of ampicillin and gentamicin or cefuroxime alone until microbiological advice is available.

Sternotomy infection and mediastinitis

Median sternotomy is used for most cardiac surgical procedures and the reported incidence of deep sternal infection varies from 0.5 per cent to 4.5 per cent (9) while superficial disturbances of wound healing may be present in up to 16 per cent of patients (43). The latter is a minor cause of morbidity in contrast to deep sternal infections which can produce mediastinitis, generalized sepsis, disruption of coronary grafts or of the whole sternal wound, with infection of prosthetic valves resulting in significant morbidity and prolonged hospital stay or, indeed, the death of the patient.

Post-operative infections following valve replacement operations and CABG operations differ (13, 14). Sternal infection after valve replacement is uncommon and predominantly staphylococcal, whereas after CABG it is more common and caused by *Staph. aureus* or endogenous coliforms. Contamination of the graft from the skin of the leg is suggested as the source of these coliforms. When coliforms are isolated, the significance may be uncertain and often debridement is required to prove infection. Sternotomy infections are most commonly seen with slow-healing wounds which become infected. Primary sternotomy infection is usually due to *Staph. aureus* and flucloxacillin is the recommended antibiotic. Isolation of CNS and diphtheroids from sternal wounds is often of doubtful clinical significance. However, Bor *et al.* (9) believe that CNS may be a pathogen at the sternotomy site, which contains sawn bone debris, haematoma, wire, and bone wax.

In addition to the general factors which may predispose to wound infection already outlined, re-operation for bleeding is probably the most important contributor to subsequent deep wound infection. A comprehensive review of this topic is presented by Bor *et al.* (9).

Treatment of deep wound infection and sternal dehiscence is complex and may include debridement and delayed wound closure, debridement, sternal closure, and closed irrigation, or debridement and closure with muscle flaps as a primary or delayed procedure. Such treatment is complex and beyond the scope of this chapter but has been discussed by Scully *et al.* (44).

Post-operative chest infections

Respiratory complications can occur after any major operation but after cardiac surgery patients are ventilated for several hours and also have a sternotomy wound. The wound is a source of discomfort and coughing is often difficult for several days. This inevitably leads to some sputum retention and can give rise to respiratory tract infection in some 10–15 per cent of patients. Physiotherapy can help significantly and there are seldom serious clinical problems. However patients with pre-existing lung disease and patients who require prolonged assisted ventilation are more likely to develop respiratory infections. Those infections are usually manifest by pyrexia, production of purulent secretions and deranged blood gases. The commonest micro-organisms isolated from sputum or tracheal secretions are *H. influenzae* and *Strep. pneumoniae*. The antibiotic of choice is ampicillin or erythromycin. If there is no response to antibiotics, a respiratory screen for atypical causes of pulmonary infection such as *Mycoplasma* sp., *Legionella* sp., and viruses should be considered. There is no evidence that specific antibiotic prophylaxis reduces the incidence of post-operative chest infections. The adult respiratory distress syndrome (ARDS) may develop after cardiopulmonary bypass. It is characterized by diffuse bilateral pulmonary infiltrates, hypoxaemia, and respiratory distress (45). The pathogenesis of ARDS is poorly understood and there is no clinical or laboratory test for its diagnosis.

Line-associated infection

Management of intravenous and intra-arterial catheter lines is very important after cardiac surgery. These lines may become colonized with skin micro-organisms such as CNS and diphtheroids which can cause transient bacteraemia and early prosthetic valve endocarditis. With meticulous attention to aseptic techniques, line-associated infections should not be a significant problem.

Early recognition of catheter line-associated infection is important. Often the patient has a pyrexia, with a positive blood culture and no obvious source of infection. To confirm catheter line-associated bacteraemia, blood cultures must be taken from the catheter itself and from a peripheral vein. The latter is most important since it will confirm a bacteraemia whereas the line culture may simply reflect colonization of the line. When catheter sepsis is suspected or confirmed by blood cultures, the catheter should be removed and the tip sent for culture. There is no evidence to support the routine changing of non-infected lines.

Daily dressings of 'Opsite' on the skin around the catheter have been shown to be beneficial in removing the local skin bacteria at the insertion site (46). One simple method of reducing line sepsis may be the routine addition of 0.05% sodium metabisulphate as described by Freeman *et al.* for left atrial catheters (47).

Urinary tract infection

The monitoring of renal function in cardiac surgical patients requires urinary catheterization. This may be necessary for prolonged periods and daily bacteriological examination of urine should be performed in these patients since it is well-known that nosocomial urinary tract infections are related to the time the catheter is *in situ* (48). The organisms most commonly isolated from urinary tract infection are coliforms.

Infected implants

In addition to prosthetic valves, other implants which may become infected are pacemakers (49) or vascular conduits, particularly those used in replacement of sections of the aorta. Infection of such implants usually necessitates their removal (see Chapter 23).

Summary and conclusions

The general principles of preventing and treating infection in cardiothoracic surgery are, with a few exceptions, similar to those for other branches of surgery. The cardiac surgical patient may, however, be more susceptible to infection because of the need for extracorporeal perfusion, and the transplant patient even more so because of the need for immunosuppression. In the thoracic patient, pre-existing lung infection is frequently present which necessitates rigourous pre-and post-operative physiotherapy.

Antibiotic prophylaxis is now considered to be an essential part of the management of the cardiac patient and the thoracic patient but is not a substitute for punctilious surgical practice. It is not yet established, however, whether broad or narrow spectrum antibiotics provide optimal prophylaxis or whether single dose therapy is as effective as multiple dose therapy. For established infection, antibiotics should be used in a discriminating fashion based on the organism microbiologically proven to be responsible.

References

1. Kirklin, J.K., Westaby, S., Blackstone, E.H., Kirklin, J.W., Chenoweth, D.E., and Pacifico, A.D. (1983). Complement and the damaging effects of cardiopulmonary bypass. *J. Thorac. Cardiovasc. Surg.*, **86**, 845–7.
2. Utley, J.R. (1982). The immune response to cardiopulmonary bypass. In *Pathophysiology and techniques of cardiopulmonary bypass*, Vol 1 (ed. J.R. Utley), pp. 132–44. Williams & Wilkins, Baltimore.
3. Freeman, R. and Hjersing, N. (1980). Bacterial culture of perfusion blood after open heart surgery. *Thorax*, **35**, 754–8.
4. Morran, C.G., Finlay, I.G., Mathieson, M., McKay, A.J., Wilson, N., and McArdle, C.S. (1983). Randomized controlled trial of physiotherapy for post-operative pulmonary complications. *Br. J. Anaesth.*, **55**, 1113–7.
5. Brown, R.B., Hosmer, D., Chen, H.C., Teres, D., Sands, M., Bradley, S., *et al.* (1985). A comparison of infections in different ICUs within the same hospital. *Crit. Care Med.*, **13**, 472–6.
6. Ledingham, I.McA., Alcock, S.R., Eastaway, A.T., Mcdonald, J.C., McKay, I.C., and Ramsey, G. (1988). Triple regimen of

selective decontamination of the digestive tract, systemic cefotaxime, and microbiological surveillance for prevention of acquired infection in intensive care. *Lancet*, **i**, 785–90.

7. Van Saene, H.K., Stoutenbeek, C.A.P., Miranda, D.R., Zandstra, D.F., and Langrehr, D. (1986). Recent advances in the control of infection in patients with thoracic injury. *Injury*, **17**, 332–5.
8. Linder, J. (1988). Infection as a complication of heart transplantation. *J. Heart Transplant*, **7**, 390–4.
9. Bor, D.H., Rose, R.M., Modlin, J.F., Weintraub, R., and Friedland, G.H. (1983). Mediastinitis after cardiovascular surgery. *Rev. Infect. Dis.*, **5**, 885–97.
10. Fong, I.W., Baker, C.B., and McKee, D.C. (1979). The value of prophylactic antibiotics in aorta-coronary bypass operations. A double-blind randomized trial. *J. Thorac. Cardiovasc. Surg.*, **78**, 908–13.
11. Penketh, A.R.L., Wansbrough-Jones, M.H., Wright, E., Imrie, F., Pepper, J.R., and Parker, D.J. (1985). Antibiotic prophylaxis for coronary artery bypass graft surgery (letter). *Lancet*, **i**, 1500.
12. Sutherland, R.D., Martinez, H.E., Guynes, W.A., and Miller, L. (1977). Post-operative chest wound infections in patients requiring coronary bypass: a controlled study evaluating prophylactic antibiotics. *J. Thorac. Cardiovasc. Surg.*, **73**, 944–7.
13. Wells, F.C., Newsom, S.W., and Rowlands, C. (1983). Wound infection in cardiothoracic surgery. *Lancet*, **i**, 1209–10.
14. Farrington, M., Webster, M., Fenn, A., and Phillips, I. (1985). Study of cardiothoracic wound infection at St Thomas' Hospital. *Br. J. Surg.*, **72**, 759–62.
15. Wilson, A.P.R., Treasure, T., Sturridge, M.F., and Gruneberg, R.N. (1986). Antibiotic prophylaxis in cardiothoracic surgery in the United Kingdom: current practice. *Thorax*, **41**, 396–400.
16. Hillis, D.J., Rosenfeldt, F.L., Spicer, W.J., and Stirling, G.R. (1983). Antibiotic prophylaxis for coronary bypass grafting. Comparison of a five-day and a two-day course. *J. Thorac. Cardiovasc. Surg.*, **86**, 217–21.
17. Soteriou, M., Recker, F., Geroulanos, S., and Turina, M. (1989). Perioperative antibiotic prophylaxis in cardiovascular surgery: a prospective randomized comparative trial of cefazolin versus ceftriaxone. *World J. Surg.*, **13**, 798–802.
18. Herr, R., Starr, A., McCord, C.W., and Wood, J.A. (1965). Special problems following valve replacement. Embolus, leak, infection, red cell damage. *Ann. Thorac. Surg.*, **1**, 403–15.
19. Calderwood, S.B., Swinski, L.A., Waternaux, C.M., Karchmer, A.W., and Buckley, M.J. (1985). Risk factors for the development of prosthetic valve endocarditis. *Circulation*, **72**, 31–7.
20. Goodman, J.S., Schaffner, W., Collins, H.A., Battersby, E.J., and Koenig, M.G. (1968). Infection after cardiovascular surgery: clinical study including examination of antimicrobial prophylaxis. *N. Engl. J. Med.*, **278**, 117–23.
21. Ilves, R., Cooper, J.D., Todd, T.R.J., and Pearson, F.G. (1981). Prospective randomized, double-blind study using prophylactic cephalothin for major, elective, general thoracic operations. *J. Thorac. Cardiovasc. Surg.*, **81**, 813–7.
22. Walker, W.S., Faichney, A., Raychaudhury, T., Prescott, R.J., Calder, M.A., Sang, C.T.M., *et al.* (1984). Wound prophylaxis in thoracic surgery a new approach. *Thorax*, **39**, 121–4.
23. Mannell, A., Plant, M., and Frolich, J. (1983). The microflora of the oesophagus. *Ann. R. Coll. Surg. Engl.*, **65**, 152–4.
24. Finlay, I.G., Wright, P.A., Menzies, T., and McArdle, C.S. (1982). Microbial flora in carcinoma of oesophagus. *Thorax*, **37**, 181–4.
25. Bartlett, J.G., Gorbach, S.L., Thadepalli, H., and Finegold, S.M. (1974). Bacteriology of empyema. *Lancet*, **i**, 338–40.
26. Little, G., Alvins, E., and Matthews, H.R. (1981). Prophylactic antibiotics in oesophageal resection. *Thorax*, **36**, 73.
27. Freedman, L.R. (1987). The pathogenesis of infective endocarditis. *J. Antimicrob. Chemother.*, **20** (Suppl A), 1–6.
28. Cates, J.E. and Christie, R.V.. (1951). Subacute bacterial endocarditis. *Q. J. Med.*, **20**, 93–130.
29. Schnurr, L.P., Ball, A.P., Geddes, A.M., Gray, J., and McGhie, D. (1977). Bacterial endocarditis in England in the 1970s, a review of 70 patients. *Q. J. Med.*, **46**, 499–512.
30. Bain, R.J., Geddes, A.M., Littler, W.A., and McKinlay, A.W. (1987). The clinical and echocardiographic diagnosis of infective endocarditis. *J. Antimicrob. Chemother.*, **20** (Suppl A), 17–27.
31. Shanson, D.C., and Littler, W.A. (1989). Infective endocarditis. In *Septicaemia and endocarditis. Clinical and microbiological aspects*, (ed. D.C. Shanson), pp. 143–71. Oxford University Press, Oxford.
32. Werner, A.S., Cobbs, C.G., Kay, D., and Hook, E.W. (1967). Studies on the bacteraemia of bacterial endocarditis. *J. Am. Med. Assoc.*, **202**, 195–203.
33. Working Party of the British Society for Antimicrobial Chemotherapy. (1985). Antibiotic treatment of streptococcal and staphylococcal endocarditis. *Lancet*, **ii**, 815–7.
34. Coleman, D.L., Horwitz, R.I., and Andriole, V.T. (1982). Association between serum inhibitory and bactericidal concentrations and therapeutic outcome in bacterial endocarditis. *Am. J. Med.*, **73**, 260–7.
35. Stratton, C.W. (1987). The role of the microbiology laboratory in the treatment of infective endocarditis. *J. Antimicrob. Chemother.*, **20** (suppl. A), 41–9.
36. McCartney, A.C., Orange, G.V., Pringle, S.D., Wills, G., and Reece, I.J. (1988). Serum C—reactive protein in infective endocarditis. *J. Clin. Path.*, **41**, 44–8.
37. Pringle, S.D., McCartney, A.C., Marshall, D.A.S., and Cobbe, S.M. (1989). Infective endocarditis caused by *Streptococcus agalactiae*. *Int. J. Cardiol.*, **24**, 179–83.
38. Richardson, J.V., Karp, R.B., Kirklin, J.W., and Dismukes, W.E. (1978). Treatment of infective endocarditis: A 10 year comparative analysis. *Circulation*, **58**, 589–97.
39. Karchmer, A.W. (1984). Treatment of prosthetic valve endocarditis. In *Endocarditis* (ed. M.A. Sande, D. Kaye, and R.K. Root), pp. 163–82. Contemporary issues in infectious diseases Series, Vol. 2. Churchill Livingstone, New York.
40. Mayer, K.C. and Schoenbaum, S.C. (1982). Evaluation and management of prosthetic valve endocarditis. *Prog. Cardiovasc. Dis.*, **25**, 43–8.
41. Braimbridge, M.V., and Eykyn, S.J. (1987). Prosthetic valve endocarditis. *J. Antimicrob. Chemother.*, **20** (Suppl A), 173–80.
42. Karchmer, A.W. and Caputo, G.M. (1986). Endocarditis due to coagulase-negative staphylococci. In *Coagulase-negative staphylococci* (ed. P.A. Mårdh and K.H. Schleifer), pp. 179–87. Almqvist & Wiksell, Stockholm.
43. Wilson, A.P., Gruneberg, T.N., Treasure, T., and Sturridge, M.F. (1988). *Staphlococcus epidermidis* as a cause of post-operative wound infection after cardiac surgery: assessment of pathogenicity by a wound-scoring method. *Br. J. Surg.*, **75**, 168–70.
44. Scully, H.E., Leclerc, Y., Martin, R.D., Tong, C.P., Goldman, B.S., Weisel, R.D., *et al.* (1985). Comparison between antibiotic irrigation and mobilization of pectoral muscle flaps in treatment of deep sternal infections. *J. Thorac. Cardiovasc. Surg.*, **90**, 523–31.
45. Shale, D.J. (1987). The adult respiratory distress syndrome—20 years on (editorial). *Thorax*, **42**, 641–5.
46. Jarrard, M.M., Olson, C.M., and Freeman, J.B. (1980). Daily dressing change effects on skin flora beneath subclavian catheter

dressings during total parenteral nutrition. *J. Parent. Ent. Nutr.* **4**, 391–2.

47. Freeman, R., Holden, M.P., Lyon, R., and Hjersing, N. (1982). Addition of sodium metabisulphite to left atrial catheter infusates as a means of preventing bacterial colonization of the catheter tip. *Thorax*, **37**, 142–4.
48. Kunin, C.M. (1984). Genitourinary infections in the patient at risk: extrinsic factors. *Am. J. Med.*, **76**, 131–9.
49. Heimberger, T.S. and Doma, R.J. (1989). Infections of prosthetic heart valves and cardiac pacemakers. *Infect. Dis. Clin. North Am.*, **3**, 221–45.

Further Reading

Freeman, R. and Gould, F.K. (1987). *Infection in cardiothoracic intensive care*. Edward Arnold, London.

30

Orthopaedic surgery

SEAN P.F. HUGHES

Infection following total joint replacement

Total joint replacement is now commonplace. The number of total hip replacement operations performed in the UK each year is around 60 000. Total knee replacement is also widely practised and these amount to approximately 40 000 each year. Combined with other joint replacement operations undertaken for shoulders, elbows, toes and hands, the number of joints replaced is probably in excess of 150 000 per annum.

Historically, the incidence of infection following these procedures ranged from 5 to 10 per cent, producing horrendous problems and disability. Indeed, Sir John Charnley, the founder of modern total joint replacement, stated in 1982 that 'if post-operative infection continues between 1 and 5 per cent this operation can be justified only for the elderly and grossly disabled patients' (1). Clearly, if infection had continued at these high rates there would be a monumental problem. For example an orthopaedic surgeon undertaking 200 joint replacements each year would have up to 20 patients requiring extensive revision surgery, with prolonged hospitalization and disability of the patient. If this occurred in patients under the age of 60 years these patients would probably need to have several further operations and perhaps end up with disability far worse than their original complaint.

Therefore, there have been extensive programmes to prevent infection following joint replacement. This has been broadly along two main fronts:

1. Clean air
2. Antibiotic prophylaxis

Clean air

The concept of clean-air systems in the operating theatre is well established. Pathogenic organisms settle on debris greater than 12 μm diameter (2), circulate in the theatre, and can then enter a wound at the time of surgery. Air filters should remove particles greater than 5 μm. This is particularly important in hip or knee surgery where the area of exposure is large and the potential for infection is subsequently great. Blowers and Crew established the basis of clean operating theatre design and showed that there needs to be 15–20 air changes per hour in order to control this problem (3). Charnley developed the concept further and established the principles of the ultra clean air operating environment.

Charnley believed that in an ultra clean air environment all debris is removed from the operating field by the increased flow of air which is usually vertical in direction. The air changes are increased to 300 or more per hour. He combined this approach with the use of specially constructed suits which remove contaminants from the surgeons and assistants and reduced the rate of infection to less than 1 per cent (4).

This concept has been adopted widely and is the basis of modern orthopaedic practice. The Medical Research Council conducted a prospective trial involving over 8000 operations, in the UK and Sweden, and were able to demonstrate the efficacy of this method of reducing wound infection following total joint replacement (5).

Antibiotic prophylaxis

Another, or complementary approach, is the use of prophylactic antibiotics to prevent infection following total joint replacement. In a controlled trial Ericson *et al.* demonstrated that the incidence of infection was significantly reduced from 10 per cent in controls to 0 per cent in patients who received prophylactic cloxacillin (6).

In 1975, Benson and Hughes, in a retrospective review, demonstrated the range the pathogenic organisms encountered in infected total joint replacement (7). These are shown in Table 30.1.

Table 30.1. Organisms isolated from infected total joint replacements.

Staphylococcus aureus
Streptococcus faecalis
Escherichia coli
Proteus species
Pseudomonas aeruginosa
Coagulase negative staphylococcus
Anaerobic bacteria

Armed with this information and with the results of Ericson's study, cephalosporins were assessed as appropriate antibiotics to prevent infection after total joint replacements. Effective levels of cephalosporins were found in the bone and surrounding tissues at the time of operation following an intravenous dose (8) and in a prospective trial Pollard *et al.* were able to demonstrate that a short, high-dose regimen of cephaloridine was as effective in reducing infection following joint replacement as a two-week course (9).

This regimen was similar to that used by others in general surgery (10, 11) and laid the basis for short, high-dose regimens in the prevention of infection following total joint replacement. In the authors unit cefuroxime 1.5 g is given intravenously at induction of anaesthesia, followed by 750 mg intramuscularly 6 and 12 h post-operatively.

Antibiotics in bone cement

An alternative method of delivering antibiotics to patients who are undergoing total joint replacement is to place the antibiotic in the bone cement. This idea was first promoted by Buchholz and Engelbrecht who demonstrated the value of adding the antibiotic, gentamicin, to bone cement (12). Since then several studies have been undertaken to show that antibiotic can be placed in cement and can be recovered from the surrounding fluid *in vitro* and *in vivo* (13, 14).

The rationale of giving antibiotics by this route has recently been questioned in patients who are undergoing elective surgery for primary joint replacement. Although the method is effective, there is a real risk that by releasing relatively low doses of antibiotic over a prolonged period of time, resistant pathogenic organisms may multiply. Recently, Elson and his colleagues reported the alarming presence of the coagulase negative staphylococcus, *Staphylococcus epidermidis*, in patients undergoing revision surgery who had had antibiotics inserted into the bone cement as prophylaxis at their original operation (15).

This fact needs careful attention and perhaps detracts from the use of antibiotics in bone cement as prophylaxis, particularly as McQueen *et al.* have shown that there is no difference in the incidence of infection if antibiotics are given intravenously or in the bone cement in patients undergoing total joint replacement (16).

Hence, at the present time, it is probably safest to combine the principles of clean air in the operating theatre with a short regimen of a parenteral cephalosporin in order to prevent infection following total joint replacement.

Treatment

Infection following total joint replacement may present early or late (Fig. 30.1). Early infection is that which occurs and is diagnosed within the first three months after operation. The patient has a discharge from the wound, which is red and inflamed. The patient has pain at rest. There is a fever, which may be accompanied by an elevated erythrocyte sedimentation rate (ESR) and/or a raised white cell count. At this stage there are unlikely to be any radiological change.

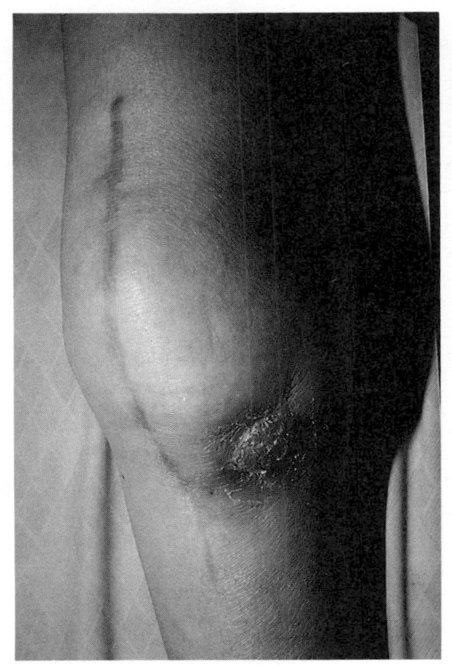

Fig. 30.1. An infected total knee replacement. (See plate section.)

Late infection is diagnosed in a patient following total joint replacement by pain at rest, the isolation of a pathogenic organism from the infected joint, radiological evidence of bone infection and an ESR that is 30 mm/h above the pre-operative level (7). C-reactive protein is a useful diagnostic test in patients with an infected total hip replacement, particularly when over 20 mg/L (17).

Treatment of the patient with an early infection

Once the diagnosis of infection is made it is important to start immediate treatment. Infection at this stage may be superficial or deep. If the infection is superficial there is a red wound and a serous discharge, but only a minimal fever. In this situation it is reasonable to give high dose antibiotics for a limited period of time and, for example, cefuroxime can be given intravenously for three to five days.

However, if there is really any suggestion from clinical examination that there is deep infection, because of the presence of pus, pain and fever, the patient should be returned to the operating theatre for proper and adequate wound debridement. This can be combined with appropriate high dose antibiotic therapy for a longer period of time—up to 14 days (Fig. 30.2). It is very unwise to treat a patient with an established infection with antibiotics alone.

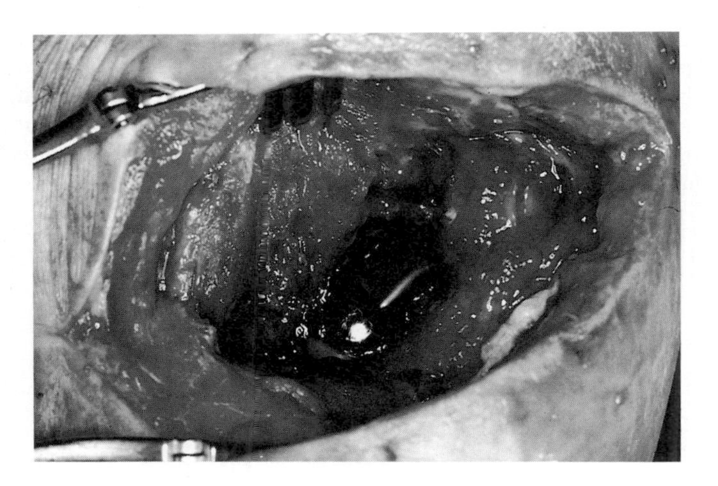

Fig. 30.2. An infected total hip replacement showing pus at the operation site. (See plate section.)

Treatment of late infection

Once it is clear that a patient has an established deep infection following total joint replacement, surgical treatment is essential. The diagnosis is made by history and examination and is supplemented by radiological investigations (Fig. 30.3).

Bone scanning techniques using technetium-labelled phosphate compounds, gallium-labelled reticulocytes, or indium-labelled white cells are helpful. Arthrography can be used to demonstrate loosening and, when the arthrogram is performed, aspirate from the joint can be sent for culture.

Current opinion suggests that an exchange total joint replacement can be undertaken at the initial operation provided that *Pseudomonas* spp. are not isolated (18, 19). The procedure involves removal of the prosthesis and removing all infected tissue followed by either:

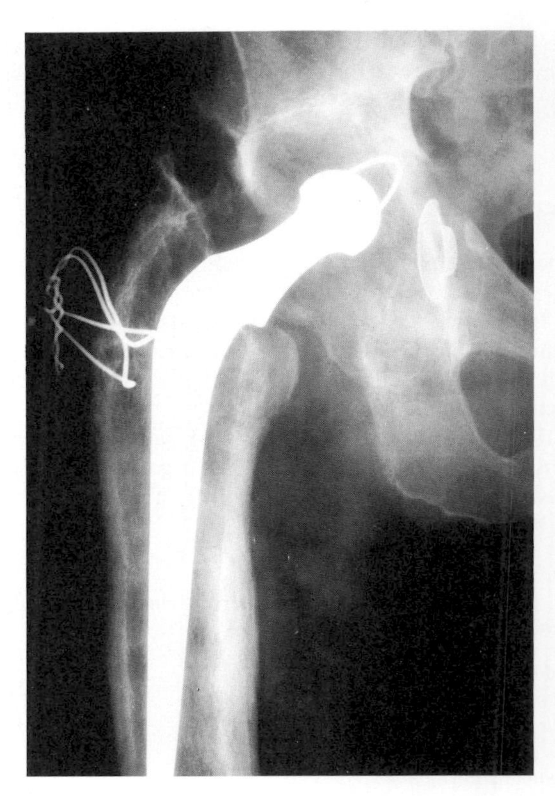

Fig. 30.3. Radiograph of an infected total hip replacement: showing periosteal reaction and bone destruction.

(a) immediate insertion of a new prosthesis, with or without bone cement into which antibiotic has been added, or
(b) leaving the excision arthroplasty alone for a period of time until the tissues have settled, and then delayed insertion of the exchange prosthesis some 6–12 months later. During this period bone cement beads, loaded with gentamicin, are inserted to provide a high concentration of antibiotic in the tissues for a period of time, and hence cleanse the infected site (Fig. 30.4).

Delayed replacement is advocated for patients who have *Pseudomonas* spp. isolated from the infected joint as these infections have a particularly bad reputation. In certain elderly, unfit patients prolonged antibiotic therapy can be used with limited success (20).

Acute haematogenous osteomyelitis

Acute haematogenous osteomyelitis occurs primarily in young children after pathogenic organisms enter the blood-stream and settle in areas of high vascularity in the bone. Classical sites are the metaphysis of growing bones such as the upper end of the tibia. In the past, such infections were lethal, but in

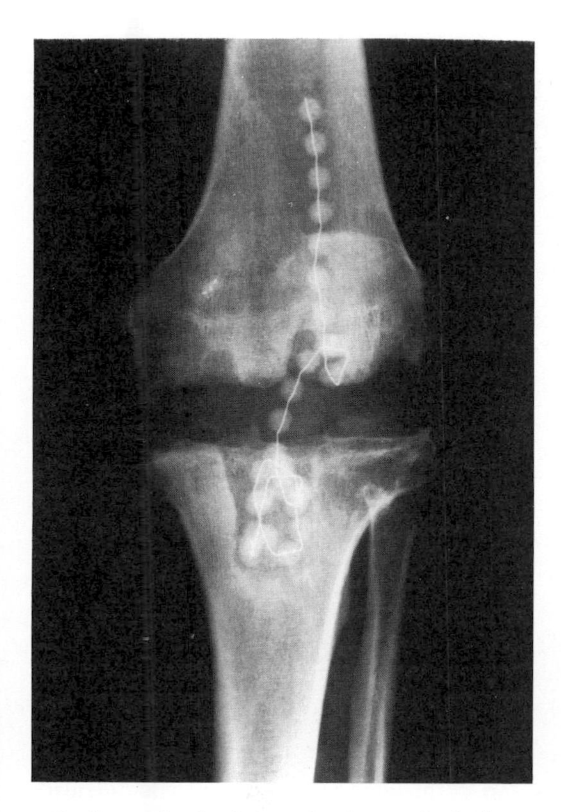

Fig. 30.4. Radiograph of a knee joint from which the prosthesis has been removed and gentamicin beads have been inserted.

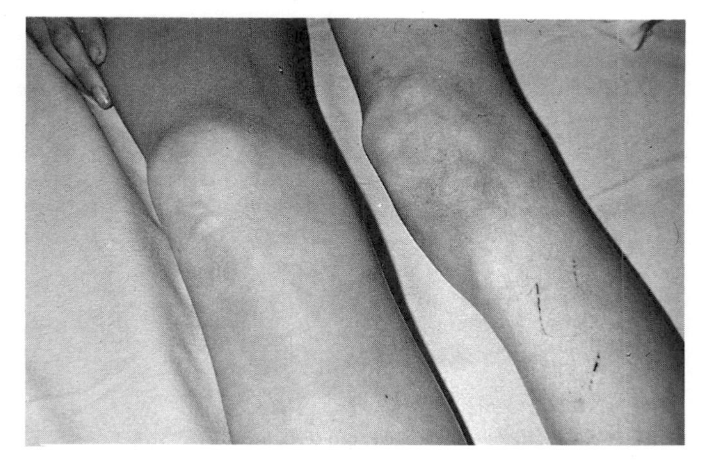

Fig. 30.5. Acute osteomyelitis of the upper tibia in a boy of 10 years of age. (See plate section.)

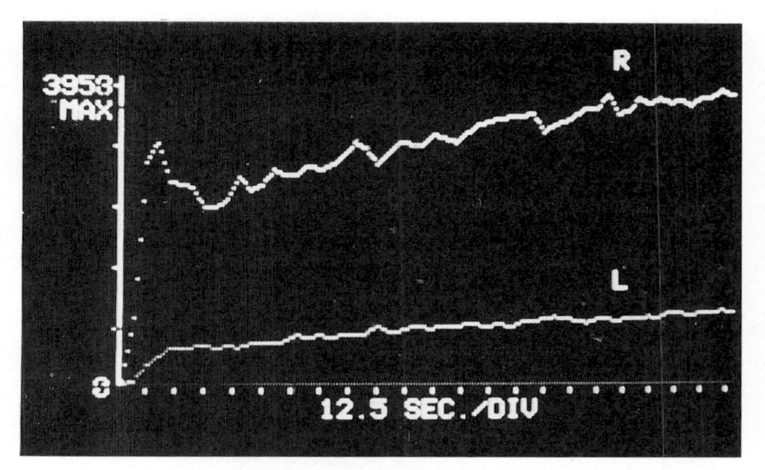

Fig. 30.6. A bone scan showing the increased uptake of ^{99m}Tc-MDP in the vascular phase of the scan. This patient had osteomyelitis of the right tibia.

developed countries these infections are now usually diagnosed and treated successfully.

It is currently believed that, because of its structure, pathogens are unable to pass the growth plate and hence it is likely that a subperiosteal abscess will form when infection occurs at the upper end of the tibia. In those patients who sustain an infection of the upper end of the femur, which lies within the capsular attachment of the hip joint, the pus will pass into the hip joint, producing a septic arthritis.

Diagnosis

The diagnosis of acute haematogenous osteomyelitis is made from the history, examination, and investigation. There is usually a short history of pain and fever and the child is ill. There may be a history of recent trauma, but this is not always present. On examination the child may have the signs of infection: redness, tenderness, and swelling. Infection may localize with fluctuation suggesting a collection of pus (Fig. 30.5).

Investigations include ESR, C-reactive protein, total and differential white cell count, and a haemoglobin estimation. Blood cultures must be taken at this stage. Radiographs invariably show little in the early stages, but the vascular phase of a bone scan is usually of value (Fig. 30.6).

An indium-labelled bone scan may also be undertaken and can help if there is a localized collection of pus.

The pathogenic organisms most commonly isolated are *Staphylococcus aureus*, *Streptococcus pyogenes*, *Haemophilus influenzae*, Gram-negative organisms and *Pneumococcus* spp., and *Salmonella typhi* may be isolated particularly when the patient has sickle-cell disease. Anaerobic organisms may also be cultured.

Treatment

A variety of different antibiotic regimens are advocated: fucidic acid and erythromycin (21); fucidic acid and oxacillin (22); and benzyl penicillin and flucloxacillin (23).

The regimen used by the author is intravenous cefuroxime combined with benzyl penicillin until such time as the pathogens are known. The treatment can be continued for up to six weeks, as originally advocated by Trueta in 1968 (24).

If at any time during the course of this treatment there is evidence of pus collecting, then the pus must be drained. This should be done by open operation, and the periosteum must be incised to allow the pus to be evacuated. If this practice is not followed, not only will the infection fail to resolve, but the vascular supply to the area of bone will be damaged and the result will lead to established osteomyelitis.

It is essential to monitor these patients at regular intervals, and to proceed to early surgery as soon as a subperiosteal collection of pus is identified. However, the need to drill the bone is unproven (25) as there is good evidence that bone has a centrifugal blood flow (26). In addition, there is fluid in bone, which is free and unbound (27) and it has been shown that large molecules move across bone (28). McCarthy *et al.* have demonstrated that there is a fluid flow within bone (29) and Montgomery *et al.* have confirmed that the movement of fluid is centrifugal (30). Therefore it is rational to expect pathogens and pus to move to the surface of bone where the pus can be evacuated by incising the periosteum.

Chronic osteomyelitis

Chronic osteomyelitis can be the sequelae of acute osteomyelitis or can arise *de novo*. It can follow acute haematogenous osteomyelitis which has failed to respond to treatment and can also be a sequelae of open fractures.

Chronic bone infections can occur following infection from tuberculosis, syphilis; brucellosis and, more recently, the human immunodeficiency virus (HIV). Chronic bone infection is in itself a disability for the patient which, apart from the continuous skin breakdown and discharge from of pus from the bone, can also lead to local squamous cell carcinoma, pathological fractures of the bone and amyloid disease, which may in turn lead to renal failure (Fig. 30.7).

The particular problem of this chronic infection is that inside the bone there may be a host of pathogenic organisms encased in a glycocalyx. This may be within a sequestrum and, therefore, isolated from the rest of the bone (Fig. 30.8).

The diagnosis of chronic osteomyelitis is made on clinical grounds and pathogenic organisms must be identified from as near to the depth of the source infection as possible. Radiological changes are the most helpful and can demonstrate bone destruction. Standard tomography is particularly helpful in identifying the presence of a sequestrum.

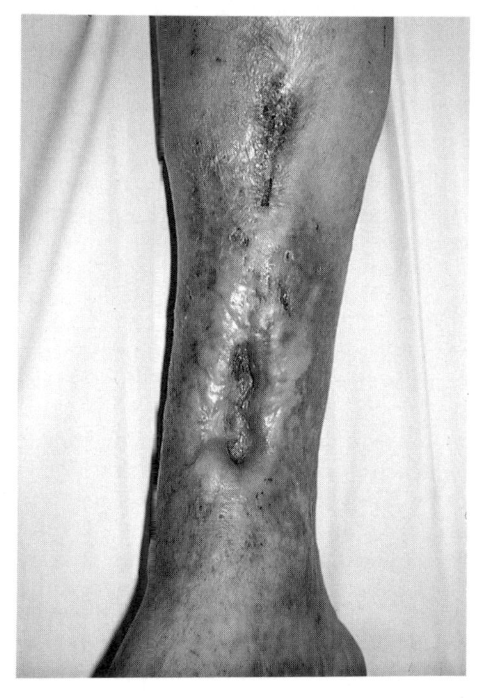

Fig. 30.7. Chronic osteomyelitis of the tibia. (See plate section.)

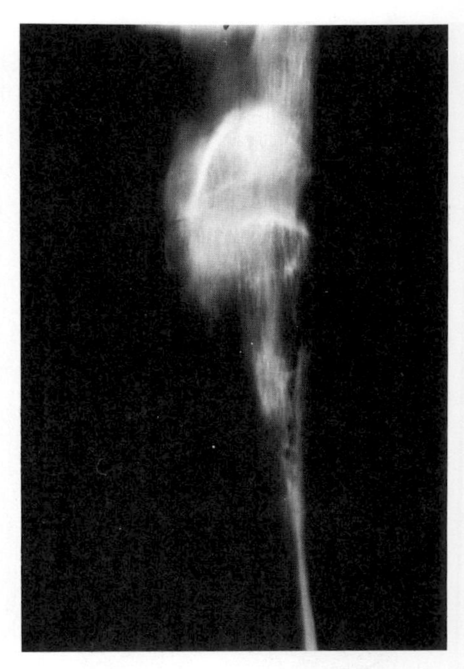

Fig. 30.8. A tomogram demonstrating a sequestrum in the tibia.

Treatment consists of antibiotic therapy for a prolonged period of time. Antibiotics can be given systemically and later changed to the oral route. The choice of antibiotic depends on the pathogens isolated, but it is the author's practice to give cephalexin 500 mg 6-hourly (31). Antibiotics can also be placed in bone cement beads and have been shown to control the infection effectively (32) (Fig. 30.9).

The surgical treatment needs to be extensive, particularly in long standing bone infection. All the dead tissue must be removed and this may then be followed by some form of fixation to stabilize the bone. It can be accompanied by either a bone graft using small cancellous chips (33), vascularized bone graft (34), or by means of bone transport to close a defect. A myocutaneous flap may also be necessary to cover the defect in the soft tissue that has arisen after the extensive surgery.

If all else fails amputation of the infected part may be necessary.

Infective arthritis

Bacteria can gain entry to a joint by a variety of routes. Infective arthritis may occur as the result of bacteria entering a joint through the blood-stream from a distant focus, as the result of an associated acute haematogenous osteomyelitis such as occurs in neonatal septic arthritis where there may be a damaging effect on the development of the infant femoral head, after direct innoculation, or as a result of a metal implant into the joint. Infective arthritis can occur from chronic infection such as tuberculosis and brucellosis.

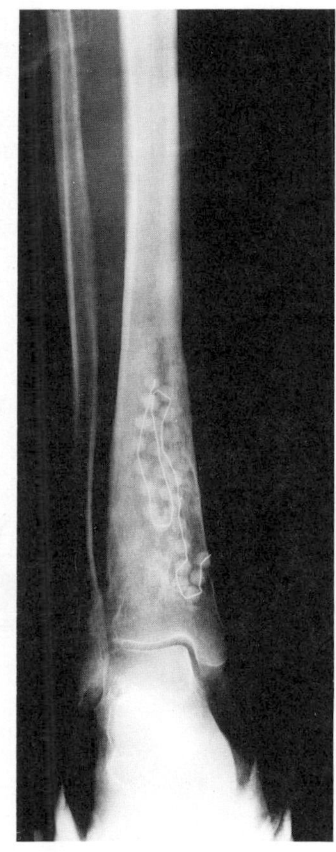

Fig. 30.9. Chronic osteomyelitis treated by excision of the dead bone and insertion of gentamicin bone cement beads.

The principles of treatment have already been outlined. It is first necessary to establish the diagnosis by clinical examination demonstrating a hot swollen joint with severe pain on movement. The presence of the infection is confirmed by aspiration of the joint followed identification of the pathogenic organism. There may be systemic effects and blood should be cultured to identify a bacteraemia or septicaemia.

Radiographs are of value, especially if bone has been destroyed or the joint surface is damaged. Bone scanning may be useful, particularly an indium-labelled white cell scan.

Treatment consists of intravenous high-dose antibiotic therapy combined with surgical drainage of the pus. Open surgical drainage is an important part of the treatment and is to be preferred to aspiration, although arthroscopic washout of the joint has been reported with limited success (35). It is of paramount importance that the pus is evacuated once infection has been diagnosed because pus destroys hyaline cartilage resulting in a stiff and painful joint.

References

1. Charnley, J. (1982). *The future of total hip replacements*. Proceedings of the Tenth Open Scientific Meeting of the Hip Society. Mosby, St. Louis, Missouri.
2. Noble, W.C., Lidwell, C.M., and Kingston, D. (1963). The size distribution of airborne particles carrying micro-organisms. *J. Hygiene*, **61**, 385–91.
3. Blowers, R. and Crew, B. (1960). Ventilation of operating theatres. *J. Hygiene*, **58**, 427–48.
4. Charnley, J. and Eftekhar, N. (1969). Post-operative infection in total prosthetic replacement arthroplasty of the hip joint. *Br. J. Surg.*, **56**, 641–9.
5. Lidwell, O.M., Lowbury, E.J.L., Whyte, W., Blowers, R., Stanley, S.J., and Lowe, D. (1982). Effect of ultraclean air in operating rooms on deep sepsis in the joint after total hip or knee replacement: a randomised study. *Br. Med. J.*, **285**, 10–14.
6. Ericson, C., Lidgren, L., and Lindberg, L. (1973). Cloxacillin in the prophylaxis of post-operative infection of the hip. *J. Bone Joint Surg. (Am.)*, **55**, 808–13.
7. Benson, M.K.D. and Hughes, S.P.F. (1975). Infection following total hip replacement in a general hospital with special orthopaedic facilities. *Acta Orthop. Scand.*, **46**, 968–78.
8. Hughes, S.P.F., Dash, C.H., Benson, M.K.D., and Field, C. (1978). Infection following total hip replacement and the possible prophylactic role of cephaloridine. *J. R. Coll. Surg. Edinb.*, **23**, 9–12.
9. Pollard, J.P., Hughes, S.P.F., Scott, J.E., Evans, M.J., and Benson, M.K.D. (1979). Antibiotic prophylaxis in total hip replacement. *Br. Med. J.*, **1**, 707–9.
10. Polk, H.C. and Lopez-Mayor, J.F. (1969). Post-operative wound infection; a prospective study of determinant factors and prevention. *Surgery*, **66**, 97–103.
11. Evans, C. and Pollock, A.V. (1973). The reduction of surgical wound infections by prophylactic parenteral cephaloridine. *Br. J. Surg.*, **60**, 434–7.
12. Buchholz, H.W. and Engelbrecht, H. (1970). Über die Deporwirkun einiger. Antibiotica bei Vermschung mit dem Kunslharz Palacos. *Chirurgie*, **41**, 511–515.
13. Hughes, S.P.F., Field, C.A., Kennedy, M.K.R., and Dash, C.H. (1979). Cephalosporins in bone cement. *J. Bone Joint Surg. (Br.)*, **61**, 96–100.
14. Innes, A., Hughes, S.P.F., Robertson, S., and Dash, C.H. (1985). Cefuroxime in CMW bone cement: a clinical study. *Int. Orthop.*, **9**, 265–9.
15. Hope, P.G., Kristinsson, K.G., Norman, P., and Elson, R.A. (1989). Deep infection of cemented total hip arthroplasties caused by coagulase negative staphylococci. *J. Bone Joint Surg. (Br.)*, **71**, 851–5.
16. McQueen, M.M., Hughes, S.P.F., May, P., and Verity, L. (1990). Cefuroxime in total joint arthroplasty. *J. Arthroplasty*, **5**, 169–72.
17. Sangen, L., Carlsson, A.S. (1989). The diagnostic value of C-reactive protein in infected total hip arthroplasties. *J. Bone Joint Surg. (Br.)*, **71**, 638–41.
18. McDonald, D.J., Fitzgerald, R.H., and Ilstump, D.M. (1989). Two stage reconstruction of a total hip arthroplasty because of infection. *J. Bone Joint Surg. (Am.)*, **71**, 828–34.
19. Morrey, B., Westholm, F., and Schoifer, S. (1989). Long term results of various treatment options for infected total knee arthroplasty. *Clin. Orthop.*, **248**, 120–8.
20. Goulet, J.A., Pellicci, P.M., Brause, B.D., and Salvati, J. (1988). Prolonged suppression of infection in total hip arthroplasty. *J. Arthroplasty*, **3**, 109–16.
21. Blockey, N.J. and McAllister, T.A. (1972). Antibiotics in acute osteomyelitis in children. *J. Bone Joint Surg. (Br.)*, **54**, 299–309.
22. Mollan, R.A.B. and Piggott, J. (1977). Acute osteomyelitis in children. *J. Bone Joint Surg. (Br.)*, **59**, 1–7.
23. Cole, W.G., Dalziel, R.E., and Leith, S. (1982). Treatment of acute osteomyelitis in childhood. *J. Bone. Joint Surg. (Br.)*, **64**, 218–23.

24. Trueta, J. (1968). *Studies in the development and decay of the human frame*. Saunders, Philadelphia.
25. Blockey, N.J. (1976). *Children's orthopaedics. Practical problems*, Chapter 2. Butterworths, London.
26. Brookes, M., Elkin, A.C., Harrison, R.G., and Heald, C.B. (1961). A new concept of capillary circulation in bone cortex. *Lancet*, **i**, 1078–81.
27. Hughes, S.P.F., Davies, R., and Kelly, P. (1978). Fluid space in bone. *Clin. Orthop.*, **134**, 332–41.
28. Owen, M., Howlett, C.R., and Triffitt, J.T. (1977). Movement of albumin and polyvinylpyrolidone through bone tissue fluid. *Calcif. Tiss. Res.*, **23**, 103–12.
29. McCarthy, I.D., Bronk, J.T., and Kelly, P.J. (1989). The measurement of interstitial fluid flow in cortical bone. Presented at the British Microcirculation Society, April.
30. Montgomery, R.T., Sutker, B.D., Bronk, J.T., Smith, S.R., and Kelly, P.J. (1988). Interstitial fluid flow in cortical bone. *Microvasc. Res.*, **35**, 295–307.
31. Hughes, S.P.F., Nixon, J., and Dash, C.H. (1981). Cephalexin in chronic osteomyelitis. *J.R. Coll. Surg. Edinb.*, **26**, 335–9.
32. Hedstrom, S., Lidgren, L., Torholm, C., and Onnerfalt, R. (1980). Antibiotic containing bone cement beads in the treatment of deep muscle and skeletal infections. *Acta Orthop. Scand.*, **51**, 863–9.
33. Papineau, L.J., Alfageme, A., Dalcourt, J.P., and Pilon, L. (1979). Osteomyelite chronique: excision et graffe de spongieux a l'air libre après mises a plat extensives. *Int. Orthop.*, **3**, 165–76.
34. Pho, R.W.H., Levack, B., Satku, K., and Patrudul, A. (1985). Free vascularised fibular graft in the treatment of congenital pseudarthrosis of the tibia. *J. Bone Joint Surg. (Br.)*, **67**, 64–70.
35. Flood, J.N. and Kolarik, D.B. (1988). Arthroscopic irrigation and debridement of infected total knee arthroplasty: report of two cases. *J. Arthroplasty*, **4**, 182–6.

Further reading

Coombs, R. and Fitzgerald, R.H. Jr. (ed.) (1989). *Infection in the orthopaedic patient*. Butterworths, London.

Gillespie, W.J. and Nade, S. (1987). *Musculoskeletal infections*. Blackwell Scientific Publications, Melbourne.

Gustilo, R.B. (1989). *Orthopaedic infection: diagnosis and treatment*. Saunders Harcourt Brace Jovanovich, Philadelphia.

Hughes, S.P.F., and Fitzgerald, Jr, R.H. (1986). *Musculoskeletal infections*. Year Book Medical Publishers, Inc, Chicago.

31

Surgical infection in obstetric practice

MICHAEL J. TURNER and DENIS F. HAWKINS

Introduction

Despite the advent of antibiotics, infection during pregnancy continues to pose major problems for the mother and her baby. This is particularly true in developing countries. In obstetrics, infection presents two additional considerations. What effect will pregnancy have on the infection and its treatment, and what effect will the infection and its treatment have on the course of the pregnancy and the puerperium? While the risk to the fetus of antimicrobial drugs in pregnancy is small (1) certain drugs, for example, the tetracyclines, should be avoided (2, 3). Fortunately, the risk to the breast-fed newborn of such drugs, given to the mother, is extremely small (4).

The normal vaginal flora is difficult to define (5); microbial species that can be isolated vary from time to time in the same individual, from individual to individual, and from population to population. Important variables which influence flora include ovarian hormone production, sexual activity, hormone or antibiotic treatment, and surgery. The normal adult flora in pregnancy consists of both aerobic and anaerobic organisms and can be examined by qualitative or quantitative analysis (5). Incidences cited (6) (Table 31.1) are a non-quantitative measure, as to whether the organism is present or absent. Thus, apparent distinctions depend on the techniques employed in specimen collection, the culture techniques and the expertise of those using them. Quantitative studies reflect the dynamics of the flora but are difficult and time-consuming. Selective media studies are required to isolate some organisms.

The presence of *Neisseria gonorrhoeae* in the vagina is always pathogenic. The pathogenicity of other vaginal organisms may depend on the patient's immune reactions, the number of bacteria present, and the clinical circumstances.

There are physiological alterations in humoral and cellular immune function during pregnancy (7). In general, cellular immunity is depressed, which explains why pregnant women are more susceptible to viral, bacterial, protozoal, and fungal infections.

The structural integrity of the genital tract may be broken by labour itself or by surgical intervention. A caesarean section incision is an important aetiological factor in the development of uterine infection. Careful attention to surgical technique can help to reduce the risk of post-operative infection (7). The tissues should be handled gently to avoid compromising the blood supply and devitalization; haemostasis should be secured to prevent the development of haematomata which can become infected; and the amount of suture material remaining in the operative bed should be minimized. The use of prophylactic antibiotics should be regarded as complementary to good surgical technique rather than as a substitute.

Another important mechanical barrier against infection during pregnancy is the chorio-amniotic membrane. Once the membranes have been ruptured, either spontaneously or surgically, the patient runs a higher risk of an intrauterine infection. This is not only due to removal of the mechanical

Table 31.1. Flora of the posterior fornix of the vagina in 200 women in the first trimester of pregnancy (6).

Organism	Patients (No.)	Incidence (%)
Staphylococcus epidermidis	134	67
Lactobacilli	118	59
Anaerobic streptococci	86	43
Faecal streptococci (including Lancefield group D streptococci)	64	32
Coryneform organisms	62	31
Microaerophilic streptococci	44	22
Candida albicans	29	15
Other yeasts	5	3
Streptococcus agalactiae (Lancefield group B)	33	17
Bacteroides group	33	17
Escherichia coli	33	17
α-haemolytic streptococci (aerobic)	24	12
Mycoplasma hominis	10	5
Ureaplasma ureolyticum	0	–
Staphylococcus aureus	5	3
Other β-haemolytic streptococci (Lancefield groups C or G)	3	2
Clostridium perfringens	0	–
Trichomonas vaginalis	4	2

barrier to passage of vaginal organisms into the uterus. Potentially pathogenic organisms, both aerobic and anaerobic, have been cultured from amniotic fluid in over 50 per cent of women in labour with intact membranes (8). It is likely that antimicrobial substances in amniotic fluid, particularly β-lysin (9) and the low molecular weight substance described by Schlievert *et al.* (10) normally prevent bacterial proliferation and are diluted by fluid transfer into the amniotic cavity after the membranes are ruptured. The activity of both of these substances is zinc dependent (11, 12).

Pregnancy may also alter the pharmacokinetics of drugs prescribed to treat infections. Maternal serum levels of antibiotics are lower in the pregnant patient compared with levels in non-pregnant patients (2). This is due to diminished absorption of drugs given orally, the increased intravascular volume of pregnancy, an increased glomerular filtration rate which increases renal excretion, and transfer of antibiotics to the fetal compartment (13). Thus, antibiotics need to be given in higher doses to obtain tissue levels similar to those outside pregnancy. Fetal drug distribution differs from that of the adult, with functional shunting of blood away from the lungs (2). Some antibiotics (for example, choramphenicol) are subject to more plasma protein binding in the fetus than in the mother, which reduces the levels of free drug available to the tissues. High maternal serum levels, therefore, may not be effective in preventing fetal respiratory tract infections in the presence of intrauterine infection.

Sources of surgical infection in obstetrics

Urinary infections

Urinary tract infections (UTI) occur either as an exacerbation of latent pyelonephritis or from the use of urinary catheters pre-operatively or in labour.

Between two and seven per cent of antenatal women have 'asymptomatic bacteriuria', that is, more than 100 000 colony-forming units/ml (cfu/ml) can be cultured from their urine (14). A much smaller proportion have undiagnosed loci of pyelonephritis in their kidneys. Pregnancy predisposes to UTI because there is a tendency to urinary stasis due to dilation of the calyces and the ureters are dilated, relaxed and sometimes kinked under the influence of enormously increased progesterone and perhaps corticosteroid levels. Surgical manipulations and labour itself enhance the risk.

Catheters are frequently used without clear exposure and adequate cleansing of the urethral orifice. The transfer of bacteria from the lower urethra into the bladder is inevitable (15). Infection is maintained if the catheter is left indwelling, and chemotherapy cannot be relied upon to cure it (16). The use of catheters has diminished somewhat—for example, 'difficult' forceps deliveries have been abandoned and few obstetricians now believe that routine catheterization is necessary before a forceps delivery. It may be desirable to empty the bladder before a caesarean section. Unnecessarily, many surgeons leave the catheter in during the operation and thereafter, to make sure the urine is not bloodstained at the end and to relieve themselves of the responsibility of checking that the patient has passed urine some hours later. Indwelling catheters are inserted to measure hourly urine output in, for example, severe pre-eclampsia and eclampsia. This adds urinary infection to the patient's problems and serves only to make the doctors feel they are doing something and to ensure that at least a nurse looks at the patient each hour. If oliguria occurs this becomes apparent soon enough without the aid of a catheter (17).

Vaginal operations

The vagina resembles the mouth in that both have endogenous, and often potentially pathogenic, bacterial flora (see Table 31.1), and both cavities are impossible to sterilize completely. Merely to insert an antiseptic solution, often of some striking colour, optimistically is of little value, as it does not penetrate between the rugae, into the vaginal sebaceous glands or into the crypts of the cervical canal. The function of cleaning the vagina with a simple antiseptic solution before a vaginal operation such as cerclage, is primarily to remove the debris of vaginal and other secretions, and to prevent that debris being incorporated into incisions in the vaginal skin or carried up through the cervix. Some more extensive procedures probably do more harm than good. Enthusiastic scrubbing around the cervix can dislodge the protective cervical mucus plug and introduce contaminated fluid from the vaginal vault. Pre-operative antiseptic douches are potentially lethal in pregnancy. Apart from introducing contaminated fluid into the uterus and tubes, a fatal air embolus can result.

For intrauterine manipulation, a hand must be passed through the vagina into the uterus. Long-sleeved surgeons' gloves used to be available for this; economy often now dictates that they are not. The risk of infection varies with the extent of the manipulation, its duration, and associated trauma. Simple manual removal of the placenta within a very few minutes after delivery of the baby has a very low morbidity. When numerous external attempts to remove a retained placenta, culminating one or several hours later in a formal removal under general anaesthesia was in vogue there is a risk of serious infection.

When an episiotomy or laceration is being repaired the likely source of contamination is bacteria from the perineal skin or the anus—it is common for instruments or suture materials to touch these areas during manipulations to expose the vaginal wound. In America, a 'spreader'—a self-retaining instrument providing lateral traction on the sides of the incision at the fourchette—is widely used. It is scorned by English obstetricians who fear it might cause discomfort. In fact, it is more comfortable for the patient, as all the manipulations to expose the vaginal incision are avoided, and it exposes clean edges of the wound to be sutured.

Caesarean section

The sources of wound infection and genital tract infection after caesarean section are primarily bacteria from the patient's abdominal skin introduced during or after the incision, and bacteria ascending from the vagina before, during or after the operation.

In our own study from two London hospitals (18) the skin pathogens found in 187 patients are shown in Table 31.2. *Staphylococcus aureus* predominated. Of 19 patients from whom this organism was grown from the skin before the operation, 13 developed post-operative wound infection or endometritis (5 of 10 with antibiotic prophylaxis, 8 of 9 without). *Staph. aureus* was cultured from 6 of the 19 patients who developed post-operative infection. It is evident that current procedures intended to sterilize the skin before an abdominal operation are relatively ineffective. This may be the reason a higher incidence of post-operative infection is found after emergency caesarean sections compared with elective procedures in some studies. It may also be a factor in the higher incidence of infection after caesarean section in obese women (19) and in women living in poor circumstances.

In other studies, an association between bacteria causing infections after caesarean section and the vaginal flora (Table 31.3) have been found. In particular, the group B haemolytic streptococci carried in the vagina can give rise to a high pyrexia 24 h after caesarean section, and anaerobic organisms from the vagina can cause an endomyometritis developing days after the operation. The practice of passing a finger or dilator down through the cervix before closing the uterus to verify patency has largely been abandoned. If it is felt essential, the instrument should be recovered vaginally.

Table 31.2. Abdominal skin cultures taken before caesarean section in 187 women.

Staphylococcus aureus	19
Other staphylococci	55
Streptococcus faecalis	2
Group B streptococci	1
Coliforms	1
No bacterial growth	109

Table 31.3. Vaginal cultures taken before caesarean section in 187 women.

Staphylococcus aureus	4
Group B streptococci	4
Other haemolytic streptococci	3
Streptococcus faecalis	7
Lactobacilli	19
Candida albicans	5
No significant growth	145

Another potential source of contamination is the surgeon. In a recent report (20), gloves were found to be punctured after 54 per cent of caesarean sections, and the surgeon was aware of the puncture in only half of these. About half the punctures occurred during suture of the uterine incision and were attributed by the authors to grasping the edge of the incision with the fingers. In another context it has been shown that wearing two pairs of gloves much reduces the number of punctures through to the surgeon's fingers. Surgical technique is usually thought to be important. Draping and skin towels are felt to be important by some; others feel that when warm and sodden with tissue fluid, blood and amniotic fluid (or when a fluid film covers impermeable drapes) they can be an effective incubator for skin bacteria. Industrial action in a hospital laundry has sometimes provided the opportunity to test the hypothesis that a careful, and fairly swift, surgeon wearing an apron and sterile gloves, operating on a patient whose skin has been washed with soap and water and not draped at all, could achieve as low infection rates as are obtained with all the usual paraphernalia.

Infection after caesarean section has been found by multivariate analysis to be related, independently, both to the duration of the operation and to the amount of blood loss (21). The time factor suggests that the less time available to airborne bacteria in operating theatres to drift down on to the open wound the better. Even bacterial filters in air supplies to operating theatres do not help if trolleys straight from hospital corridors are pushed through between operations, and ten or more people are in the theatre during an operation. The relationship to blood transfusion may just reflect the complexity of the procedure or it may signal a patient with low resistance to infection (see Chapter 8).

Normal puerperium

It has been thought that the endometrial cavity is free from bacterial contamination for approximately six hours after normal labour and delivery (22), but Calman and Gibson (23) found the incidence of positive uterine cultures to be 33 per cent after one day, increasing to 66 per cent after four days. Using shielded swabs to prevent contamination from the cervix, Laros *et al* (24), found an average of 40 per cent positive endometrial cultures, the organisms being mainly *Staph. epidermidis*, diphtheroids, and streptococci (non-haemolytic, viridans, and anaerobic). Whether or not this invasion of the uterine cavity is always responsible for puerperal endomyometritis is doubtful. There is no correlation between the presence of these organisms and the incidence of uterine infection (24), and the route of infection may be lymphatic or haematogenous.

Of particular relevance to puerperal sterilization is the penetration of bacteria to the lumen of the fallopian tubes. Hellman (25) found that the histological appearances of salpingitis occur in an increasing proportion of patients in the days after delivery, being present in 50 per cent by day eight. The concomitant appearance of bacteria in the tubes was not detected by Rubin *et al* (25), but Laros *et al* (24) found positive cultures from the tubes in 14 per cent of patients at 12 to 36 h after delivery, increasing to 40 to 41 per cent at 3 to 5 days. The organisms were mainly *Staph. epidermis*, diphtheroids and coliforms. Again, the presence of bacteria did not correlate with the occurrence of infection.

Antimicrobial drugs and pregnancy

This topic has been reviewed recently (1, 27–29). The practical use of antimicrobial drugs in pregnancy is described in detail by Ledward *et al* (3).

The overall risk to the fetus of using these drugs in pregnancy is, at the most, very small. In the Collaborative Perinatal Project (31), a study of 50 282 mother–child pairs yielded 8088 mothers who had been exposed to antimicrobial and antiparasitic drugs in the first 16 weeks of pregnancy. The standardized relative risk of a baby with any congenital malformation was 0.95 (95 per cent confidence limits 0.87–1.05).

Penicillins, erythromycin, cephalosporins, metronidazole, nitrofurantoin, and local antifungals are apparently harmless to the fetus at all stages of pregnancy, though a woman with real allergic sensitivity to a penicillin (which is rare) can convey that sensitivity to the newborn, by transplacental passage of antibiotics. The combination of clavulanic acid with amoxycillin (Augmentin) seems to be harmless, but the number of patients so far studied is relatively small. Information on the more recent penicillins has failed to reveal adverse effects on the fetus, but in pregnant patients it is wise to prefer the use of older, widely used drugs. Antenatal women are representative of the general, rather than the hospital population. As such they are a low-risk group for the carriage of resistant organisms and it is seldom necessary to resort to recently developed antibiotics.

Cephalosporins have been widely used in pregnancy in recent years and no specific risk to the fetus has emerged in practice. There is a theoretical risk that latamoxef and cefamandole, which contain *N*-methyltetrazole groups, might interfere with vitamin K metabolism. If these drugs are used it is reasonable to check the mother's prothrombin ratio at the completion of the course, and restore any defect with phytomenadione.

Erythromycin has been widely used and has not been found to convey any toxicity to the fetus. Prolonged courses of the estolate are usually avoided, as pregnant women are particularly susceptible to intrahepatic cholestasis.

Tetracyclines given in pregnancy were not found to be associated with dysmorphic fetal abnormalities in three major studies. They are chelating agents which bind divalent metal ions and are incorporated into the dentine of developing teeth, causing discoloration; only small amounts are found in enamel. Even small doses given to the mother are capable of staining the fetal teeth. Discoloration of the deciduous teeth can be caused any time after the first four months of pregnancy for the maxillary and mandibular incisors and after five months for the maxillary and mandibular canines. The severity of the staining depends on drug dose, duration of treatment, the time of treatment in relation to odontogenesis and the drug involved. Staining occurs with greater frequency if the total dose given to the mother exceeds 3 g or if treatment is continued for more than 10 days. Tetracycline and dimethylchlortetracycline produce the most severe staining whilst oxytetracycline and doxycycline stain the least. The tetracyclines are also deposited in the fetal long bones, and it has been suspected that they might affect bone growth, but there is at present no clear evidence of this. Nonetheless, there is no common indication for the use of tetracyclines where they cannot be replaced with another antibiotic, and the former drugs should not be used in pregnant women.

The use of both lincomycin and clindamycin in pregnancy has been studied and no fetal ill-effect found.

Chloramphenicol is not a popular drug in Great Britain – the memory of patients with aplastic anaemia is too strong, and some of the early cases occurred in pregnant women. The postulated risk that the drug given to a mother in later pregnancy might cause the grey baby syndrome in the newborn has not been substantiated.

Streptomycin given to a pregnant woman is well known to have a potential for causing newborn deafness. The risk has been exaggerated – in the days when tuberculosis was treated throughout pregnancy with the drug, without assessment of blood levels, the incidence of actual hearing loss in the babies was less than 5 per cent. Most of the defects detected in the children were high-frequency hearing loss above the speech frequencies, and vestibular function defects which had been compensated. None the less, indications for using streptomycin in pregnancy are now very rare. A very few cases of infant hearing-loss have been reported after the use of kanamycin in pregnancy but none has yet occurred after using gentamicin, tobramycin, or amikacin.

Sulphonamides have been used in many millions of pregnant women and there is no evidence of teratogenesis from the major surveys. Co-trimoxazole contains sulphamethoxazole and trimethoprim. The sulphonamide interferes with para-aminobenzoic acid in the synthesis of folates in bacteria, and trimethoprim interferes with the reduction of folates in the biosynthesis of pyrimidines and purines. Human cells do not synthesise folates and have a different folate reductase which is less sensitive to trimethoprim. The manufacturers of co-trimoxazole say that the drug is contraindicated in pregnancy, but this is probably just self-protective. Both co-trimoxazole and trimethoprim have been widely used in pregnancy and there has been no report of associated fetal abnormalities. None the less, it is reasonable to prescribe a small supplement of folinic acid with these drugs. There were one or two anecdotal cases of fetal abnormality reported in association with the use of long acting sulphonamides in pregnancy and it cannot be said that their use was sufficiently wide as to establish safety. The use of sulphonamides in pregnancy might predispose to defective albumin binding of bilirubin, and to free hyperbilirubinaemia and hence kernicterus in the newborn, but in practice this does not occur. The reason is that soluble sulphonamides have quite a short half-time in mother and fetus, and the chance of significant quantities remaining in the newborn after delivery is small. Perhaps administration to a mother should be avoided if premature delivery is anticipated.

The claim that metronidazole might be teratogenic came about the time that an oral preparation was introduced to the American market. There is no sound evidence from animal work that this is the case, and there is ample evidence from human studies that use of the drug in pregnancy is not associated with any harm to the fetus. Metronidazole has a disulfiram-like effect and alcohol should be avoided whilst it is being taken, or the combination will make the mother feel ill.

Both nitrofurantoin and nalidixic acid are in general harmless in pregnancy. Both drugs, and for that matter, chloramphenicol, should be avoided in late pregnancy if there is any risk of glucose-6-phosphate dehydrogenase deficiency in the fetus, or a newborn haemolytic anaemia might develop.

Breast-feeding mothers (4)

The risks to the breast-fed newborn of giving antimicrobial drugs to the mother are very small indeed. The only risk with penicillins and cephalosporins, where only low concentrations pass into breast milk, is the very rare possibility that an allergic mother may have transferred antibodies to the baby; at least one case of a newborn skin rash has been reported. Erythromycin passes freely into breast milk but no adverse newborn reaction has been reported. There is a theoretical risk of predisposing to oral candidal infections. Aminoglycosides pass into breast milk but are very poorly absorbed by the fetus and the theoretical risk of ototoxicity is remotely small. Similar considerations apply to tetracyclines, which are chelated by milk and not absorbed by the fetus; there has been no case of newborn dentition being affected by this route.

With sulphonamides, which pass into milk and are absorbed by the baby, the risks are again small and theoretical. Perhaps breast milk should be avoided with jaundiced premature babies if the mother is taking a sulphonamide, just in case albumin binding of bilirubin in the baby might be affected. Sulphisoxazole was the drug most likely to cause such interference, sulphonilamide the least likely. If the mother is taking co-trimoxazole or trimethoprim it is reasonable that the baby should have folic acid as part of the routine vitamin supplementation.

Chloramphenicol is usually avoided; the risk of newborn bone marrow depression is very small, but other antibiotics are nearly always appropriate. There is a little evidence that clindamycin and lincomycin may be concentrated in breast milk; again the risk to the baby is very small indeed, but other antibiotics are available. If the mother is taking metronidazole the newborn intake is of the order of 5 mg/day, a fraction of a therapeutic dose, but babies clearly indicate that there is an unpleasant taste to the milk.

The only significant risk of maternal antimicrobial treatment is to glucose-6-phosphate dehydrogenase deficient babies. In this situation, feeding breast milk containing sulphonamide, chloramphenicol, nalidixic acid, or nitrofurantoin should be avoided, or a newborn haemolytic anaemia may result.

Prevention and management of infections

Urinary tract infection

Symptomatic bacteriuria complicates between 3 and 8 per cent of pregnancies (32). The generally accepted criterion for a bacteriologically proven UTI is 100 million or more cfu/litre (10^5 cfu/ml) in a mid-stream urine sample (33). The sensitivity of this criterion in predicting the occurrence of symptomatic infection in a non-pregnant patient is 95 per cent. No data is available on its predictive sensitivity during pregnancy (32).

Available evidence suggests that sulphonamides, nitrofurantoin, ampicillin and the first generation cephalosporins are equally effective in treating asymptomatic UTIs caused by organisms reported to be sensitive to these drugs. Single-dose treatment is rarely effective clinically if the patient is symptomatic. Patients with symptomatic pyelonephritis should be treated promptly, parenterally initially, with either ampicillin or a cephalosporin (34), as high pyrexia can affect the fetus adversely, or cause a miscarriage or pre-term delivery. Pyrexias over 38 °C should be treated with tepid sponging or paracetamol. The idea that the signs of infection may thus be masked is ridiculous.

If there is clinical response within 24 to 36 h it is a mistake to change the antibiotic when laboratory sensitivities are reported, but the addition of an antibiotic appropriate for a resistant organism is advised to prevent perpetuation of resistant strains and the spread of resistance factors. If there is no clinical response, the choice of a second antibiotic should be guided by laboratory sensitivities. An overlap of 24 h is desirable as the first drug may have been causing some bacteriostasis, and tissue levels have to be achieved with the drug to which the organism is sensitive (35).

Cervical cerclage

In a small number of patients, pre-term labour may be due to cervical incompetence and a cervical cerclage may be performed to prevent pre-term delivery. While the insertion or removal of cervical sutures may be complicated by infection, there is no evidence that the risk of infection in these patients is reduced by the use of prophylactic antibiotics. None the less, antibiotic prophylaxis has been recommended for all patients undergoing cerclage after 17 weeks of pregnancy (36).

When cervical cerclage is planned with 24 hours' notice it is wisest to take a cervical and vaginal bacterial culture and to use antibiotic prophylaxis appropriate to any pathogens isolated. Antibiotic prophylaxis is also desirable when there is a history of circlage becoming infected in a previous pregnancy, and it may be indicated if there is a history of pre-term rupture of the membranes in a previous pregnancy associated with infection. When cerclage is performed in an acute situation with bulging membranes (37) those membranes have already been exposed to vaginal flora and antibiotic prophylaxis with a cephalosporin and metronidazole should be used. If a patient with a cervical suture in place develops a uterine infection, most authorities would favour removal of the suture, treatment with systemic antibiotics and delivery of the fetus.

Pre-term rupture of the membranes

Whilst attention is focused on the role of intracervical infection as the cause of pre-term rupture of the membranes, it should not be forgotten that, in at least half the cases of early spontaneous membrane rupture, no evidence of infection can be obtained by sophisticated microbiological or histopathological techniques. It is, therefore, of great importance to prevent these patients becoming affected by ascending infection.

In some environments, one of the reasons for hospital admission is to prevent these patients becoming infected as a consequence of sexual intercourse. In all environments the commonest factor contributing to intra-amniotic infection is vaginal examination, manipulating vaginal flora into an open cervix. Rectal examinations are associated with a greater risk of this happening, and provide less information. Even the passage of a sterile vaginal speculum is bound to convey bacterial flora from the lower vagina to the cervix.

The earlier the membranes rupture pre-term the greater the hazard to the fetus if intra-amniotic infection occurs—the baby may not survive if it has to be delivered before 30 weeks because of intrauterine infection. A few obstetricians forbid any form of vaginal examination of these patients, and their juniors soon learn, to their surprise, that this restriction has little or no effect on management or outcome. It is reasonable to permit a single examination with a speculum, taking care not to disturb the cervix, if there is doubt if the membranes are ruptured, and to take a high vaginal swab for culture at the same time. The widely held concept that it is necessary to ascertain the exact state of the cervix before making every decision on management of pre-term rupture of the membranes is fallacious.

The use of prophylactic antibiotics after pre-labour pre-term rupture of membranes has been examined in a number of studies (38). In none of these was there any good evidence of benefit to the fetus by reduction in the incidence of newborn infection (39, 40). A benefit shown was a decreased incidence of maternal infectious morbidity post-partum (38). Similar benefit might have been achieved by deferring antibiotics until after the baby had been delivered.

It is now accepted that intracervical infection and chorionamnionitis are major factors in the onset of pre-term delivery and in pre-term labour with spontaneous rupture of the membranes.

Pathogens may be isolated directly from the uterus by amniocentesis or they may be cultured from the lower genital tract following a speculum examination. It is open to question whether such microbiological information alters the clinical management of patients with pre-term membrane rupture. There is no evidence that the clinical outcome is improved by treatment, except in the case of group B streptococcal infection, where parenteral benzylpenicillin or ampicillin given to the mother is likely to protect the baby from infection.

The differentiation between chorionamnionitis and overt intrauterine infection with its risk of fetal infection is far from easy to make. With a low-grade maternal pyrexia, perhaps settling to normal, chorionamnionitis alone may be the problem, and delay in effecting delivery may give an uninfected, very pre-term baby an increased chance of survival. Regrettably, neither maternal white cell counts nor C-reactive protein measurements are effective in making the distinction in practice. The use of amniocentesis, with white cell counts, examination of amniotic fluid for the presence of bacteria and measurement of dextrose content, is being studied as an aid to the diagnosis of intra-amniotic infection. Sustained maternal pyrexia, even if low grade, the development of uterine tenderness, or the discharge of purulent amniotic fluid, all suggest amniotic fluid, and hence fetal, infection.

When the diagnosis is of early pre-term rupture with chorionamnionitis alone, and another week or two *in utero* will improve the chances of survival of the fetus, there is a case for treating the mother with antimicrobial drugs, such as a cephalosporin and metronidazole. The use of a double catheter with two balloons, sutured into the cervix in these circumstances has been described (41). The amniotic cavity is then perfused with normal saline containing a cephalosporin.

When a diagnosis of intrauterine infection is established, the patient should be delivered. The mother is usually commenced on an antibiotic combination such as metronidazole and a cephalosporin. If the fetus is delivered for intrauterine infection, full investigation for sepsis should be initiated and the baby started on systemic antibiotics at birth. Neonatal death from infection can occur within 24 h if this is not done.

Normal labour and delivery

Infection during normal labour is not very common. If pyrexia occurs it is likely to be due to genital tract infection, UTI, or an incidental cause like influenza. Urine and vaginal swabs are sent for microscopy and culture, and a parenteral antibiotic, usually amoxycillin, is given; rectal or intravenous metronidazole is often given in addition.

After surgical induction of labour, only about 1 per cent of patients delivered within 24 h were found to develop intrapartum infection (42). If uterine infection does occur during labour, consideration should be given to caesarean section to remove the baby from a septic environment.

More recently, there has been concern about vaginal carriage of group B streptococci. Invasion of the fetus can take place any time between membrane rupture and delivery of the baby, and is responsible for a small number of intrapartum and neonatal perinatal deaths every year. The organism is difficult to eradicate permanently during pregnancy, even with repeated courses of amoxycillin, but there is good evidence that the baby can be protected by parenteral benzylpenicillin or ampicillin given to the mother during labour, and continued in the newborn. A rapid screening test for Group B streptococci is available (43) and has been shown to be cost-effective in preventing perinatal deaths (44). Universal screening of women admitted in labour may not be feasible, but there is a good case for screening women in whom the organism has been detected during pregnancy; those in premature labour, particularly if the membranes are ruptured; those with pre-labour or prolonged rupture of the membranes; and those for whom induction of labour is planned.

Caesarean section

The incidence of infection after caesarean section is greatly underestimated by surgeons who do not maintain a careful audit of infection rates in their practice. It ranges between 25 and 85 per cent (45). The wide variation in reported incidence is due, in part, to differences in the definition of infection and differences in the populations studied. Over the last twenty years, there has been a dramatic increase in the number of women in developed countries who are delivered by caesarean section. This has resulted in considerable attention being devoted, particularly in North America, to the use of prophylactic antibiotics in an attempt to reduce maternal morbidity.

In a review of 31 placebo controlled studies, prophylactic antibiotics reduced the average incidence of febrile morbidity from 46 to 19 per cent in the patients treated (46). Prophylactic antibiotics decreased the incidence of febrile morbidity and endometritis in all 31 studies, decreased the incidence of UTI in all but one study, and decreased the incidence of wound infection in all but five studies. Thus, patients given prophylactic antibiotics are less likely to require other antibiotics post-operatively and they spend less time in hospital. In a review of over 90 controlled trials it was concluded that the evidence justified far wider adoption of antibiotic prophylaxis than currently exists (45). It was also argued that, on balance, the available evidence favours shorter or single dose regimens over longer or multiple dose regimens for prophylaxis (45). There is no documented evidence that prophylactic antibiotics for caesarean section prevent occassional serious infectious complications such as a pelvic abscess, but it is reasonable to expect that decreasing the overall incidence of infection post-partum should tend to prevent the development of serious infections.

In our own study examining the efficacy of cephradine prophylaxis for caesarean section we used stepwise logistic regression analysis to isolate primary predictive factors which are of importance in their own right (18). The results in 201 patients showed that the important primary variables in reducing the incidence of infection were the pre-operative absence of skin pathogens ($p < 0.05$) and the prophylactic administration of cephradine ($p < 0.001$). Other studies have indicated that variables such as whether or not the patient was in labour and whether or not the membranes were ruptured are important independent factors in determining the risk of post-operative infection (45), and obesity (19), low social class, duration of the operation, and need for blood transfusion (21) should be borne in mind as predisposing factors for infection if a selective policy of antibiotic prophylaxis is to be applied.

Theoretically, the maximum benefit from prophylactic antibiotics should be gained if high tissue levels of antibiotic precede the surgical incision (47). In practice, administering intravenous antibiotics after clamping the cord appears to be equally effective in preventing post-partum infection (48). This avoids the antibiotic crossing the placenta to the fetus. There is no increase in the rate of neonatal sepsis in consequence (49), and it has the logistic effect of reducing the paediatricians' desire to subject the baby to investigation for infection (49). If neonatal investigations do prove necessary, they are not complicated by the presence of a low level of antibiotic in the baby.

No single drug has been shown to be superior in the prevention of infection after abdominal delivery but the simpler cephalosporins are probably the most cost-effective. The broad-spectrum penicillins are as effective as the cephalosporins but there is no convincing evidence that metronidazole conveys any additional benefits (45). The general consensus is that the optimum method for prophylaxis is an intravenous perioperative loading dose followed by a second dose 6 h after the operation and third dose 6 h after that (46). There is no evidence that one particular route is more effective than another but intravenous administration is probably the most feasible. With short duration of antibiotic prophylaxis, there is less risk of a resistant micro-organism flourishing, but the higher the risk of infection, the longer the time the prophylactic treatment should be continued. Infection after antibiotic prophylaxis may be due to resistant organisms (50) and consideration should be given to changing the patient's antibiotic from that used for prophylaxis.

In addition to the clinical benefits, there is strong evidence that antibiotic prophylaxis after caesarean section results in financial savings. In our study, cephradine prophylaxis resulted in savings of the order of £1000–3000 per hundred patients having a caesarean section (18). These savings are similar to those found by others (51).

Post-partum infection

Puerperal infections related to the confinement include perineal infection, endomyometritis, septicaemia, wound infection, and UTI. Rupture or torsion of an unsuspected ovarian cyst can result in peritoneal symptoms. Respiratory infections may be precipitated by general anaesthesia for operative delivery; breast infections may complicate lactation. Incidental causes of infection such as influenza, gastroenteritis, and malaria and other tropical infections should not be forgotten in the differential diagnosis of pyrexia.

Genital tract infection is not common after a normal labour and delivery (52). Patients at particular risk are those who have had a prolonged labour or an operative delivery. The commonest sites are the uterus, the parametria and the adnexa; and the wound following caesarean section.

Diagnosis is based on the classical triad of history, physical examination and investigation. A mid-stream urine sample is examined microscopically and sent for culture, and a high vaginal swab sent for culture. Patients with a confirmed pyrexia of 38°C or more should have blood cultured. Micro-organisms identified on the high vaginal swab may not be those responsible for the infection. Transabdominal sampling of the uterine cavity has not been shown to be of value in clinical management.

Treatment is usually initiated at once, without waiting for the results of investigations, and antibiotics are used parenterally, at least initially, and in high doses. The reason for this is to secure a prompt therapeutic response, bearing in mind the potential consequences for the patient's future fertility if resolution is delayed and involves fibrosis; and the sensitivity of the puerperal women to early spread of infection.

Infections of mild or moderate severity are usually treated with amoxycillin or a cephalosporin, often with metronidazole. If there is failure is to respond after 24 to 36 h, additional antibiotics are given, guided by the results of investigations. If the involvement of Gram-negative organisms is suspected, either co-trimoxazole or gentamicin is added, according to the severity of the situation. High pyrexias within 24 hours of delivery are usually due either to haemolytic streptococci, which require benzylpenicillin, or to acute pyelonephritis, which may need gentamicin. A seriously ill patient with a modest or even subnormal temperature may have anaerobic septicaemia, and metronidazole should then be incorporated in the regimen.

Serious, life-threatening infections require management in an intensive care situation, with full system support available and attention paid to all the ancillary measures necessary (35). Parenteral antibiotic treatment should be broad spectrum from the start, with a penicillin like flucloxacillin, gentamicin, and metronidazole; precautions against vaginal mycosis with nystatin or clotrimazole, and similar care to infusion sites should be taken from the start. Subsequent antimicrobial management depends primarily on clinical response—laboratory sensitivities are a guide to selection of alternative antibiotics and to detect a resistant organism which may require a particular drug. It is unwise to change an antibiotic to another drug abruptly, without any overlap.

Post-partum sterilization

The morbidity of this procedure performed within 48 h of delivery should be quite low—in one study there was a 2 per cent incidence of endometritis, 3 per cent wound infections, 4 per cent urinary infections, and 2 per cent respiratory problems (53). Some of these may have been consequences of the pregnancy and confinement rather than the sterilization operation.

There is thus little case for giving prophylactic antibiotics, except to patients who have had a complicated labour and delivery, or who have medical complications which render them at high risk if infection occurs.

References

1. Bloomfield, T.H. and Hawkins, D.F. (1991). The effects of drugs on the human fetus. In *Scientific foundations of obstetrics and gynaecology*, (4th edn.) (ed. E.E. Philips and M.E. Setchell), Chapter 28. Heinemann Medical, London.
2. Stewart, K.S. (1981). Bacterial infections. *Clinics in Obstetrics and Gynaecology*, **8**, 315–32.
3. Ledward, R.S., Hawkins, D.F., and Stern, L. (1991). Drug treatment in obstetrics. *A handbook of prescribing* (2nd edn.), pp. 194–6. Chapman & Hall, London.
4. Hawkins, D.F. (1989). Antibiotics and breast feeding. *Int. J. Feto-Maternal Med.*, **2**, 223–6.
5. Hammill, H.A. (1989). Normal vaginal flora in relation to vaginitis. *Obstet. Gynecol. Clin. North Am.*, **16**, 329–36.
6. de Louvois, J., Grant, A.N., Arandle, J., Toplis, P.J., Callen, P.J., and Hurley, R. (1980). Bacteraemia following suction termination of pregnancy. *J. Obstet. Gynaecol.*, **1**, 40–5.
7. Larsen, B. (1989). Host defence mechanisms in obstetrics and gynaecology. *Clinics in Obstetrics and Gynaecology*, **10**, 37–64.
8. Miller, J.M., Pupkin, M.J., and Hill, G.B. (1980). Bacterial colonization of amniotic fluid from intact fetal membranes. *Am. J. Obstet. Gynecol.*, **136**, 796–804.
9. Ford, L.C., DeLange, R.J., and Lebherz, T.B. (1977). Identification of a bactericidal factor (β-lysin) in amniotic fluid at 14 and 40 weeks' gestation. *Am. J. Obstet. Gynecol.*, **127**, 788–92.
10. Schlievert, P., Johnson, W., and Galask, R.P. (1970). Isolation of a low molecular weight antibacterial system from human amniotic fluid. *Infect. Immun.*, **14**, 1156–66.
11. Ford, L.C., Kasha, W., Heins, Y., *et al.* (1981). Identification of β-lysin as a zinc-dependent antibacterial protein in the amniotic fluid. *J. Obstet. Gynaecol.*, **2**, 79–84.
12. Scane, T.M.N. and Hawkins, D.F. (1986). Antibacterial activity in human amniotic fluid: dependence on divalent cations. *Br. J. Obstet. Gynaecol.*, **93**, 577–81.
13. Ledger, W.J. (1987). Antibiotics in pregnancy. *Clin. Obstet. Gynecol.*, **20**, 411–21.
14. Cunningham, F.G. (1987). Urinary tract infections complicating pregnancy. *Baillière's Clin. Obstet. Gynaecol.*, **1**, 891–908.
15. Gillespie, W.A., Linton, K.B., Miller, A., and Slade, N. (1960). The diagnosis, epidemiology and control of urinary infection in urology and gynaecology. *J. Clin. Path.*, **13**, 187–94.
16. Wargo, J.D., Teichner, R., and Ferguson, J.H. (1960). Sulfamethoxypyridazine (Kynex)—an evaluation in urinary tract infections. *Am. J. Obstet. Gynecol.*, **80**, 490–4.
17. Derham, R.J., Hawkins, D.F., De Vries, L.S., Aber, V.R., and Elder, M.G. (1984). Outcome of pregnancies complicated by severe hypertension and delivered before 34 weeks; stepwise logistic regression analysis of prognostic factors. *Br. J. Obstet. Gynaecol.*, **96**, 1173–81.
18. Turner, M.J., Egan, D.M., Qureshi, W.A., *et al.* (1990). Use of cephradine prophylaxis of infection after caesarean section; stepwise logistic regression analysis of relevant factors. *J. Obstet. Gynaecol.*, **10**, 204–9.
19. Moir-Bussy, B.R., Hutton, R.M., and Thompson, J.R. (1984). Wound infection after caesarean section. *J. Hosp. Infect.*, **5**, 359–70.
20. Smith, J.R. and Grant, J.M. (1990). The incidence of glove puncture during caesarean section. *J. Obstet. Gynaecol.*, **10**, 317–8.
21. Wolfe, H.M., Gross, T.L., Sokal, R.J., Bottoms, S.F., and Thompson, K.L. (1988). Determinants of morbidity in obese women delivered by cesarean section. *Obstet. Gynecol*, **71**, 691–6.
22. Wilson, J.R. (1961). *Management of obstetrical difficulties*, p. 524. C.V. Mosby, St. Louis, Missouri.
23. Calman, R.M. and Gibson, J. (1954). The bacteriology of the puerperal uterus. *Journal of Obstetrics and Gynaecology of the British Commonwealth*, **61**, 623–7.
24. Laros, R.K., Zatuchni, G.I., and Andros, G.J. (1973). Puerperal tubal ligation morbidity, histology and bacteriology. *Obstet. Gynecol.*, **41**, 397–403.
25. Hellman, L.M. (1949). Morphology of the human fallopian tube in the early puerperium. *Am. J. Obstet. Gynecol.*, **57**, 154–65.
26. Rubin, A. and Czernobilsky, B. (1970). Tubal ligation: a bacteriologic, histologic and clinical study. *Obstet. Gynecol.*, **36**, 199–203.
27. Hawkins, D.F. (1986). Antimicrobial drugs in pregnancy and adverse effects on the fetus. *J. Obstet. Gynaecol.* **6**, (suppl. 1), S11–S13.
28. Ledward, R.S. (1987). Antimicrobial drugs in pregnancy. In *Drugs and pregnancy. Human teratogenesis and related problems* (2nd edn.) (ed. D.F. Hawkins), pp. 148–65. Churchill Livingstone, Edinburgh.
29. Hawkins, D.F. (1989). Drugs used to treat medical disorders in pregnancy and fetal abnormalities. In *Reviews in perinatal medicine*, Vol. 6 (ed. E.M. Scarpelli and E.V. Cosmi), pp. 91–131. Alan R. Liss, New York.

30. Ledward, R.S., Hawkins, D.F., and Stern, L. (1991). Infections. *Drug treatment in obstetrics. A handbook of prescribing*, pp. 147-225. Chapman & Hall, London.
31. Heinonen, O.P., Slone, D., and Shapiro, S. (1977). *Birth defects and drugs in pregnancy*, pp. 296-313. Publishing Sciences Group, Littleton, Massachusetts.
32. Wang, E. and Smaill, F. (1989). Infection in pregnancy. In *Effective care in pregnancy and childbirth* (ed. I. Chalmers, M. Enkin, and M.J.N.C Keirse), Chapter 24, pp. 534-64. Oxford University Press, Oxford.
33. Kass, E.H. (1960). The role of asymptomatic bacteriuria in the pathogenesis of pyelonephritis. In *Biology of pyelonephritis* (ed. E.L. Quinn and E.H. Kass), pp. 399-412. Little Brown, Boston.
34. Chow, A.W. and Jewesson, P.J. (1985). Pharmacokinetics and safety of antimicrobial agents during pregnancy. *Rev. Infect. Dis.*, **7**, 287-313.
35. Gaya, H. and Hawkins, D.F. (1981). Pelvic infection. In *Gynaecological therapeutics* (ed. D.F. Hawkins), pp. 142-210. Baillière Tindall, London.
36. Faro, S. (1989) Antibiotic prophylaxis. *Obstet. Gynecol. Clin. North Am.*, **16**, pp. 279-90.
37. Novy, M.J., Haymond, J., and Nichols, M. (1990). Shirodkar cerclage in a multifactorial approach to the patient with advanced cervical changes. *Am. J. Obstet. Gynecol.*, **162**, 1412-20.
38. Keirse, M.J.N.C., Ohisson, A., Treffers, P.E., and Kanhai, H.H.H. (1989). Prelabour rupture of the membranes pre-term. In *Effective care in pregnancy and childbirth* (ed. I. Chalmers, M., Enkin, and M.J.N.C. Keirse), Vol. 1, pp. 666-93. Oxford University Press, Oxford.
39. Dunlop, P.D.M., Crowley, P.A., Lamont, R.F., and Hawkins, D.F. (1986). Pre-term ruptured membranes, no contractions. *J. Obstet. Gynaecol.*, **7**, 92-96.
40. Amon, E., Lewis, S.V., Sibai, B.M., Villar, M.A., and Arheart, K.L. (1988). Ampicillin prophylaxis in pre-term premature rupture of membranes; a prospective randomized study. *Am. J. Obstet. Gynecol.*, **159**, 539-43.
41. Ogita, S., Mizuno, M., Takeda, Y., *et al.* (1988). Clinical effectiveness of a new cervical indwelling catheter in the management of premature rupture of the membranes: a Japanese collaborative study. *Am. J. Obstet. Gynecol.*, **159**, 336-41.
42. Muldoon, M.J. (1968). A prospective study of intrauterine infection following surgical induction of labour. *Journal of Obstetrics and Gynaecology of the British Commonwealth*, **75**, 1144-50.
43. Stiller, R.J., Blair, E., Clark, P., and Tinghitella, T. (1989). Rapid detection of vaginal colonization with group B streptococci by means of latex agglutination. *Am. J. Obstet. Gynecol.*, **160**, 566-8.
44. Strickland, D.M., Yeomans, E.R., and Hankins, G.D.V. (1990). Cost-effectiveness of intrapartum screening and treatment for maternal group B streptococci colonization. *Am. J. Obstet. Gynecol.*, **163**, 4-8.
45. Enkin, M., Enkin, E., Chalmers, I., and Hemminki, E. (1989). Prophylactic antibiotics in association with caesarean section. In *Effective care in pregnancy and childbirth* (ed. I. Chalmers, M. Enkin, and M.J.N.C. Keirse), Vol. 2, pp. 1246-69. Oxford University Press, Oxford.
46. Rayburn, W.F. (1983). Prophylactic antibiotics during caesarean section: an overview of prior clinical investigations. *Clin. Perinatol.*, **10**, 461-72.
47. Cartwright, P.S., Pittaway, D.E., Jones, H.W., and Entman, S.E. (1984). The use of prophylactic antibiotics in obstetrics and gynaecology. A review. *Obstet. Gynecol.*, **39**, 537-54.
48. Gordon, H.R., Phelps, D., and Blanchard, K. (1979). Prophylactic caesarean section antibiotics: maternal and neonatal morbidity before or after cord clamping. *Obstet. Gynecol.*, **53**, 151-6.
49. Cunningham, F.G., Leveno, K.J., De Palma, R.T., Roark, M., and Rosenfeld, C.R. (1983). Perioperative antimicrobials for caesarean delivery: before or after cord clamping? *Obstet. Gynecol.*, **62**, 151-4.
50. Faro, S., Cox, S.M., Phillips, L., and Baker, J. (1986). Influence of antibiotic prophylaxis on vaginal microflora. *J. Obstet. Gynaecol.*, **6**, suppl. 1, S4-S6.
51. Mugford, M., Kingston, J., and Chalmers, I. (1989). Reducing the incidence of infection after caesarean section: implications of prophylaxis with antibiotics for hospital resources. *Br. Med. J.*, **299**, 1003-6.
52. Gibbs, R.S. (1980). Clinical risk factors for puerperal infection. *Obstet. Gynecol.*, **55**, supplement, 178S-83S.
53. Wilson, E.A., Dilts, P.V., Jr., and Simpson, T.J. (1973). Comparative morbidity of postpartum sterilization procedures. *Am. J. Obstet. Gynecol.*, **115**, 884-9.

32

Infections in gynaecological surgery

ALLAN B. MACLEAN

Infection that may complicate gynaecological surgery

Range of procedures and sites of infection

The definition of post-surgical infection can be difficult. It is not enough to demonstrate the presence of bacteria; nor can the diagnosis be based on a collection of clinical signs. Some of these difficulties are illustrated in the definition of infection complicating gynaecological surgery. Post-hysterectomy pelvic infection, pelvic cellulitis, parametritis, or vault/cuff infection are all defined as being associated with lower abdominal or pelvic pain, tenderness to deep palpation, and an elevation of temperature. Pain and tenderness are frequent findings after surgery, and are difficult to quantitate or interpret. The use of an elevated temperature (usually greater than 38 °C) is included in the definition of terms such as 'fever index' or 'febrile morbidity' in the gynaecological literature. It must be recognized that post-operative pyrexia may also be due to tissue ischaemia or crushing, absorption of blood from the peritoneal cavity, or even due to blood transfusion.

The lower genital tract is colonized with a wide variety of organisms. One of the better reviews is that by Larsen and Galask (1) who have reported their own microbiological findings, and have reviewed the literature. The majority of women will have a mixed bacterial flora within the vagina. Lactobacilli and diphtheroids will be present in 75 per cent of women, but are of low pathogenicity and unlikely to have clinical significance. A mixture of aerobic and anaerobic streptococci are present. The majority of women are colonized by one or more species of anaerobic cocci, predominantly peptococcus and peptostreptococcus species. The aerobic streptococci will be alpha, beta, and non-haemolytic. The predominant group among the beta haemolytic are Lancefield's group B. Group D Streptococci will be present in approximately one-third. Other aerobic cocci include enterococcus (formerly known as *Streptococcus faecalis*), *Staphylococcus aureus*, and *Staph. epidermidis*. Gram-negative bacilli will be found in approximately 30 per cent of healthy women, the predominant organism being *Escherichia coli*. Gram-negative anaerobic organisms present are bacteroides, including *B. bivius*, *B. disiens*, and *B. fragilis*. Other anaerobes will be members of the *Clostridium* and *Fusobacterium* species.

Many factors influence the prevalence of these organisms including pregnancy, postmenopausal status, concurrent use of hormone replacement therapy, oral contraception, antibiotic therapy, foreign bodies such as a ring pessary and the presence of necrotic tumour, etc. Additional organisms introduced through sexual activity may also be found including *Neisseria gonorrhoeae*, *Chlamydia trachomatis*, and *Mycoplasma* species. Thus, to demonstrate the presence of any of these organisms at the top of the vagina after surgery does not equate necessarily with post-operative infection. Infection after gynaecological surgery may involve sites other than the surgical wounds. Up to 40 per cent of women will have post-operative bacteriuria (2), and of these some, but not all, will be symptomatic. Organisms are introduced during pre-operative bladder catheterization; if pain or other factors prevent complete bladder emptying post-operatively, these organisms will proliferate in the residual urine to reach significant numbers (greater than 10^5 organisms per millilitre).

Infection may also occur within the chest, at sites of venous access (phlebitis) or rarely phlebitis in lower leg veins, or infection complicating spinal or epidural anaesthesia.

Abdominal surgery

Any incision of the abdominal wall will allow the entry of skin organisms, or those exogenous contaminants from the theatre environment or surgical team (see Chapters 2 and 3). Procedures on the uterine tube (either at laparoscopy or laparotomy) may liberate tubal organisms, including sexually transmitted *N. gonorrhoeae* or *C. trachomatis*. Conditions associated with haemoperitomeum, such as ruptured tubal pregnancy or haemorrhage from ovarian cysts may leave residual amounts of blood suitable to act as a culture medium for any inoculated organisms, unless drainage is efficient.

Total abdominal hysterectomy is associated with an abdominal wound and one where the upper vagina is opened to remove the cervix. Sub-total hysterectomy is rarely performed nowadays, but had the advantage in pre-antibiotic days of leaving the vagina unopened. Vaginal organisms will contaminate this wound producing pelvic or vault infection. Davey *et al.* (3) in a Dundee study reported an incidence of wound plus pelvic infection of 29 per cent in patients undergoing abdominal hysterectomy. Dicker *et al.* (4) reported an incidence of 'febrile morbidity' of 32 per cent after abdominal hysterectomy, with 4.4 per cent pelvic infection.

The risk of infection increases with more radical procedures such as for cervical or ovarian carcinoma. This increase is due to longer operating time (3), more extensive dissection with tissue damage, collection of haematomata or lymphocysts, and impairment of immunological responses in these debilitated patients (5). The risk of surgical infection is further increased if the large bowel is opened, intentionally or otherwise, during surgery for gynaecological malignancy.

Vaginal surgery

Vaginal surgery carries the risk of post-operative infection because of the many potentially pathogenic organisms present in the operative field, because of ascending spread when the peritoneum is opened during vaginal hysterectomy and because of the increased need for post-operative bladder drainage. Davey *et al.* (3) reported an incidence of wound/pelvic infection of 27 per cent in patients undergoing vaginal hysterectomy, similar to that for abdominal hysterectomy in their study. White *et al.* (6) reported 'febrile morbidity' rates of 55 per cent for vaginal and 36 per cent for abdominal hysterectomy. Amirikia and Evans (7) reported 'febrile morbidity' rates of 26 per cent for vaginal and 16 per cent for abdominal hysterectomy. Dicker *et al.* (4) reported a 'febrile morbidity' incidence of only 15 per cent after vaginal hysterectomy with pelvic infection occurring in 3.3 per cent. It is interesting to note that, in this latter series, post-hysterectomy infection was higher after abdominal rather than vaginal surgery; however, prophylactic antibiotics had been given to 82 per cent of the women who underwent vaginal surgery but to only 32 per cent of women who underwent abdominal hysterectomy.

Procedures involving the cervix

Infection can complicate cone biopsy and cause secondary haemorrhage or fibrosis with subsequent stenosis (8). The infective complications of radical hysterectomy with lymphadenectomy for cervical carcinoma are increased due to prolonged surgical time and disruption of lymphatics. Radiotherapeutic management of cervical carcinoma often had infective complications because radium sources were left within the uterus and endocervix for up to 72 h. The presence of necrotic tumour encouraged proliferation of anaerobic organisms and a pyometra was often encountered. The increasing use of caesium sources and remote afterloading techniques to deliver high dose rates have lessened these risks.

Even diagnostic dilatation and curettage appears to have a risk of post-operative infection, probably from the introduction of vaginal or cervical organisms at the time of uterine instrumentation. Taylor and Graham (9) described the laparoscopic appearances in patients with unexplained infertility where tubal damage from infection was seen more frequently in those women who had not had previous pelvic inflammatory disease but had undergone diagnostic curettage, than in women who had not.

Procedures involving injection of dye or contrast to assess tubal patency

Approximately one-third of women who present with infertility will have tubal damage. One way of assessing this is to inject radio-opaque contrast. Injection of contrast may introduce infection, or may produce spillage of infected tubal content into the peritoneal cavity. Pyper *et al.* (10) described the risk of infection associated with laparoscopy and hydrotubation, and recommend that the dye should not be injected if bilateral hydrosalpinges are clearly seen; if a unilateral hydrosalpinx is seen and dye is injected to confirm the patency of the other tube post-operative antibiotic treatment should be given for 5 days. If the tubes appear patent and healthy prophylactic antibiotics were not recommended.

Procedures on the pregnant uterus

Since the Abortion Act came into operation in April 1968, the number of deaths from therapeutic abortion in Scotland, England, and Wales has been small. Although criminal abortion is no longer a major problem, maternal mortality from septic abortion and associated with spontaneous abortion, mid-trimester abortion, missed abortion, and occasionally therapeutic abortion still occurs. Further, septic abortion remains a major problem in the third world.

Pelvic infection with abortion is linked with previous pelvic inflammatory disease, the gestation at which abortion occurs, the technique used in the management of missed abortion or therapeutic abortion, and the presence of retained tissue. The causative organisms may be multiple, but infection with anaerobic bacteria and in particular *Clostridium perfringens* may be associated with significant sequelae. Their presence may be of no clinical consequence, but may cause gas gangrene or systemic illness with haemolysis, haemoglobinaemia, haemoglobinuria, acute renal failure, disseminated intravascular coagulopathy, and death. This particular form of pelvic infection occurs when the clostridia are introduced from the vagina into the uterus, when the uterus contains non-viable or necrotic tissue, and when this tissue remains in the uterus for sufficient time to allow incubation of organisms.

Post partum infection is more likely to be seen following caesarean section and if retained tissue is present within the uterus. These problems are discussed in the previous chapter and by MacLean (11).

How to avoid infection in gynaecological surgery

Patient preparation

The endogenous organisms found within the vagina have been described earlier. In normal circumstances little pre-operative preparation is required. However, where there is an increased likelihood of sexually transmitted disease appropriate swabs should be taken before surgery. Patients with a ring pessary should have this removed well in advance of surgery. The use of oestrogen cream will encourage the healing of vaginal ulceration associated with prolapse or use of a ring, but increase mucosal vascularity and should be stopped two weeks pre-operatively.

Formerly, Bonney's blue solution was splashed liberally into the vagina to reduce bacterial presence prior to abdominal hysterectomy. There are concerns that this dye may be carcinogenic and the current recommendations are to use methylene blue, aqueous chlorhexidine, or povidone–iodine.

The patient's bowel should be empty at the time of surgery: this is important for vaginal surgery and where regional anaesthesia is used, as the latter is associated with sphincteric relaxation. If the bowel has not moved the evening before theatre, glycerin suppositories or a phosphate enema are usually effective. Patients requiring a more thorough bowel preparation, e.g. prior to surgery for ovarian tumour, can be given magnesium sulphate or sodium picosulphate (Picolax) elixir (providing there is no evidence of bowel obstruction).

Some patients with moderate to marked cystocele or with procidentia will have difficulty with micturition. Incomplete emptying of the bladder will encourage a residual urine pool to become infected. A midstream urine specimen should be cultured pre-operatively; if the urine is infected, sensitivities should be sought and the most appropriate antibiotic used as soon as the result is available.

Smoking among our patients is an unfortunate, but frequent reality. Smokers should be encouraged to stop before planned elective procedures—it is their wound that will hurt with post-operative coughing. Pre-operative chest physiotherapy to clear mucus plugs may help to reduce post-operative respiratory infection. Major surgery should be deferred in patients with pharyngitis as the endotracheal intubation increases the risk of chest infection. The use of regional anaesthesia for vaginal surgery has an advantage over general anaesthesia in reducing the risk of post-operative chest infections.

Patients with a history of rheumatic valvular disease or corrected congenital cardiac anomaly and who are at risk of bacterial endocarditis should be given an appropriate prophylactic antibiotic regimen, which should include activity against Gram-negative organisms. Ampicillin 1 g (or 1 g vancomycin, if the patient is allergic to penicillin) and gentamicin 120 mg intramuscularly should be given with the premedication.

Theatre preparation and operative techniques to reduce the risks of infection

Kitchener and Kingdom (12) have described how these aspects can reduce the risks of infection. The theatre environment at the beginning of the list should be as clean and as dust-free as is practicable. Thus, cases requiring laparotomy are normally placed first on the list, and heavily contaminated or infected cases, such as septic abortion, Bartholin's abscess etc are done last. However, where the operating theatre has adequate ventilation that is little evidence that such an arrangement has any great influence on the incidence of infection. The operating gynaecologists and assistants should start each list with a two-minute surgical scrub with soap or chlorhexidine, but before minor cases use 0.5 per cent chlorhexidine plus 1 per cent glycerine solution for hand rinsing prior to gloving. The wearing of gowns for surgery such as suction termination may not significantly reduce infective complications for the patient, but may be protective for the surgeon.

The risks of wound infection are increased not only by the inoculation of organisms, but by the provision of conditions conducive to bacterial proliferation and the impairment of host resistance. Abdominal wall infection will be encouraged by failure to achieve haemostasis, excessive use of electrodiathermy, careless use of retractors, and excessively tight or inappropriately positioned sutures. Pelvic infection will be encouraged by damage during bladder dissection, excessive size of ovarian or uterine pedicles, large amounts of chromic catgut suture material in the vaginal vault, or inadequate haemostasis. The indications for surgical drainage in gynaecological procedures have recently been defined (13): closed-system suction drainage of the retropubic space and groin wounds at radical vulvectomy, and open, passive drainage of abscesses and haematomata. It is not necessary to drain the peritoneum or rectus sheath of every hysterectomy, but prophylactic suction drains placed in areas of increased vascularity and removed 24–48 h later are beneficial. Swartz and Taneree (14) showed that the use of suction drainage of the vaginal vault to prevent haematoma collection was as effective as prophylactic antibiotics in preventing pelvic infection. An alternative is to leave the vault open to allow adequate drainage, but using a continuous locking suture to achieve haemostasis.

Finally, the time to perform the necessary surgery should be minimized without sacrificing safety. Davey *et al.* (3) showed an increase in the incidence of wound and pelvic infection according to the duration of hysterectomy, from less than 10 per cent if the procedure took less than 45 min to 50 per cent if greater than 90 min.

The use of prophylactic antibiotics in gynaecological surgery

Antibiotics have been used for years in high risk patients to reduce the risk of serious infection such as bacterial endocarditis, in neutropenic patients, and where there is a risk of meningococcal meningitis. Their use in surgery dates from the observations of Burke (15) that staphylococci inoculated into experimentally inflicted wounds would be less likely to cause infection if antibiotic was already present in the tissues. The general principles of the use of prophylactic antibiotics are reviewed in Chapter 8 and Ledger *et al.* (16) have given guide-lines for their use in gynaecology:

(a) the operation should carry a significant risk of post-operative infection;
(b) the operation should cause significant bacterial contamination;
(c) the antibiotic used for prophylaxis should have laboratory evidence of effectiveness against the contaminating micro-organisms and there should be evidence of clinical effectiveness;
(d) the antibiotic should be present in the wound, in effective concentration, at the time of incision;
(e) a short-term, low toxicity regimen of antibiotics should be used;
(f) antibiotics needed to combat resistant infections should be reserved and not used for prophylaxis;
(g) the benefits of prophylactic antibiotics must outweigh the dangers of antibiotic use.

Subsequent studies (almost all being performed in North America) have suggested that prophylactic antibiotics have an important contribution in preventing infection after vaginal hysterectomy in pre-menopausal women, perhaps post-menopausal women, and perhaps also for abdominal hysterectomy. The uncertainty exists because serious post-hysterectomy infections such as pelvic abscess and pelvic vein thrombophlebitis are uncommon events, and therefore other indices of delayed recovery or infection such as 'bed days' or 'febrile morbidity' have been used to show the differences between treated and untreated groups. Some of these differences will disappear when other parameters including cost are used. In the Dundee study it was shown that when the cost of antibiotics prescribed by the general practitioner were added to those of treatment in hospital, the placebo group was cheaper than cephradine and mezlocillin for vaginal hysterectomy, but the cephradine group was cheaper than either placebo or mezlocillin for abdominal hysterectomy (3).

This study also highlighted the effect that duration of surgery has on infection rates, and the likely benefits of prophylactic antibiotics. In the Dundee study (3) only 5 per cent of the operations lasted more than 1.5 h, compared with a similar study of vaginal and abdominal hysterectomy where 66 per cent of the operations lasted more than 1.75 h (17). This difference may explain, partly, why prophylactic antibiotic usage is almost compulsory in the US, but infrequent or inconsistent in the UK. Until recently, gynaecologists in the UK have been less concerned with cost-effectiveness or litigation; these and other factors, including increased promotion by the pharmaceutical companies, may increase antibiotic use in gynaecology in the future (18).

Prophylactic antibiotics have been advocated in other areas of gynaecological surgery. Although there has been no study to show advantage over placebo, antibiotics have been given to women undergoing laparotomy for malignant disease, especially when there is the likelihood that large bowel may be opened. Patients undergoing hysterosalpingography, or laparoscopy with chromo (hydro) tubation and with a past history, or operative evidence, of pelvic inflammatory disease should have antibiotic cover (10). There are recommendations, although no prospective studies to confirm benefit, that women undergoing tubal surgery to restore patency should have antibiotics. Sonne-Holm *et al.* (19) have presented data to support the suggestion that a woman undergoing suction termination of pregnancy should receive antibiotics if she had earlier had pelvic inflammatory disease. Other studies have suggested that such therapy must be effective against chlamydia. Alternatively, patients can be tested for *Chlamydia trachomatis*, and treated if positive, prior to the termination.

As has already been described, the flora of the genital tract is polymicrobial, with a mixture of anaerobic and aerobic organisms. Further, many of the aerobic bacilli can produce beta-lactamase and other enzymes to reduce the antibiotic effect. Therefore, there is no simple, first line antibiotic that will cover all potential pathogens. Recommendations for suitable choices include ampicillin and other synthetic, broad spectrum penicillins including piperacillin and mezlocillin, co-amoxyclav, cephalosporins and the anti-anaerobic drug metronidazole. The need to cover anaerobic organisms, except where the large bowel has been opened or where necrotic tissue remains with septic abortion, remains unclear. A report from Cardiff (20) showed that co-amoxyclav had advantages over metronidazole as prophylaxis for hysterectomy, and recommended the use of an agent, or combination of agents, with activity against both aerobic and anaerobic bacteria. Although second and third generation cephalosporins are effective against many anaerobic bacteria there is evidence that cephradine (first generation with reduced activity against anaerobic bacteria) is just as effective for hysterectomy prophylaxis, and less expensive (21).

Prophylactic antibiotics were often given for prolonged courses, but today most recommendations are that the drug should be given with the pre-medication, and not continued post-operatively. There is evidence that prophylactic antibiotics can alter the genital tract flora, with an increase in enterococcus colonization and the development of resistance when three doses of cephalosporin were given (22, 23). In view of the alarming reports of development of antibiotic resistance occurring in many places, antibiotics must be used wisely and not as a panacea to cover lapses in surgical technique.

The following guide-lines are given on the use of prophylactic antibiotics in gynaecological surgery:

1. If antibiotics are to be used to cover vaginal hysterectomy, a simple and inexpensive drug such as nitrofurantoin or trimethoprim should be given that will be effective against the significant incidence of post-operative bacteriuria (2).
2. Antibiotics should only be given in selected patients undergoing abdominal hysterectomy, where previous pelvic surgery or infection may prolong the procedure (more than 1.5–2 h) or increase the risk of further infection.
3. Patients undergoing surgery for malignant disease such as cervical or vulval carcinoma, should receive prophylactic antibiotics when the procedure is likely to be prolonged. Cover with a long-acting cephalosporin should be given and metronidazole added only if the bowel is opened.

4. Patients undergoing termination of pregnancy, tests of tubal patency or tubal surgery should be covered, if thought to be at increased risk, with an antichlamydial agent, e.g. doxycycline.

How to recognize infection

Clinical features

Pyrexia is the principal clinical feature of infection. However, its presence, in the first 24 h following surgery may not be due to infection, as has been discussed earlier. Rarely is major infection seen in the first day following gynaecological surgery, it is usually due to infection that pre-dates the surgery, as with septic abortion, pelvic or urinary tract infection.

Between day 1 and 3 post-operatively pyrexia is usually due to development of infection in the urinary or respiratory tracts, and rarely within the peritoneum as a result of operative damage to a viscus. Pyrexia that occurs more than three days after surgery is likely to be due to wound infection (superficial or deep, and including fasciitis), pelvic infection (especially if the temperature spikes up to 39 °C or higher), phlebitis, endometritis (with the development of infection in retained tissue after an evacuation) as well as urinary and respiratory tract infections.

In addition to the timing of the pyrexia, the signs and symptoms will suggest the sources of infection. Complaints of urinary frequency or dysuria, comments from the physiotherapist about the colour of the sputum or presence of mucoid plugs and reduced air entry, or observations by the nursing staff on the appearance of the wound may all be relevant. Endometritis will be associated with abnormal vaginal bleeding, perhaps with offensive odour.

Pelvic infection may have no feature apart from a spiking pyrexia and tachycardia. There may be symptoms of frequency of micturition and increased bowel activity, or urine volumes may be reduced due to hypovolaemia and the bowel may be quiet due to ileus. The impression of a vault collection may be perceived on vaginal examination, but may be more obvious to the finger on rectal examination.

Septicaemia may have the associated features of rigors, tachycardia, hypotension, poor peripheral perfusion, and oliguria. Confusion may arise as to the underlying cause, and to whether these features are due to concealed blood loss, cardiogenic shock, or pulmonary embolism.

Appropriate investigations

If infection is suspected, appropriate microbiological specimens should be taken for culture before further management is initiated. Such specimens may include midstream urine, sputum, blood culture, endocervical swab, or wound swab for culture. Occasionally, when managing septic abortion or after infertility investigations, an endocervical swab should be taken specifically for chlamydia.

Blood investigations should include haemoglobin, (as a fall between the first post-operative day and the development of pyrexia may be associated with an infected vault collection), white blood count, and serum urea and electrolyte estimations if infection is systemic or if treatment with aminoglycosides may be indicated. C-reactive protein levels or erythrocyte sedimentation rates are unlikely to be helpful in the immediate post-operative period, as they may rise in response to the surgical trauma.

Where indicated a chest radiograph may confirm the clinical suspicion of respiratory tract infection. Pelvic ultrasound can be useful to demonstrate residual tissue within the uterus after incomplete abortion or suction termination, or may demonstrate pelvic fluid with pelvic infection. The use of vaginal ultrasound to investigate post-operative pelvic infection is still being evaluated.

Management of post-operative infection

Once the diagnosis of infection has been made the following steps should be taken:

(a) Obtain appropriate specimens for a bacteriological diagnosis, if this has not already been done.

(b) Consider the need for surgical intervention.

(c) Consider the choice of antibiotics.

The need for further surgery

The need to re-operate on a patient because of post-operative complications may be obvious, or may require a difficult decision based on the balance of multiple factors.

Retained uterine tissue after earlier evacuation, for example after suction termination, or wide excision of necrotic areas involved with necrotizing fasciitis obviously need surgical intervention. Although antibiotic therapy is administered when each of these procedures must be done, neither surgery nor antibiotic will prove effective if used alone.

The more difficult situations include pelvic abscess after hysterectomy, cellulitis following a pregnancy, or secondary haemorrhage after a cone biopsy. Where a vault collection is suspected it may be possible to pass a finger through the sutures in the vaginal vault, and release the infected haematoma. If drainage is inadequate, or if the patient's condition deteriorates further, laparotomy, peritoneal toilet with saline or tetracycline solution, and passive drainage with a wide-bore tube becomes necessary. The anatomy within the pelvis may be distorted by collections of pus, or omental and bowel adhesions. The source of the bleeding has usually settled and identification may not be possible. Careless dissection of pedicles, or of the vaginal vault, may produce further haemorrhage which may be difficult to control in the midst of friable tissues.

When infection occurs after an abortion or post-partum, hysterectomy may be necessary to control uterine bleeding and to remove the source of infection. When haemorrhage occurs some five to ten days after a cone biopsy, initial attempts to control the situation may require re-suturing of the cervix, under general anaesthesia. If there is significant lysis of clot because of infection and sutures tear out of the cervix because of its friability, abdominal hysterectomy may be the only way to control blood loss. The vaginal vault is better left open and a wide bore tube drain positioned through it to allow drainage and to reduce further the risk of infection.

The choice of antibiotic

The selection of an antibiotic appropriate for post-operative infection will be influenced by:

(a) Information on the host, including a history of allergy, the presence of underlying renal or hepatic disease, the possibility of interaction with other drugs, or possibility of immunosuppression.

(b) An awareness of the likely source of the infection and of the causative organisms, e.g. *Staph. aureus* in a skin wound, or Gram-negative bacilli in urine.

(c) The antibiotic's spectrum of activity, its pharmacokinetics and adverse effects, its availability for oral or parenteral administration, and its cost.

Recommendations

Infection of the wound requires adequate drainage, irrigation, and an oral anti-staphylococcal antibiotic, such as flucloxacillin, is recommended. Urinary tract infection should be treated with oral trimethoprim, cotrimoxazole, nitrofuration, amoxycillin, cephradine, ciprofloxacin, or co-amoxyclav. Chest infection should be treated by physiotherapy plus oral amoxycillin, co-amoxyclav, cephradine, or tetracycline.

When infection follows termination of pregnancy or fertility investigations, oral tetracycline will cover the aerobic and many anaerobic organisms as well as chlamydia. Alternatively, erythromycin can be used. If clostridia are suspected, high doses of intravenous penicillin should be given. If pelvic infection occurs, oral tetracycline, amoxycillin, co-amoxyclav or a cephalosporin can be given, and if the patient is debilitated with vomiting the antibiotic (such as a second of third generation cephalosporin, piperacillin, or co-amoxyclav) must be given intravenously.

If there has been contamination of the pelvis with bowel content, or the patient is seriously ill, metronidazole should be given, initially intravenously and subsequently by suppository, together with intravenous gentamicin. If gentamicin is given care should be taken to measure peak and trough levels after the first 24 h, and the dose adjusted accordingly. If the patient has septicaemia she may require the monitoring and care of an intensive therapy unit.

Gynaecological infections requiring surgery

Bartholin's abscess (greater vestibular gland)

Infection may cause a primary obstruction of the duct of the gland, producing a cystic swelling or abscess. Alternatively, the duct may have been previously distorted by an episiotomy or sexual trauma and subsequent infection or oedema may occlude the duct totally, allowing an abscess to develop. Bartholin's abscess is usually found in sexually active women, and is uncommon after the menopause. Any swelling of this area in postmenopausal women should be biopsied to exclude malignancy.

The organisms isolated include *E. coli*, *Staph. aureus*, *Staph. epidermidis*, *N. gonorrhoeae*, *Pseudomomas* spp., *Enterococcus faecalis*, anaerobic cocci, and mycoplasma. Bacteriology swabs should always be taken: up to one-third of woman with gonorrhoea will have these organisms present in the Bartholin's gland duct.

Management requires adequate surgical drainage. A cruciate incision is made over the point of maximal fluctuation, but preferably allowing drainage into the vestibule; incisions over vulval skin will produce scarring and lead to dyspareunia. The corners of the cruciate incision are excised to allow adequate de-roofing of the abscess, and the skin edges are sutured with chromic catgut to the pericyst edges, to ensure haemostasis and allow subsequent drainage of the gland. The cavity should not be packed—it is painful to remove the next day. Antibiotic therapy should be started if *N. gonorrhoeae* is isolated, or if cellulitis is present. Excision of the gland should not be attempted as this anatomical area can be vascular. If the surgery is inadequate, recurrence of obstruction with cyst formation will occur.

Endometritis

The diagnosis of endometritis is based on a history of abnormal uterine bleeding, pain (dysmenorrhoea and dyspareunia), and a predisposing event such as a recent pregnancy, abortion, or the presence of an intrauterine contraceptive device (IUCD). The clinical findings are of pyrexia, tachycardia, pelvic pain, and uterine tenderness. If extension of infection occurs, with spread to the tubes (salpingitis) or parametrium (parametritis, cellulitis) the systemic signs will be more spectacular and there will be the features of pelvic peritonitis (i.e. the woman will be unable to move her abdominal wall freely) and cervical excitation pain will be present.

Management

An IUCD may cause this problem with sexually transmitted organisms, organisms of the vaginal flora, and occasionally with actinomyces. Management consists of removing the device which should be sent for bacteriological culture, and commencing appropriate antibiotics.

Infection with retained tissue

Patients will present with bleeding (secondary post-partum haemorrhage or incomplete abortion), and in addition to the findings of endometritis the cervix may be open. Ultrasound scan (vaginal or abdominal) will show retained tissue or absence of a clear endometrial echo. Management is by uterine evacuation under general anaesthesia, either by digital curage (if the uterine size is more than 16 weeks) or curettage.

Septic abortion

The management of septic abortion depends on the early recognition of infection, the use of parenteral antibiotics that will cover clostridia and anaerobic cocci as well as aerobic bacteria, and the removal of retained tissue soon after antibiotics have been started. This latter procedure requires care and experience; over vigorous curettage will produce uterine perforation or result in Ashermann's syndrome (intrauterine synechiae) while incomplete removal will allow infection to continue. If infection is advanced, support to the systemic circulation and treatment of renal failure may be required. Occasionally, hysterectomy will be necessary to control uterine haemorrhage (24).

Pelvic sepsis

The diagnosis of pelvic inflammatory disease is based on history, clinical findings in the pelvis, and microbiological identification of a causative organism. Increasingly, the diagnosis is confirmed by laparoscopic findings. The choice of antibiotic should cover the possibilities of chlamydia, gonococci, and Gram-negative bacilli. If the infection is chronic or recurrent, involvement with anaerobic organisms must also considered.

If the patient is significantly unwell and has failed to show any response to 24 h of parenteral antibiotics, reappraisal of the diagnosis is necessary. This may require diagnostic laparoscopy, when the need to proceed to laparotomy may be recognized. If a laparotomy is undertaken this should be via a vertical incision which will give sufficient access to manage a tubo-ovarian abscess (especially if ruptured) or peritonitis secondary to acute appendicitis. Careful division of adhesions and loculations, peritoneal toilet and the use of one or more wide-bore tube drains placed in the pelvis or iliac fossa may be necessary. Attempts to remove the appendix, tubes, or uterus in the presence of diffuse peritonitis can be associated with serious morbidity or mortality (24). More definitive surgery may be required later, once the infection has been controlled.

Chronic cervicitis

There was previously a vogue for treating by cautery or diathermy those patients who complained of chronic vaginal discharge and were found to have a cervical 'erosion'. Colposcopy has shown that 'erosions' should be considered as visible columnar epithelium (known as 'ectopy' or 'eversion' now). Providing *N. gonorrhoeae* and *C. trachomatis* have been excluded, 'cervicitis' does not require treatment except by increasing vaginal acidity (with Aci-jel) to promote squamous metaplasia.

Over the last twenty-five years the availability of broad spectrum antibiotics, changes in abortion laws, and general improvement in health have reduced the problems of infection after gynaecological surgery, and gynaecological problems requiring surgery. However, infection still occurs; resident doctors must know of the potential for problems, and how to manage them.

References

1. Larsen, B. and Galask, R. P. (1980). Vaginal microbial flora: practical and theoretical relevance. *Obstet. Gynecol.*, **55**, 100S–113S.
2. Kingdom, J. C. P., Kitchener, H. C., and MacLean, A. B. (1990). Post-operative urinary tract infection in gynecology: implications for an antibiotic prophylaxis policy. *Obstet. Gynecol.*, **76**, 636–8.
3. Davey, P. G., Duncan, I. D., Edward, D., and Scott, A. C. (1988). Cost-benefit analysis of cephradine and mezlocillin prophylaxis for abdominal and vaginal hysterectomy. *Br. J. Obstet. Gynaecol.*, **95**, 1170–7.
4. Dicker, R. C., Greenspan, J. R., Strauss, L. T., Cowart, M. R., Scally, M. J., Peterson, H. B. *et al.* (1982). Complications of abdominal and vaginal hysterectomy among women of reproductive age in the United States. *Am. J. Obstet. Gynecol.*, **144**, 841–8.
5. Brooker, D. C., Savage, J. E., Twiggs, L. B., Adcock, L. L., Prem, K. A., and Sanders, C. C. (1987). Infectious morbidity in gynecologic cancer. *Am. J. Obstet. Gynecol.*, **156**, 513–20.
6. White, S. C., Wartel L. J., and Wade, M. E. (1971). Comparison of abdominal and vaginal hysterectomies. *Obstet. Gynecol.*, **37**, 530–7.
7. Amirikia, H. and Evans, T. N. (1979). Ten year review of hysterectomies: trends, indications, and risks. *Am. J. Obstet. Gynecol.*, **134**, 431–7.
8. Sharp, F. and Cordiner, J. W. (1985). The treatment of CIN: cone biopsy and hysterectomy. *Clin. Obstet. Gynaecol.*, **12**, 133–48.
9. Taylor, P. J. and Graham, G. (1982). Is diagnostic curettage harmful in women with unexplained infertility? *Br. J. Obstet. Gynaecol.*, **89**, 296–8.
10. Pyper, R. J. D., Ahmet, Z., and Houang, E. T. (1988). Bacteriological contamination during laparoscopy with dye injection. *Br. J. Obstet. Gynaecol.*, **95**, 367–71.
11. MacLean, A. B. (1990). Puerperal pyrexia. In *Clinical infection of obstetrics and gynaecology* (ed. A. B. MacLean), pp. 195–209. Blackwell, Oxford.
12. Kitchener, H. C. and Kingdom, J. C. P. (1990). Sepsis in gynaecological surgery. In *Clinical Infection in obstetrics and gynaecology* (ed. A. B. MacLean), pp. 313–24. Blackwell, Oxford.
13. Hilton, P. (1988), Surgical wound drainage; a survey of practices among gynaecologists in the British Isles. *Br. J. Obstet. Gynaecol.*, **95**, 1063–9.
14. Swartz, W. H. and Tanaree, P. (1975). Suction drainage as an alternative to prophylactic antibiotics for hysterectomy. *Obstet. Gynecol.*, **45**, 305–10.
15. Burke, J. F. (1961). The effective period of preventive antibiotic action in experimental incisions and dermal lesions. *Surgery*, **50**, 161–8.
16. Ledger, W. J., Gee, C., and Lewis, W. P. (1975). Guide-lines for antibiotic prophylaxis in gynecology. *Am. J. Obstet. Gynecol.*, **121**, 1038–45.
17. Shapiro, M., Munoz, A., Tager, I. B. Schoenbaum, S. C., and Polk, B. F. (1982) Risk factors for infection at the operative site after abdominal or vaginal hysterectomy. *N. Engl. J. Med.*, **307**, 1661–6.
18. Kennedy, R. and Duncan, I. D. (1990). Antibiotic prophylaxis in gynaecology. In *Clinical infection in obstetrics and gynaecology* (ed. A. B. MacLean), pp. 325–38. Blackwell, Oxford.
19. Sonne-Holm, S., Heisterberg, L., Hebjorn, S., Dyring-Andersen, K., Andersen, J. T., and Hejl, B. L. (1981). Prophylactic antibiotics in first trimester abortions: a clinical, controlled trial. *Am. J. Obstet. Gynecol.*, **139**, 693–6.
20. Brown, E. M., Depares, J., Robertson, A. A., Jones, S., Hughes, A. B., Coles, E. C., *et al.* (1988). Amoxycillin-clavulanic acid (Augmentin) versus metronidazole as prophylaxis in hysterectomy: a prospective, randomized clinical trial. *Br. J. Obstet. Gynaecol.*, **95**, 286–93.
21. Hemsell, D. L., Heard, M. C., Nobles, B. J., Bawden, R. E., and Hemsell, P. G. (1987). Single dose prophylaxis for vaginal and abdominal hysterectomy. *Am. J. Obstet. Gynecol.*, **157**, 498–501.
22. Stiver, H. G., Forward, K. R., Tyrrell, D. L., *et al.* (1984). Comparative cervical microflora shifts after cefoxitin or cefazolin prophylaxis against infection following cesarean section. *Am. J. Obstet. Gynecol.*, **149**, 718–21.

23. Hemsell, D. L., Heard, M. C., Hemsell, P. G., Nobles, B. J., and Bawdon, R. E. (1988). Alterations in lower reproductive tract flora after single-dose piperacillin and triple-dose cefoxitin at vaginal and abdominal hysterectomy. *Obstet. Gynecol.*, **72**, 875–80.

24. Rivlin, M. E. and Hunt, J. A., (1986). Surgical management of diffuse peritonitis complicating obstetric/gynecologic infections. *Obstet. Gynecol.*, **67**, 652–6.

33

Surgery and AIDS

C. JOSEPH CAHILL

Introduction

The epidemic spread of the acquired immune deficiency syndrome (AIDS) in the ten years since the first patients were reported (1) leaves over 288 000 affected world-wide, and 3433 in the UK by June 1990 (2). Over 60 per cent have already died, and millions more are infected with the AIDS virus but have not yet developed the syndrome.

The virus is believed to have arisen in central Africa, probably Zaïre, by spontaneous mutation from another human or green monkey retrovirus. It spread rapidly amongst men and women, and into neighbouring countries. Zaïre, formerly the Belgian Congo, sought French speaking technical advisors, many of whom came from Haiti. Both homosexual and heterosexual transmission of virus into this group occurred, and when Haiti became popular as a holiday resort among homosexual men from California in the 1970s, the virus was introduced into the Western world. The mobility and promiscuity of this group resulted in very rapid spread in the gay community, with spillover into drug addicts, female partners of bisexual men, and recipients of transfused blood products.

The human immunodeficiency virus (HIV)

The causative agent was not identified until 1983, when Barre-Sinoussi and her colleagues at the Institut Pasteur in Paris, and Gallo at the National Institute of Health in the United States simultaneously isolated the same retrovirus. Initial difference in nomenclature was resolved, and the virus is now known as HIV (Human Immunodeficiency Virus). A second agent, HIV2, was identified in Africa in 1987.

Until antibody tests became available in 1984, and universally applied to blood donors (October 1985 in the UK), HIV was transmitted by blood transfusion, particularly of concentrated products such as Factor VIII pooled from multiple donations. Consequently, haemophiliacs have a high incidence of HIV disease acquired at that time.

HIV is now endemic in subsaharan Africa in men, women, and children, but in the UK remains, at present, largely confined to identifiable high-risk groups (Table 33.1).

HIV infection

The HIV viruses 1 and 2, and simian immunodeficiency virus (SIV) with which much of the experimental work towards a vaccine is performed, are members of the Lentivirus subgroup of retroviruses. The retroviruses convert their RNA genome into a DNA copy using reverse transcriptase enzymes for incorporation into the nuclear DNA of the infected cell. HIV binds to the CD4 receptor on helper/inducer T lymphocytes with subsequent passage into the cell and incorporation of nuclear material. Replication follows with conversion back via

Table 33.1. Patients at risk of HIV infection.

Homosexual men
Bisexual men
Intravenous drug abusers
Haemophiliacs
Recipients of blood or blood products before universal testing
Indigenous population of subsaharan Africa
Sexual partners or children of the above

messenger RNA to viral genome and protein. New HIV particles are released, with progressive destruction of the T4 lymphocytes and the development of opportunist infections and malignancies which characterize AIDS.

Course of HIV infection

Following infection with HIV, antigen is detectable for one to four weeks in many individuals before antibody becomes detectable. This 'seroconversion' usually occurs within two to three months. ELISA (enzyme linked immunosorbent assay) detection of antibody to intact virus is followed by detection of antibodies to p24 core protein and gp41 envelope glycoprotein. Seroconversion is often accompanied by the acute viral illness characterizing CDC Group I disease (Table 33.2). Following a very variable period of symptomless antibody production (CDC Group II), p24 antibody disappears with re-emergence of antigen in serum. This correlates with fall in CDIV lymphocyte numbers and progression to AIDS (CDC Groups III and IV) (3). HIV antibodies do not neutralize virus, and the individual must be considered infective at all times.

Table 33.2. CDC classification of HIV infection.

Group			
(I)	Acute infection		
(II)	Asymptomatic infection		
(III)	Persistent generalized lymphadenopathy		
(IV)	Other disease:	(A)	constitutional disease
		(B)	neurological disease
		(C)	secondary infectious disease
			(1) as defined for AIDS
			(2) others
		(D)	secondary malignancy
		(E)	other conditions

Occupational transmission of HIV

The surgeon may encounter patients at any stage of HIV infection. Those in CDC groups I and II may present with any surgical problem, but often with the septic complications of intravenous drug abuse, or the anorectal complaints of male homosexuals. Those in Groups III and IV require surgery in a variety of situations (see below).

Although the risk of transmission of HIV from an infected patient to a health care worker appears to be very small, additional precautions are necessary to avoid transmission, particularly by needlestick injury. The Centers for Disease Control, Atlanta (CDC) recommend universal precautions—treating every patient as a potential innoculation risk from HIV, hepatitis B, and other blood borne pathogens (4–6). This may be the counsel of perfection, but has major consequences financially and logistically, and is probably unnecessary in the UK where the prevalence of HIV is low and sustantially within identifiable high risk groups (Table 33.1). Nevertheless, the HIV pandemic has resulted in general modification of our surgical practice (see below), and it is not now acceptable for a surgeon to come into contact with blood or other body fluids.

Risk of HIV transmission to health care workers

By December 1990 there had been 19 documented seroconversions in health care workers following a specific exposure, and a further 16 presumptive occupationally acquired HIV infections in individuals without other exposure. Three seroconversions have occurred in individuals involved in the home care of HIV patients. These 38 seroconversions in health care workers reflect an unknown number of exposures, but nine are included in the 14 prospective studies of transmission in the US, Canade, UK, Italy, and Spain following percutaneous occupational injury. In 1852 patients at risk, this represents a seroconversion rate of 0.48 per cent (upper 95 per cent confidence limit = 0.8 per cent).

Risk to the surgeon

The risk of seroconversion for surgical personnel in a high prevalence area (San Francisco) has been calculated at one case every eight years (7). This falls to one every 80 years where the prevalence is 3 per cent (8), or to one every 800 years at 0.3 per cent—nearer the estimated prevalence in the UK of 50 000 (9). Much of this calculation is arbitrary, and the risk is not uniform. Certain surgical procedures carry greater risk than others, and some surgeons have a far higher rate of personal needlestick injury than others. Major abdominal and pelvic surgery with prolonged duration and significant blood loss carries an increased risk (7). Orthopaedic surgery with potential aerosol formation from power tools and reamers might increase the risk, but this has not been confirmed. No increase in HIV transmission has been shown in dentists, also subject to aerosol formation (10).

HIV infection, with almost certain eventual progression to AIDS and death, is devastating, and engenders fear in health care workers (11). Although the risk is small, the consequences merit considerable precaution as no curative treatment is available.

Risk to the patient

The risk of transmission of HIV from an infected health care worker to a patient is low. Nearly a thousand patients operated upon by an American surgeon who developed AIDS, and by a British surgeon found to be HIV positive, underwent antibody testing. Only one patient, an intravenous drug abuser, proved positive (32). However, an American dentist probably infected five patients during their treatment, as two female patients had no other risk factor and the provirus nucleotide sequences in dentist and patients were remarkably similar (33).

The UK expert advisory panel on AIDS has accepted the recommendation of the joint HIV advisory panel of the Royal Colleges that an HIV infected health care worker should seek specialist guidance, which will normally preclude further involvement in major invasive surgery (12, 13).

Precautions to prevent HIV transmission

Identification of 'at risk' groups permits additional precautions to be taken. Most individuals asked about their sexual orientation or substance misuse will respond honestly if the questions are posed in a non-threatening way during the course of routine history taking. They should be raised once rapport with the patient has been established. Even if it is not possible to pursue direct questioning an evasive or obfuscating response may permit evaluation of the likelihood of risk. Some groups have attempted to obtain this information by means of a questionnaire (14), but the author's view is that this may place unnecessary strain on the subsequent clinical interview.

HIV antibody testing

The considerable emotional, ethical, and practical problems surrounding HIV antibody testing have received much publicity. The Royal College of Surgeons of Edinburgh has advocated wider antibody testing with consent of high risk groups, and even without consent in emergencies. The British Orthopaedic Association have advocated universal antibody testing, reflecting the high level of anxiety among orthopaedic surgeons about the risk for them of operating upon HIV positive patients (15). The Royal College of Surgeons of England have suggested that antibody testing without consent may be permissible following injury to one of the operating team (12).

These responses are largely emotional, and not well supported in fact. The belief that knowledge of the HIV antibody status of an individual decreases the risk of injury to the surgeon has not been substantiated. In San Francisco, against a background of universal precautions, prior knowledge did not decrease the risk (7). Further, a negative antibody test does not exclude HIV infection. Infected individuals who have not yet produced antibody, in the seroconversion window, may have circulating antigen and be particularly capable of transmitting infection. This window is of uncertain length, and may, exceptionally, extend up to three years (16). The 'reassurance' of a negative HIV antibody test is inappropriate, and the author prefers to manage all patients in risk groups as if they have HIV disease. If HIV moves further into the female population, identification of risk cases will become increasingly difficult. Increased reliance on universal precautions and, possibly, on the use of both antigen and antibody tests will be necessary.

Antibody testing has been advocated following needlestick injury (12). If this proves negative, it must be repeated once or twice at three monthly intervals before the health care worker can be reassured. If positive, it has been advocated that prophylactic zidovudine be offered immediately to the health care worker to prevent viral incorporation by blocking reverse transcriptase. The CDC have concluded that current studies are inadequate to establish the efficacy or safety of zidovudine for prophylaxis after occupational exposure to HIV, and that its use cannot be considered a necessary component of postexposure management (17). This takes account of the risk of seroconversion, and the efficacy and toxicity of zidovudine. Knowledge of antibody status is of little help in deciding whether or not zidovudine should be used. In the Westminster Hospital, London, zidovudine prophylaxis is offered following exposure to a CDC group IV patient, a group who frequently express antigen in blood and body fluids. Recently, use of CDIV monoclonal antibody to block cell receptor antigen, and to minimise receptors available to HIV, have been proposed after occupational exposure (19).

Specific precautions in surgical practice

Universal measures

Although the full extent of measures used in 'at risk' patients is impractical universally, wise modifications to standard surgical practice in the authors unit include the following.

Out-patients

Gloves are worn for all proctoscopic and sigmoidoscopic examinations, and the first glove changed after preliminary rectal examination. Disposable proctoscopes and sigmoidoscopes are always used. Gloves are worn for gastrointestinal endoscopy and venesection.

Operating theatre

1. No sharp instrument is ever passed by hand between the surgeon and scrub nurse. Scalpels, needles, biopsy needles, and sharp tube drain introducers are placed beside the surgeon in a kidney dish. They are returned to the dish immediately after use, and removed without delay by the nurse. Sharp instruments are not laid down in the operative field.
2. Needles are never re-sheathed.
3. Fingers are never used to guide a needle point during suturing in accessible areas.

Orthopaedic surgeons in the author's unit now always wear eye protection.

Precautions in innoculation risk patients

A dedicated theatre is not necessary, but innoculation risk patients are generally placed at the end of operating lists, as all unnecessary equipment is removed from theatres for these patients, and contamination of the theatre may involve delay before the next operation is started. Inevitably this means that operation on those patients become more prone to cancellation.

Portering, anaesthesia, and recovery

Porters, anaesthetic staff, and recovery staff wear impervious gowns, gloves, eye-protection if necessary. Anaesthesia is induced in the operating room to minimize the areas contaminated, and disposable equipment and circuits are used where possible.

Contaminated endotracheal tubes and laryngeal airways are removed before the patient moves to the recovery area. Soiled dressings are changed before transfer of the patient through the hospital to the ward.

Operating theatres

Staff with open wounds, abrasions, or eczema of the hands and forearms should not operate on HIV patients. Pregnant theatre staff should be excluded as many HIV and homosexual patients carry cytomegalovirus (CMV).

All unnecessary equipment is removed from the operating theatre and anaesthetic machines, and unnessary staff are excluded. The operating table is covered with an impervious plastic sheet, and anaesthesia is induced on the table. Surgeons and scrub staff wear a plastic disposable apron, glasses, impervious disposable gowns, double gloves, and plastic overshoes to minimize contamination of theatre footwear. The larger pair of gloves is more comfortable on the inside.

Disposable drapes are preferred, and a disposable Caesarian section drape (3M UK) is used for laparotomies. This incorporates a large plastic circumferential gutter which contains blood, fluid, and resected tissue, minimizing contamination of personnel and theatre. Disposable liners for suction bottles are routinely employed.

Sharps are disposed of immediately. Ideally sutures are tied after the needle has been removed, but the needle point is closed into the needle-holder if this is not possible. Some surgeons prefer to use diathermy for incision and dissection to avoid scalpels altogether, and laser and ultrasonic dissectors have been proposed. The latter are unproven, and the CO_2 laser at least has been implicated in transmission of viable papilloma virus in the plume (18).

Staplers are preferred for bowel anastomosis, and are used routinely for skin closure in innoculation risk patients. At the conclusion of the operation the gown, outer gloves, apron, overshoes, and inner gloves are discarded, in that order, at the theatre door into a yellow alginate disposal bag. Contaminated footwear is also discarded for cleaning in the theatre. Instruments are washed in hot soapy water to remove gross contamination, and then placed in a clear plastic bag. They are then autoclaved before being handled by TSSU staff who clean, pack and re-autoclave in the usual way.

Any spillage of blood or body fluid is covered with sodium dichlorocyanurate granules which are left for two minutes before being wiped up with disposable towels. All other surfaces are cleaned with 1 per cent hypochlorite.

Ward management

The innoculation risk patient may be nursed on any ward. Gloves and aprons are worn for medical and nursing procedures, and the disposal of waste. Particular care is required for the disposal of sharps.

Surgery on patients with HIV

CDC Group I and II patients

Patients in CDC group I undergoing acute infection and seroconversion seldom present to the surgeon. Group II patients may present with any surgical problem, and should be identified by routine questioning and antibody testing, with counselling and consent if their status is not already known. Many of our HIV patients are referred by HIV and sexually transmitted disease physicians, so their status is known. Common procedures include the following.

Ano-rectal conditions

Anal warts and perianal infection are common in male homosexuals, regardless of their HIV status, though perianal infection is more common in patients with HIV disease than those who are not affected. Simple infection may be associated with herpes simplex ulceration, and non-Hodgkin's lymphoma may be confused with perianal abscess (20). In AIDS patients, Kaposi's sarcoma may present in the anorectum with secondary ulceration, and *Mycobacterium avium intracellulare* (MAI) may cause chronic infection.

Fissure and fistula in ano in HIV patients are treated in the usual ways, with the emphasis on conservatism, as CDC group IV patients (those with AIDS) may have impaired healing (21). Continence of the 'gay anus' may be impaired, and division of the internal sphincter is best avoided. The key to successful management of perianal infection in these patients is careful evaluation, with biopsy and adequate microbiological information to permit treatment on otherwise conventional lines.

Anal warts are common in male homosexuals, and very uncommon in other groups. Therefore we have included men with anal warts in our classification of innoculation risk patients (22). Warts in the HIV patients may be more dysplastic and aggressive than those in other patients, but the papilloma subtypes are the same (23). There is an increased incidence of carcinoma *in situ*, and squamous carcinoma of the anus is more common in homosexual men. However, no progression from *in situ* to invasive disease has been seen in the author's patients, all treated by local excision and diathermy or laser coagulation.

Adequate biopsies must be taken, and warts are then treated conventionally, though eradication is more difficult and healing may be impaired.

Painful anal ulceration in male homosexuals is common, and due to trauma and infection in most cases. Herpes simplex may be involved and must be sought. CMV is extremely common in the gastrointestinal (GI) tract of HIV patients, and its presence is not necessarily important. Biopsy is essential, not least to exclude squamous carcinoma. Treatment is conventional, with antiviral agents such as acyclovir if appropriate, stool softeners, and analgesia. True fissures respond well to sphincterotomy in CDC group II patients, but conservatism must be exercised with groups II and IV (23). Local excision of ulcers has achieved good results in some refractory ulcers in our patients, with good healing in all cases.

Lymph node biopsy

Lymph node biopsy may be required if uncertainty occurs about the nature of swelling in a single node or groups of nodes. Generalized lymphadenopathy almost invariably represents progression to stage III disease—persistent generalized lymphadenopathy, and biopsy to confirm this should be unnecessary. Localized lymphadenopathy is frequently due to mycobacterial infection or lymphoma, both of which represent CDC group IV disease (AIDS).

CDC Group III and IV, PGL and AIDS

Laparotomy

Twelve to fifteen per cent of AIDS patients experience abdominal pain, which is sometimes severe, but only about 5 per cent of these will require surgery (24). The commonest disease processes leading to emergency laparotomy in the author's experience (24) are CMV colitis, appendicitis (also sometimes associated with CMV), intra-abdominal lymphoma and atypical mycobacterial infection (MAI). This series comprised 28 patients from the Westminster (19), St Mary's (6), and Middlesex (3) hospitals. The perioperative mortality (7 per cent) rose to 11 per cent in 30 days, due to disease progression of AIDS, but compares well with other series with hospital mortalities of 46 per cent (25) and 57 per cent (26) in Los Angeles. This may be due to aggressive early intervention in CMV colitis megacolon, but surgery in our hands conferred little benefit in patients with MAI infection or lymphoma. Sixty-four per cent of these patients were alive at three months and 48 per cent at six months, so emergency surgery in AIDS patients must not be withheld on the grounds of excessive morbidity and mortality.

Laparotomy may also arise from obstruction due to Kaposi's sarcoma, for abdominal tuberculosis, for acalculous cholecystitis due to *Cryptosporidium*/CMV, and for GI Bleeding (27–29). Splenectomy may be necessary for HIV associated thrombocytopaenia, and is beneficial in raising platelet counts, but not in prevention of progression of HIV disease (30, 31).

The HIV infected patient presenting with abdominal pain should be assessed like any other patient, but in CDC group IV patients early CT scanning may detect focal hepatic or biliary disease and intra-abdominal lymphadenopathy. These are conditions which have derived little benefit from laparotomy, and many AIDS patients require careful conservative management of severe abdominal pain. Patients with intestinal obstruction and severe GI bleeding require early surgery, and those with right iliac fossa pain should be treated as normal, i.e. if the signs warrent appendicectomy, it should be performed. Patients with diarrhoea, a common manifestation of HIV disease, who develop abdominal pain require careful observation, and serial plain abdominal radiography. Colonic dilatation has been successfully treated by total colectomy in our patients.

It has been suggested that healing is impaired after major surgery in AIDS patients. This has not been substantiated, and outcome appears to be related more to the CDIV T-cell count, nutritional status and haemoglobin level than any single hallmark of HIV infection.

Vascular access

CDC group IV patients require regular vascular access for antimicrobial chemotherapy of opportunist infection, and for treatment with ganciclovir (DHPG) or foscarnet to prevent blindness due to CMV retinitis. Hickman lines and totally implanted vascular access ports have a high incidence of infection in these patients, and multiple placement is often required. In the authors unit construction of arteriovenous fistulae is being considered as an alternative.

Orthopaedic, cardiac, and neurosurgical procedures

HIV patients in all CDC groups may require these procedures. Haemophiliac patients need a variety of orthopaedic operations, and any HIV-infected patient may present to the traumatologist. With awareness of risk, appropriate surgery should be performed. Intravenous drug abusers have an increased incidence of infective endocarditis, and, in the presence of controlled infection, those with HIV infection respond well to valvular surgery. AIDS has multiple neurological manifestations, and the neurosurgeon may be called upon to drain cerebral abscess in particular.

Nutrition

Terminal CDC group IV patients may require nutritional support if free from other active illness, and percutaneous endoscopically assisted gastrostomy has proved ideal for this group.

The surgeon has much to offer patients with HIV disease, and should not allow personal anxiety about limited risk, or inappropriate nihilism to dissuade him.

References

1. Gottlieb, M.S., Schroff, R., Schanker, H.M. *et al.* (1981). *Pneumocystis carinii* pneumonia and mucosal candidiasis in previously healthy homosexual men: evidence of a new acquired cellular immunodeficiency. *N. Engl. J. Med.*, **305**, 1425–31.
2. Statistics from the World Health Organisation and the Centers for Disease Control. (1990). *AIDS*, **4**, 1173–7.
3. Lange, J.M., Paul, D.A., Huisman, H.G. *et al.* (1986). Persistent HIV antigenaemia and decline of HIV core antibodies associated with transition to AIDS. *Br. Med. J.*, **293**, 1459–62.
4. Center for Disease Control. (1987). Recommendations for prevention of HIV transmission in health care settings. *MMWR*, **36**, 18–35.
5. Centers for Disease Control. (1988). Update: universal precautions for prevention of transmission of human immunodeficiency virus, hepatitis B virus, and other blood borne pathogens in health care settings. *MMWR*, **37**, 377–88.
6. Centers for Disease Control. (1989). Guide-lines for prevention of transmission of human immunodeficiency virus and hepatitis B virus to health care and public-safety workers. *MMWR*, **38**(s6).
7. Gerberding, J.L., Littel, C., Tarkington, A, Brown, A., and Schecter, W.P. (1990). Risk of exposure of surgical personnel to patients blood during surgery at San Francisco General Hospital. *N. Engl. J. Med.*, **322**, 1788–93.
8. Leentvar-Kuijpers, A., Keeman, J.N., Dekker, E. *et al.* (1989). HIV: occupational risk of surgical specialists and operating room personnel in the St Lucas hospital in Amsterdam. *Ned. Tidschr. Geneeskd.*, **133**, 238–91.
9. AIDS in the UK. (1990). *Lancet*, **336**, 1000.

10. Klein, R.S., Fehelan, J.A., Freeman, K. *et al.* (1988). Low occupational health risk of human immunodeficiency virus amongst dental professionals. *N. Engl. J. Med.*, **318**, 86–90.
11. Gazzard, B.G. and Wastell, C. (1990). HIV and Surgeons. *Br. Med. J.*, **301**, 1003–4.
12. Royal College of Surgeons of England. (1990). *Statement on AIDS and HIV infection*. December.
13. *AIDS: HIV infected health care workers: Report of the recommendations of the DHSS Expert Advisory Committee on AIDS.* (1988). HMSO ISBN 011321140 6.
14. Vipond, M.N., Tyrrell, M.R., Gatzen, C. *et al.* (1990). Questionnaire identification of surgical patients at risk of HIV infection. *J. R. Coll. Surg. Edinb.*, **35**, 305–7.
15. Arnow, P.M., Pottenger, L.A., Stocking, C.B. *et al.* (1989). Orthopaedic surgeons' attitudes and practices concerning treatment of patients with HIV infection. *Public Health Rep.*, **104**, 121–9.
16. Lee, M.H., Waxman, H., and Gillooley, J.F. (1986). Primary malignant lymphoma of the anorectum in homosexual men. *Dis. Colon Rectum*, **29**, 413–6.
17. Centers for disease control. (1990). Statement on occupational exposure to Human Immunodeficiency Virus, including considerations regarding zidovudine postexposure use. *MMWR*, **39**, 1–14.
18. Garden, J.M., O'Banion, M.K., Shelnitz, L.S. *et al.* (1988). Papillomavirus in the vapour of carbon dioxide laser treated verrucae. *J. Am. Med. Assoc.*, **259**, 1199–202.
19. Rieber, E.P., Reiter, C., Gurtler, L. *et al.* (1990). Monoclonal CD4 antibodies after accidental HIV infection. *Lancet*, **336**, 1007–8.
20. Miles, A.J.G., Mellor, C.H., Gazzard, B.G., *et al.* (1990). The surgical treatment of anorectal disease in HIV positive homosexual males. *Br. J. Surg.*, **77**, 869–71.
21. Wakeman, R., Johnson, C.D., and Wastell, C. (1990). Surgical procedures in patients at risk of human immunodeficiency virus infection. *J. R. Soc. Med.*, **8**, 315–8.
22. Cahill, C.J. and Wastell, C. (1987). HIV and the homosexual in the surgical rectal clinic. *Br. J. Surg.*, **74**, 540–1.
23. Gottesman, L., Miles, A.J.G., Milsom, J. *et al.* (1990). The management of anorectal disease in HIV positive patients. *Int. J. Colon. Dis.*, **5**. 6[illegible]–72.
24. Davidson, T., Allen Mersh, T., Miles, A.J.G. *et al.* (1991). Emergency laparotomy in AIDS. *Br. J. Surg.* **78**, 924–6.
25. Wilson, S.E., Robinson, G., Williams, R.A. *et al.* (1989). Acquired immune deficiency syndrom (AIDS)—indications for abdominal surgery, pathology and outcome. *Ann. Surg.*, **210**, 428–34.
26. Robinson, G., Wilson, S.E., and Williams, R.A. (1987). Surgery in patients with acquired immunodeficiency syndrome. *Arch. Surg.*, **122**, 170–5.
27. Deziel, D.J., Hyser, M.J., Doolas, A. *et al.* (1990). Major abdominal operations in acquired immunodeficiency syndrome. *Am. Surg.*, **56**, 445–50.
28. Wolkomir, A.F., Barone, J.E., Hardy, H.W., and Cottone, F.J. (1990). Abdominal and anorectal surgery and the acquired immune deficiency syndrome in heterosexual intravenous drug abusers. *Dis. Colon Rectum*, **33**, 267–70.
29. LaRaja, R.D., Rothenberg, R.E., Odom, J.W., and Mueller, S.C. (1989). The incidence of intra-abdominal surgery in acquired immunodeficiency syndrome: a statistical review of 904 patients. *Surgery*, **105**, 175–9.
30. Tyler, D.S., Shaunak, S., Bartlett, J.A., and Iglehart, J.D. (1990). HIV1 associated thrombocytopenia. The role of splenectomy—review. *Ann. Surg.*, **211**, 211–7.
31. Ravikumar, T.S., Allen, J.D., Bothe, A., and Steele, G. (1989). Splenectomy. The treatment of choice for human immunodeficiency virus associated related immune thrombrocytopenia? *Arch. Surg.*, **124**, 625–8.
32. Bird, A.G., Gore, S.M., Leigh-Brown, A.J., and Carter D.C. (1991). Escape from collective denial: HIV transmission during surgery. *Br. Med. J.*, **303**, 351–2.
33. Centers for Disease Control. (1991). Transmission of HIV infection during an invasive dental procedure. *MMWR*, **40**, 21–7, 377–81.

Further reading

Sim, A.J.W. and Jeffries, D.J. (1990). *AIDS and Surgery*. Blackwell, Oxford.

34

Post-splenectomy infection

ERIC W. TAYLOR

Introduction

Splenectomy is performed for many reasons. The most common indication is after trauma in which the spleen is damaged but, not infrequently, the trauma may be iatrogenic and splenectomy may become necessary in the course of some other surgical procedure such as pancreatic, gastric, or left colonic operations. In addition, there is a number of medical conditions for which splenectomy is indicated: the hereditary haemolytic anaemias, Hodgkin's disease and idiopathic thrombocytopenic purpura (ITP) are perhaps the most common, although, with the advent of computerized tomography, splenectomy is now rarely performed as part of a staging laparotomy for lymphoma. The spleen has also been removed in patients undergoing renal transplantation to reduce the problem of rejection.

In 1919 Morris and Bullock first suggested that the patient who has undergone splenectomy is at an increased risk of septicaemia (1). In 1952 King and Schumaker (2) reported five patients who developed overwhelming infection after splenectomy and since then an increasing number of patients have been reported to have developed the syndrome that has become known as the overwhelming post-splenectomy infection (OPSI) syndrome.

Surgeons are involved in the care of patients after trauma and are frequently called upon to perform a splenectomy. They are involved in the management of these patients both immediately after the operation and occasionally when the patient subsequently develops OPSI. More rarely, surgeons of all specialties have to perform some other operative procedure on patients who have previously undergone splenectomy. The risk of infection in each of these three situations will be reviewed together with the changes to the immune system which occur after splenectomy. The value of vaccines and prophylactic antibiotics in preventing post-splenectomy infections will be discussed.

The risk of immediate post-operative infection

Immediately after any operation there are risks of infection occurring in the wound specific to the operation site, and less specifically to the chest and urinary tract. The urinary tract is particularly liable to infection if the patient has been catheterized which is common practice in the management of most badly traumatized patients. The more specific infections of a subphrenic abscess, septicaemia, or pancreatitis may occur in patients who have undergone splenectomy. Numerous reports have suggested that patients undergoing splenectomy are at an increased risk of immediate post-operative infection.

Sekikawa and Shatney (3) have shown that, as the severity of injury increases, the incidence of wound infection, intra-abdominal infection and death due to infection also increase in patients who have undergone splenectomy. But these results merely confirm that severely injured patients sustain more infective complications than less severely injured patients, and do not in themselves implicate splenectomy as a factor in the aetiology of infection. However, if the incidence of a fulminant infection and septicaemia (22.7 per cent) and of death with infection (7.2 per cent) as reported by Sekikawa and Shatney is compared with another major series in which all trauma is considered, including some patients who required splenectomy (4), fulminant infection might be anticipated in only 12 per cent and death with infection in 2.3 per cent. These differences would suggest that splenectomy is associated with an increased risk of infection immediately after the traumatic episode. Standage has reported a morbidity incidence of 29.6 per cent and mortality of 9.4 per cent in a series of 277 patients who underwent splenectomy (5). The majority of the deaths were from infective complications and death occurred in 15 per cent of patients after incidental splenectomy.

However, Willis has compared a series of 80 patients who had had splenectomy with 80 patients with a similar injury severity score, but who did not need a splenectomy (6). He found no difference in the incidence of early post-operative septicaemia, pneumonia, empyema, wound infection, urinary tract infection, or subphrenic abscess.

In a retrospective study Rao has assessed the factors associated with local infection after splenectomy and has shown that both wound infection and subphrenic abscess occur more frequently when a drain is placed in the splenic bed (7). In addition, it has been suggested that the incidence of infection immediately after splenectomy is in part dependent upon the reason for splenectomy. Klaus *et al.* have shown that both pneumonia and subphrenic abscess occurred with greater frequency in patients who underwent splenectomy for malignant disease than when splenectomy was performed for trauma (8).

The long-term risk of infection

Definition

The overwhelming post-splenectomy infection syndrome has become well recognized since the term was first used by Diamond in 1969 (9). OPSI has been defined as a fulminant bacteria with meningitis or pneumonia occurring weeks or years after splenectomy (10). The syndrome presents with nausea, vomiting, and confusion with coma, and death is reported to occur in 50 to 75 per cent (2, 11–14). Electrolyte imbalance is seen with severe hypoglycaemia, together with a bacteraemia, which may be in excess of 10^6 organisms per millilitre. No obvious focus of infection may be identifiable. The high bacterial count of the blood compares with less than 10^3 organisms per millilitre of blood in non-splenectomized individuals who present with the clinical signs of bacteraemia and septicaemia. Disseminated intravascular coagulation occurs and this may lead to adrenal haemorrhage (Waterhouse–Friederickson syndrome).

Incidence

OPSI is not a common event and may occur many years after splenectomy. Therefore any estimate of its incidence is likely to be conservative—patients may suffer the signs and symptoms and these could be attributed to some other cause without recognition that the patient had previously undergone a splenectomy. Age and the underlying cause leading to the splenectomy influence the subsequent incidence of infection and these factors must be accounted for when assessing the incidence compared with controls. In addition, the lag between splenectomy and OPSI may be many years and it is difficult to follow patients, often children at the time of operation, for long enough to assess fully the incidence of OPSI.

Singer reviewed 2975 children who had undergone splenectomy and showed that OPSI occurred in 4.25 per cent, which is a sixtyfold increase over the normal incidence, and that death from sepsis occurred in 2.5 per cent, a fiftyfold increase (10). There has been some doubt as to whether this raised incidence is seen in adult patients but O'Neal and McDonald compared 256 patients who had undergone splenectomy with 250 control patients (12). In a follow-up period of four to five years, seven patients in the splenectomy group had died due to sepsis compared with no patient in the control group ($p<0.05$). They estimated the increased prevalence at 540-fold after reviewing 256 adult patients with median follow up of 45 months. OPSI had occurred in 2.7 per cent.

In 234 lymphoma patients reported by Hays only four episodes of bacterial infection, as confirmed by blood culture, had occurred during 3.8 year mean follow up (15). This is a 1.7 per cent risk of infection but 83 per cent of these patients had been given pneumococcal vaccination and 74 per cent were receiving prophylactic antibiotics.

Others have reported a much higher incidence of infection, Green *et al.* reported a 9 per cent incidence of major infection and a 30 per cent incidence of minor infection in 144 patients followed for an average of 61 months (16). In data collected from a number of reports, Francke and Neu have reported 3.9 per cent infection occurring in 4846 patients, with death occurring in 2.4 per cent of 5485 patients (17).

Microbiology

Whilst the pneumococcus is the organism isolated most frequently from blood cultures in patients presenting with OPSI, particularly serotypes XII, XXII, and XXIII, *Neisseria meningitides*, *Escherichia coli*, *Haemophilus influenzae*, *Salmonella* spp., *Streptococcus haemolytica*, and *Staphylococcus aureus* have all been isolated from patients with this syndrome. Viruses may also play a part in the pathology: cytomegalovirus (9), herpes (18), and influenza virus (19) have all been reported and splenectomy has been reported to predispose to malaria (20).

Predisposing factors

Just as malignant disease may be associated with a higher incidence of immediate post-splenectomy infection so the underlying disease process may influence the incidence of later

OPSI. Eraklis and Filler have shown that patients with idiopathic thrombocytopenic purpura (ITP) and thalassaemia have a higher incidence of infection than patients whose splenectomy was performed for spherocytosis or trauma, but that leukaemia, Hodgkin's disease, and portal hypertension have a much higher incidence of OPSI at 6.19 per cent (21). In the paper by O'Neal and McDonald (12) three (4.3 per cent) of the 69 patients who had undergone splenectomy for haematological malignant disease died compared with four (2.2 per cent) of the 187 whose splenectomy was necessitated by trauma.

Keil and Bennett have compared 56 patients who underwent splenectomy for Hodgkin's disease with 28 patients with similar disease, but who had not had splenectomy (22). They found that splenectomy in Stage II and III disease did not increase the risk of infection, but that the use of chemotherapy was a more important predisposing factor.

Age is also important. The majority of infections after splenectomy have occurred in patients who underwent the operation whilst less than two years of age.

Time of maximum risk

In a review of 540 children Horan and Colebatch (23) suggested that most infections occurred within two years of splenectomy and similar results have been published by Pimpl *et al.* who have reported the results of a study to compare the post-mortem findings of 202 patients who had had a splenectomy with a group of 403 similarly injured patients who had not (24). Pulmonary embolism, pyelonephritis, and death-related pneumonia were all significantly more frequent in the splenectomy group as was the incidence of patients dying of infection following multiple organ failure. However, perhaps of most interest is their finding that 50 per cent of the patients in the splenectomy group had died within three months of the operation and 78.7 per cent within three years, clearly indicating that this is the period of maximum risk.

In addition to the altered state of resistance to bacterial infection which accompanies splenectomy, Barbuie *et al.* have published a review of HIV positive patients who have had a splenectomy performed for ITP (25). They have suggested that splenectomy has an effect on the development of AIDS in HIV positive patients. In their review 9 (25 per cent) of 36 post-splenectomy patients developed signs of AIDS compared with 6 (8 per cent) of 65 who did not have a splenectomy.

The risk of infection when undergoing subsequent operations

It is reasonable to assume that the splenectomized patient is at greater risk of infection when undergoing a subsequent operation but this question does not appear to have been addressed in the literature and there would appear to be no study or series of patients to confirm or refute this hypothesis. If an assessment of the risk is to be made it might be of value to review the function of the spleen following bacterial challenge.

Ellison and Fabri (26) have identified three reticulo-endothelial functions of the spleen which are: the production of opsonins, the clearance of micro-organsims and phagocytosis, and the elaboration of a specific immune response.

Opsonin production

The spleen produces two proteins which serve as opsonins: tuftsin and properdin (27). Tuftsin promotes phagocytosis by polymorphonuclear leucocytes (28). The C3 and C5 fraction of complement are reduced following splenectomy, and properdin is a vital component of the alternative complement pathway. After splenectomy properdin is reduced for as long as 20 years (17), but, as Hosea has noted (29) 'the complement system has so much reserve that only after 99 per cent depletion of serum C3 are severe opsonic effects noted'. It is possible that this is the reason that the loss of the ability to clear organisms from the blood appears to be short-lived. Almdahl has shown that the ability to clear bacteria from the blood is lost after splenectomy, but that by week 15 there is no difference between sham laparotomy and splenectomized rats (30).

Phagocytosis and clearance of micro-organisms

Dahl *et al.* have shown that there is abnormal polymorphonuclear leucocyte function in patients who had undergone splenectomy and who then demonstrate an increased susceptibility to infection (31). The spleen acts as as a clearance organ for bacteria and Pouché has shown that splenectomy reduces the clearance of encapsulated organisms such as pneumococci from the blood (32). Cheslyn-Curtis *et al.* has shown that splenectomy also reduces the clearance of Gram-negative bacteria, which are not encapsulated (33). In addition she has demonstrated a reduced fibronectin concentration in the splenectomized rat. The clearance of pneumococcus from the bloodstream has been shown to be significantly reduced in splenectomized rats compared with normal animals, and this is thought to be because the liver can only clear well opsonised bacteria from the blood, poorly opsonized bacteria are cleared by the spleen alone (34).

Splenectomy also reduces the delayed type hypersensitivity reaction to *Bacillus* Calmett-Guérin vaccine in animals (35), reduces amplifier T-cell activity (36) and the production of memory cells (29). Other organisms are also removed from the blood by the spleen and this may be why splenectomy reduces the body's defences to malarial parasites (20).

Alteration of immune system function

The IgM antibody response that occurs after exposure to an antigen is initiated in the white pulp of the spleen and is, therefore, reduced after splenectomy (17). This reduced antibody response may be part of the reason why the ability of the liver to remove bacteria from the blood is reduced after splenectomy. Encapsulated organisms must be opsonized before phagocytosis can occur in the liver, and this does not occur in the absence of sufficient antibody response.

For these reasons it would seem logical to conclude that the patient, however long after splenectomy, is at increased risk of infection after a subsequent operative procedure, but testing this in a clinical trial would be logistically extremely difficult.

In the meantime it would seem wise to administer a prophylactic antibiotic to a splenectomized patient undergoing a further operation.

Splenic trauma—the surgical options

Splenic conservation

Surgeons have become increasingly aware of the benefits of a conservative approach to the traumatized spleen. Repair of the spleen may be possible (37) and polyglycolic acid mesh nets have been introduced onto the market which may help to enclose the damaged spleen, to apply a degree of compression and thus to encourage thrombosis (38). A successful conservative approach has been claimed in 80 per cent of 205 patients by the Papua New Guinea Splenic Injury Study Group (20).

A partial splenectomy should be considered rather than a total splenectomy and, if the whole spleen does have to be removed, small slivers of splenic tissue should be implanted either into the omentum or be left to lie free in the peritoneum—a procedure known as splenosis or autotransplantation. Estimates of the amount of spleen that need to remain if the patient is to be protected from infection have varied. Ellison and Fabri have indicated that splenic immune function will remain if one-third of the spleen is conserved (26), but they suggest that insufficient splenic tissue would remain viable via collateral blood supply if the splenic artery were ligated.

Autotransplantation

When total splenectomy is performed slivers of splenic tissue can be reimplanted freely into the peritoneal cavity, between the layers of the omentum, into the abdominal wall or the splenic tissue can be injected into the liver. Whilst these techniques have been found effective in experimental animals, partial splenectomy probably gives better splenic function (29).

Autotransplantation is not without problems. The normal sequence of regeneration is for the implanted spleen to necrose, but within three or four weeks revascularization occurs and the tissue regenerates. Within two or three months a moderate body of tissue may be present to take up splenic function. However, if infection occurs at the time of necrosis the patient may have a persistent pyrexia and the splenic graft will fail (39).

Medical management of post-splenectomy patients

Although the incidence of OPSI would appear to be debatable there would seem to be little doubt that patients are at an increased risk of infection after splenectomy and that there is a high mortality associated with that infection. If splenectomy cannot be avoided can the patient be protected from OPSI by any other means? Attempts to reduce the incidence of OPSI have progressed along two lines: vaccination and the administration of prophylactic antibiotics.

Vaccination

The organism most commonly isolated from the blood of patients with septicaemia after splenectomy is *Strep. pneumoniae*, particularly serotypes XII, XXII, and XXIII. Vaccines have been shown to be effective in preventing pneumococcal pneumonia and bacteraemia in South African goldminers who are at risk of this infection (40, 41). The vaccine given consists of purified capsular polysaccharide antigen of the 23 most common serotypes of *Strep. pneumoniae* (42) (Pneumovax 23, Merck Sharp and Dohme, USA).

When the splenectomy is to be performed as an elective procedure the vaccine should be given two weeks before the operation, but a single dose only should be given because a second dose may be associated with systemic reactions. In addition, the safety of this vaccine has not been established in children below the age of two years and vaccination of young children is not recommended. This is particularly relevant to the post-splenectomy situation where the greatest risk of OPSI would appear to be in children who needed to undergo splenectomy below this age.

The efficacy of vaccination is not fully proven and in a prospective, double-blind, placebo-controlled trial of 2295 high-risk patients over the age of 55, using 14 valent pneumococcal capsular polysaccharide vaccine, the value of vaccination was not established (43). Despite the possibility of failure the Immunisation Practices Advisory Committee of the USA still recommends vaccination after splenectomy (44).

The failure of vaccination may, in part, be because the response to the vaccine is greater with an intact spleen (45)—an added reason for pre-operative vaccination where splenectomy is performed electively.

Vaccination against *Haemophilus* spp. and meningococcal infection is also available and all three vaccines may be given simultaneously without loss of effect (46).

Prophylactic antibiotics

The alternative method of protecting patients from OPSI is to administer prophylactic antibiotics. Francke and Neu have recommended antibiotic prophylaxis for patients with low levels of pneumococcal antibodies, those who subsequently require chemotherapy for malignancy, and for children under the age of 5 years (17). Others have recommended their use for the first two or three years after splenectomy (26), or until the child is 5 years old (47).

Penicillin is usually recommended but pneumococci may become resistant to penicillin, and other organisms which may cause OPSI may not be sensitive to this antibiotic (10, 48). Amoxycillin has been advocated because it is also active against *H. influenzae* (17). Rotation of antibiotics has been suggested to prevent the development of resistance, and low dose therapy may prevent other side-effects, particularly changes in gastrointestinal flora.

Prophylactic antibiotics have not always been effective in preventing attacks of OPSI (49, 50) and therefore it would seem that constant vigilance is necessary even if the patient has been vaccinated and is receiving antibiotics.

Summary

The asplenic patient is at an increased risk of infection both immediately and long term. Post-splenectomy infection is associated with an increased mortality, and splenectomy for malignancy or haematologous disease carries an especially high risk of infection. The spleen should be preserved completely or in part whenever possible and a constant vigilance should be maintained in the management of patients who have undergone a splenectomy, particularly in the first three years of their subsequent life.

References

1. Morris, D.H. and Bullock, F.D. (1919). The importance of the spleen in resistance to infection. *Ann. Surg.*, **70**, 513–21.
2. King, H. and Schumaker, H.B. (1952). Splenic studies: I: Susceptibility to infection after splenectomy performed in infancy. *Ann. Surg.*, **136**, 239–41.
3. Sekikawa, T. and Shatney, C.H. (1983). Septic sequelae after splenectomy for trauma in adults. *Am. J. Surg.*, **145**, 667–73.
4. Caplan, E.S. and Hoyt, N. (1981). Infection surveillance and control in the severely traumatized patient. *Am. J. Intern. Med.*, **70**, 638–40.
5. Stadage, B.A. and Goss, J.C. (1982). Outcome and sepsis after splenectomy in adults. *Am. J. Surg.*, **143**, 545–8.
6. Willis, B.K., Deitch, E.A., and McDonald, J.C. (1986). The influence of trauma to the spleen or post-operative complications and mortality. *J. Trauma.*, **26**, 1073–6.
7. Rao, G.N. (1988). Predictive factors in local sepsis after splenectomy for trauma in adults. *J. R. Coll. Surg. Edinb.*, **33**, 68–70.
8. Klaus, P., Eckert, P., and Kern, E. (1979). Incidental splenectomy: Early and late post-operative complications. *Am. J. Surg.*, **138**, 296–300.
9. Diamond, L.K. (1969). Splenectomy in childhood and the hazard of overwhelming infection. *Paediatrics*, **43**, 886–9.
10. Singer, D.B. (1973). Post-splenectomy sepsis. In *Perspective in pediatric pathology* (ed. H.S. Rosenberg and R.P. Bolande), pp. 285–311. Year Book Medical Publishers, Chicago.
11. Gopal, V. and Bisno, A.L. (1977). Fulminant pneumococcal infections in 'normal' asplenic hosts. *Arch. Intern. Med.*, **137**, 1526–30.
12. O'Neal, B.J. and McDonald, J.C. (1981). The risk of sepsis in the asplenic adult. *Ann. Surg.*, **194**, 775–8.
13. Leonard, A.S., Giebink, G.S., Baesl, T.S., and Krivit, W. (1980). The overwhelming post-splenectomy sepsis problem. *World J. Surg.*, **4**, 1423–32.
14. Schwartz, P.E., Sterioff, S., Mucha, P.E. *et al.* (1982). Post-splenectomy sepsis and mortality in adults. *J. Am. Med. Assoc.*, **248**, 2279.
15. Hays, D.M., Turnberg, D.L., Chen, T.T. *et al.* (1986). Post-splenectomy sepsis and other complications following staging laparotomy for Hodgkin's disease in children. *J. Pediatr. Surg.*, **21**, 628–32.
16. Green, J.B., Schackford, S.R., and Fridlund, P. (1986). Late septic complications in adults following splenectomy for trauma: a prospective analysis in 144 patients. *J. Trauma*, **26**, 999–1004.
17. Francke, E.L. and New, H.C. (1981). Post-splenectomy infection. *Surg. Clin. North Am.*, **61**, 135–155.
18. Manning, D.M., Luparello, F.J., and Arena, V.C. (1980). Herpes Zoster after splenectomy. *J. Am. Med. Assoc.*, **243**, 56–8.
19. Roberts, G.T. and Roberts, J.T. (1976). Post-splenectomy sepsis due to influenzal viraemia and pneumococcaemia. *Can. Med. Assoc. J.*, **115**, 435–7.
20. Papua New Guinea Splenic Injury Study Group. (1987). Ruptured spleen in the adult. An account of 205 cases with particular reference to non-operative management. *Aust. NZ J. Surg.*, **57**, 549–53.
21. Eraklis, A.J. and Filler, R.M. (1972). Splenectomy in childhood. A review of 1413 cases. *J. Pediatr. Surg.*, **4**, 382–8.
22. Keel, A. and Bennett, T. (1983). Splenectomy and infection in Hodgkins disease. *Br. J. Surg.*, **70**, 278–80.
23. Horan, M. and Colebatch, J.H. (1962). Relation between splenectomy and subsequent infection: A clinical study. *Arch. Dis. Child.*, **37**, 398–414.
24. Pimpl, W., Dapunt, O., Kaindl, H., and Thalhamer, J. (1989). Incidence of septic and thrombo-embolic related deaths after splenectomy in adults. *Br. J. Surg.*, **76**, 517–21.
25. Barbui, T., Cortelazzo, S., Minetti, B., Galli, M., and Buelli, M. (1987). Does splenectomy enhance risk of AIDS in HIV-positive patients with chronic thrombocytopenia? *Lancet*, **ii**, 342–3.
26. Ellison, E.C. and Fabri, P.J. (1983). Complications of splenectomy, etiology, prevention and management. *Surg. Clin. North Am.*, **63**, 1313–30.
27. Eichner, E.R. (1979). Splenic function: normal, too much, and too little. *Am. J. Med.*, **66**, 311–20.
28. Constantopoules, A., Najjar, V.A., Wish, J.B., Necheles, T.H., and Stolbach, L.L. (1973). Defective phagocytosis due to tuftsin deficiency in splenectomized patients. *Am. J. Dis. Child.*, **125**, 663–5.
29. Hosea, S.W. (1983). Role of the spleen in pneumococcal infection. *Lymphology*, **16**, 115–20.
30. Almdahl, S.M., Osterud, B., and Brox, J.H. (1987). Splenectomy in the rat. *Acta Chir. Scand.*, **153**, 287–90.
31. Dahl, M., Hakenson, L., Kreugar, A., Olsen, L., Nilsson, U., and Venge, P. (1986). Polymorphonuclear neutrophil function and infections following splenectomy in childhood. *Scand. J. Haematol.*, **37**, 137–43.
32. Pouché, A., Saroldi, F., Colombi, A., Tiberio, G., and Turano, A. (1987). Effects of splenectomy and hemisplenectomy on pneumococcal infection and bacterial clearance in the rat. *Eur. Surg. Res.*, **19**, 86–90.
33. Cheslyn-Curtis, S., Aldridge, M.C., Bigli, J.E.J., Dye, J., Chadwick, S.J.D., and Dudley, H.A.F. (1988). Effect of splenectomy on Gram-negative bacterial clearance in the presence and absence of sepsis. *Br. J. Surg.*, **75**, 177–80.
34. Scher, K., Wroczynski, M., and Jones, C. (1983). Protection from post-splenectomy sepsis: effect of prophylactic penicillin and pneumococcal vaccine on clearance of type-3 Pneumococcus. *Surgery*, **93**, 792–9.
35. Neveu, P.J. (1984). Immune responses to a hapten-carrier conjugate in splenectomized and BCG treated guinea pigs. *Int. Arch. Allergy Appl. Immunol.*, **73**, 104–7.
36. Amsbaugh, B.F., Prescott, B., and Baker, P.J. (1978). Effect of splenectomy on the expression of regulatory T-cell activity. *J. Immunol.*, **121**, 1483–5.
37. Cooper, M.J. and Williamson, R.C.N. (1981). Splenectomy: indications, hazards and alternatives. *Br. J. Surg.*, **71**, 173–80.
38. Delaney, H.M., Porreca, F., Mitsudos, J., *et al.* (1981). Splenic capping. An experimental study of a new technique for splenorrhaphy using woven polyglycolic acid mesh. *Ann. Surg.*, **196**, 187–93.
39. Greco, R.S. and Alvarez, F.G. (1981). Protection against pneumococcal bacteraemia by partial splenectomy. *Surg. Gynecol. Obstet.*, *152*, 67–9.
40. Rhodes, M., Lennard, T.W.J., and Venables, C.W. (1988). Omental abscess: a rare complication after implantation of

autologous splenic tissue into the omentum. *Br. J. Surg.*, **75**, 288.

41. Smith, P., Oberholzer, D., Hayden-Smith, S., Koornhof, H. J., and Hilleman, M. R. (1977). Protective efficacy of pneumococcal polysaccharide vaccine. *J. Am. Med. Assoc.*, **238**, 2613–6.
42. Robbins, J. B., Austrian, R., and Lee, C. J. (1983). Consideration for formulating the second generation pneumococcal capsular polysaccharide vaccine with emphasis on the cross-reactive types within groups. *J. Infect. Dis.*, **148**, 1136–59.
43. Simberkoff, M. S., Cross, A. P., Al-Ibrahim, M., *et al.* (1986). Efficacy of pneumococcal vaccine in high risk patients. *N. Engl. J. Med.*, **315**, 1318–27.
44. Immunization Practices Advisory Committee (Centre for Disease Control). (1984). Update: pneumococcal polysaccharide vaccine usage—United States. *Morbidity and Mortality Weekly Report*, **33**, 273–81.
45. Hosea, S. W., Brown, E. J., Burch, C. G., Berg, R. A., and Franck, M. M. (1981). Impaired immune response to polyvalent pneumococcal vaccine. *Lancet*, **i**, 804–7.
46. Ambrosino, D. M. (1986). Simultaneous administration of vaccines for *Haemophilus influenzae* type b, pneumococci and meningococci. *J. Infect. Dis.*, **154**, 893–6.
47. Ammann, A. J. and Diamond, L. K. (1978). Indications for pneumococcal vaccination in patients with impaired splenic function. *N. Engl. J. Med.*, **299**, 778–9.
48. Editorial. (1985). Splenectomy—a long term risk of infection. *Lancet*, **ii**, 928–9.
49. Brivet, F., Herer, B., Fremaux, A., *et al.* (1984). Fatal post-splenectomy pneumococcal sepsis despite pneumococcal vaccine and penicillin prophylaxis. *Lancet*, **i**, 456–7.
50. Evans, D. (1984). Fatal post-splenectomy sepsis despite prophylaxis with penicillin and pneumococcal vaccine. *Lancet*, **i**, 1124.

Further reading

Shaw, J. H. F. and Print, C. G. (1989). Post-splenectomy sepsis. *Br. J. Surg.*, **76**, 1074–81.

Francke, E. L. and New, H. C. (1981). Post-splenectomy infection. *Surg. Clin. North Am.*, **61**, 135–55.

West, K. W. and Grosfeld, J. L. (1985). Post-splenectomy sepsis: Historical background and current concepts. *World J. Surg.*, **9**, 477–83.

35

Intensive therapy units

A. PETER R. WILSON and GEOFFREY L. RIDGWAY

Introduction

The surgical patient who needs intensive care is at risk of infection from many sources. In addition to the operative procedure he will require invasive monitoring and intravenous fluids; his trachea will be intubated, and his urine will be drained via a urethral or suprapubic catheter. The patient's own immune system is compromized by the anaesthesia, the breaching of normal anatomical defences, the underlying illness, and by complement activation. Immunosuppressive agents may be used in transplant recipients. The high staff to patient ratio and the open structure of the intensive therapy unit (ITU) readily permit the transmission of pathogens between patients, particularly when pressure of work leads to a breakdown of aseptic technique.

Rates of infection in ITUs vary between 7 and 45 per cent (1), and are particularly high in units admitting multiple trauma or burns patients. The rate increases with duration of stay in the unit. Infection is predominantly associated with venous catheterization, the respiratory and urinary tracts, and wounds.

Many patients will receive broad spectrum antibiotics that alter the endogenous bowel flora resulting in loss of colonization resistance. Antibiotic resistant organisms, usually Gram-negative bacilli or yeasts, can then colonize the mucous surfaces and predispose to respiratory, urinary and wound infections. Superinfection by *Clostridium difficile* may result in toxin-induced pseudomembranous colitis. Organisms from a symptomatic patient readily contaminate bedpans, floors, and the hands of staff. Outbreaks can occur unless the index case is adequately source isolated.

Bacterial resistance to commonly used antibiotics ensures the increasing use of extended spectrum agents; for example, the quinolones, monobactams, and thienamycins. However, the pressure for selection of resistance can be reduced by restriction of the choice and spectrum of the antibiotics used and by reserving treatment for infection rather than colonization. Thus, the involvement of the microbiologist in the daily management of the critically ill surgical patient is important.

Two-thirds of respiratory infections are caused by pathogens colonizing the oropharynx; others are exogenous and potentially preventable. The most likely route of cross-infection is via the hands of the nurses, physiotherapists, and medical staff; yet doctors wash their hands after only 28 per cent of contacts with patients, nurses after 43 per cent of contacts, and physiotherapists after 76 per cent of contacts (2). Hand-washing between patient contacts must be enforced and sinks should be conveniently located within the unit, and available in every side room. Facilities for source isolation, including gloves and plastic aprons, must be available for use when required. The design of the unit should provide ample space between beds to allow access without increasing the chance of transmission by direct contact. Staff must be educated in proper hand washing techniques and discouraged from reusing disposable items.

The surgical patient in the ITU

Although all surgical patients are prone to develop infection, diagnosis is often difficult in the critically ill patient. The duration of vascular catheterization and the presence of pus in sputum or wound drainage may be helpful. Whenever sepsis is suspected, wound dressings should be taken down to look for erythema, serous discharge and wound separation. Fever may be caused by an administered drug or blood product, a collagen vascular disease, vasculitis, deep venous thrombosis, pulmonary embolism, neoplasia, or anaesthesia rather than by infection. Signs in the lungs may be non-specific: arterial hypoxaemia and changes on the chest radiograph are often caused by pulmonary oedema and adult respiratory distress syndrome (ARDS) without infection. Abdominal pain and fever may be caused by acute acalculous cholecystitis (3) or mesenteric infarction, and abdominal signs are easily missed in the elderly or in patients receiving opiates.

Culture should be made of urine, sputum or tracheal aspirate, blood (drawn from two sites), and of any fluid collections in the joints, abdomen, or pleura. Neurosurgical patients or those with head injury may require examination of the cerebrospinal fluid. Most patients will already have received or be receiving antibiotics for the prophylaxis of wound infection or for the treatment of infection found at operation. If the patient's condition allows, antibiotics should be stopped for 24 h before sampling.

Multiple trauma patients are highly susceptible to infection, particularly if they require assisted ventilation. Stoutenbeek *et al.* (4) found that 48 of 59 (81 per cent) of these patients developed infection during a mean stay of 14 days in the ITU. Respiratory tract infections occurred in 35 (59 per cent), septicaemia in 25 (42 per cent), urinary tract infections in 19 (32 per cent), and wound infections in 15 (25 per cent).

Antibiotic therapy and prophylaxis

Over 80 per cent of patients in the ITU receive antibiotics during their stay and the routine use of a single broad spectrum antibiotic is likely to result in a rising prevalence of infection by resistant bacteria. Antibiotics such as ampicillin, imipenem, or cefoxitin are potent inducers of beta-lactamase in Gram-negative bacteria and resistance to cephalosporins may persist after treatment is completed. Genetic material coding for antibiotic resistance can be transferred between bacterial strains or even species as has been outlined in Chapter 7.

Empirical antibiotic therapy should always be chosen in the knowledge of the likely sensitivity pattern of pathogens isolated in each ITU. Ideally, a narrow spectrum antibiotic should be used when the organism is known to be susceptible. Antibiotics should be used to decontaminate the gastrointestinal tract selectively only as part of a formal protocol under close microbiological surveillance (5) (see Chapter 35). Although emergence of resistance does not appear to be a problem in units using selective decontamination, topical and aerosol antibiotics are probably best avoided.

Initial treatment will usually be a combination of antibiotics which should be made with the specific intention of widening the spectrum, providing synergistic activity, discouraging the emergence of resistance during treatment or of ensuring optimal activity in the patient with septic shock. For example, flucloxacillin or cefuroxime may be given with an aminoglycoside to act against *Staphylococcus aureus* and the enterobacteriaceae, and metronidazole against anaerobic bacteria. Whenever a patient fails to respond, all intravascular lines should be replaced and intra-abdominal collections of pus should be sought and, if present, drained.

Benzyl penicillin (7.2–10.8 g/day IV) remains the treatment of choice for pneumococcal pneumonia or necrotizing fasciitis caused by *Streptococcus* pyogenes. Benzyl penicillin, or ampicillin (500 mg IV every 6 h), should be used in combination with an aminoglycoside in the treatment of enterococcal infections. An isoxazolyl penicillin, for example flucloxacillin, is resistant to staphylococcal beta-lactamase, and is used for most infections caused by *Staph. aureus*. Indications are empyema, post-operative abscesses and osteomyelitis. High doses (up to 12 g/day IV in 6 doses) or administration with probenecid may be required in severe illness. Combination with an aminoglycoside or fusidic acid may improve antibacterial activity at the site of infection. Clindamycin or trimethoprim/rifampicin are alternatives. Most hospital strains of *Staph. epidermidis* and a few strains of *Staph. aureus* are resistant to methicillin/flucloxacillin but are susceptible to vancomycin (1 g IV every 12 h by infusion) or teicoplanin (400 mg IV 24 h by bolus).

With the exception of enterococcal infections, ampicillin is rarely useful in the ITU as most nosocomial Gram-negative pathogens are resistant. The ureidopenicillins, such as mezlocillin or azlocillin, are active against *Pseudomonas aeruginosa* and most isolates of the enterobacteriaceae, but they should only be used in combination with an aminoglycoside as resistance develops if they are used alone. Mezlocillin (5 g IV every 6 h) is effective in pneumonia, peritonitis, soft tissue infections and urinary and biliary tract infections caused by susceptible pathogens (6).

Cefuroxime (750 mg–1.5 g IV every 8 h) is stable to many beta-lactamases and is widely used to treat septicaemia, urinary infections and respiratory tract infections caused by Gram-negative bacilli, including those caused by *Haemophilus influenzae* (7). It is active against staphylococci and streptococci (not enterococci) but penicillins are to be preferred if a Gram-positive pathogen is isolated. Cefotaxime (2 g IV every 8 h) has a similar range of activity and is a suitable alternative. For severe pseudomonal infections, ceftazidime, (but not cefuroxime or cefotaxime), can be used. Although ceftazidime (1–2 g IV every 8 h) has less antistaphylococcal activity than cefuroxime, it is highly active against the enterobacteriaceae, including multi-resistant strains. It may be indicated in severe surgical infections, for example peritonitis, acquired during a stay on the ITU.

Despite an increasing number of resistant strains, the aminoglycosides, such as gentamicin, remain the drugs of choice in severe Gram-negative bacterial infections in ITU patients. They are active against *Staph. aureus* and *Ps. aeruginosa* and they are commonly used in a synergistic combination with penicillins or cephalosporins. Aminoglycosides are not effective against enterococci or streptococci, except when given with a penicillin. Otoxicity and nephrotoxicity are the main disadvantages and monitoring of serum levels is required every 1–2 days to judge the correct dosage.

Ciprofloxacin (200 mg IV every 12 h) is active against most Gram-negative species, including *Ps. aeruginosa* and staphylococci, but streptococci are less susceptible. It is effective in complicated urinary tract infections, Gram-negative bacterial pneumonias and osteomyelitis but should be reserved for use as an alternative to beta-lactams where resistance occurs. Resistance to ciprofloxacin may emerge on treatment, notably in *Pseudomonas* spp. infecting the respiratory tract (8).

Metronidazole (1 g p.r. every 12 h or 500 mg IV every 8 h) is active against strictly anaerobic bacteria and is as effectively administered by the rectal as the intravenous route. It is usually given in combination with beta-lactams for up to seven days, in addition to surgical drainage of intra-abdominal abscess. Clindamycin (600 mg every 6 h by infusion) is effective against Gram-positive bacteria and Gram-negative anaerobic bacteria and can be used to treat aspiration pneumonia, anaerobic pulmonary infections and, in combination with gentamicin, intra-abdominal sepsis.

Imipenem/cilastatin (500 mg IV every 6 h) is a potent inhibitor of most aerobic and anaerobic bacteria including enterococci and *Pseudomonas* spp. Its efficacy is similar to that of the combination of gentamicin and clindamycin in the treatment of sepsis following abdominal surgery.

Septicaemia and septic shock

Most patients dying in the ITU have at least one episode of infection but it is the patient's response to sepsis rather than uncontrolled infection which determines outcome (9). Commonly caused by Gram-negative bacteraemia, 'septic shock' is similar whether it follows invasion by bacteria, viruses, or fungi and is not distinguishable from shock due to soft tissue damage, ruptured aneurysm, or pancreatitis. Multiple organ failure is a common complication of operations for severe intra-abdominal sepsis and of emergency operations (10). Mortality is determined by the number of systems involved; prolonged ventilation and severe renal failure carrying the worst prognosis (see Chapter 12).

Escherichia coli was the organism isolated in 20 per cent of 2518 hospital-acquired septicaemias in one series (11). The organism is derived from the urinary, biliary, and gastrointestinal tracts, usually after manipulation or instrumentation, and from wounds. Other Gram-negative isolates were less common, for example *Pseudomonas* spp. (9 per cent), *Klebsiella* spp. (9 per cent) or *Proteus mirabilis* (6 per cent). *Staph. aureus* was isolated in 19 per cent and coagulase negative staphylococci in 7 per cent of nosocomial septicaemias, coming from intravascular cannulae or clean surgical wounds (11). The risk of death from septic shock is highest when the primary focus of infection is a wound, burn or an abscess, or the respiratory tract. A mixed growth of organisms from the blood carries a high mortality.

The poor prognosis of septic shock due to Gram-negative bacteraemia has been attributed to the role of endotoxin, a lipopolysaccharide released from the bacterial cell wall. It is capable of stimulating many mediators needed for the development of shock, including histamine, complement, coagulation factors, vasoactive polypeptides, prostaglandins, and leukotrienes, and probably acts by releasing cytokines from macrophages. These cytokines, for example interleukins, tumour necrosis factor (TNF) and interferon gamma, given intravenously can reproduce the host response to infection in a dose-dependent fashion, probably by acting on the hypothalamus. The appearance of TNF in the blood is predictive of death in severe sepsis. In baboons, death may be prevented by administration of antibodies to TNF two hours before experimental bacteraemia (9).

The onset of shock is characterized by decreased total peripheral resistance as arterial smooth muscle relaxes, and by a rise in cardiac output and oxygen consumption. The patient is warm but hypotensive. Later venous smooth muscle also relaxes and plasma leaks into the tissues reducing venous return and cardiac output. The hypotension results in sympathetic activation, a rise in peripheral vascular resistance, decreased perfusion of the kidneys and lungs, and lactic acidosis. Fibrinolysis may result in disseminated intravascular coagulation and bleeding at venepuncture sites and from mucous membranes. The patient is now cyanotic, cold and confused. Death may then supervene. Although fever is the commonest sign of bacteraemia, it may be absent in severely ill patients.

Up to 72 h after onset of bacteraemia, damage to pulmonary vasculature, probably by the superoxide radical anion, $\cdot O_2^-$, released from phagocytes, results in worsening hypoxia, diffuse pulmonary infiltration and loss of lung compliance (ARDS). The clinical signs are often indistinguishable from a diffuse infective pneumonia but a search for and eradication or drainage of an infective focus, may be curative (12).

In any patient in whom septic shock is suspected, two blood cultures, preferably from separate sites must be performed before antibiotic treatment starts or is changed. Gram-negative bacteria are rarely contaminants and coagulase negative staphylococci may be significant if in at least two culture bottles.

Resuscitation involves careful administration of fluids and of pressor agents, such as dobutamine, while monitoring the pulmonary artery wedge pressure. Mechanical ventilation and oxygen supplementation are used to correct hypoxia. Haemofiltration is started if acute renal failure has developed. Any collection of pus should be drained and gut perforation repaired or exteriorized.

Initial antibiotic treatment of septicaemia should always be guided by known or expected antibiotic susceptibility patterns. Following abdominal surgery, a combination of cefuroxime and metronidazole for up to one week may be used, subject to local resistance patterns. After clean surgery, flucloxacillin and gentamicin should be used to cover *Staph. aureus*, and after urological operations, or prolonged urinary catheterization, a ureidopenicillin and an aminoglycoside will ensure treatment of Gram-negative bacteria and enterococci. Ureidopenicillins are used in ascending cholangitis. A change to specific treatment should be made as soon as the antibiotic sensitivities of the relevant infecting organism are known. For the enterobacteriaceae, cefuroxime, with or without aminoglycosides, is suitable and for *Ps. aeruginosa*, a common choice is a ureidopenicillin or ceftazidime combined with an aminoglycoside.

Bacteraemia with *Staph. aureus* may be associated with metastatic abscesses, and aggressive treatment is justified with a high dose of flucloxacillin (2 g IV 6 h) and fusidic acid or gentamicin. Benzyl penicillin should be used in preference to flucloxacillin if the isolate is sensitive. Anaerobic organisms in the blood are usually associated with infection of intestinal origin and may be treated with clindamycin or metronidazole.

A reduction in mortality has been observed with the prophylactic administration of antibodies to endotoxin core glycolipid (13) and monoclonal preparations are now available for therapeutic use (29).

Pneumonia

Pneumonia in the surgical intensive care unit accounts for more deaths than infection at any other site (14). Colonization of the oropharynx with Gram-negative bacilli occurs rapidly in the critically ill patient receiving broad spectrum antibiotics. Tracheal intubation encourages colonization of the lower respiratory tract and pneumonia may follow. The longer the period of ventilation the greater the likelihood of pneumonia. Post-operative pain, reduced cough reflex, and poor cilial function contribute to the development of pneumonia, particularly in patients with chronic obstructive airways disease, a history of smoking, prolonged surgery, thoracic or upper abdominal operations, and tracheostomy. Aspiration is the likely route of infection, particularly when secretions are profuse and the patient's level of consciousness is reduced.

A definitive diagnosis of pneumonia may be difficult in the ITU (14). The isolation of organisms from respiratory secretions is useful in determining the spectrum of antibiotic to be used but not for diagnosis. Culture of the sputum does not distinguish colonization from pathogenic bacteria unless the organism is present in the blood or pleural fluid. Isolates may simply reflect the selection pressure of the current antibiotic regimen. In one series of 55 patients, common isolates were *Enterobacter* spp. (29 per cent), *E. coli* (24 per cent), *Ps. aeruginosa* (24 per cent), *H. influenzae* (22 per cent), *Klebsiella* spp. (18 per cent), *Strep. pneumoniae* (13 per cent), *Staph. aureus* (24 per cent) and yeasts (40 per cent) and they were often obtained in mixed culture (15). Fibreoptic bronchial brush biopsy may not provide more reliable results than blind bronchial aspiration (16).

Ideally, antibiotic treatment should be of narrow spectrum to limit overgrowth by resistant flora, including yeasts and other respiratory fungi. However, broad spectrum regimens are commonly used as the true pathogen is rarely known. Nosocomial pneumonia should be treated with cefuroxime with or without gentamicin, reserving ceftazidime or ureidopenicillins for resistant infections (Fig. 35.1). The need for an aminoglycoside is uncertain as the concentration in respiratory secretions is low but there is an *in vitro* synergistic interaction with broad spectrum penicillins against *Ps. aeruginosa*. Aspiration pneumonia and lung abscess are associated with mixed *Bacteroides* spp. and anaerobic cocci and they are best treated with clindamycin or benzyl penicillin and metronidazole. The risk of aspiration can be reduced by the use of small feeds, intravenous feeding, intubation, or posture.

Hand-washing by the nurses and physiotherapists should be encouraged, and bronchial aspiration should be performed aseptically, wearing gloves, and inserting tracheal catheters only once. Ventilation equipment should have disposable tubing, which can be changed between patients or every two weeks. Filters are used to retain both moisture and bacteria and should be changed daily. If filters are not available, the humidifier reservoir should be filled with distilled water and cleaned daily.

Selective decontamination eradicates carriage of aerobic Gram-negative bacilli from the gastrointestinal tract and reduces the number of patients developing pneumonia after general surgery (see Chapter 36). However, overall mortality is not affected.

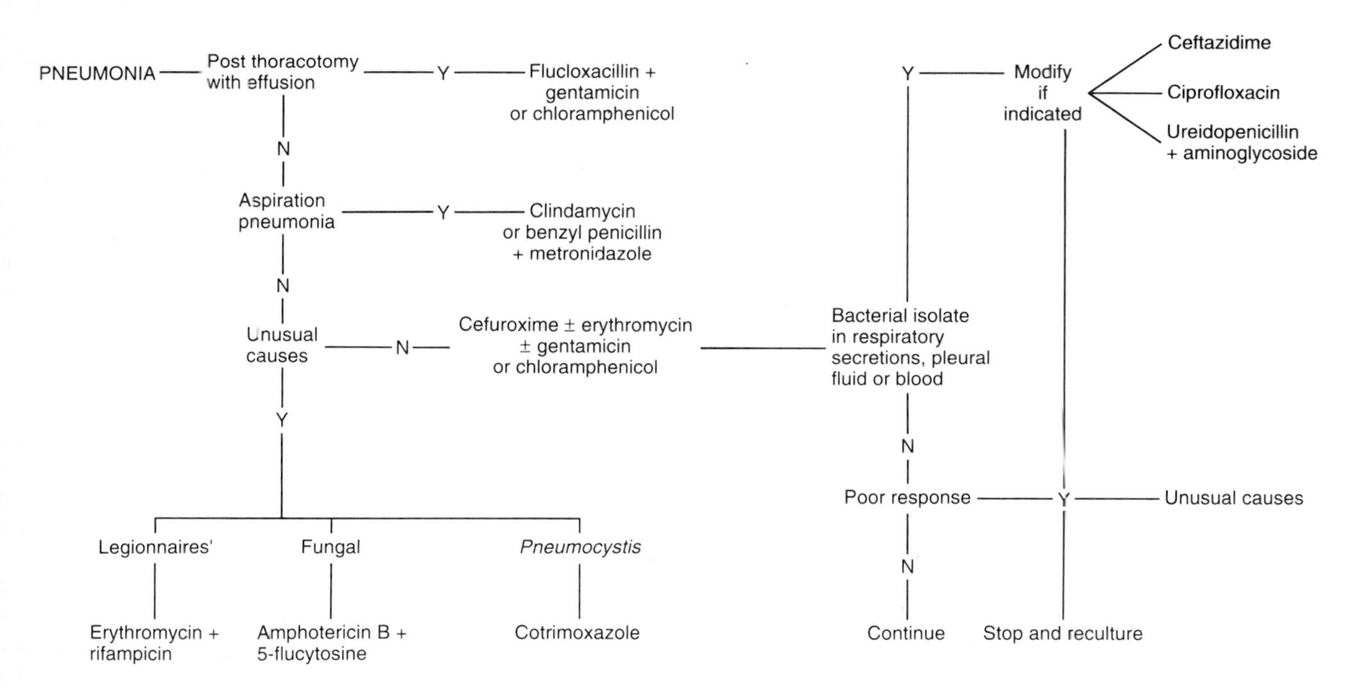

Fig. 35.1 Antibiotic management of post-operative pneumonia.

Infection and prostheses

Intravascular catheters are a potential source of bacteraemia in intensively monitored patients, but the incidence depends on the definition of infection and method of culture (17). In a series of 440 patients (780 catheter tips) colonization increased with the duration of use but varied with different sites (18). At the femoral site 24 (29 per cent) of 84 catheters were colonized compared with 59 (13 per cent) of 467 at the subclavian site. There were 14 patients with catheter-related bacteraemia, representing 1.6 per cent of all catheters and 9 per cent of colonized ones. Bacteraemia from arterial cannulae is rare. Superficial signs of inflammation may be suggestive of infection but are not specific and examination should be made for retinal lesions, splinter haemorrhages and signs of embolism.

When catheter-related infection is suspected, a blood culture should be obtained via the catheter, and a second blood culture taken from a site well away from the catheter insertion. In addition a swab should be obtained from the insertion site. When possible, the catheter should be removed and the tip sent for semiquantitative culture. *Staph. aureus* is the commonest cause of catheter related bacteraemia, 91 (55 per cent) of 182 episodes in one series, but coagulase-negative staphylococci account for an increasing proportion (38 (23 per cent) of 182 episodes), as their significance is more recognized. *Klebsiella* spp. and *Ps. aeruginosa* accounted for 6 per cent and 5 per cent of bacteraemias. Infection probably derives from the skin flora, by contamination during insertion or by subsequent colonization from the patient or staff (19).

Infection of catheters used for total parenteral nutrition can be predicted by detection of skin colonization and confirmed by culture of blood taken through the catheter. Breaks of aseptic technique are frequently associated with infection, for example, the use of the feeding line for central venous pressure readings, or disconnection and contamination of the line.

Coagulase-negative staphylococci isolated in catheter-related infections are usually resistant to flucloxacillin and often to the aminoglycosides. Immediate removal of the cannula is usually the only effective treatment and is mandatory in Gram-negative infections, proven bacteraemia or if pus discharges from the entry site. In other patients, treatment with IV vancomycin may be attempted but not for more than three days unless the fever resolves. Infections with *Candida* spp. should be treated with amphotericin B. The possibility of endocarditis should be considered in patients who develop a catheter-related bacteraemia.

Hands should be washed before insertion of any catheter and the site should be cleaned with skin disinfectant and allowed to dry. Sterile gloves should be worn for placing central venous lines. Cannulae should be secured and covered with a sterile dressing. The site should be inspected in the event of any pain or an unexplained fever and all cannulae and tubing should be changed preferably every 48 hs. Injection of drugs should be through a designated site (a rubber sleeve or diaphragm) after cleaning with a skin disinfectant. Intravenous fluids should be discarded after 24 h.

Infections of prosthetic valves and vascular grafts are caused by staphylococci or Gram-negative bacilli. Infections may appear at any time after surgery and a high index of suspicion is needed as there may be few signs other than fever. Prolonged treatment with bactericidal antibiotics, for example vancomycin plus gentamicin or rifampicin for staphylococci, may be effective. Surgical replacement of the graft is usually necessary. Mortality is high but less than that of medical treatment alone.

Wound infection

The surgical wound must not be overlooked in the management of metabolic, respiratory, or cardiovascular failure. Open wounds or burns are rapidly colonized with bacteria from the environment or from the patient's own flora and infection, inflammation and necrosis may trigger ARDS and multiple organ failure. Following abdominal surgery, fever in the absence of localizing signs suggests an intra-abdominal abscess and the need for surgical drainage.

The discharge of pus is the most obvious sign of infection and is the main criterion in most studies. However, serous discharge, erythema, and wound separation may indicate underlying sepsis. In most cases, daily dressings or debridement are adequate treatment. Appropriate antibiotics (flucloxacillin or cefuroxime with metronidazole) are needed only if the patient has signs of a spreading cellulitis, bacteraemia or purulent dehiscence. In the ITU, all unhealed wounds should be covered with a dry sterile dressing and only exposed for inspection or for renewal of the dressing by using aseptic technique.

Necrotizing fasciitis is a rapidly progressive infective necrosis of superficial and deep fascia and subcutaneous fat. It usually occurs after a minor injury in a limb but can occur after ischiorectal infection or abdominal surgery. Haemolytic streptococci are present, often with *Bacteroides* spp. and coliforms. Progressive bacterial gangrene is a slowly spreading gangrene of the skin and superficial fat which can occur in ischaemic tissue following drainage of a deep abscess or other surgery. Microaerophilic streptococci and *Staph. aureus* are responsible. In either condition, a cardinal sign is dusky purple patches within an area of cellulitis. Septic shock rapidly supervenes. Management involves blood and wound cultures, intravenous fluids, and parenteral antibiotics, initially gentamicin and clindamycin, or benzyl penicillin, gentamicin, and metronidazole. Within 24 h, all necrotic tissue should be excised with the overlying skin, and dressings subsequently changed every 48 h. Skin grafts may be performed when the wound shows healthy granulating tissue. Gas gangrene is a rare but frequently fatal complication of traumatic or surgical wounds caused by toxigenic *Clostridium* spp. (see Chapter 18).

Severe intra-abdominal sepsis may complicate trauma, large bowel surgery or pancreatitis and carries a mortality of 60 per cent or more. Repeated laparotomies are required for debridement and lavage or the abdomen may be left open and irrigated with saline. A covering mesh with a zipper has practical advantages but further abscesses may form if lavage is curtailed prematurely (20). Pancreatic abscess is treated by appropriate parenteral antibiotics, distal pancreatectomy and packing of the wound as lesser procedures have a higher risk of mortality. Blood cultures should be obtained whenever fever or hypotension develops and often yield a mixed bacterial growth. Cultures of fluid from drains are usually mixed and do not distinguish colonization of the catheter from infection of the patient. One or more Gram-negative bacilli are usually present but anaerobes may go undetected if transport of specimens to the laboratory is delayed. Choice of antibiotic will depend on *in vitro* susceptibilities but initially a second generation cephalosporin (for example, cefuroxime), metronidazole and possibly gentamicin are appropriate.

Mediastinitis follows cardiac surgery in 1 to 2 per cent of cases and may require intensive care (21). Staphylococci or mixed Gram-negative organisms are isolated and treatment consists of surgical debridement and mediastinal irrigation. Parenteral antibiotics may be used to treat bacteraemia, particularly if a prosthetic valve is present, but are less effective in treating the wound infection itself.

Urinary infection

The majority of urinary tract infections in the surgical patient are related to urethral catheterization and other urological procedures, such as cystoscopy. Colonization of the catheter and the incidence of bacteriuria increases with the age of catheter and almost all will be infected after two weeks. Approximately one per cent of catheter infections are associated with bacteraemia (22). Disconnection of the catheter and collecting tube permits ascending colonization of the catheter. Alternatively, organisms entering the urethral meatus may pass up towards the bladder between catheter and wall of the urethra. The patient's own perineal flora is the most common source of infecting organisms.

Diagnosis of infection may be clinical rather than microbiological, and all other possible sources of infection should be excluded. Blood should be cultured in patients with abdominal pain, rigors, confusion, and/or fever in the presence of a urinary catheter. 'Significant' bacteriuria (greater than 10^5 cfu/ml) is probably helpful only in identifying the possible source of an organism in the blood or when cross-infection may have occurred. *Escherichia coli* is the most common isolate (58 per cent), the remainder equally divided between *P. mirabilis*, *Klebsiella-Enterobacter* spp., staphylococci, *Ps. aeruginosa*, and enterococci (23).

Organisms colonizing the urinary catheter are often multiply resistant and antibiotic treatment may encourage other more resistant organisms to proliferate. Treatment is unnecessary in asymptomatic infections and removal of the catheter is sufficient in most other patients. If a bacteraemia infection is suspected, treatment should be started empirically and the catheter removed. Colonization of the catheter can be delayed by strict aseptic technique during insertion, closed sterile drainage, and ensuring free flow of urine. The catheter should be fixed securely to prevent accidental trauma to the urethra and removed as soon as it is no longer needed.

Diarrhoea

Diarrhoea is a frequent occurrence in the critically ill and may be associated with mucosal damage due to ischaemia, shock, and hypoxaemia. Ileus is a common sign of multiple organ failure. Pre-operative diarrhoea, use of purgatives, faecal impaction, and post-operative pelvic abscess need to be excluded by the history and examination. A stool sample should be cultured for *Salmonella* spp., *Shigella* spp., and *Campylobacter* spp. Up to 50 per cent of patients given enteral feeds have diarrhoea associated with lactose intolerance, high osmolality, low residue, and too rapid administration (24). Villous atrophy after prolonged fasting and bacterial overgrowth following the use of H_2 histamine receptor antagonists may also be important.

The majority of antibiotics used in the management of the debilitated patient predispose to antibiotic associated colitis. Disruption of the normal bowel flora and the presence of other beta-lactamase producing bacteria promote the growth of *C. difficile*. Cytotoxic agents, nasogastric tubes, enemata and inflammatory bowel disease are contributory factors. A specimen of stool should be obtained for the detection of *C. difficile* cytotoxin B. If possible, a sigmoidoscopy should be performed to confirm the diagnosis and to obtain a biopsy. Symptoms will usually recede within a week of withdrawal of antibiotics but this is often impractical in the critically ill patient. Oral vancomycin (125 mg p.o. every 6 h for 7–10 days) or metronidazole must then be used. Replacement of fluid and electrolytes is important in all patients with diarrhoea. Symptomatic patients should be nursed in source isolation (stool/urine) to reduce the risk of transmission to other patients via attendants.

Renal and liver failure

Renal and liver failure are common consequences of septic shock. When failure of these organs occurs the chances of survival are reduced and the patient is rendered more susceptible to infection. Mortality is highest among those patients developing acute renal failure after operations on the large bowel (25). Vigorous cardiovascular resuscitation, vasopressor agents, and loop diuretics may reduce or prevent acute renal failure if started before it is well established. It is important to find and eliminate any deep infection by repeat laparotomy and antibiotic treatment.

The only reliable method of administration of antibiotics is by the intravenous route but it may be difficult to estimate the correct dose in the critically ill. Elimination is often impaired and cerebral permeability is increased so that neurotoxicity and other adverse effects are more likely. Hypoalbuminaemia affects the free level of antibiotic in the serum. Many antibiotics, such as vancomycin, gentamicin, the cephalosporins and penicillins, are excreted through the kidneys and will accumulate when creatinine clearance falls below 30 ml/min. Vancomycin and aminoglycoside dosage should be altered on the basis of daily serum assays by increasing the dosage interval rather than by changing the individual dose. Nephrotoxicity arises when serum levels have not been adequately monitored or when a nomogram has been used alone. The dose of ciprofloxacin should be halved when creatinine clearance is less than 20 ml/min. Antipseudomonal penicillins, such as piperacillin, should be given in half or a third of the normal dosage to avoid prolongation of the bleeding time. Erythromycin, clindamycin, chloramphenicol, fusidic acid, and rifampicin are mainly metabolized in the liver and can be given in normal dosage. However, in the presence of liver failure, they should be avoided or given in reduced dosage. The clearance and protein binding of chloramphenicol is also decreased and serum levels should be assayed. Modification of the dosage of metronidazole is probably unnecessary in renal or hepatic failure.

Clearance of antibiotics in haemodialysis depends on the type of machine, the flow rates, and on urine output. Cephalosporins and aminoglycosides are slowly eliminated and the dosage of aminoglycosides must be determined by the level of antibiotic in the serum (26, 27). Amphotericin B, vancomycin, clindamycin, fusidic acid, and rifampicin are poorly dialysed and no supplementary doses are needed. There are few studies of haemofiltration but the recommended dose of cefotaxime is 1 g every 24 h depending on the fluid replacement rate (28).

Conclusions

The surgical patient in the intensive care unit is highly susceptible to nosocomial infection, particularly septicaemia and pneumonia caused by Gram-negative bacteria. Clinical and radiological signs and bacterial culture are often of limited help in the diagnosis. Broad spectrum antibiotics are used initially but the spectrum should be narrowed if a pathogen is identified and older well-tried agents are to be preferred. Septic shock and multiple organ failure present the greatest therapeutic challenge and sources of infection, such as a wound infection, should never be neglected. ARDS may be part of this presentation or the result of an infective pneumonia. Fever without obvious source might be resolved by changing all intravascular cannulae or by detection and drainage of an abscess. Antibiotics with potentially toxic adverse effects, like the aminoglycosides, should be frequently assayed and not continued in the face of a rapidly falling urine output.

References

1. Daschner, F. (1985). Nosocomial infections in intensive care units. *Intensive Care Med.*, **11**, 284–5.
2. Daschner, F. (1985). Useful and useless hygienic techniques in intensive care units. *Intensive Care Med.*, **11**, 280–3.
3. Howard, R. J. (1981). Acute acalculous cholecystitis. *Am. J. Surg.*, **141**, 194–8.
4. Stoutenbeek, C. P., van Saene, H. K. F., Miranda, D. R., Zandstra, D. F., and Binnendijk, B. (1984). The prevention of superinfection in multiple trauma patients. *J. Antimicrob. Chemother.*, **14**, Suppl. B, 203–11.
5. Ledingham, I. M., Alcock, S. R., Eastaway, A. T., McDonald, J. C., McKay, I. C., and Ramsay, G. (1988). Triple regimen of selective decontamination of the digestive tract, systemic cefotaxime, and microbiological surveillance for prevention of acquired infection in intensive care. *Lancet*, **i**, 785–90.
6. Konopka, C. A., Arcieri, G., and Schacht, P. (1982). Clinical experience with mezlocillin in Europe—overview. *J. Antimicrob. Chemother.*, **9**, Suppl A, 267–72.
7. Mehtar, S., Parr, J. H., and Morgan, D. J. R. (1982). A comparison of cefuroxime and cotrimoxazole in severe respiratory tract infections. *J. Antimicrob. Chemother.*, **9**, 479–84.
8. Lewin, C. S., Allen, R. A., and Amyes, S. G. B. (1990). Potential mechanisms of resistance to the modern fluorinated 4-quinolones. *J. Med. Microbiol.*, **31**, 153–61.
9. Michie, H. R. and Wilmore, D. W. (1990). Sepsis, signals and surgical sequelae (A Hypothesis). *Arch. Surg.*, **125**, 531–6.
10. Carrico, C. J., Meakins, J., Marshall, J., Fry, D., and Maier, R. (1986). Multiple organ failure syndrome. *Arch. Surg.*, **121**, 196–208.
11. Eykyn, S. J., Gransden, W. R., and Phillips, I. (1990). The causative organisms of septicaemia and their epidemiology. *J. Antimicrob. Chemother.*, **25**, Suppl C, 41–58.
12. Bell, R. C., Coalson, J. J., Smith, J. D., and Johanson, W. G. (1983). Multiple organ system failure and infection in adult respiratory distress syndrome. *Ann. Intern. Med.*, **99**, 293–8.
13. Baumgartner, J. D., Glauser, M. P., McCutchan, J. A., *et al.*, (1985). Prevention of Gram-negative shock and death in surgical patients by antibody to endotoxin core glycolipid. *Lancet*, **ii**, 59–63.
14. Tobin, M. J. and Grenvik, A. (1984). Nosocomial lung infection and its diagnosis. *Crit. Care Med.*, **12**, 191–9.
15. Mock, C. N., Burchard, K. W., Hasan, F., and Reed, M. (1988). Surgical intensive care unit pneumonia. *Surgery*, **104**, 494–9.
16. Papazian, L., Martin, C., Albanese, J., Saux, P., Charrel, J., and Gouin, F. (1989). Comparison of two methods of bacteriologic sampling of the lower respiratory tract: A study in ventilated patients with nosocomial bronchopneumonia. *Crit. Care Med.*, **17**, 461–4.
17. Plit, M. L., Lipman, J., Eidelman, J., and Gavaudan, J. (1988). Catheter related infection. A plea for consensus with review and guidelines. *Intensive Care. Med.*, **14**, 503–9.
18. Collignon, P., Soni, N., Pearson, I., Sorrell, T., and Woods, P. (1988). Sepsis associated with central vein catheters in critically ill patients. *Intensive Care Med.*, **14**, 227–31.
19. Eykyn, S. J. (1984). Infection and intravenous catheters. *J. Antimicrob. Chemother.*, **14**, 203–8.
20. Hedderich, G. S., Wexler, M. J., McLean, A. P., and Meakins, J. L. (1986). The septic abdomen: open management with Marlex mesh with a zipper. *Surgery*, **99**, 399–407.
21. Bor, D. H., Rose, R. M., Modlin, J. F., Weintraub, R., and Friedland, G. H. (1983). Mediastinitis after cardiovascular surgery. *Rev. Infect. Dis.*, **5**, 885–97.
22. Turck, M. and Stamm, W. (1981). Nosocomial infection of the urinary tract. *Am. J. Med.*, **70**, 651–4.
23. Grüneberg, R. N. (1984). Antibiotic sensitivities of urinary pathogens. *J. Antimicrob. Chemother.*, **14**, 17–23.
24. Dobb, G. J. (1988). Diarrhoea in the critically ill. *Intensive Care Med.*, **12**, 113–5.
25. Cameron, J. S. (1986). Acute renal failure in the intensive care unit today. *Intensive Care Med.*, **12**, 64–70.
26. Mann, H. J., Fuhs, D. W., and Cerra, F. B. (1987). Pharmacokinetics and pharmacodynamics in critically ill patients. *World J. Surg.*, **11**, 210–7.
27. Keller, F., Wagner, K., Borner, K., Kemmerich, B., Lode, H., Offerman, G., and Distler, A. (1986). Aminoglycoside dosage in hemodialysis patients. *J. Clin. Pharmacol.*, **26**, 690–5.
28. Hasegawa, H., Takahashi, K., Imada, A., and Horiuchi, A. (1988). Pharmacokinetics of cefotaxime and desacetylcefotaxime in renal failure patients undergoing arteriovenous haemofiltration. *Drugs.*, **35**, Suppl. 2, 78–81.
29. Zeigler, E. J., Fisher, C. J., Sprung, C. L., *et al.* (1991). Treatment of Gram-negative bacteremia and septic shock with HA-1A human monoclonal antibody against endotoxin. *N. Engl. J. Med.*, **324**, 429–36.

Futher reading

Gantz, N. M. (1985). Nosocomial infections in the intensive care unit. In *Intensive care medicine* (ed. J.M. Rippe, R.S. Irwin, J.S. Alpert, and J.E. Dalen), Chapter 67, pp. 639–47. Little Brown, Boston.

Kucers, A. and Bennett, N. M. (1987). *The use of antibiotics. A comprehensive review with clinical emphasis* (4th edn). Heinemann Medical Books, London.

Michie, H. R. and Wilmore, D. W. (1990). Sepsis, signals and surgical sequelae (a hypothesis). *Arch. Surg.*, **125**, 531–6.

Miranda, D.R. and Langrehr, D. (1988). The control of Gram-negative bacterial infection in the ICU. In *Recent advances in critical care medicine*, Vol. 3 (ed. I.M. Ledingham), Chapter 9, pp. 135–58. Churchill Livingstone, Edinburgh.

Stoddart, J.C. (1983). Hospital-acquired infections. In *Care of the critically ill patient* (ed. J. Tinker and M. Rapin), Chapter 52, pp. 873–97. Springer-Verlag, Berlin.

36

The role of selective decontamination of the digestive tract

GRAHAM RAMSAY

Introduction

The practice of intensive care is increasingly recognized as a separate and distinct speciality. This is due partly to an increasing trend towards specialization and partly to technological advances within the intensive therapy unit (ITU). Currently, in the UK most ITUs are run by anaesthetists. While this is not inappropriate, it is to be hoped that the recent development of a Joint Advisory Committee on Intensive Therapy (JACIT) will lead interested individuals in specialities other than anaesthesia to enter intensive care practice. A 'multidisciplinary' approach to intensive care has much to recommend it, particularly since the pooled skills and expertise of a group from differing specialist backgrounds can significantly enhance both the care and understanding of different patients. There are relatively few surgeons who take an active clinical role in the daily management of patients within an ITU and surgical trainees in particular need to be encouraged to seek training in the speciality. This is appropriate since in a general ITU up to 60 per cent of all patients are surgical (1). Acquired infection is a common problem in an ITU, particularly in the group of patients admitted following surgery or trauma in whom there is a significant attendant morbidity and mortality (2).

This chapter will focus primarily on the use of selective decontamination of the digestive tract (SDD) within a general ITU setting, but extension of the principles of SDD to high-risk surgical groups outwith ITU will also be discussed. The philosophy underlying SDD and the precise details of the drug regimen will be described in a subsequent section of this chapter. Critically ill patients within an ITU are prone to abnormal colonization of the gastrointestinal tract (GIT) with potentially pathogenic Gram-negative aerobic bacilli (GNAB), as will be discussed in the following section. SDD is primarily a drug regimen aimed at preventing this abnormal colonization. It is, therefore, a prophylactic regimen. However, it is common for a systemic antimicrobial agent to be administered for the first four days of the ITU stay, in addition to the SDD drugs. The full reasons for the use of a systemic agent will be discussed later but it does mean that some infected patients can be treated with SDD, plus the systemic agent, without the addition of any further therapeutic antimicrobials. Therefore, rather than thinking of SDD as a purely prophylactic regimen it may be more correct to consider it as a means of preventing abnormal colonization by GNAB, whilst preserving the patient's own indigenous gastrointestinal tract flora, which is in turn important in the prevention of colonization.

The incidence of infection in the ITU has been reported from 19 per cent to 36 per cent (2–5). There is a high incidence of unit-acquired infection, the incidence rising with the length of stay and exceeding 80 per cent in patients admitted for five or more days (2). This high incidence of infection appears to be associated with increased mortality rates (6) and, until recently, it was thought that infection contributed directly to the patients' death from multiple organ failure (MOF). This is now open to debate.

Unit-acquired pneumonia is a particularly troublesome problem in ITU and accounts for up to 60 per cent of all episodes of infection (2, 4, 7); endotracheal intubation and ventilation being the major risk factors. It is difficult to make precise statements regarding the pathogenesis of ITU infections because of the complexity of the problems. A break-through in our understanding of this area came in 1969 when Johanssen reported that illness *per se* predisposes to oro-pharyngeal carriage of GNAB (8). Subsequently, further evidence has made it clear that many ITU acquired infections are 'endogenous', with abnormal colonization of the patient's GI tract by GNAB preceding colonization and infection of the major organ systems (9–12).

The incidence of infection in different types of ITU can vary widely (4, 5). Clearly a regimen such as SDD may be appropriate in a general ITU with an infection rate above 30 per cent but would be inappropriate in a coronary care or cardiac ITU with an infection rate below 2 per cent. Therefore, before considering the introduction of SDD into a particular ITU it is first necessary to undertake a prospective assessment of the unit's infection rate, in particular the incidence of acquired infection, together with the attendant morbidity and mortality. The introduction of SDD would then only be indicated if the unit's infection rate was sufficiently high, or if identifiable subgroups of patients, treated within the unit, could be identified in whom the infection rate was high; in which case SDD should be selectively given to that particular patient group. It should be stressed at this stage that SDD is not a replacement for good traditional methods of preventing infection such as adequate asepsis and antisepsis measures, and good barrier techniques. Traditional infection prevention manoeuvres have been fully described in Chapter 35.

SDD is gaining in popularity and is being adopted with increasing frequency as a routine practice. In addition there are many trials of SDD currently in progress. This chapter is based on a review of current publications in which SDD has been used within a trial protocol and which contained sufficient data to allow adequate evaluation of the results.

Pattern of colonization and infection in traditionally managed intensive therapy units

Altered host defence mechanisms and susceptibility to surgical infection have already been discussed in Chapter 4. Critically ill patients in the ITU should be thought of as immunodeficient hosts. It is this compromized state that is the key factor in the pathogenesis of colonization and infection in ITU. Factors such as underlying disease (13, 14) and skeletal, thermal, or surgical trauma (15–18) all contribute to abnormalities of host defence. Where these factors are pertinent to an understanding of SDD, they will be discussed later.

Definition and diagnosis of colonization and infection in ITU

The following definitions will be generally, but not universally, accepted. *Colonization* is the isolation of an identical micro-organism in at least two consecutive samples (spanning one week) without clinical signs of infection. The microbial concentration in the sample is equal to or less than 10^4 colony forming units (cfu) per millilitre or per gram of specimen, accompanied by no more than five leucocytes per low power field. *Infection* is usually a microbiologically proven *clinical* diagnosis. [This may be debated, see Chapter 8: Ed.]. The number of micro-organisms must be greater than 10^5 cfu per ml or gram of specimen, accompanied by 25 or more leucocytes per low power field.

However, there are genuine problems which arise when these classical definitions are used in an ITU setting. Critically ill patients are often subject to invasive monitoring and therapeutic devices, including endotracheal intubation. The presence of these foreign bodies can be associated with inflammatory reactions to the device itself, resulting in samples containing leucocytes with sterile cultures. Furthermore, conditions such as adult respiratory distress syndrome can, in the absence of infection, mimic the clinical signs of pneumonia: purulent sputum, infiltrates on chest radiology, and deterioration in gas exchange.

Similarly, antibiotic administration prior to admission to ITU can make the microbiological findings difficult to interpret in a patient with suspected infection. It is always conceivable that the antibiotics, either topical or systemic, might remove organisms from the site of sampling giving a false-negative result. For instance, topical antisepsis may render the oro-pharynx and upper trachea sterile in a patient who is harbouring pathogenic organisms in the lower airways. It is important to remember these difficulties in the diagnosis of infection, particularly nosocomial pneumonia, when interpreting trials of SDD or other antisepsis regimens in the ITU. In one trial of SDD clinical criteria only were used for the diagnosis of respiratory infection (1) removing the possibility that poor sampling techniques or local antisepsis were responsible for negative microbiological results (see Table 36.1). Of course, this will have the effect of over-diagnosing respiratory tract infection but, when applied in an equal manner to both control and SDD groups, any reduction seen in infection rates should be clinically meaningful.

Table 36.1. Clinical criteria for the diagnosis of respiratory tract infection in ITU.

Categories	Criteria
All categories	Two temperature spikes >38.5°C/24 h White cell count $>12 \times 10^9$/L or $<4 \times 10^9$/L
Respiratory	Purulent sputum New pulmonary infiltrates on radiograph Increase in inspired O_2 fraction of 0.15 or greater to maintain oxygenation

Pattern of colonization and infection

In a traditionally managed ITU control of colonization and infection is based on aseptic technique and a restrictive antibiotic policy. Antibiotics tend to be withheld until good clinical and microbiological evidence of infection exists. An appropriate antibiotic is then given according to sensitivity testing. The principle of careful aseptic technique is clearly a good one, since regardless of whether infections are endogenously or exogenously acquired, it should, in theory, be possible to prevent them by good aseptic technique and thus avoid initial bacterial contamination. However, it is patently obvious from the high infection rates already quoted that such regimens fail to control colonization and infection in a large proportion of patients admitted to a general ITU. Colonization of the GIT by GNAB occurs rapidly following admission to ITU, usually within 48 to 72 h (1). In a number of trials it has been observed that following initial colonization of the GIT by GNAB, subsequent colonization and then infection of adjacent major organ systems occurs in a sequential fashion (Fig. 36.1).

In day-to-day life the GIT is constantly exposed to large numbers of potentially pathogenic GNAB. A variety of factors, together constituting 'colonization defence' (12), act to prevent colonization of the mucosal surfaces of the digestive tract except in situations of extremely high bacterial concentrations. In health motility, an anatomically intact mucosal surface, and the indigenous flora are probably the most important factors. Colonization and infection defence factors have been described elsewhere in this textbook and a full description

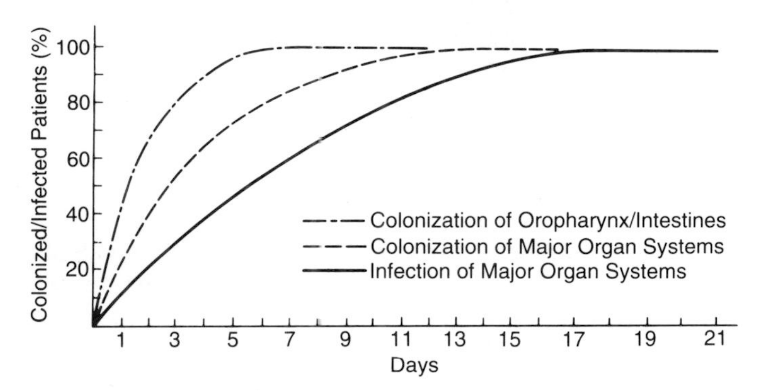

Fig. 36.1 Percentage of colonized and infected patients in ITU versus length of stay. (Results pooled from several studies).

here would be inappropriate. However, a few points, which are relevant to the understanding of the reasons, behind the introduction of SDD into ITU practice, are worthy of re-emphasis.

Impaired host defences in critically ill patients

As already indicated, a critically ill patient in ITU should be considered as an 'immunosuppressed host'. Such patients are prone to develop abnormal colonization of their GIT by GNAB; colonization and infection of adjacent major organ systems may occur subsequently. 'Colonization defence' is a concept which describes the factors which, in health, constitute the first line of defence of the GIT against colonization. The factors contributing to colonization defence are listed in Table 36.2.

Many factors contribute to a decrease in colonization defence in a critically ill patient; the effect of invasive instrumentation and underlying disease have already been mentioned (15–18). In addition, a number of factors have particular relevance to the philosophy behind the introduction of SDD.

Usage of broad-spectrum antimicrobial agents

It has long been postulated that the widespread use of broad-spectrum antibiotics can predispose to colonization by GNAB as a result of alteration to the normal indigenous flora of the GIT. Such an effect was shown to occur after large dose penicillin therapy (19) and the same group were able to prevent abnormal colonization by inducing a state of resistance in the normal flora of the GIT (20). Other workers have produced results which support the concept that colonization resistance occurs in humans and is diminished by antibiotic administration (21). Currently, increasing importance has been attached to the role of the anaerobic flora, which are numerically predominant, in the preservation of colonization resistance of the GIT (22). Parenterally administered therapeutic antibiotics tend to reach the GIT lumen in varying concentrations, depending on the degree of excretion in saliva, bile, and intestinal mucus. Such antibiotics, together with orally administered agents, can have a profound effect on the indigenous anaerobic flora of the GIT, depending on the therapeutic spectrum of the agent. Under the philosophy of SDD one of the principles is that therapeutic drugs with an anaerobic antibiotic spectrum should be avoided if they have significant excretion in either saliva, bile, or intestinal mucus.

Effect of age

There is some evidence to suggest that colonization resistance is decreased in elderly patients; colonization of the GIT and oropharynx by GNAB has been found in a proportion of this group, especially if they are institutionalized (23).

Abnormal gut motility

Lack of oral food intake, the inability of an intubated patient to swallow or chew, and decreased or absent peristalsis all tend

Table 36.2. Seven factors contributing to the defence of the oropharyngeal cavity and the gastrointestinal tract against colonization.

Factor	Local expression	
	Oropharyngeal cavity	Gastrointestinal tract
1 Anatomical integrity		
2 Normal physiology	pH of saliva	pH of gastric secretion
3 Motility	chewing, swallowing	peristalsis
4 Secretions	saliva	gastric juice, bile, mucous
5 Immunoglobulin A secretion	in saliva	in bile and mucus
6 Shedding and replacement of mucosal cells		
7 Indigenous flora (mostly anaerobic)		

to predispose to abnormal colonization. In paralytic ileus fluid accumulates within the bowel lumen and stagnant fluid in this situation, as in any other, tends to become heavily colonized.

Gastric pH, colonizations and nosocomial pneumonia

It is well recognized that gastric colonization is a preceding and predisposing factor for tracheal colonization (9) and that treatment with antacids can predispose to gastric colonization (10). In addition, ambulant patients with peptic ulcer disease show significant bacterial colonization of gastric aspirate after one month of treatment with an H_2 receptor antagonist such as cimetidine (24), again suggesting a significant relationship between pH and bacterial counts in gastric juice. This same relationship has been shown in critically ill patients (25) with an apparent cut off at pH 4; colonization of gastric juice being rare when the pH is less than 4.

In the past it has been common practice in ITU to give H_2 receptor antagonists on a routine basis for prophylaxis against stress ulceration. There is now good evidence to suggest that aggressive and complete resuscitation, thus avoiding mucosal ischaemia, is more important in the prevention of stress ulceration. Nevertheless, the widespread use of H_2 receptor antagonists in the ITU remains a substantial risk factor for gastric colonization and subsequent nosocomial pneumonia. This has been highlighted by two controlled studies comparing the mucosal protective agent sucralfate with antacids and/or H_2 receptor antagonists (26, 27). Both studies showed a lower incidence of nosocomial pneumonia in the sucralfate treated group. It is worthy of note that, in the study by Tryba (31), 53 per cent of patients in the sucralfate group had a pH above 4. Many critically ill patients have a high gastric pH and colonization of gastric juice may occur, even in the absence of antacids or H_2 receptor antagonists.

Another study has compared sucralfate with SDD in a group of patients undergoing cardiac surgery. Gastric pH was less than 4 in only 25 per cent of sucralfate-treated patients, leaving the majority without the benefit of gastric acidity as a barrier to bacterial overgrowth in the stomach (28). This study showed that gastric colonization with GNAB was significantly less in the SDD group than in the sucralfate group (12 per cent v. 55 per cent, $p < 0.001$). In addition, the rate of Gram-negative infection was significantly lower in the SDD group (6 per cent v. 20 per cent, $p = 0.02$).

Selective decontamination

Background and philosophy

Prior to the introduction of SDD into ITU practice a large background literature existed dealing with the moderately successful use of SDD in neutropaenic patients (29–31). Many different regimens for both selective and 'complete' decontamination have been used in neutropaenic patients, and, on occasion, their use was associated with the development of microbial resistance. This was particularly seen with regimens which included gentamicin. Retrospectively, it has been claimed that bacterial resistance and therapeutic failure using these regimens can be explained on the basis of flaws in the regimen chosen (32). One potentially important point is that gentamicin appears to be moderately inactivated by faeces, while this is not the case with tobramycin (33). The SDD regimen currently in use in the management of patients in the ITU should be thought of as a logical extension of, and improvement on, previous regimens used in the care of neutropaenic patients.

There are three basic principles underlying the philosophy of SDD:

1. Micro-organisms can be broadly grouped according to their intrinsic pathogenic potential. The indigenous (mostly anaerobic) flora of the GIT live in a symbiotic relationship with the host, and have a low pathogenic potential. Close examination of the microbiology indicates that virtually all nosocomial infections in the ITU are due to a limited number of aerobic micro-organisms: six micro-organisms that may

be carried by patients on admission—so-called 'community' micro-organisms (*Streptococcus pneumoniae*, *Haemophilus influenzae*, *Branhamella catarrhalis*, *Escherichia coli*, *Staphylococcus aureus*, and *Candida* species), and eight species of bacteria that are commonly acquired during ITU stay—so-called 'hospital' bacteria (*Klebsiella*, *Proteus* and *Morganella*, *Enterobacter*, *Citrobacter* and *Serratia* species, *Pseudomonas*, and *Acinetobacter* species).

2. The indigenous flora are rarely involved in infections, have important physiological functions (34) and, indeed, contribute to defence against aerobic colonization of the GIT (35).

3. Colonization and infection of major organ systems usually occurs after a previous stage of oropharyngeal and/or gastrointestinal colonization by identical aerobes, i.e. most ITU infections are 'endogenously' acquired.

The three prime aims of an SDD regimen can be summarized as follows:

1. To eliminate from, or to prevent colonization of the GIT by the potentially pathogenic aerobic bacteria.
2. To preserve the indigenous, predominantly anaerobic, flora in order to maintain colonization resistance.
3. To prevent fungal overgrowth of the GIT, since immunosuppressed patients are prone to fungal infection.

SDD regimen

To be suitable for use in an SDD regimen antimicrobial agents should ideally meet the following criteria. The antimicrobial spectrum should cover all enterobacteriaceae (including *Serratia* species, pseudomonads, and *Acinetobacter* species). The spectrum should not include anaerobic organisms, in order to establish a *selective flora elimination*. The antimicrobials should ideally have a low minimum bactericidal concentration for the GNAB listed above, because leucocytes are not present in the lumen of the intestinal canal to assist microbial killing. The agents should be non-absorbable (or absorbed only to a minimal extent) both in order to achieve high intraluminal levels and also to avoid having fluctuating levels of plasma and tissue antimicrobial concentration. The agents should show a minimal inactivation by food and faecal compounds and no degradation by faecal enzymes. The interactions between faeces, bacteria, and antimicrobial agents are of potentially great importance in deciding the success of a given SDD regimen (33).

The first use of SDD in an ITU setting was reported from Groningen (36, 37) where the regimen included the topical application of polymixin E, tobramycin, and amphotericin B (PTA regimen) details of which are given in Table 36.3. As can be seen from Table 36.3, in addition to the topical PTA regimen, systemic cefotaxime was administered to the patients for the first four days of their stay in ITU. The reasons for the addition of a short-term parenteral antibiotic as a supplement to SDD have been fully discussed elsewhere (38). A parenteral agent is deemed necessary to treat early infections due to the community bacteria listed above and also to provide cover against hospital bacteria during the two or three days required for the effect of the topical regimen to be established. The Groningen group, in a separate publication, examined the relative importance of the component parts of the SDD regimen—confirming that both oropharyngeal and gastrointestinal decontamination were required, together with a short term systemic agent (39).

Table 36.3. Prophylactic regimen based on a combination of topical and systemic antimicrobials.

Topical antimicrobials (PTA regimen)
These are administered throughout the ITU stay.

(a) Oropharyngeal cavity: A small volume of a 2 per cent mixture of polymixin E, tobramycin and amphotericin B in a paste with carboxy methyl cellulose (Orobase) is applied to the buccal mucosa with a gloved finger 4 times daily.

(b) Gastrointestinal canal: 9 ml of a suspension of polymixin E 100 mg, tobramycin 80 mg and amphotericin B 500 mg is administered via the gastric tube 4 times daily.

Systemic antimicrobial
Administered for the first 4 days of the ITU stay.
Cefotaxime 50–100 mg/kg body weight/day given intravenously

A number of the trials conducted since the original Groningen work have used variations on the original PTA regimen. Such changes may, in the future, be proven to be appropriate but, for the time being, caution should be exercised when interpreting results from trials using other than the original PTA regimen. In particular any apparent failure of decontamination or emergence of resistance should lead one to examine the agents used bearing in mind the criteria listed above regarding the suitability of agents for inclusion in an SDD regimen.

In the regimen listed in Table 36.3 the topical application of PTA to the oropharyngeal cavity is carried out with the drugs contained in a paste with carboxy methylcellulose. This is to ensure adequate contact time with the buccal mucosa but has the disadvantage of an unpleasant taste and appearance. One apparently worthwhile adaptation of the regimen is to mix the PTA drugs in a peppermint flavoured gel (40). The gel has the advantage of being palatable and has been successfully used by the author with no loss of efficacy compared with the oro-base formulation.

The role of the clinical microbiologist

Workers planning to implement an SDD regimen in their ITU must first secure the co-operation of an interested and committed clinical microbiologist. The diagnosis of infection, particularly pneumonia, can be extremely difficult in ITU and joint discussions, on a daily basis, between a clinical microbiologist and the intensive care physician can be extremely useful in deciding when additional therapeutic antibiotics are indicated.

Surveillance cultures are taken from all patients on admission as an integral part of the regimen, and thereafter cultures are taken twice weekly from the oropharynx, tracheal aspirate, gastric aspirate, rectal swab, and urine. Careful and regular monitoring of these cultures is required for several reasons.

First, it is imperative to monitor for possible emergence of resistance to either the topical or parenteral agents, although this has not yet been reported as a problem with the PTA regimen. Second, any breakdown in aseptic technique or administration of the SDD regimen can be detected by the microbiologist through monitoring of samples from the decontaminated patients.

Trials of SDD in intensive therapy units

Since the Groningen publication (37) eleven other centres have published results of SDD trials within an ITU environment: Glasgow (1), Göttingen (41), Münster (42), Munich (43), Nijmegen (44), Ulm (45), Utrecht (46), Lyon (47), The Hague (48), Lübeck (49), and the Mayo Clinic, Rochester (50). The Groningen group studied only long-stay trauma patients but all the other trials have studied a mixed ITU population. Groningen, Göttingen, Munich, and Rochester excluded all patients who were infected at the time of admission to the ITU. The Glasgow and Lyon studies analysed all patients admitted to the ITU regardless of length of stay, while the other studies examined only patients who required, or were expected to require, prolonged ventilation. Groningen, Göttingen, Glasgow, and Lübeck utilized consecutive trial designs while all the other studies were prospective with concurrent control groups. The Münster study utilized two ITUs, one using a control regimen while the other used a SDD regimen with cross-over after six months so that control and SDD patients were not mixed.

Six of the 12 studies listed above utilized the original SDD regimen as contained in Table 36.3. Variations on this regimen were used in Munich, Nijmegen, Lyon, Hague, Lübeck, and Rochester (43, 44, 47–50). In Munich the regimen differed in several ways—gentamicin replaced tobramycin; an aqueous solution of drugs was used and not a paste; gentamicin and polymyxin were applied to the nasopharynx, oropharynx, and stomach while amphotericin B was applied only to the oropharynx. In Nijmegen and The Hague, the quinolone, norfloxacin, replaced tobramycin and, in The Hague only, trimethoprim was used systemically instead of cefotaxime. In Lyon, both SDD and control groups received amphotericin B enterally and oropharyngeal and nasopharyngeal disinfection was achieved with povidone iodine, whilst, in addition, the SDD group received tobramycin and polymyxin enterally. In Lübeck both neomycin and bacitracin were added to the topical PTA regimen. In Rochester nystatin replaced amphotericin B and gentamicin replaced tobramycin. Finally, in Munich, Lyon, and Lübeck systemic prophylaxis with cefotaxime was not used.

In Nijmegen the study contained two control groups. Patients in the first group, who developed infection, received antibiotics which may have affected the indigenous, anaerobic flora, whereas the second group received only antibiotics thought to have minimal influence on the indigenous anaerobic flora (i.e. did not disturb colonization resistance). In Lübeck the study contained two treatment groups, both of which received SDD. The first group received ranitidine for stress ulcer prophylaxis whilst the second group received sucralfate.

Colonization rates

All twelve studies confirmed the rapid increase in GNAB colonization of the upper GIT in the control groups, rising from 0 to 40 per cent on admission to 50 to 100 per cent by one week. SDD achieved a consistent reduction in colonization by GNAB, usually within 48 h, and all studies reported a colonization rate of only 0 to 5 per cent by seven days. In Munich (43) a worrying percentage of organisms resistant to gentamicin was found amongst the isolates screened but this has not been reported from any of the trials utilizing the PTA regimen.

Rectal colonization by GNAB was also consistently reduced, but the effect required considerably longer to achieve, particularly in trials containing large numbers of post-operative patients. Paralytic ileus meant that rectal colonization was not abolished for in excess of two weeks (1).

Therefore, in these trials, SDD has been uniformly successful in eliminating GNAB carriage, particularly in the upper GIT, but how selective was this effect? In the Glasgow study (1) careful attention was paid to the isolation rates of normal flora from the screening samples, as well as the isolation rates for GNAB. In the control group the isolation rate of normal flora decreased steadily as GNAB colonisation increased. By contrast, in the SDD group, normal flora isolation rates dropped for the first four days, during the time that systemic cefotaxime was administered, but thereafter isolation rates of normal flora returned to the levels seen at the time of admission to ITU. Therefore, it would appear that the decontamination effect of the regimen is selective.

Infection rates

SDD had a statistically significant beneficial effect on infection rates in all twelve studies (Table 36.4). The greatest impact was on Gram-negative respiratory tract infections though infection rates in other organ systems were also reduced. The infection rates reported from the different centres vary widely, especially for the control groups. This can largely be explained by differing patient populations, differing criteria for the diagnosis

Table 36.4. Acquired infection rates in SDD trials (%).

Centre	Respiratory tract bacteraemia		Urinary tract			
SDD	Control	SDD	Control	SDD	Control	SDD
Groningen (37)	59	8	32	2	42	3
Glasgow (1)	18	3	3	1	11	8
Göttingen (41)	75	7	30	10	8	6
Münster (42)	46	10	16	10	–	–
Munich (43)	70	21	–	–	–	–
Nijmegen (44)	78/62*	6	8	0	–	–
Ulm (45)	42	6	8	0	–	–
Utrecht (46)	40	6	6	3	57	30
Lyon (47)	21	3	–	–	–	–
The Hague (48)	44	6	27	4	15	0
Lübeck (49)	49	14/7†	–	–	–	–
Rochester (50) (Mayo)	62	4‡				

* 2 control groups † 2 treatment groups ‡ total infections

of infection, and differing criteria for the separation of pre-existing from acquired infections.

In the Nijmegen study (44), with two control groups, no apparent difference was seen in infection rates. As mentioned above, the groups differed according to whether the therapeutic antibiotics used would, or would not, be expected to have an effect on indigenous, anaerobic, GIT flora. In Lübeck, the SDD groups was split into two according to whether the patients received H_2 receptor antagonists or sucralfate for stress ulcer prophylaxis. SDD significantly reduced the respiratory tract infection rate from the level seen in the control group. Sucralfate appeared to confer an additional advantage with a respiratory infection rate of 7 per cent compared with 14 per cent in patients receiving SDD with H_2 receptor antagonists.

Mortality rates

The results as assessed by mortality rates have been a little less consistent (Table 36.5). Göttingen, Lyon, Hague, and Lübeck all reported a significant reduction in mortality in their SDD groups (41, 47–49) while the remaining eight trials show no significant difference in overall mortality rates. However, Munich and Utrecht (43, 46) reported a significant reduction in infection-related mortality with SDD, and Glasgow (1) reported a significant benefit in trauma patients. It should be mentioned that in Lübeck the significant reduction in overall mortality was only seen when SDD was combined with sucralfate.

Cost implications and work-load

Only the Groningen group have studied the effects on SDD on the total running costs of an ITU and the supporting laboratory services (51); they reported a large saving following the introduction of SDD. In Glasgow, the original estimate of additional antibiotic costs after introducing SDD was £6000 per annum. Current costings (1990) have been accurately calculated at £6.45 per patient per day; this is utilizing a gel for the oro-pharyngeal decontamination rather than paste and includes all staff and equipment costs as well as drug costs. Although not fully evaluated there should be a large reduction in the cost of disposible items such as venous lines and pulmonary artery catheters resulting from the reduction in the incidence of infection. The workload of the microbiology service is certainly decreased because the vast majority of surveillance cultures produce 'no growth' results and there has been a significant reduction in the number of clinical samples submitted for microbiological examination (51).

Table 36.5. Mortality rates in SDD trials (%).

Centre		Control	SDD	p value
Groningen	(37)	8	3	NS
Glasgow	(1)	24	24	NS
(Trauma)		26	0	0.002
Göttingen	(41)	14	0	<0.05
Münster	(42)	–	NS	–
Munich	(43)	30	24	NS
(Infection related deaths)		15	0	<0.05
Nijmegen	(44)	22/10*	12	NS
Ulm	(45)	22	30	NS
Utrecht	(46)	32	29	NS
(Infection related deaths)		NS	(SDD < control)	<0.05
Lyon	(47)	18	6	<0.05
The Hague	(48)	54	31	0.02
(Infection related deaths)		15	0	0.004
Lübeck	(49)	54	35/18†	0.01
Rochester (Mayo)	(50)	NS	NS	–

* = 2 control groups † = 2 treatment groups

Microbial resistance

There is an understandable concern, often expressed, that because SDD represents the generalized prophylactic use of antibiotics in ITU there must be a high risk of microbial resistance developing. Such concern misses the point: that in a traditionally managed ITU very large quantities of parenteral, therapeutic antibiotics are administered to treat suspected or proven infections. Therefore SDD should not be compared with a situation in which no antibiotics are used. In fact, the introduction of SDD produces a reduction in the usage of therapeutic antimicrobials (1, 46, 49) and therefore will reduce the selection pressure for resistance—since fluctuating antibiotic levels within the GIT after parenteral administration is one of the recognized factors in the emergence of resistance. All units have isolated GNAB which are resistant to one or other of the agents used but these tend not to persist, often disappearing without a change in the antibiotic regimen. In Groningen, the pattern of microbial resistance over a thirty month period, during which an SDD regimen was used, has been the subject of a separate publication (52) which reported no increase in resistance to any of the agents used.

Even organisms which are partially resistant to the drugs contained in the regimen on standard disc testing are often successfully eliminated because of the very high concentrations of topical agents used.

Some of the studies have reported that surveillance cultures during the SDD regimen have shown an increase in the frequency of isolation of *Staphylococcus epidermidis* and enterococci (45).

Eastaway (53) has reported that GNAB have reappeared in rectal swabs after a mean of five days in patients who were followed after discharge from the ITU back to a general surgical ward. GNAB resistance to SDD agents was low and did not correlate with resistance present at the time of ITU admission.

Utilization of SDD to control an outbreak of microbial resistance

Brun-Buisson *et al.* (54) reported the use of SDD in the control of a nosocomial outbreak of intestinal colonization and infection with multi-resistant enterobacteriaceae. During a ten-week incidence study it was found that 19.6 per cent of patients were colonized with multi-resistant strains. Isolation of these strains occurred at a mean of 16 days after admission, and preceded detection in clinical samples by a mean of 11 days. Patients were then randomly allocated to either a control group or an SDD group. During the decontamination trial, intestinal colonization rates decreased to 10 per cent in the control group and 3 per cent in the SDD group, with corresponding infection rates of 3 per cent and 0. Following the eight-week trial period no new case of colonization with the multi-resistant strains was seen.

The intestinal colonization rate with Gram-positive cocci was higher in the SDD group than in the control group, and the overall rate of nosocomial infections was 33 per cent in the control group and 32 per cent in the SDD group. The authors concluded that SDD can help to control an outbreak of intestinal colonization and infection with multi-resistant Gram-negative bacilli but should not be recommended for routine prevention of endemic nosocomial infections. There are several good reasons why the authors failed to confirm the overall effect on nosocomial infections seen in all the other studies. First, their regimen was neomycin, polymyxin E, and nalidixic acid given enterally only. Second, no SDD drugs were applied to the oropharynx, although oropharyngeal disinfection with povidine iodine was used. Third, no systemic agent was used. There are, therefore, considerable differences between the regimen used here and the classical regimen described in Table 36.3. In particular, it is likely that the omission of oropharyngeal decontamination is important with regard to the prevention of nosocomial pneumonia, which is the commonest nosocomial infection in ITU.

In summary it would appear that, even in units not using SDD routinely, its introduction for a short period may be useful in the control of an outbreak of colonization with resistant GNAB.

SDD in high-risk surgical groups, and other potential applications of the regimen

In addition to its usage in ITU, SDD is increasingly being adopted for use in high risk surgical groups outwith ITU. In a mixed ITU many patients are infected at the time of admission. Since SDD is essentially a prophylactic regimen against colonization its use in high-risk surgical groups, prior to surgery or ITU admission, is entirely appropriate.

Oesophageal surgery

Tetteroo *et al.* (55) have reported the successful use of SDD, utilizing the PTA regimen, to reduce Gram-negative colonization and infections after oesophageal resection. Patients undergoing oesophageal resection have a particularly high frequency of lower respiratory tract infections with GNAB. In their trial they observed that 32 of 58 control patients acquired 51 infections while only 12 of 56 SDD treated patients acquired 18 infections; a significant difference. In addition, the requirement for post-operative therapeutic antibiotics was significantly lower in the SDD group and no endogenous infection caused by GNAB was seen in the SDD patients.

Transplantation

Transplantation patients are at increased risk for infection because of the immuno-suppressive treatment given to prevent rejection of the transplant. Consequently all patients have T-cell suppression. Amongst the most severely compromised of transplant patients are those receiving allogeneic bone marrow transplantation, who require strong immunosuppression in order to mitigate or prevent graft versus host disease. SDD has been reported to have been successful in preventing infection in bone marrow transplant patients (56, 57).

Liver transplant patients are also extremely prone to infection. In addition to the immunosuppression these patients also have a two to three week period before the Kupffer cells repopulate the sinusoids. During this period spill-over of GIT organisms is likely. The successful use of SDD as a prophylactic regimen has been reported in patients undergoing liver transplantation (58, 59), while encouraging early results have also been reported from other centres, including Birmingham, UK.

Burns patients

Severely burned patients are often treated within an ITU, where they suffer from the same nosocomial infection problems as other patients. In addition, burn patients are extremely prone to infection of the burn-wound, particularly with endogenous GNAB (60). Organisms drived from the upper GIT contaminate burn wounds of the upper limbs and trunk, while organisms derived from the lower GIT and rectum tend to contaminate the lower limbs and lower half of the trunk. Again, SDD has been shown to be of benefit to burn patients (61).

Head and neck cancer

Head and neck cancer patients undergoing radiotherapy are prone to develop a reactive inflammatory-like process of the oropharyngeal mucous membrane, a problem known as irradation mucositis. Mucositis causes serious complaints such as pain and difficulties with swallowing, eating, and speech. This can lead to serious systemic toxicity and weight loss (62).

It is now known that colonization of the oropharyngeal tissues with GNAB significantly contributes to the process. It has also been shown that SDD led to a highly significant reduction in mucositis compared with a control group (63).

Cardiothoracic surgery

In general, infection rates in cardiac surgery ITUs are rather low. However, the successful introduction of SDD into a cardiac ITU, leading to a significant reduction in infection, has been reported (28, 64).

Other potential applications

The number of potential applications for SDD is increasing rapidly. It has been suggested that the high incidence of endogenous infections with GNAB in neonatal surgical units might well be favourably affected by the introduction of SDD (65). Colonic surgery, major vascular, and chemotherapy—for solid tumours as well as for leukaemias—are other potential areas where SDD might usefully be employed. In some of these cases the use of the gel formulation for the oropharynx would be particularly useful because its palatability makes it ideal for ambulant patients.

Effect of SDD on multiple organ failure

SDD was introduced to the ITU setting because of the very high incidence of unit-acquired infection, and there can be little doubt that SDD does have a significant impact on the incidence of acquired Gram-negative infections, with all 12 trials showing a statistically significant reduction. As can be seen from Table 36.5, SDD also appears to have an impact on mortality rates, with seven centres quoting a significant reduction in mortality, either overall or in subgroups.

However, it has become clear that despite the SDD regimen many patients still die of MOF in the absence of infection. Therefore, it has to be assumed that the previously observed link between infection, MOF and late deaths in ITU was not necessarily a causative one. Patients may die of MOF secondary to 'non-bacterial sepsis' whilst treated with SDD. There is now increasing evidence to suggest that such patients are suffering from absorption of mediators such as endotoxin from the GIT (66). If gut-origin endotoxin is a major mediator (67), then SDD may have a role in reducing the gut load of endotoxin, by reducing GNAB colonization. However, as presently administered, the reduction of lower bowel GNAB with SDD is both slow and incomplete (particularly in post-operative surgical patients) suggesting that further synergistic therapy may be required if gut-mediated MOF is to be prevented (67, 68).

Comments and conclusions

Despite the problems mentioned earlier with the definition and diagnosis of nosocomial infection in the ITU (in particular respiratory tract infection), SDD does appear to be of proven benefit as a method of reducing the incidence of ITU-acquired infection, particularly Gram-negative infections. It takes two to three days for the decontamination effect to be achieved, even in the oropharynx, and therefore short-stay patients, in particular those admitted for overnight observation post-operatively, are unlikely to benefit from the regimen. There is, therefore, a strong argument for the selective administration of SDD; there would appear to be clear evidence of a significant benefit in trauma patients and a strong suggestion that other long-stay groups in general ITUs would also benefit. SDD should not be utilized in areas with a low risk of infection such as coronary care units.

Not all trials have reported an effect of SDD on mortality. However, given the relatively small size of some of the study groups it is impressive that 7 of the 12 trials reviewed in this chapter do show a reduction, either in overall, or sub-group, mortality. Meta-analysis of the trial results is probably inappropriate because of the differing regimens, different ITU types and different criteria for patient inclusion. There is now a large multi-centre trauma trial in progress which should give a definitive answer to the effect of SDD on mortality.

Any intensive care physician who intends to adopt SDD must first of all gain the support of all clinicians likely to admit patients to the unit. It is also important that the intensive care physician has a large degree of control over the antibiotic policy of the unit, since inappropriate use of prophylactic antibiotics may adversely affect the indigenous flora of the bowel and colonization resistance. It is imperative that all units using the regimen have close contact with a clinical microbiologist, and even outside a trial situation it is imperative that surveillance cultures are performed in order to detect the development of resistance to the SDD agents. To date there has been no significant problem with antibiotic resistance but careful surveillance must continue.

Finally, SDD is not a substitute for careful aseptic technique in the ITU. Regardless of whether infections are deemed to be endogenous or exogenous, they are in theory preventable if initial contamination and subsequent colonization is prevented.

References

1. Ledingham, I. McA. Alcock, S. R., Eastaway, A. T., McDonald, J. C., MacKay, I. C., and Ramsay, G. (1988). Triple regimen of selective decontamination of the digestive tract, systemic cefotaxime, and microbiological surveillance for prevention of acquired infection in intensive care. *Lancet*, **i**, 785–90.
2. Thorp, J. M., Richards, W. C., and Telfer, A. B. M. (1979). A survey of infection in an intensive care unit. *Anaesthesia*, **68**, 457–67.
3. Donowitz, L. G., Wenzel, R. P., and Hoyt, J. W. (1982). High risk of hospital acquired infection in the ICU patient. *Crit. Care Med.*, **10**, 335–7.
4. Brown, R. B., Hosmer, D., Chen, H. C., *et al.* (1985). A comparison of infections in different ICUs within the same hospital. *Crit. Care Med.*, **13**, 472–6.
5. Chandrasetar, P. M., Kruse, J. A., and Matthews, M. F. (1986). Nosocomial infection among patients in different types of intensive care unit at a city hospital. *Crit. Care Med.*, **14**, 508–10.
6. Machiedo, G. W., LaVerme, P. J., McGovern, P. J., and Blackwood, J. M. (1981). Patterns of mortality in a surgical ICU. *Surg. Gynecol. Obstet.*, **152**, 757–9.
7. Kerver, A. J. H., Rommes, J. H., Mevissen-Verhage, E. A. E., *et al.* (1987). Colonization and infection in surgical intensive care patients—a prospective study. *Intensive Care Med.*, **13**, 347–51.
8. Johannsen, W. J., Pierce, A. K., and Sanford, J. P. (1969). Changing pharyngeal bacterial flora of hospitalised patients. *N. Engl. J. Med.*, **281**, 1137–40.
9. Atherton, S. T. and White, D. J. (1978). Stomach as a source of bacteria colonizing respiratory tract during artificial ventilation. *Lancet*, **ii**, 968–9.
10. du Moulin, G. C., Paterson, D. G., Hedley-Whyte, J., and Lisbon, A. (1982). Aspiration of gastric bacteria in antacid treated patients: a frequent cause of post-operative colonization in the air-way. *Lancet*, **i**, 242–5.
11. Flynn, D. M., Weinstein, R. A., Nathan, C., Gaston, M. A., and Kabins, S. A., (1987). Patients endogenous flora as the source of nosocomial Enterobacter in cardiac surgery. *J. Infect. Dis.*, **156**, 363–8.
12. van Saene, H. K. F., Stoutenbeek, C. P., Zandstra, D. F., Gilbertson, A. A., Murray, A., and Hart, C. A. (1987). Nosocomial infections in severely traumatized patients: magnitude of problem, pathogenesis, prevention and therapy.

Acta Anaesth. Belg., **38**, 347–53.
13. Rayfield, E.J., Ault, M.J., Keusch, G.T., *et al.* (1982). Infection and diabetes: the case for glucose control. *Am. J. Med.*, **72**, 439–50.
14. van Epps, D.E., Strickland, R.G., and Williams, R.C. (1975). Inhibitors of leukocyte chemotaxis in alcoholic liver disease. *Am. J. Med.*, **59**, 200–7.
15. Howard, R.J. and Simmons, R.L. (1974). Acquired immunologic deficiences after trauma and surgical procedures. *Surg. Gynecol. Obstet.*, **139**, 771–82.
16. Münster, A.M. (1976). Post-traumatic immunosuppression is due to activation of suppressor T-cells. *Lancet*, **i**, 1329–30.
17. Ninnemann, J.L., Condie, J.T., Davies, S.E., and Crocket, R.A. (1982). Isolation of immunosuppressive serum components following thermal injury. *J. Trauma*, **22**, 837–44.
18. van Dijk, W.C., Verbrugh, H.A., van Rijswijk, R.E.N., Vos, A., and Verhoef, J. (1982). Neutrophil function, serum opsonic activity, and delayed hypersensitivity in surgical patients. *Surgery*, **92**, 21–9.
19. Sprunt, K. and Redman, W. (1968). Evidence suggesting importance of role of interbacterial inhibition in maintaining balance of normal flora. *Ann. Intern. Med.*, **68**, 579–80.
20. Sprunt, K., Leidy, G.A., and Redman, W. (1971). Prevention of bacterial overgrowth. *J. Infect. Dis.*, **123**, 1–10.
21. Barza, M., Giuliano, M., Jacobus, N.V., and Gorbach, S.L. (1987). Effect of broad spectrum parenteral antibiotics on colonization resistance of intestinal microflora of humans. *Antimicrob. Ag. Chemother.*, **31**, 723–7.
22. van Der Waaij, D., Berghuis-Devries, J.M., and Lekkerkerk-van Der Wees, J.A.C. (1971). Colonization resistance of the digestive tract in conventional and antibiotic treated mice. *J. Hyg.*, **69**, 405–11.
23. Valenti, W.M., Trundell, R.G., and Bentley, D.W. (1978). Factors predisposing to oralpharyngeal colonization with gram-negative bacilli in the aged. *N. Engl. J. Med.*, **298**, 1108–11.
24. Ruddell, W.S.J., Axon, A.T.R., Findlay, J.M., Bartholomew BA, and Hill M.J. (1980). Effector of cimetidine on the gastric bacterial flora. *Lancet*, **i**, 672–4.
25. Hillman, K.M., Riordan, T., O'Farrell, S.M., and Tabaqchal, S. (1982). Colonisation of the gastric contents in critically ill patients. *Crit. Care Med.*, **10**, 444–7.
26. Tryba, M. (1987). Risk of acute stress bleeding and nosocomial pneumonia in ventilated intensive care unit patients: Sucralfate versus antacids. *Am. J. Med.*, **83** (Suppl 3b), 117–24.
27. Driks, M.R., Craven, D.E., Celli, B.R., *et al.* (1987). Nosocomial pneumonia in intubated patients given sucralfate as compared with antacids or histamine type 2 blockers: the role of gastric colonization. *N. Engl. J. Med.*, **718**, 1376–82.
28. Flaherty, J., Kabins, S.A., and Weinstein, R.A. (1989). New approaches to the prevention of infection in Intensive Care Unit patients. In *Infection control by selective decontamination* (ed. H.K.F. van Saene, C.P. Stoutenbeek, P. Lawin, and I.McA. Ledingham), pp. 184–8. Springer-Verlag, Berlin.
29. Storring, R.A., Jameson, B., McElwain, T.J., Wilshaw, E., Speirs, A.S.D., and Gaya, H. (1977). Oral absorbed antibiotics prevent infection in acute lymphoblastic leukaemia. *Lancet*, **ii**, 837–40.
30. Bodey, G.P. (1981). Antibiotic prophylaxis in cancer patients: regimens of oral non-absorbable antibiotics for prevention of infection during induction or remission. *Rev. Infect. Dis.*, **3**, S259–68.
31. Rozenberg-Arska, M., Dekker, A.W., and Verhoef, J. (1983). Colistin and trimethoprim-sulfamethoxazole for the prevention of infection in patients with acute lymphocytic leukaemia. *Infection*, **11**, 167–9.
32. van Saene, H.K.F. and Stoutenbeek, C.P. (1987). Selective decontamination (editorial). *J. Antimicrob. Chemother.*, **20**, 462–5.
33. van Saene, H.K.F., Stoutenbeek, C.P., and Lerk, C.F. (1985). Influence of faeces of the activity of antimicrobial agents used for decontamination of the alimentary canal. *Scand. J. Infect. Dis.*, **17**, 295–300.
34. Mackowika, P.A. (1982). The normal microbial flora. *N. Engl. J. Med.*, **307**, 83–93.
35. Buck, A.C. and Cooke, E.M. (1969). The fate of ingested *Pseudomonas aeruginosa. J. Med. Microbiol.*, **2**, 521–5.
36. van Saene, H.K.F., Stoutenbeek, C.P., Miranda, D.R., and Zandstra, D.F. (1983). A novel approach to infection control in the intensive care unit. *Acta Anaesthesiol. Belg.*, **3**, 193–208.
37. Stoutenbeek, C.P., van Saene, H.K.F., Miranda, D.R., and Zandstra, D.F. (1984). The effect of selective decontamination of the digestive tract on colonization and infection rate in multiple trauma patients. *Intensive Care Med.*, **10**, 185–92.
38. Alcock, S.R. (1989). Use of a short term parenteral antibiotic as a supplement to SDD. In *Infection control by selective decontamination* (ed. H.K.F van Saene, C.P. Stoutenbeek, P. Lawin, and I.McA. Ledingham), pp. 102–8. Springer-Verlag, Berlin.
39. Stoutenbeek, C.P., van Saene, H.K.F., Miranda, D.R., Zandstra, D.F., and Langrehr, D. (1987). The effect of oropharyngeal decontamination using topical non-asborbable antibiotics on the incidence of nosocomial respiratory tract infections in multiple trauma patients. *J. Trauma*, **27**, 357–64.
40. Crome, D. (1989). Pharmaceutical technology in selective decontamination. In *Infection control by selective decontamination* (ed. H.F.K. van Saene, C.P. Stoutenbeek, P. Lawin, and I.McA. Ledingham), pp. 109–12. Springer-Verlag, Berlin.
41. Sydow, M., Burchardi, T., Fraatz, T., Crozier, T.A., Seyde, W., and Ruchel, R. (1988). Prevention of nosocomial pneumonia in mechanically ventilated patients in a respiratory intensive care unit. *Intensive Care Med.*, **14**, S310.
42. Thülig, D., Hartenauer, U., Diemer, W., Lawin, P., Fegeler, W., and Ritzerfeld, W. (1989). Infection control by selective flora suppression in critically ill patients. *Anaesth. Intensivther. Notfallmed.*, **24**, 345–54.
43. Unertl, K., Ruckdeschel, G., Selbmann, H.K., *et al.* (1987). Prevention of colonization and respiratory infections in long-term ventilated patients by local antimicrobial prophylaxis. *Intensive Care Med.*, **13**, 106–13.
44. Aerdts, S.J.A., van Dalen, R., Calsener, H.A.L., and Vollaard, D.J. (1989). The effect of a novel regimen of selective decontamination on the incidence of unit-acquired lower respiratory tract infections in mechanically ventilated patients. In *Infection control by selective decontamination* (ed. H.F.K. van Saene, C.P. Stoutenbeek, P. Lawin, and I.McA. Ledingham), p. 123. Springer-Verlag, Berlin.
45. Konrad, F., Schwalb, E.B., Heeg, K., *et al.* (1989). Frequency of bacterial colonization and respiratory tract infections and resistance behaviour in patients subjected to long-term ventilation with selective decontamination of the digestive tract (expanded abstract translated to English). *Der Anaesthetist*, **38**, 99–109.
46. Kerver, A.J.H., Rommes, J.H., Mevissen-Verhage, E.A.E., *et al.* (1988). Prevention of colonization and infection in critically ill patients: a prospective randomized study. *Crit. Care Med.*, **16**, 1087–93.
47. Guillaume, C., Godard, J., Bui-Xaun, B., Bachmann, P., Reverdy, M.E., and Motin, J. (1989). Selective digestive tract decontamination in a polyvalent intensive care unit: a double blind study. *ICAAC*, Abstract No. 325.
48. Ulrich, C., Harinck-De Weerd, J.E., Bakker, N.C., Jacz, K., Doornbos, L., and de Ridder, V.A. (1989). Selective decon-

tamination of the digestive tract with norfloxacin in the prevention of ICU-acquired infections: a prospective randomized study. *Intensive Care Med.*, **15**, 424–31.

49. Schardey, M., Meyer, G., Kern, M., Marre, R., Hohlbach, G., and Schildberg, F. W. (1989). Nosocomial respiratory tract infections: preventive measures in surgical intensive care patients (English abstract translation). *Intensive Med.*, **26**, 242–9.
50. Cockerill, F. R., Muller, S. M., Anhalt, J. P., and Thompson, R. L. (1989). Reduction of nosocomial infections by selective digestive tract decontamination in the ICU. *ICAAC*, Abstract No. 785.
51. Miranda, D. R., van Saene, H. K. F., Stoutenbeek, C. P., and Zandstra, D. F. (1983). Environment and costs in surgical intensive unit. The implication of selective decontamination of the digestive tract. *Acta Anaesthesiol. Belg.*, **3**, 223–2.
52. Stoutenbeek, C. P., van Saene, H. K. F., and Zandstra, D. F. (1987). The effect of oral non-absorbable antibiotics on the emergence of resistant bacteria in patients in an intensive care unit. *J. Antimicrob. Chemother.*, **19**, 513–20.
53. Eastaway, A. T., Clark, J., and Martindale, E. (1989). Reappearance of aerobic gram negative bacilli and the emergence of resistance following SDD. In *Infection control by selective decontamination* (ed. H. F. K. van Saene, C. P., Stoutenbeek, P. Lawin, and I. McA. Ledingham), p. 154. Springer-Verlag, Berlin.
54. Brun-Buisson, C., Legrand, P., Raus, A., *et al.* (1989). Intestinal decontamination for control of nosocomial multi-resistant gram-negative bacilli. *Ann. Intern. Med.*, **110**, 873–81.
55. Tetteroo, G. W. M., Wagenvoort, J. A. T., Castelein, A., Tilanus, H. W., Ince, C., and Bruining, H. A. (1990). Selective decontamination to reduce gram-negative colonization and infections after oesophageal resection. *Lancet*, **335**, 704–7.
56. Schmeiser, T. H., Kurrle, E. Arnold, R., Kriger, D., Heit, W., and Heimpel, H. (1988). Antimicrobial prophylaxis in neutopenic patients after bone marrow transplantation. *Infection*, **16**, 19–24.
57. Heimbahl, A., Gahrton, G., Groth, C. G., *et al.* (1984). Selective decontamination of the alimentary tract microbial flora in patients treated with bone marrow transplantation. A microbiological study. *Scan, J. Infect. Dis.*, **16**, 51–60.
58. Rosman, C., Klompmaker, I. J., Bonsel, G. J., Bleichrodt, R. P., Arends, J. P., and Sloof, M. J. (1990) The efficacy of selective decontamination as infection prevention after liver transplantation. *Transplant. Proc.* **22**, 1554–5.
59. Wiesner, R. H., Hermans, P. E., Rakela, J., *et al.* (1988). Selective bowel decontamination to decrease Gram-negative aerobic bacterial and candida colonization and prevent infection after orthotopic liver transplantation. *Transplantation*, **45**, 570–4.
60. van Saene, H. K. F. and Nicolay, G. P. A. (1979). The prevention of wound infection in burn patients. *Scand. J. Plast. Reconstr. Surg.*, **13**, 63–7.
61. Manson, W. L., Westerveld, A. W., Klasen, H. J., and Sauer, E. W. (1987). Selective intestinal decontamination of the digestive tract for infection prophylaxis in severely burned patient. *Scand. J. Plast. Reconstr. Surg.*, **21**, 269–72.
62. Spijkervet, F. K. L., van Saene, H. K. F., Panders, A. K., Vermey, A., and Mehta, V. M. (1989). Scoring irradiation mucositis in head and neck cancer patients. *J. Oral. Pathol.*, **18**, 167–71.
63. Spijkervet, F. K. L. (1989). *Irradiation mucositis and oral flora* (Thesis) Rijksuniversiteit, Groningen, pp. 95–104.
64. Thülig, B., Hartenour, U., Diemer, W. *et al.* (1989). *Der Anaesthetist*, **38**, S352 (Abstract).
65. Leonard, E. M., van Saene, H. K. F., Shears, P., Walker, J., and Tam, P. K. H. (1990). Pathogenesis of colonisation and infection in a neonatal surgical unit. *Crit. Care Med.*, **18**, 264–9.
66. Meakins, J. L. and Marshall, J. C. (1989). The gastrointestinal tract: the 'motor' of multiple organ failure. *Arch. Surg.*, **121**, 197–201.
67. Ramsay, G. and Ledingham, I. McA. (1989). Management of multiple organ failure: control of the microbial environment In *Multiple organ failure* (ed. D. J. Bihari and F. D. Cerra, pp. 327–36. New Horizons Series: No. 3. Society of Critical Care Medicine, Fullarton, California.
68. Ramsay, G. (1989). Endotoxaemia in multiple organ failure: a secondary role for SDD? In *Infection control by selective decontamination*, (ed. H. F. K. van Saene, C. P. Stoutenbeek, P. Lawin, and I. McA. Ledingham). pp. 135–42. Springer-Verlag, Berlin.

Further reading

Editorial. (1988). Microbial selective decontamination in intensive care patients. *Lancet*, **i**, 803–4.

Johanson, W. G. (1989). Infection prevention by selective decontamination in intensive care (Editorial) *Intensive Care Med.*, **15**, 417–9.

Sanderson, P. J. (1989). Selective decontamination of the digestive tract (Editorial) *Br. Med. J.*, **299**, 1413–14.

Van Saene, H. K. F., Stoutenbeek, C. P., Lawin, P., and Ledingham, M. A. (ed.) (1989). *Infection control by selective decontamination*. Springer-Verlag, Berlin.

Index